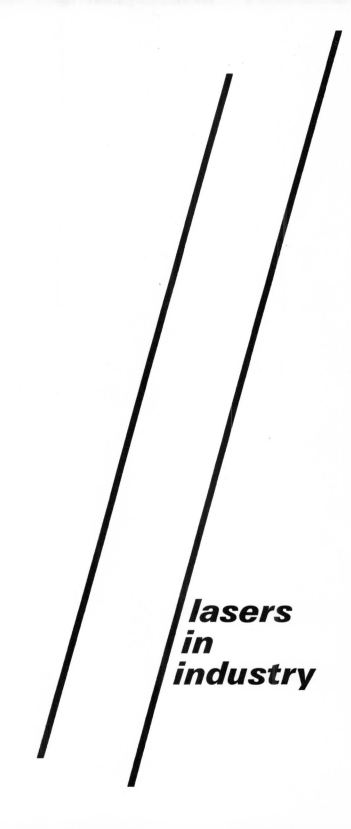

lasers
in
industry

WESTERN ELECTRIC SERIES

lasers in industry, edited by **S. S. Charschan**

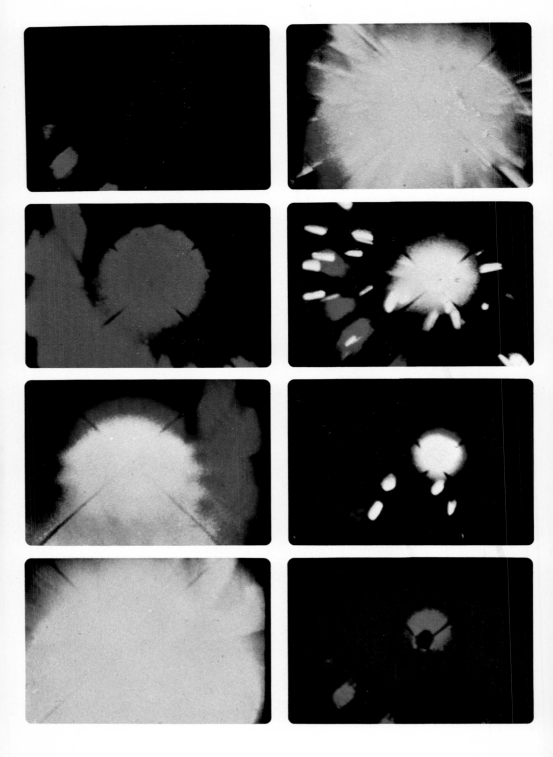

lasers in industry

edited by **S. S. Charschan**
Member of Research Staff
Western Electric

Van Nostrand Reinhold Company

New York / Cincinnati / Toronto / London / Melbourne

Van Nostrand Reinhold Company Regional Offices:
New York   Cincinnati   Chicago   Millbrae   Dallas

Van Nostrand Reinhold Company International Offices:
London   Toronto   Melbourne

Library of Congress Catalog Card Number: 75–182397

ISBN 0–442–21516–9

Manufactured in the United States of America

Published by Van Nostrand Reinhold Company
450 West 33rd Street, New York, N. Y. 10001

Published simultaneously in Canada by Van Nostrand Reinhold Ltd.

15   14   13   12   11   10   9   8   7   6   5   4   3   2   1

Library of Congress Cataloging in Publication Data

Lasers in industry.

   (Western Electric series)
   Includes bibliographical references.
   1. Lasers. I. Charschan, S. S., 1922–   ed.
II. Series: Western Electric Company, Inc. Western
Electric series.
TK7871.3.L35   621.36′6   75–182397
ISBN 0–442–21516–9

contributors

J. F. Carr
S. S. Charschan
R. O. De Nicola
F. P. Gagliano
R. J. Klaiber

A. Kestenbaum
J. Longfellow
M. A. Saifi
L. S. Watkins
V. J. Zaleckas

All members of Research Staff, Western Electric (at time of writing).

preface

In 1960, the scientific world was electrified by news of the world's first laser action. Only five years later, at a rate surpassing the accelerating pace of modern technology, industry had harnessed the laser. On December 14, 1965, Western Electric announced the first use of laser light in a mass production application: a laser system had been developed for piercing holes in diamond dies for drawing wire.

Since then, the laser has proven to be an effective tool in numerous other industrial applications, and increasing numbers of engineers are encountering this new technology in their work. Lasers in industry are being used to measure process parameters and to scribe, drill, evaporate, and weld a wide variety of materials in a wide variety of applications. As a result, more and more engineers are finding that they need reliable information on subjects such as interferometry, thermal processing, holography, detection, and laser safety procedures. This book has been written for those engineers who want to apply lasers to the solution of industrial problems.

Its blend of theory and application is designed to help such engineers solve most, if not all, of the laser problems they will run into. Review material is included, particularly in the first three chapters covering laser fundamentals, the interaction of laser radiation with materials, and fundamentals of laser processing. In addition, the book is heavily cross-indexed for the convenience of those who are using it eclectically. The reader is referred to material elsewhere in the book and to reference sources wherever this may prove helpful.

There are ten chapters plus a glossary. The glossary contains many essential definitions and illustrative examples of optical components used in conjunction with laser systems for industrial applications. The material contained in the chapters is described as follows:

Chapter 1 Different types of lasers and the fundamental theories of laser operation are emphasized. Descriptions of pulsing arrangements and mirror configurations, outlines of laser construction, and characteristics of laser light are included. Treatment of the subject matter requires only a basic knowledge of physics and is presented in this manner to facilitate understanding by engineers of various disciplines.

Chapter 2 Models are developed which describe the interaction of electromagnetic radiation with materials. In the first section both classical and quantum aspects of electromagnetic fields are discussed. A review of the concepts of solid-state physics is included to develop a better understanding of the interaction models. Optical properties of metals and semiconductors, scattering theory, and second harmonic generation are discussed in a manner appealing to all engineers.

Chapter 3 This chapter provides working definitions and illustrations for focusing optics required in laser processing. The thermodynamic and metallurgical phenomena which apply to thermal processing of materials are presented and models are developed to explain typical laser-material interactions. Experimental data are introduced which corroborate the basic assumptions of the models.

Chapter 4 Practical comparisons are made of theoretical power needs versus actual process requirements for laser welding, drilling, and micromachining. System parameters, advantages and disadvantages, processing speeds, and limitations are profusely illustrated by examining the implementation of typical laser systems used for industrial processing.

Chapter 5 Permanent changes in materials which may be effected with a laser beam are described in this chapter. Heat treating with its attendant recrystallization, grain growth, and microstructures are described in depth along with the diffusion phenomena in metals, insulators, and semiconductors. Zone melting by conventional means and by laser are compared. The possibilities of chemical reactions are discussed in preparing for future applications.

Chapter 6 Reflection and scattering of light from different classes of materials are discussed. Measurement techniques relying on the reflection or scattering of laser radiation are then described. Applications of ellipsometry, Doppler velocity measurements, Rayleigh light scattering, and other techniques are illustrated.

Chapter 7 An introduction to diffraction theory is developed to clarify the presentation of industrial applications of diffraction effects. Discussions progress from the simple slit and wire measurement to the use of complex spatial filters useful in pattern recognition and inspection of integrated circuit photomasks.

Chapter 8 The subjects of interferometry and holography are introduced by a germane discussion on temporal and spatial coherence, with a subsequent step-by-step development of the theory of interferometry. Laser interferometer applications are described. This is followed by an explanation of holography. Three-dimensional image recording and reconstruction capabilities and applications are illustrated and discussed.

Chapter 9 Systems that apply to detection and measurement of various lasers operating in CW, pulsed, or Q-switched modes are described in detail, and representative systems are illustrated to provide a guide for the instrumentation needs of practicing engineers. The physical laws that govern operation of the different kinds of detectors are presented in an easily understood fashion. Limitations imposed upon operations by noise are examined.

Chapter 10 Hazards that exist due to the unique character of laser beams are described. Safety levels of radiation from the laser are listed, and sample calculations are performed for determining radiation levels.

In addition, recommended safety programs for industrial applications, together with equipment needed to provide a safe working environment, are presented.

It is intended that all of this material, heretofore not available in a single text, will be helpful to members of the academic community wanting to enter this rapidly growing field, as well as to practicing engineers.

The ten authors who collaborated in the preparation of *Lasers in Industry* have all drawn upon years of experience as members of the Laser Studies Group at Western Electric's Engineering Research Center in Princeton, New Jersey. All are specialists in the areas covered in their chapters. The book is truly a collaborative effort in that all authors reviewed each of the other contributions and made significant comments which resulted in revisions or expansions.

In addition to my fellow authors, whose untiring efforts made this book possible, several other people have been extremely helpful in its preparation. For such help, I offer my thanks and gratitude to Tom P. Long for guidance and, in particular, to Ron L. Whalin who reviewed most of the chapters. Helpful technical comments and criticisms have been supplied by fellow engineers and scientists at the Western Electric Engineering Research Center and at the Bell Telephone Laboratories, whose help I can scarcely acknowledge individually. The additional critiques furnished by members of the Corporate Education Center deserve a separate thanks.

S. S. CHARSCHAN, Editor
Princeton, N. J.

contents

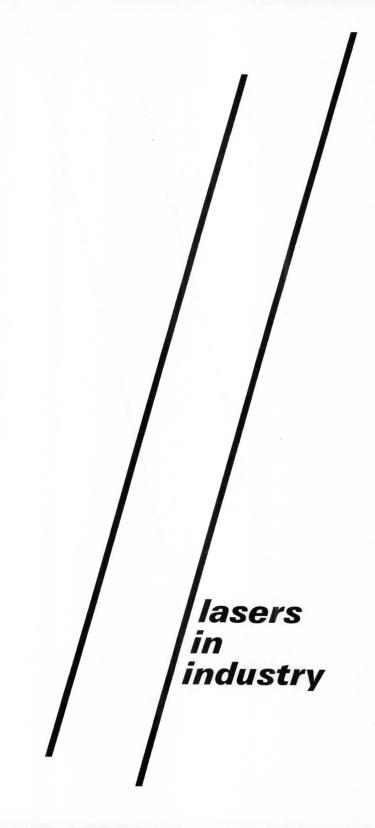

lasers
in
industry

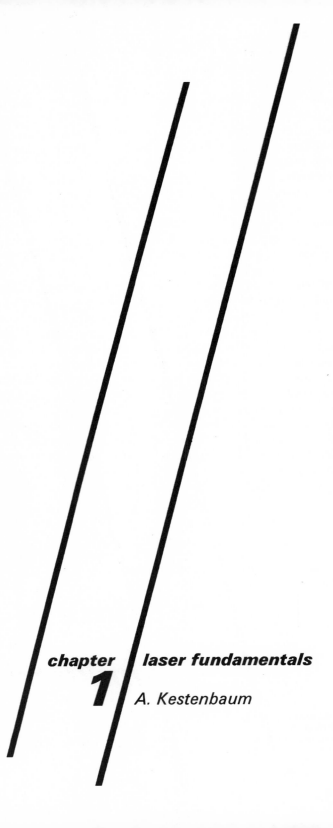

chapter

1

laser fundamentals

A. Kestenbaum

1·0 introduction

The laser is a unique source of radiation capable of delivering intense coherent electromagnetic fields in the spectral range between the ultraviolet and the far infrared. This laser beam coherence is manifested in two ways: (1) it possesses good temporal coherence qualities since it is highly monochromatic, and (2) it is spatially coherent—as evidenced by the nearly constant phase wavefront and directionality of the emitted light.* The temporal coherence of the laser is a measure of the ability of the beam to produce interference effects as a result of differences in path lengths and is, therefore, important for such applications as interferometry and holography. The spatial coherence is particularly important for power applications where it provides the capability of focusing all the laser's available output energy into an extremely small spot size. Thus, power densities, which are unattainable with any other source of light, can be attained.

Spatial and temporal coherence are properties that have long been recognized as indispensable for various industrial and laboratory applications. Long before the advent of the laser, light possessing various degrees of coherence could be obtained by filtering ordinary light. However, the filtering process resulted in an output beam of such low intensity as to render such techniques useless in most practical applications. It remained for the laser, with its inherent properties of coherence and high intensity, to demonstrate the applicability of optical electromagnetic radiation to numerous new technologies.

The special characteristics of laser radiation are directly attributable to the phenomenon of stimulated emission and to the feedback mechanism provided by the cavity structure. Figure 1-1, a schematic diagram of a typical gas laser, highlights the major elements of a laser system. Such a

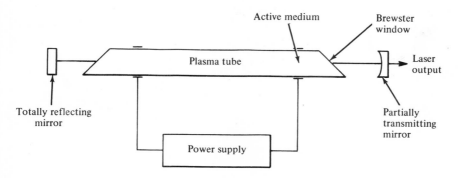

Figure 1-1   Schematic of a gas laser.

* The use of the acronym laser, which stands for Light Amplification by Stimulated Emission of Radiation, has been expanded to include frequencies in the ultraviolet and infrared in addition to the visible part of the spectrum. It is within this broader context that the term "light" will be used throughout this book.

system consists of an active medium (lasing material), which in this case is gas, but may consist of a solid or a liquid. A power supply pumps energy into the active medium, exciting the active atoms* and rendering amplification possible. The laser, however, normally functions as an oscillator rather than an amplifier and is consequently a source of coherent light rather than an amplifier of existing light signals. To achieve oscillation, mirrors are placed perpendicular to the axis of the active medium to form an optical resonant cavity. Stimulated emission in the active medium results in the required amplification, whereas the mirrors supply the feedback required for regenerative action and oscillation. These features combine to differentiate the lasers from other sources of light and lead to the singularly intense light typical of lasers. The first part of this chapter explains these concepts in greater detail.

1·1 spontaneous and stimulated emission and absorption

Since the initial demonstration of laser operation using ruby in 1960,[1] lasing action has been achieved in gases, liquids, and solid materials, at wavelengths ranging from approximately 110 nm to more than a millimeter. Pulsed as well as continuous wave (CW) output can be obtained from these lasers, with pulse durations as short as a fraction of a picosecond. Output power for continuous operation may exceed ten thousand watts, with peak power of several gigawatts possible in a pulsed mode of operation. Despite this great diversity in wavelength, pulse length, and output power, the physical processes which underlie the generation of laser radiation are common to all lasers, with only minor modifications.

The interaction between an electromagnetic wave and matter is an intrinsic quantum mechanical process. Thus, a rigorous quantitative analysis of such interaction requires quantum mechanical formulation and treatment. However, in many instances, an elementary qualitative description may be adequate to illustrate the general concepts without the need for quantum mechanical techniques. Accordingly, our treatment of the electromagnetic field will be an entirely classical (nonquantum mechanical) one. (Basic concepts of energy, material, and their interactions are discussed and elaborated in Chapter 2.)

The atoms, ions, or molecules involved in the interaction must be viewed as a quantum mechanical system and will possess numerous discrete energy levels. When the system interacts with an electromagnetic

---

* Ions and molecules may also comprise the active elements in a laser medium.

field, transitions between these various energy levels will occur, and energy will be emitted or absorbed at a frequency characteristic to the material. Energy levels due to the quantized nature of electronic orbits are the initial and final states that often participate in a laser transition. However, transitions between other types of levels such as those in molecules due to vibrational and rotational motion may also be employed to achieve laser action, as is, indeed, the case with one of the most important lasers, the CO_2, at wavelengths approximating 10.6×10^3nm.

A simple and yet meaningful model representing such an atomic system* may consist of a large number of identical, infinitely sharp two energy-level atoms, each with an upper energy-level E_n and a lower energy-level E_m, and one of which is depicted in Figure 1-2. Although it is true that this model is a gross simplification of the atomic system, it contains the essential features for describing the interaction process between the electromagnetic field and the atoms. Electromagnetic

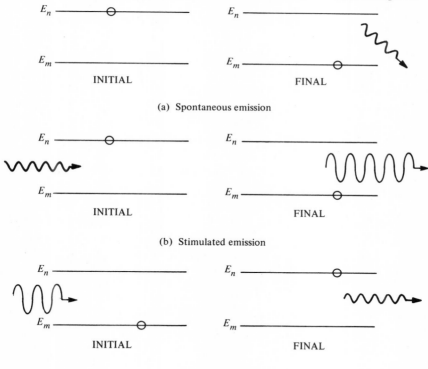

(a) Spontaneous emission

(b) Stimulated emission

(c) Absorption

Figure 1-2   Interaction of a two-level system with electromagnetic field.

* From here on, we will use the term atomic system in a generic sense, whereby it can represent a system made up of atoms as well as ions or molecules.

radiation may be absorbed or emitted by the atoms at a characteristic frequency v_{nm} satisfying the relation

$$v_{nm} = \frac{E_n - E_m}{h} \tag{1-1}$$

where $h = 6.626 \times 10^{-34}$ Js is Planck's constant.

There are numerous and quite varied methods by which an atom may be raised from a lower to a higher energy level, several of which will be discussed later; but when an atom finds itself in an excited state, there are only two independent processes through which its excess energy may radiatively be emitted. The atom may decay spontaneously, even in the absence of an external electromagnetic field, emitting an electromagnetic wave in a random manner shown in Figure 1-2a, or it may be induced to emit radiation by an already existing electromagnetic field. In the latter case, the radiated wave is in the same direction as the inducing field, has the same phase, and possesses identical polarization. This is illustrated in Figure 1-2b. This second form of emission is recognized as stimulated emission and may be utilized to provide phase-coherent amplification of light, similar to the lower frequency phase-coherent amplification provided by various electronic devices.

The rate of stimulated (induced) emission is proportional to the energy density (J/m^3Hz) of the inducing field $\rho(v_{nm})$ at the characteristic frequency, as well as to the number of atoms or population of the excited state N_n. The total power radiated through the process is, therefore, given by the expression,

$$P_{\text{induced}} = hv_{nm} N_n B_{nm} \rho(v_{nm}) \tag{1-2}$$

where B_{nm} is a proportionality constant that represents the strength of the induced downward transition between the two levels. Since spontaneous emission occurs equally well in the presence or absence of external radiation, the rate of the process will be independent of any existing field. But (as in the case of stimulated emission), the rate here is also proportional to the population of the excited state. The total power radiated spontaneously by the collection of atoms is thus given by

$$P_{\text{spontaneous}} = hv_{nm} N_n A_{nm} \tag{1-3}$$

where A_{nm} is once more a proportionality constant and represents the rate of the spontaneous transition between the two levels. The proportionality constants A_{nm} and B_{nm}, which are called the *Einstein coefficients of spontaneous and induced emission*, respectively, are related to each other and may be calculated on the basis of quantum mechanical considerations. If there are any atoms in the lower energy state, simultaneous with stimulated emission, an opposite process of induced absorption where an atom is stimulated to undergo a transition from the lower to the upper state will also occur. The rate of absorption of this process, which is schematically depicted in Figure 1-2c, is once more directly proportional to the energy density of the field. In this case it is also proportional to population of the lower state. The power absorbed from the electromagnetic field is thus

$$P_{absorbed} = h\nu_{nm} B_{mn} N_m \rho(\nu_{nm}) \tag{1-4}$$

where B_{mn} is the proportionality constant representing the strength of the upward transition. It can be shown[2,3] that $B_{nm} = B_{mn}$, and therefore the ratio of the power absorbed to the power radiated through stimulated emission is given by the ratio of the population of the lower state to that in the upper state.*

In thermal equilibrium, the populations of the two energy levels are related by means of a Boltzmann distribution given by

$$\frac{N_n}{N_m} = \exp\left(-\frac{E_n - E_m}{kT}\right) \tag{1-5}$$

where k is Boltzmann's constant equal to 1.3806×10^{-23} J/°K, and T is the absolute temperature. At room temperature $kT \simeq 1/40$ eV, so that for optical transitions in the visible or near-infrared range where $E_n - E_m \geq 1$ eV, the upper level population is vanishingly small in comparison with the lower energy level.

Since under normal conditions the population of the lower state will be greater than that of the upper one, the power absorbed by the collection of atoms will exceed the power radiated into the field through stimulated emission. This situation will obviously result in the attenuation of the field. But, if we somehow succeed in establishing a state of population inversion where $N_n > N_m$, the relative magnitudes of the two processes will be reversed, the power radiated by stimulated emission will exceed the power absorbed by the atoms, and the net effect of the stimulated processes will be a phase coherent amplification of the incident beam.

The Einstein A and B coefficients are related through the equation[3]

$$A_{nm} = \frac{8\pi h\nu_{nm}^3}{c^3} B_{nm} \tag{1-6}$$

where $c = 2.9979 \times 10^8$ m/s is the velocity of light, which may be viewed as a fundamental relationship between spontaneous and induced emission. Once the excited state is populated, both stimulated and spontaneous emission will occur simultaneously and, for a given rate of stimulated emission, the power radiated spontaneously will increase rapidly with

---

* We have assumed that the two energy levels are nondegenerate, i.e., only one state of the atom may have the energy level specified by E_n or E_m. If the energy levels are degenerate with degeneracies given by g_n and g_m, respectively, then $B_{mn} = B_{nm}(g_n/g_m)$ and the ratio of the power absorbed to the power radiated through stimulated emission will be similarly modified to include the ratio of the degeneracies. For the sake of simplicity, we would continue under the assumption of nondegeneracy of the two energy levels.

frequency (Equation 1-6), which makes the attainment of amplification through stimulated emission exceedingly difficult for frequencies in the ultraviolet and higher.

1·2   population inversion and pumping

It is evident that, to obtain amplification of the electromagnetic wave through interaction with the laser material, a state of population inversion has to be created between the levels partaking in the optical transition. Furthermore, the net power gain will be proportional to the population difference since upward and downward radiative transitions corresponding to stimulated absorption and emission are allowed and will take place simultaneously.   The operation leading to population inversion is called *pumping*, and involves numerous other energy levels besides the two directly participating in the lasing action.   Despite the complexity of the energy structure of laser materials, many common lasers essentially operate as three or four energy-level systems, and a brief analysis of such pumping schemes will illustrate the basic principles of achieving population inversion in practice.

1·2·1   three-level laser system

The first successful laser operation used ruby (aluminum oxide in which Cr^{3+} ions replace about 0.05% of the Al^{3+} ions) as the active medium. In view of its historical significance and practical importance as a present day solid-state laser, it is instructive to examine the mechanism responsible for the operation of such a laser system.   Due to the energy band structure of ruby, a three-level laser model is quite adequate for describing the optical pumping action leading to population inversion and will be employed here.

With the aid of the energy-level diagram of a typical three-level laser, as illustrated in Figure 1-3, we may proceed to explain the conditions necessary for the attainment of population inversion.   In thermal equilibrium, the majority of atoms are found in the ground state.   The initial step in the pumping operation consists of raising some atoms from the ground state into a broad energy band, which in Figure 1-3 is denoted by 2. A flash lamp is commonly used to provide the incident broadband electromagnetic radiation required for the optical transition.   Once an atom exists in the broad energy level 2, it may relax to either the upper laser level (marked energy level 1) or back to the ground state.   But, if the primary relaxation mechanism is a fast, nonradiative decay into the upper laser level, most atoms will cascade down into that level, spending a relatively short time in the broad excited level 2.   The upper laser level is a metastable level with a rather long relaxation time, and, consequently, an

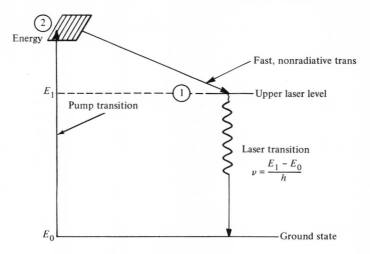

Figure 1-3   Three-level laser system.

accumulation of atoms in that state is possible. If the rate with which atoms are pumped from the ground state to the broad energy level is sufficiently high, a situation can occur when the number of atoms reaching and remaining in the metastable level exceeds the number of atoms still occupying the ground state. The result is population inversion. Amplification by means of stimulated emission may now take place at a frequency of $v = (E_1 - E_0)/h$, where the metastable and ground states participate in the stimulated transition. To obtain a quantitative idea of the rate of pumping required for achieving population inversion, we note that the rate of increase in the population of the broad excited level 2 is given by

$$\frac{dN_2}{dt} = WN_0 - WN_2 - \frac{N_2}{\tau_{21}} \tag{1-7}$$

where N_0 and N_2 are the populations of the respective energy levels, W is the pump-stimulated transition probability, and τ_{21} is the fast non-radiative relaxation time. In (1-7), of the three terms on the right, the first represents the rate of increase in the population of level 2 due to absorption of energy from the incident pump; the second represents the rate of decrease of the population due to stimulated emission back to the ground state, and the third takes into account the loss in population as a result of the primary relaxation mechanism to level 1.

In the steady state, $dN_2/dt = 0$, and the ratio of the populations is given by

$$\frac{N_2}{N_0} = \frac{W\tau_{21}}{1 + W\tau_{21}} \simeq W\tau_{21} \tag{1-8}$$

where the last approximation assumes a fast relaxation time satisfying the condition $\tau_{21} \ll 1/W$.

Similarly, the rate of increase in the population of level 1 is given by the equation

$$\frac{dN_1}{dt} = \frac{N_2}{\tau_{21}} - \frac{N_1}{\tau_{10}} \qquad (1\text{-}9)$$

where the first term on the right represents the rate of increase in the population due to relaxation from the higher, broad energy level, and the second denotes the rate of decrease in the population of level 1 as a result of atomic decay from level 1 to the ground state. In the steady state $dN_1/dt = 0$ and

$$N_2 = \frac{\tau_{21}}{\tau_{10}} N_1 \qquad (1\text{-}10)$$

and relating N_1 to N_0 by means of the previously derived (1-8), we obtain

$$\frac{N_1}{N_0} = W\tau_{10} \qquad (1\text{-}11)$$

Population inversion in the nondegenerate case will, therefore, be achieved when $W > 1/\tau_{10}$, or when the pumping rate from the ground state to the broad energy level exceeds the relaxation rate from level 1 back to the ground state. This result could have been derived directly, since the various assumptions regarding the relaxation mechanism between levels 2 and 1 imply that atoms pumped into level 2 rapidly cascade down to level 1, effecting an almost direct pumping from the ground state to the upper laser level. If the pumping rate is greater than the relaxation rate from level 1, atoms will accumulate in that level which will eventually lead to a population inversion. The role that level 2 plays in this pumping scheme, even though transitory in nature, is an indispensable one, since, for states with equal degeneracies $B_{nm} = B_{mn}$ and no direct pumping between the two levels can achieve more than equality in the populations of those levels.

1·2·2   *four-level laser system*

In contrast to a three-level system where at least 50 percent of the atoms have to be lifted out of the ground state if population inversion is to be realized another scheme, generically termed *four-level pumping*, permits the establishment of population inversion between specific energy levels, and only a small fraction of the atoms have to be pumped from the ground state during laser action. The simple model of such a system, as shown in Figure 1-4, constitutes a surprisingly accurate model for many complex laser systems such as rare-earth lasers, including Nd:YAG and various gas laser systems.

As in the three-level laser system, atoms are initially raised from the ground state into the broad energy level 3 by either absorbing electro-

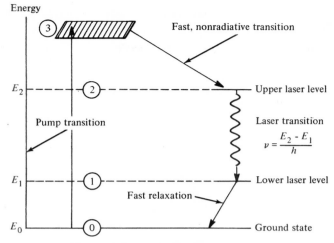

Figure 1-4 Four-level laser system.

magnetic radiation from an optical pump such as a flash lamp (as in many solid-state lasers), or through electron impact (as in many gas lasers). A fast, nonradiative relaxation from this excited state ensues—primarily into level 2 which serves as the upper laser level and is usually a metastable level. By virtue of the long relaxation time of level 2, an accumulation of atoms in that state occurs. Level 1, which serves as the lower laser level, possesses a fast relaxation time and is usually appreciably above the ground state $(E_1 - E_0 \gg kT)$. These two characteristics will ensure the existence of population inversion, since the first condition guarantees the absence of a buildup in the population of level 1, and the second implies the virtual emptiness of that level in thermal equilibrium. It is clear, therefore, that only a small percentage of the total atomic population has to be lifted out of the ground state in order to create the desired population inversion between levels 1 and 2.

To establish necessary conditions for the relative magnitudes of the various relaxation times, we note that the rate equation for level 3 assumes the form

$$\frac{dN_3}{dt} = W(N_0 - N_3) - \frac{N_3}{\tau_{32}} \tag{1-12}$$

where W is once more the pump-stimulated transition probability, N_0 and N_3 are the populations of the respective energy levels, and τ_{32} is the short relaxation time that characterizes the primary relaxation mechanism from level 3 to level 2. In the steady state $dN_3/dt = 0$, the populations of the two above-mentioned levels are related by

$$\frac{N_3}{N_0} = \frac{W\tau_{32}}{1 + W\tau_{32}} \simeq W\tau_{32} \tag{1-13}$$

where use has been made of the assumption that the relaxation time is sufficiently short to satisfy the condition $\tau_{32} \ll 1/W$. Assuming that level 2 relaxes primarily into level 1 at a very slow relaxation rate, we have as the rate equation for this metastable level

$$\frac{dN_2}{dt} = \frac{N_3}{\tau_{32}} - \frac{N_2}{\tau_{21}} \tag{1-14}$$

which, in the steady state, reduces to

$$N_3 = \frac{\tau_{32}}{\tau_{21}} N_2 \tag{1-15}$$

Similarly for level 1,

$$\frac{dN_1}{dt} = \frac{N_2}{\tau_{21}} - \frac{N_1}{\tau_{10}} \tag{1-16}$$

resulting in a steady-state population relationship of the form

$$N_2 = \frac{\tau_{21}}{\tau_{10}} N_1 \tag{1-17}$$

and we observe that population inversion between levels 1 and 2 is in this case independent of the pumping rate and will be achieved under the presently assumed model so long as $\tau_{21} > \tau_{10}$. However, as was noted before, the net power gain through stimulated processes is proportional to the difference in the population of the two participating levels, which for the present case is given by

$$N_2 - N_1 = WN_0(\tau_{21} - \tau_{10}) \simeq WN(\tau_{21} - \tau_{10}) \tag{1-18}$$

and is seen to be directly proportional to the pumping rate as well as to the population of the ground state. The last approximation relating the population difference to the total number of available atoms in the active material N employs the fact that, in most practical four-level laser systems, only a small fraction of the atoms are actually pumped into the broad energy level 3. The population of the ground state, which in view of the energy gaps between the discrete levels is initially essentially equal to the total number of atoms, will thus remain unchanged.

The preceding analysis demonstrates the lower threshold pumping power level of a four-level system as compared with a three-level system. If τ is the radiative decay time of the lasing transition, the ratio of the population difference between the laser transition levels to the total number of atoms in a three-level system is given by

$$\frac{N_1 - N_0}{N_1 + N_0} = \frac{W\tau - 1}{W\tau + 1} \tag{1-19}$$

whereas the corresponding expression for the four-level system assumes the form

$$\frac{N_2 - N_1}{N_2 + N_0} = \frac{W\tau}{W\tau + 1} \tag{1-20}$$

and we observe that to attain a prescribed population difference, which might correspond to the population difference necessary for the onset of oscillation in a real laser system, a higher pumping rate is required in a three-level system, assuming other parameters of both systems are equal.

1·3 cavity and feedback

As was stated earlier, the laser in its most common mode of operation generates coherent light and thus functions as an oscillator rather than an amplifier. Consequently, it is necessary to incorporate a suitable feedback element into the system, in addition to the active material that provides amplification by means of stimulated emission. This optical feedback circuit generally consists of mirrors placed on both ends of the lasing medium forming an open optical resonant cavity. These mirrors act on the electromagnetic field in such a way as to restrict possible sustained oscillations to a limited number of energy configurations that are denoted as the modes of the field in the cavity.

1·3·1 threshold condition

Before exploring the various field configurations imposed by the cavity, it is instructive to examine the required population inversion for attaining oscillation in a particular field configuration.

Oscillations in a laser cavity will occur whenever the amplification through stimulated emission is sufficiently high to exactly balance the attenuation suffered by the field due to various loss mechanisms which are invariably present in the system. The most significant losses in the cavity are due to (1) the scattering of light by optical inhomogeneities, (2) the absorption in the mirrors and in the laser medium, and (3) the power extracted from the cavity through a partially transmitting mirror, which is the useful output of the laser. Oscillations will consist of a wave traveling back and forth between the mirrors which is neither amplified nor attenuated upon a completion of one round trip.

The loss mechanism may be characterized by a decay time constant $\tau_c = Q/2\pi v$, where Q is the quality factor of the cavity and v the frequency of the emitted radiation. The loss in field intensity (power per unit of area) will therefore be described by

$$\left(\frac{dI}{dt}\right)_L = -\frac{I}{\tau_c} \tag{1-21}$$

The rate of net increase in intensity due to induced transitions is readily obtained by slight modification of (1-2) and (1-4) in the form

$$\left(\frac{dI}{dt}\right)_G = h\nu\left(n_n - n_m\frac{g_n}{g_m}\right)cW_i \tag{1-22}$$

where n_n and n_m are the population densities of levels n and m, g_n and g_m are the degeneracies of the respective levels and have been reintroduced for the sake of completeness, c is again the velocity of light, and W_i is the rate of induced transitions between the levels. For transitions which are induced by a nearly monochromatic radiation field of intensity I, the stimulated transition rate is given by[3]

$$W_i(\nu) = \frac{A_{nm}c^2}{8\pi h\nu^3}g(\nu)I \tag{1-23}$$

where the atomic line shape function $g(\nu)$ has been introduced to account for the finite width of the atomic line.*

For sustained oscillations, the gain in intensity must either equal or exceed the loss, which implies that

$$\left(\frac{dI}{dt}\right)_L + \left(\frac{dI}{dt}\right)_G \geq 0 \tag{1-24}$$

and upon combining (1-21) and (1-22) and (1-23), we arrive at the threshold condition for oscillation at a frequency at or near the center of the atomic line ν_0 in the form of

$$\left(n_n - n_m\frac{g_n}{g_m}\right) = \frac{8\pi\nu^2}{c^3 g(\nu_0)\tau_c A_{nm}} \tag{1-25}$$

For the most common line shapes $g(\nu_0) \sim 1/\Delta\nu$ where $\Delta\nu$ is the width of the line and we observe that the critical inversion density necessary for oscillations (Equation 1-25) will diminish with decreasing line width.

1·3·2 mode configurations

The optical resonator is usually formed by placing mirrors (either plane or curved) perpendicularly to the axis along which the laser light will propagate. This structure tends to maintain particular electromagnetic field configurations with sufficiently low loss, so that it may be compensated by the gain attained through stimulated emission. These configurations are referred to as the modes of the cavity.

---

* In our initial analysis of a two-level system, it was convenient to visualize the atomic lines as being infinitely narrow. However, due to broadening mechanisms,[4] the atomic lines are actually spread, and $g(\nu)$ is the distribution function of frequencies which constitute the shape of the line. It satisfies the relation $\int g(\nu)\,d\nu = 1$, and $g(\nu)\,d\nu$ represents the probability of finding an atom with a transition frequency between ν and $\nu + d\nu$.

Since the laser resonator is a rather elongated one with length along the laser axis (usually taken to be the z direction) much greater than the lateral dimensions in the x and y directions, it is possible to separate the field configurations into transverse and longitudinal modes which are very nearly independent of one another.   As a result, we may view the field inside the cavity as composed of particular transverse configurations propagating back and forth along the laser axis whose pattern over the surface of the mirrors is maintained upon the completion of each round trip.   Oscillation will take place only in those modes that do not sustain excessive losses upon successive reflections by the mirrors, and it is intuitively clear that geometrical and physical optics considerations will limit these modes to those whose direction of energy propagation is approximately in the z direction, and whose energy distribution in a transverse plane does not appreciably spread as a result of diffraction.   For these cases, most of the energy can be intercepted and reflected back by the opposite mirror for further amplification by the laser materials.

The transverse modes in practical laser resonators are derived by using a scalar formulation of Huygen's principle,[5] where the field at one mirror is assumed to be caused by the field distribution at the other mirror. A self-consistent analysis[6,7,8] for the most commonly used mirror structures reveals that in the vicinity of the z axis, the wavefronts are approximately spherical, and the amplitude of the electric field which is tangent to these equiphase surfaces is given by[6]

$$E_{mn} = E_0 \frac{w_0}{w} H_m\left(\sqrt{2}\,\frac{x}{w}\right) H_n\left(\sqrt{2}\,\frac{y}{w}\right)\exp\left(-\frac{x^2 + y^2}{w^2}\right) \qquad (1\text{-}26)$$

In (1-26), H_m and H_n are the Hermite polynomial of orders m and n, and w which is given by

$$w = w_0\left[1 + \left(\frac{\lambda z}{\pi w_0^2}\right)^2\right]^{1/2} \qquad (1\text{-}27)$$

defines the spot size of the lowest order ($m, n = 0$) mode, and by virtue of diffraction depends on z.   In (1-27), λ is the wavelength in the resonator medium, and w_0 is the smallest possible value that the spot size can have which is assumed at a point where the wavefront is planar, and from where the z dimension is measured.   Since a wave having an electric field component given by (1-26) will also have a transverse magnetic field which is related to it through Maxwell's equations, the modes characterized by (1-26) are designated by notation TEM_{mn} (transverse electromagnetic wave).   Since $H_0 = 1$, we observe that the fundamental mode ($n, m = 0$) possesses a Gaussian distribution with an intensity which is maximum along the laser axis gradually diminishing in the lateral direction.   For a resonator with mirrors of radii of curvature R_1 and R_2 separated by a distance d, the spot sizes or beam radii of this Gaussian beam at the respective mirrors as depicted in Figure 1-5 are given by[8]

$$w_1^4 = \left(\frac{\lambda R_1}{\pi}\right)^2 \frac{R_2 - d}{R_1 - d} \frac{d}{R_1 + R_2 - d} \qquad (1\text{-}28)$$

and

$$w_2^4 = \left(\frac{\lambda R_2}{\pi}\right)^2 \frac{R_1 - d}{R_2 - d} \frac{d}{R_1 + R_2 - d} \qquad (1\text{-}29$$

In terms of the cavity parameters, the spot size at the beam waist w_0 which may fall either inside or outside the cavity is given by[8]

$$w_0^4 = \left(\frac{\lambda}{\pi}\right)^2 \frac{d(R_1 - d)(R_2 - d)(R_1 + R_2 - d)}{(R_1 + R_2 - 2d)^2} \qquad (1\text{-}30)$$

Figure 1-6 depicts the field patterns obtained for the Gaussian mode, as well as some other low order modes.

In addition to limiting oscillation to a finite number of transverse modes, the mirrors also determine the frequencies at which sustained oscillation may take place. If oscillation at any frequency is to persist, the phase difference occurring as a result of one complete round trip must be an integer multiple of 2π. This implies that to a good approximation the resonance condition

$$d = \frac{n\lambda}{2} \qquad (1\text{-}31)$$

is satisfied, where d is the mirror separation, λ is the wavelength in the

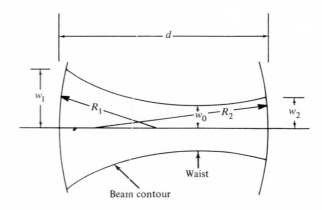

Figure 1-5   Mode parameters of interest for a resonator with mirrors of unequal curvature.

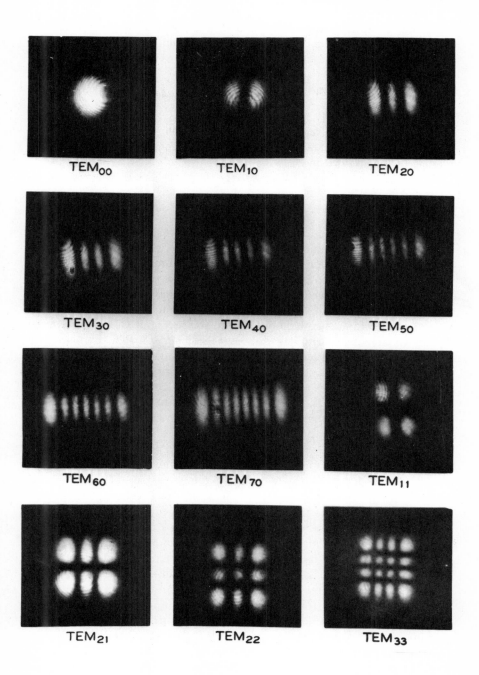

Figure 1-6 Some low-order, single-mode field patterns.[8] *(With permission of* Applied Optics.*)*

medium comprising the cavity, and n is a positive integer. When expressed in terms of the frequency, the above equation assumes the form

$$v = \frac{nc}{2d} \qquad (1\text{-}32)$$

where c is the velocity of light in the medium. Different integers n will give rise to different frequencies, which constitute the longitudinal modes of the cavity. We readily see that the frequency separation between adjacent longitudinal modes is given by

$$\Delta v = \frac{c}{2d} \qquad (1\text{-}33)$$

As was mentioned before, the atomic lines participating in the laser transition are not infinitely narrow, but in fact possess finite width, which for sufficiently high gain will permit oscillation at numerous frequencies all satisfying (1-32), while falling at or near the center of the atomic resonance line. As a result, each transverse mode will have associated with it a number of longitudinal modes whose maximum value is given by the ratio of the atomic width to the intermode spacing of (1-33). The exact number can quite accurately be controlled, and, in fact, oscillation in only one longitudinal mode is entirely feasible and may be implemented in several ways, e.g., inserting an etalon* in the cavity.

The schematic diagram of a laser cavity consisting of two plane-parallel mirrors enclosing the laser medium shown in Figure 1-7 may be used to explain the onset of laser oscillation. Initially, no electromagnetic radiation (in the classical sense of the term) is present in the cavity; therefore, once population inversion is achieved through some pumping scheme, atoms can only emit spontaneously. Since spontaneous emission is randomly distributed in all directions, a great part of this radiation propagates away from the cavity in arbitrary directions and is lost. However, the small part that has a direction of propagation perpendicular to the mirrors may stay in the cavity, and this part provides the source for stimulated emission. Upon successive reflections by the mirrors, light traveling through the laser medium is further coherently amplified. If the gain of this medium is sufficiently high, a condition described by (1-24) may be reached, where the total gain attained by the wave adequately compensates for the total loss it sustains in the cavity, and oscillation ensues. Since the population of the excited atomic state taking part in the lasing transition will be depleted by the stimulated emission process, oscillation may be possible on a continuous or pulsed-only basis, depending on the pumping mechanism employed and the properties of the atomic system. It should be noted that, due to the depopulation of the excited

* See Glossary for a description of an etalon.

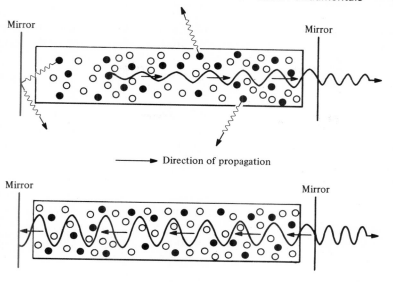

Direction of propagation

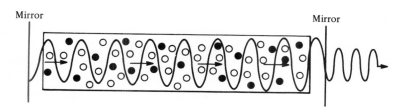

Figure 1-7 Fabry-Perot cavity and buildup of oscillation.

state by stimulated emission, the actual gain during oscillation (the so-called saturated gain) is lower than the initial gain during the buildup of oscillation, and this reduced gain has to be sufficiently high to overcome the losses in the cavity.

Losses in the cavity formed by plane-parallel mirrors will be extremely sensitive to the parallelism of the two mirrors. Slight angular misalignment might result in the reflected beam missing the opposite mirror, leading to excessive loss and difficulties in attaining oscillation. Even under perfect parallelism, it can be shown that a resonator formed by plane-parallel mirrors has higher diffraction losses than cavities formed by various combinations of plane and curved mirrors, and, for this and the previously mentioned reason, it is clear that it is indeed advantageous to use curved mirrors in constructing a laser cavity. However, only certain combinations of curvatures and mirror separations are allowed if high diffraction losses are to be avoided. These combinations are governed by a simple rule: either the center of curvature of one of the mirrors, or the mirror itself, but not both, must lie between the other mirror and its center of curvature.

Algebraically this condition may be expressed as

$$0 \le [(d/R_1) - 1][(d/R_2) - 1] \le 1,$$

where R_1, R_2, and d are illustrated in Figure 1-5. Cavities satisfying the above condition are termed stable. Figure 1-8 contains a few examples of such stable cavities including some of the widely used structures, as well as unstable (high loss) cavities. It is often desirable, and sometimes possible, to operate the laser in a single transverse mode (usually the lowest-order mode). This can generally be accomplished by limiting the radius of the resonator, and since the energy of the higher-order modes spreads much more quickly with propagation than that of the fundamental mode,[8] a proper selection of resonator radius will restrict oscillation to the mode with the least diffraction loss, i.e., the lowest order mode.

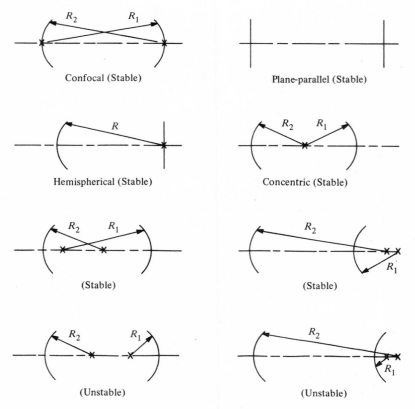

Figure 1-8   Examples of stable and unstable mirror combinations.

1·4   Q-switching, mode locking, and cavity dumping

Despite its unique nature, the light generated by the original ruby laser contained random and independent pulsations, thus rendering the reproduction of a particular pulse an impossible task. Attempts at controlling the output of the laser in both the frequency and the time domains were successful in not only modifying the shape and duration of the output pulse, but also in attaining peak power levels much higher than those obtainable under normal operating conditions. Since pulse lengths and their associated power levels play a significant role in many laser applications, it behooves us to examine the more important techniques employed in achieving increased light intensity: *Q-switching*, *mode locking*, and *cavity dumping*.

1·4·1   description of Q-switching

Since the characteristics of the cavity play an important role in determining the properties of the output beam, the quest for a better controlled, more powerful beam was initially directed toward methods that effectively altered the quality factor (Q factor) of the cavity and became known as Q-switching or Q-spoiling. The Q factor for a particular mode may be defined as

$$Q = \frac{\omega \times \text{energy stored in the mode}}{\text{energy dissipated in mode per unit of time}}$$

where ω is the angular frequency of the mode. We immediately observe that a change in Q may be effected through a change in the loss sustained by the mode.

The idea underlying Q-switching is ingenious, but quite simple,[9] and relies on the fact that oscillation in a laser occurs as soon as the stimulated emission gain is sufficiently high to overcome the various losses suffered by the electromagnetic wave in the cavity. If, through some means, losses can be maintained at a relatively large value that quenches the buildup of oscillation, continued pumping will create large population inversion, and, if at this stage the Q of the cavity is suddenly increased by an instantaneous and drastic reduction in these cavity losses, the gain will substantially exceed the losses and all of the energy accumulated and stored in the atomic system during pumping will be discharged in one giant pulse. The nonlinear characteristics of the Q-switching results in peak powers much larger than those obtained under normal lasing operation and the technique has successfully been applied to furnish pulses as short as 20–30 ns, with peak powers approaching a gigawatt.

A qualitative understanding of the process may be gained through a simple treatment of the atomic medium, the field, and the cavity. If we again view the atomic system as consisting of a large number of identical two energy-level atoms, each with an energy separation $h\nu_{nm}$, we see that the energy released by the system in a Q-switching pulse per unit of volume is given by

$$\mathscr{E} = \tfrac{1}{2} h\nu_{nm}(n_n(0) - n_m(0)) \qquad (1\text{-}34)$$

where $n_n(0)$ and $n_m(0)$ are the number of atoms per unit of volume in the upper and lower level, respectively, at the instant the Q of the cavity is being improved, and where it is assumed that the pulse terminates when population inversion has ended ($n_n = n_m$). The $\tfrac{1}{2}$ factor appearing in (1-34) accounts for the fact that the difference in population decreases by 2 with each de-excitation of an atom. Assuming that the output pulse power rises instantaneously to its peak value, and then decays exponentially with a characteristic decay time $\tau_c = Q/\omega$ of the cavity, the total energy contained in such an exponential pulse will be given by

$$E = P_p \tau_c \simeq V\mathscr{E} \qquad (1\text{-}35)$$

where V is volume occupied by the active atoms participating in the interaction process and P_p is the peak power. Using (1-34) we get a rough estimate for the available peak power in the form

$$P_p = \frac{1}{2\tau_c} h\nu_{nm} (n_n(0) - n_m(0))V \qquad (1\text{-}36)$$

In the brief analysis just concluded, the switching and its effect on the output pulse was assumed to be instantaneous. In real laser systems, the switching as well as the rise time for the pulse will take a finite amount of time, and there will be a delay from the time the switching is initiated to the appearance of a pulse in the laser output. All these realities, combined with the fact that the atomic system must be captured with a large excess of population inversion over that occurring in normal laser operation, impose a lower limit on the speed of switching. Typically required switching times are of the order of 50 ns and can be implemented by a variety of techniques that will be described in the following subsection.

1·4·2   Q-switching techniques

There are numerous methods by which the Q of the cavity may be spoiled. These methods may involve electro-optical, magneto-optical, or acousto-optical effects, as well as saturation of atomic levels in materials introduced into the laser cavity, or it may even more simply be accomplished through the rotation of one of the cavity mirrors. The principles behind the operation of some of the more important techniques are described below, where mention is also made of the merits and disadvantages inherent in each.

One possible method for mechanically altering the Q of the cavity consists of physical rotation of one of the cavity mirrors as is schematically depicted in Figure 1-9. Since the critical condition of mirror parallelism has to be achieved before oscillation can take place, we observe that during the part of the cycle when a large angle exists between the laser axis and the normal to the rotating mirror, high losses would prevent oscillation, and hard pumping during that time may create a large excess of population inversion. If the timing of the pump action is synchronized to reach a maximum at the instant the rotating mirror is returned to parallelism, laser gain will be substantially above that under normal lasing conditions, and a giant Q-switched pulse will appear at the output. The resulting pulse length (usually between 25–50 ns) is somewhat longer than the pulse lengths obtained through other means and is primarily due to the time it takes the mirror to attain the most preferential angular alignment.

In contrast to mechanical switching where relatively slow switching speed places a lower limit on pulse length, electronic switching utilizing

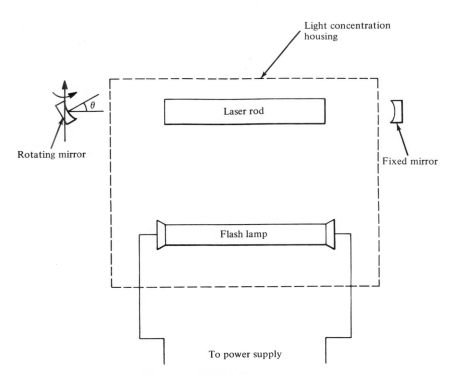

Figure 1.9   Solid-state Q-switched laser using rotating mirror.

electro-optic effects may be employed to achieve Q-switched pulses of shorter duration.   In an electro-optic Q-switched laser,[10] care is taken to obtain linearly polarized light at the output of the laser, and a birefringent material (or a material in which birefringence may be induced) and whose indices of refraction change in response to the application of an electric field is introduced into the cavity.   This material may be solid, such as KDP (potassium dihydrogen phosphate) crystal, or liquid, such as nitrobenzene.   A polarizer is also inserted into the cavity, and the two are oriented in such a way that the polarizer absorbs all the linearly polarized light that makes a double pass through the electro-optic material.   When the electro-optic material that is inserted into the cavity responds to the linear electro-optic effect, the element is called a *Pockels cell*, whereas an element containing a material responding to the quadratic electro-optic effect is termed a *Kerr cell*.*   To achieve complete blockage of light, quarter-wave voltage has to be applied to the cell, creating an electric field which rotates the polarization of the linearly polarized light by 90° upon forward and back passes through the cell.   Removal of this applied voltage appreciably reduces the losses in the cavity, and when it is timed to coincide with a state of maximum excess population inversion, a powerful Q-switched pulse will once more be produced.

Since electronic switching is inherently faster than mechanical switching, electro-optic Q-switching and similar electronically controlled methods result in shorter pulse lengths, besides easing the omnipresent synchronization problems of capturing the atomic system with maximum inverted population at the instant the pulse is initiated.   However, the insertion of additional elements into the cavity inevitably introduces optical losses and inhomogeneities which detract from the optimal coherence properties of the laser beam.   Commercial units employing Pockels cells to Q-switch solid-state (ruby, Nd:glass) lasers produce pulses 15–25 ns in duration with peak power in the region of 100 MW.

Similar to electro-optic materials where a linear electro-optic effect (Pockels effect) or a quadratic effect (Kerr effect) may be used to vary the polarization of the laser light, magneto-optic materials relying on the Faraday effect may be employed.[11]   Such a magneto-optic technique will also necessitate the use of a polarizer and usually involves magnetic fields which are difficult to obtain.

Just as Pockels, Kerr, or Faraday cells may be arranged in the cavity to produce high losses and quench oscillation for a desired length of time, an acousto-optic modulator† placed inside the cavity can similarly be used to generate a Q-switched pulse.[12]   The acousto-optic modulator usually consists of a piezoelectric transducer which is bonded to a high quality, low optical loss material.   The transducer is electrically driven to set up a

---

* See Glossary for definitions of Pockels (see Modulator) and Kerr cells.
† See Chapter 6 for a more detailed discussion on acousto-optical interactions.

traveling acoustic diffraction grating which diffracts the light away from the cavity axis, thus increasing the single pass loss beyond the single pass gain and quenching possible oscillation. A high Q oscillating state is achieved in the cavity by pulsing off the signal driving the transducer, therefore permitting the light to propagate back and forth without diffraction through the acousto-optic material and along the cavity axis. This Q-switching method possesses a high degree of reproducibility, primarily because of the availability of high quality, low loss acousto-optic materials, to which piezoelectric transducers may readily be attached, and does not depend on the availability of linearly polarized light. Commercially available, continuously pumped Q-switched Nd:YAG lasers employ the scheme described above to attain pulses 150–300 ns in length or even shorter with peak power exceeding 5 kW at a repetition rate of up to 50,000 pps.

In contrast to the various techniques described so far, where the switching speed is limited by the characteristics of the active mechanical or electronic switching device, there exists a passive and elegant method that utilizes the much shorter atomic and molecular lifetimes and is consequently both simpler and faster. The method takes advantage of properties of materials called *saturable absorbers*,[13,14] which display a change in opacity directly related to the incident radiation intensity. When such a saturable dye (e.g., cryptocyanine in acetone for ruby) is inserted in the cavity, it will inhibit the onset of oscillation by absorbing the small intensity of light present in the cavity, thus permitting the establishment of a large excess of population in the upper laser level. However, this inhibitory action is not completely effective and, when the small intensity reaches a certain level, the dye saturates, suddenly becomes transparent, and the fast buildup of oscillation culminates in the emission of a giant powerful pulse.

The Q-switching techniques are applicable to lasers where the upper level atomic state possesses a relatively long lifetime. Table 1-1 lists lifetimes of the upper laser levels of a few prominent lasers. The top three lasers have suitable lifetimes for Q-switching, whereas the bottom three have lifetimes that are too short for effective Q-switching.

TABLE 1-1   Lifetimes of Upper Laser Levels for Prominent Lasers

Laser	Line(nm)	Lifetime
CO_2	10.6×10^3	~ 4 ms
Nd:YAG	1.06×10^3	~ 230 μs
Ruby	694.3	~ 4 ms
HeNe	632.8	~ 0.1 μs
Ar	488.0	~ 0.01 μs
HeCd	325.0	~ 0.26 μs

1·4·3   description and techniques of mode locking

Regardless of the Q-switching method, pulses produced are always limited to a minimum length of a few nanoseconds, and the finite energy that can be stored in the atomic system usually restricts the power output from such a laser to several hundred megawatts.   A novel and completely different approach to the problem of producing shorter pulses was needed, and various mode-locking modulation schemes proved successful in achieving pulses of picosecond (10^{-12} s) duration and peak powers in the order of gigawatts.

In an ordinary laser, if no special precautions are taken, a number of longitudinal modes will usually oscillate simultaneously.   Because the atomic resonance line participating in the lasing transition is inhomogeneously broadened,[4] these various longitudinal modes "see" and thus interact with different atomic populations, and consequently oscillate independently of one another.   If, by some means, it were possible to eliminate the random relative phase and amplitude fluctuations that result from lack of coupling between the modes, constructive and destructive interference between these discrete frequency components might lead to a narrowing (in the time domain) of the laser output.

The introduction of definite phase and amplitude relations between the longitudinal modes may be implemented in two distinct fashions.   The initial method employs active modulation by a modulating cell that varies the losses or the optical length of the cavity at a precise frequency equal to a multiple of the intermode spacing of $c/2d$.[15,16]   Losses in the cavity may be modulated through light diffraction by an ultrasonic cell, whereas the optical length of the cavity may readily be altered by inserting and properly orienting an electro-optic crystal, such as KDP, inside the laser cavity.

When an active internal modulator is operating at a frequency $v_m = c/2d$, it would assist the longitudinal mode with the highest gain (usually the one with a frequency v_0 which is closest to the center of the atomic resonance line) in establishing sidebands at frequencies $v_0 \pm \ell\, v_m$, $\ell = 1, 2, 3, \ldots, k$, where k is the maximum positive constant which leaves the sideband within the atomic line width.   The fact that the sidebands fall on cavity resonances satisfying (1-32) couples the longitudinal modes of the cavity with definite phase and amplitude relationships.

Simple Fourier analysis[17] reveals that the greater the number of discrete Fourier components possessing definite phase relations and interfering in a wave, the shorter will be the corresponding pulse in the time domain, with a commensurate increase in peak amplitude.   The uncertainty principle between the frequency and time variables[17] limits the narrowness of a pulse to $\Delta t \simeq 1/\Delta v$, where Δt is pulse length and Δv is its corresponding bandwidth.   The broad line widths of some laser materials such as Nd^{3+}: glass (line width of 10–20 nm) permit the mode locking of thousands of longitudinal modes, and the generation of pulses of duration much shorter than those obtained by any other technique. If n is the number of coupled modes, concurrent with pulse narrowing, an n fold increase in peak power over average free running power is also achieved. It should also be noted that the pulses emitted by a mode locked laser are repetitive with a period equal to the inverse of the modulation frequency. This period is also equal to twice the time it takes light to traverse the cavity, so that periodic pulses are fed out by the cavity after each complete round trip through it.

Active modulation suffers from a disadvantage in that, during the lasing operation, drift in the longitudinal modes makes constant adjustment of parameters necessary if the required conditions are to be fulfilled. But just as in the case of Q-switching, passive modulation is possible, and saturable absorbers may be utilized to achieve this end too.[18]

With the insertion of a suitable saturable absorber into the cavity, the optical circuit contains all the ingredients necessary for the creation of an optical regenerative pulse generator.[19,20] To function properly, a saturable absorber identical to the one used for Q-switching must satisfy certain necessary conditions, the most important of which are (a) its relaxation time (the time it takes the dye to return to its original state after it has saturated) must be shorter than the round-trip transit time, and (b) it must have an absorption line of line width greater than, or equal to, the laser line width at the laser wavelength. Under these conditions, the absorber will act as a nonlinear circuit element tending to create sidebands at $v_0 \pm v_m$ in the frequency domain, while attenuating the lower light amplitudes and thus emphasizing the highest ones, in the time domain. Numerous passages through the absorber will couple the oscillating axial modes with definite phase and amplitude relations and further sharpen the pulses until, again, pulses whose minimum length is restricted by the uncertainty relation to $\Delta t \simeq 1/\Delta v$ are emitted from the cavity every $2d/c$ seconds. It is apparent that the use of a bleachable dye as a saturable absorber will result in simultaneous Q-switching and mode locking, and indeed the mode-locked train of pulses is observed to exist within the giant Q-switched pulse. A technique whereby a single pulse is selected out of the train of pulses generated by a mode-locked laser is available for applications requiring the use of a single pulse[21] and is based on the pulse transmission of mode of operation[22] where the Q of the cavity is spoiled back to its original low value once the peak radiation density is achieved in the cavity.

Mode locking in conjunction with a pulse compression technique in glass lasers has produced pulses in the sub-picosecond range[23] (4×10^{-13} s), whereas other systems consisting of a laser oscillator and several stages of laser amplifiers have attained powers of several trillion watts in picosecond pulses, a power level sufficiently high to trigger thermonuclear reactions.

1·4·4 cavity dumping

In Q-switching, the finite time needed to build up the field inside the cavity plus the time required to repump and establish the population inversion set an upper limit on the maximum repetition rate.   This maximum rate is of the order of 50 kHz for continuously pumped Q-switched YAG lasers, and lower for other systems.   Mode locking of continuously pumped lasers produces pulses at repetition rates of $c/2d$, which is usually in the hundreds of MHz range.   There exists another method which partially bridges this gap in the availability of repetition rates called *cavity dumping*,[24] which can provide repetition rates varying from 1 pps to several MHz, in pulses of duration between 15 ns and CW.   This method has successfully been applied to systems in which the atomic system possesses a relatively long lifetime (e.g., YAG) as well as some short lifetime systems (e.g., argon, HeNe).

An intracavity modulation system adopted for a YAG laser[25] is depicted in Figure 1-10.   The key element in the system is the acousto-optic modulator which consists of a ZnO transducer sputtered on a fused-silica substrate.   A folded cavity is created by three high reflectivity mirrors, and the modulator is inserted at a point in the cavity where the beam attains its smallest spot.

The laser is continuously pumped and kept above threshold, whereas the output coupling is periodically varied with time.   This is accomplished by activating the modulator which causes the acoustic beam to scatter the light beam passing through it.   The light beam thus transverses a path shown by the dashed lines in Figure 1-10.   This diffracted beam is then intercepted by another high reflectivity mirror and reflected away from the cavity as the useful output of the laser.

At repetition rates of the order of 1 MHz, the average power in the cavity dumped mode of operation is essentially the CW power obtained from the same cavity, whereas the peak power may approach a value 50–100 times greater than the average power.

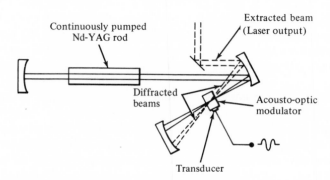

Figure 1-10   The intracavity modulation system.

1·5   coherence and interference

Undoubtedly, the most important property of laser light is its coherence, manifested in both monochromaticity (temporal coherence) and uniphase wavefront (spatial coherence).

Traditionally, the field of coherence has concerned itself with the statistical description of fluctuation phenomena in light beams, and the effects of these fluctuations on the correlations in the light between various points in the beam, in both space and time. The simplest and clearest evidence of an occurrence of correlation is revealed by interference experiments, which readily explains the long association between coherence and interference.

Classically, it is convenient to think of coherence in terms of the phase of the electromagnetic field along a particular wavefront. If at all times the light really has a constant phase across a uniphase wavefront, it is said to be completely spatially coherent. Similarly, if the phase at a particular instant of time along a traveling wavefront is identical to its phase after the wave has traveled a distance ℓ in ℓ/c seconds, for all ℓ, the field is said to be completely temporally coherent.

It is immediately obvious from the above definitions that a mono-chromatic plane wave of infinite extent will be completely coherent in both space and time. Moreover, any field whose phase is completely specified for all points in space and time by its phase along a particular surface at a particular instant of time will be completely coherent. The randomness introduced into the wave by the omnipresent noise prevents real fields from possessing complete coherence. However, lasers operating in a single transverse and longitudinal mode have outputs that are essentially mono-chromatic and uniphase, and thus possess a very high degree of both spatial and temporal coherence.

1·5·1   temporal coherence

Since the concept of coherence is associated with the possibility of obtain-ing interference effects when two fields are superposed, it is only natural to proceed and define coherence in terms of the observed interference fringes.

Interference in light beams produced as a result of time coherence may very easily be illustrated by means of a Michelson interferometer such as the one depicted in Figure 1-11. A parallel beam of light is split up and the two parts propagate in different directions. After traversing their individual paths, the two beams are recombined to create an inter-ference pattern. If the beams are made to travel paths of unequal length, the intensity will normally vary as a function of position along the obser-

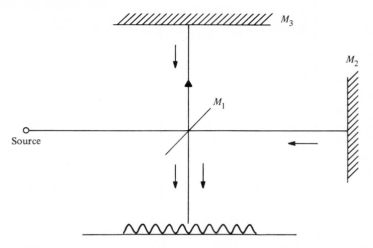

**Figure 1-11   Temporal coherence experiment using a Michelson
interferometer.**

vation screen.   A convenient parameter commonly called the *visibility* of
the interference fringes is usually defined in the form

$$V = \frac{I_{max} - I_{min}}{I_{max} + I_{min}} \tag{1-37}$$

where I_{max} and I_{min} are the maximum and minimum observed intensities,
respectively, and we immediately note that the visibility factor varies
between zero and unity.   Maximum contrast in the interference fringes
implies a visibility factor of 1 and is associated with full temporal coherence.
No contrast or complete absence of fringes implies $I_{max} = I_{min}$ and leads to
a visibility factor of zero, which is associated with complete incoherence.
Partial coherence involves a visibility factor between zero and unity.

In practice, we observe that interference fringes are produced only
when the path differences are maintained below a certain maximum
length.   For conventional light sources it might be as high as a few
centimeters, whereas for lasers it may extend to a few meters, but is
nevertheless finite.   This illustrates the fact that the laser which may
possess a higher degree of coherence than conventional light sources is
still a partially coherent light source only.   The eventual disappearance
of interference fringes for sufficiently large path differences may be
accounted for by the nonmonochromaticity of any stationary, partially
coherent light source.   The maximum path length difference under which
fringes are still observed is called the *coherence length* S_c, and the maximum
time delay corresponding to this path difference S_c/c is referred to as the
coherence time Δt.   For shorter path differences than S_c corresponding to
time delays less than Δt, fringes will be produced by the interfering light

TABLE 1-2   Line Widths of Typical Lasers

Laser	Line(nm)	Line Width
CO_2	10.6×10^3	~ 100 MHz
HeNe	632.8	~ 1500 MHz
Ar	488.0	~ 5000 MHz
Nd:YAG	1.064×10^3	~ 13 GHz
Ruby	694.3	~ 30 GHz
Nd:Glass	1.06×10^3	~ 1500 GHz

beams. The uncertainty relation between frequency and time yields $\Delta v \, \Delta t \simeq 1$, where Δv is the frequency spread (line width) of the nonmonochromatic light beam. We observe that the greater the monochromaticity of the beam, i.e., the smaller Δv is, the larger the coherence time of the light beam. Lasers operating in a single longitudinal mode have extremely narrow line widths, which accounts for the attainment of interference fringes in experiments involving path differences of several meters.

Line widths over which a few important lasers may lase (if no special precautions are taken to limit them) are presented in Table 1-2 where it is noted that the gas lasers are, in general, more monochromatic than solid-state lasers. These line widths may be reduced by limiting laser oscillation to a single or a few longitudinal modes.

1·5·2   spatial coherence

Correlation in light beams in a direction transverse to the direction of propagation may be illustrated by means of a Young-type interference experiment, as depicted in Figure 1-12. Light after passing through pinhole S is made incident upon the two pinholes, P_1 and P_2, and if the two pinholes are sufficiently close to each other, interference fringes will appear near the center point P on the screen. Whenever definite phase relations exist between light waves emanating from P_1 and P_2, the intensity at any point along the screen will depend on whether the two waves arrive in phase or out of phase, resulting in interference fringes on the screen. The visibility may once more be defined in a format analogous to (1-37), and a visibility factor of unity will again correspond to complete coherence. A visibility factor of zero will correspond to lack of correlation and complete incoherence, whereas a factor between zero and one will imply partial coherence.

It should be noted that spatial and temporal coherence of a source are essentially independent of one another, and a source may be spatially coherent while temporally incoherent and vice versa. Fortunately, the mode selection properties of the laser cavity and medium endow the laser

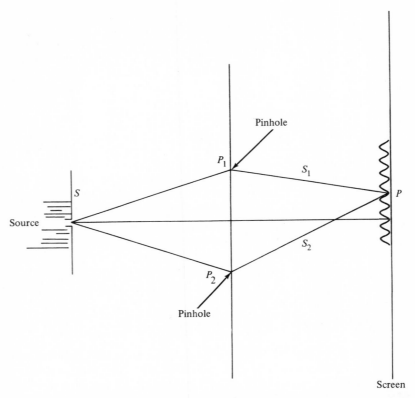

Figure 1-12 Spatial coherence exhibited by means of a Young interference experiment.

with good spatial and temporal coherence properties, thus making available for the first time intense coherent electromagnetic radiation in the visible, ultraviolet, and infrared parts of the spectrum.

The advantage of laser light over ordinary light in forming an image of high brightness arises from the nearly uniphase wavefront of the spatially coherent light emitted by the laser and is displayed in Figure 1-13. In an ordinary source (a) light is emitted randomly with the result that the total energy is, on the average, radiated in all directions. The amount of energy in a particular direction will be proportional to the solid angle subtended by the observing device. Any attempt to increase the brightness of an image over the brightness of the source with a lens cannot succeed, because even under ideal conditions the reduced area of the image just makes up for the reduced collection angle that the lens intercepts from the source.

In contrast, the coherent light produced by a laser (b) is generated over a sizable volume with the proper phase, so that when it is focused by

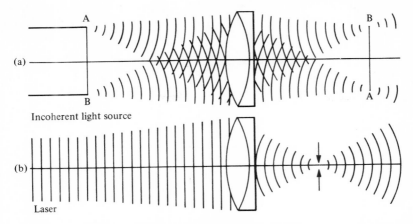

Figure 1-13 Comparison of focusing characteristics of lasers and incoherent light sources. (From **Application of Laser Light**, **by D. R. Herriott,** **copyright © Sept. 1968 by Scientific American, Inc. All rights reserved.)**

a lens, all the individual contributions by the atoms in the lasing medium are in the correct phase to add up. Accordingly, with a suitable lens, essentially all the energy of the laser can be concentrated into a very small spot, resulting in much greater energy density than the energy density of the source.

The nearly plane wavefront emanating from the laser, as depicted in Figure 1-13b, also results in higher directionality than that possessed by ordinary light. Consequently, laser light spreads out less than incoherent light and its radiance (intensity per unit of solid angle into which light is emitted) is therefore greater than that of conventional sources.

1·6 common lasers and their output characteristics

The preceding sections discussed the principles governing the operation and the general properties of all lasers. However, the diverse material properties of the lasing medium lead to numerous distinct characteristics, such as wavelength, output power, and coherence, which largely determine the usefulness of a particular laser for a specific application.

The three most important types of lasers are solid-state, gaseous, and semiconductor lasers, each type possessing unique properties while requiring differing approaches to the problems of attaining population inversion and positive feedback. The most prominent members of each of these broad classes* are listed in Figure 1-14, together with their associated

* For a fairly complete tabulation of all observed laser oscillations, the reader may consult Ref. 26.

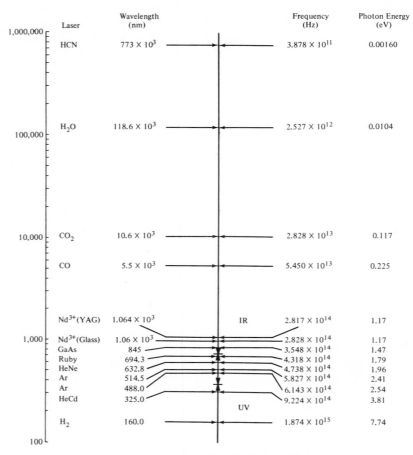

Figure 1-14   Typical available lasers.

wavelengths, frequencies, and energies of individual quanta. The solid-state lasers usually employ ions doped into a host crystal to provide stimulated emission, and flash lamps or CW lamps are used to excite optically these ions to obtain population inversion. By contrast, gaseous lasers by virtue of using a gas as the lasing medium contain fewer atoms per unit of volume and their absorption and emission lines at low pressures are much narrower than those of solid-state lasers. This generally dictates a different pumping technique (radio-frequency or dc discharges) and results in better coherence properties and lower output power. The mechanism responsible for lasing action in semiconductor lasers is different from the one encountered in conventional lasers, resulting in unique properties while requiring special pumping techniques. Before proceeding to briefly survey the operation and characteristics of several of the more important lasers, we review some basic energy and power concepts, and their relation to general modes of laser operation.

The total energy density (J/m^3) stored in an electromagnetic field is the sum of the electric and magnetic energy densities stored, which in free space assumes the form

$$\mathscr{E} = \underbrace{\tfrac{1}{2}\varepsilon_0\mathbf{E}^2}_{\substack{\text{electric}\\\text{energy}\\\text{density}}} + \underbrace{\tfrac{1}{2}\mu_0\mathbf{H}^2}_{\substack{\text{magnetic}\\\text{energy}\\\text{density}}} \tag{1-38}$$

The energy flow per unit of time (power flow) per unit of area is given by the Poynting vector* as

$$\mathbf{S} = \mathbf{E} \times \mathbf{H} \tag{1-39}$$

whose direction corresponds to the direction of energy propagation and is perpendicular to both the electric and magnetic field vectors. Finally, the field intensity is defined as the power flow across a unit area perpendicular to the direction of propagation.

Lasers are operated in one of the following modes of operation: (a) continuous wave (CW), (b) pulsed, (c) Q-switched, (d) mode locked, and (e) cavity dumped. Figure 1-15 depicts the power output shapes under several of these modes of operation.

In CW operation, as the name implies, a continuous beam of constant power is being emitted by the laser cavity (Figure 1-15a).

Pulsed operation is characterized by pulsed pumping and the emission of bursts of relatively high-energy pulses at repetition rates of from 1 pps up to hundreds of pulses per second. Pulse widths (nominally ns to several ms), repetition rates, and total energy per pulse vary depending upon the particular type system being employed. Figure 1-15b shows an idealized laser output, where the power P_1 is considered to be constant for almost the entire duration of the pulse.

As we have seen, extremely short duration, high peak power pulses can be generated using cavity dumping, Q-switching, or mode-locking techniques. The power attainable in this short pulse greatly exceeds that which can be achieved during CW or pulsed operation (Figure 1-15c), although energy is lower than that obtained in normal pulsing operations. Typical pulse widths range from several picoseconds to a few hundred nanoseconds; and repetition rates vary from one laser to another, but may range as high as 50,000 pps in Q-switched operation, and even higher in other modes of operation. The total energy per pulse is once more given by

$$E = \int_{\text{pulse}} P \, dt$$

where the integration is carried over the length of the pulse. When the

* See Chapter 2 for a more detailed discussion of electromagnetic field theory.

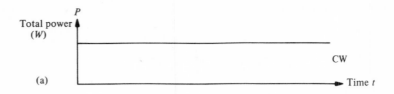

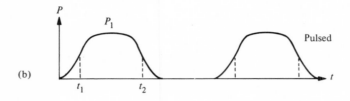

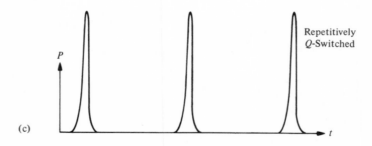

Figure 1-15   Output power shape for several modes of operation.

assumption of nearly constant power for the duration of the pulse is valid, the total energy per pulse is given by

$$E = \int_{\text{pulse}} P \, dt \simeq P_1(t_2 - t_1) \qquad (1\text{-}40)$$

1·6·1   ruby laser

In addition to possessing historical significance as the first material to demonstrate lasing action,[1] ruby $(Al_2O_3 : Cr^{3+})$ remains as one of the most widely used laser materials, primarily because of its large output power and the wavelength of its radiation.

A schematic representation of a ruby laser setup is presented in Figure 1-16, and its operation is most easily described with the help of the pertinent energy-level diagram of Cr^{3+} in Al_2O_3 crystal, given in Figure 1-17. The corresponding Cr^{3+} concentration is typically 0.05 percent by weight, and conventional spectroscopic labeling has been used

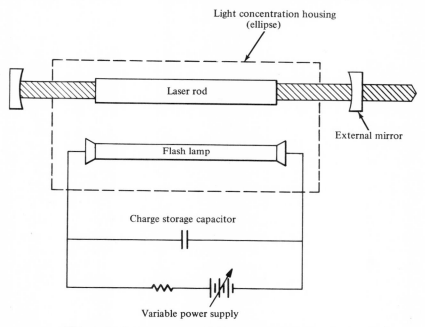

Figure 1-16 *A typical pulsed solid-state laser setup.*

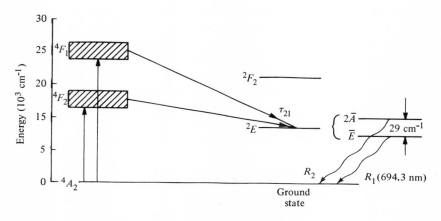

Figure 1-17 *Energy-level diagram for ruby laser.*

to denote the relevant energy levels.   At room temperature $kT \ll h\nu$ and in thermal equilibrium, most ions find themselves in the ground state.   To excite the ions into the upper laser level, a capacitor bank storing a few thousand joules is discharged into a flash lamp in a time duration of the order of a millisecond.   A large portion of the energy is converted into light, part of which is absorbed by the ruby inducing the transitions into the broad energy levels $^4F_1$ and $^4F_2$.   Essentially all ions excited into these two energy levels will immediately decay through a nonradiative process to level $\bar{E}$ which serves as the upper laser level.   Level $\bar{E}$ is a metastable one of relatively long lifetime (approximately 4 ms), and it is possible to obtain population inversion between $\bar{E}$ and the ground level, $^4A_2$.   Since the population inversion is obtained with respect to the ground level, more than 50 percent of the atoms have to be raised into level $\bar{E}$ before lasing can commence and, consequently, relatively large input energies are needed before the threshold of oscillation can be reached.   Fortunately in ruby, this problem which is common to all three-level systems is somewhat mitigated by the very high quantum efficiency (ratio of number of ions pumped into the upper laser level to the number of photons absorbed from the pump), which approaches unity.

To obtain oscillation, the ruby rod is placed between two mirrors or has its ends polished flat and coated for high reflectivity, thus providing the feedback necessary for the oscillation process.   The lasing transition, which is normally obtained between level $\bar{E}$ and $^4A_2$ (R_1 line), corresponds to a wavelength of 694.3 nm at room temperature, but laser operation between $2\bar{A}$ and $^4A_2$ (R_2 line) is possible if care is taken to suppress the R_1 line.

Even though ruby laser light is more coherent than light from conventional sources, it is nevertheless spiky and irregular.   This is partly due to inhomogeneity in the laser material, but primarily is the result of the fast buildup of oscillation and consequent depletion of the excess population of the upper laser level.   When this occurs, lasing ceases for a short time until the flash lamp again replenishes the population of the upper level.   This process continues until the pump intensity drops below the threshold value, with the overall result being a series of spikes during the lasing period.

In a typical ruby laser, the actual efficiency is rather low, and out of a total electrical input energy of a few thousand joules, only several joules appear at the output in the form of coherent laser radiation.   Since the period of oscillation is of the order of several milliseconds, output power is typically 10–20 kW.   However, due to the spiking behavior of the laser, peak power is somewhat greater and can be substantially increased by means of Q-switching and mode-locking techniques. Q-switched ruby lasers[10] are capable of producing peak powers in the range of several hundred megawatts while lasting 10–20 ns, whereas passive mode locking[20] using saturable absorbers may produce peak powers of several gigawatts in pulses of a few picoseconds in duration. In a pulsed mode of operation, repetition rates are rather low and generally do not exceed more than several pulses per second.

Finally, it should be noted that in applications requiring even greater pulsed or Q-switched powers and energies than mentioned thus far, it is possible to construct an oscillator-amplifier combinational system. In such a system, the additional amplification appreciably increases energy, power, and radiance.

1·6·2   YAG and neodymium-glass lasers

Although the ruby laser suffers from the inherent deficiency of operating as a three-level system, trivalent rare-earth ions such as Nd^{3+}, Ho^{3+} and others, in such host materials as yttrium aluminum garnet (YAG), $CaWO_4$, and glass, offer the advantage of operating as a four-level laser system and, consequently, possess much lower threshold levels than a similar ruby system. Despite the slight disadvantage of laser operation in the infrared part of the spectrum with a corresponding reduction in energy per photon, these lasers, and in particular the Nd doped YAG[27] and Nd doped glass,[28,29] are finding numerous uses in both industrial and laboratory applications, and together with the ruby lasers have become the most important solid-state lasers.

Energy-level diagrams for transitions of the trivalent neodymium ions in crystals are illustrated in Figure 1-18. Quantum mechanical notations are used to designate the individual levels.[26]

To attain population inversion in a Nd:YAG system, ions are optically pumped by a broadband, incoherent source such as a flash lamp or a CW lamp from the ground state (the $^4I_{9/2}$ level) to any or all of the energy levels lying above the $^4F_{3/2}$ level. Ions excited into these bands decay nonradiatively and with nearly unity quantum efficiency into the $^4F_{3/2}$ level. This level has a lifetime of approximately 0.25 ms and is, therefore, metastable and may serve as the upper laser level. Laser transition is normally obtained between $^4F_{3/2}$ and $^4I_{11/2}$ levels at a wavelength of approximately 1064 nm. It should be noted that the $^4I_{11/2}$ level is about 2000 cm^{-1}* above the ground level, and its population will, therefore, be negligible at normal operating temperatures. This makes the laser a four-level system and permits attainment of population inversion and oscillation at a typical threshold of a few hundred watts CW pumping power,[27] with laser output power being of the order of several watts. Efficiency may be enhanced by doping the host crystal with several different types of ions, thus broadening the absorption bands and relying

* See Glossary for a definition of a wave number (cm^{-1}).

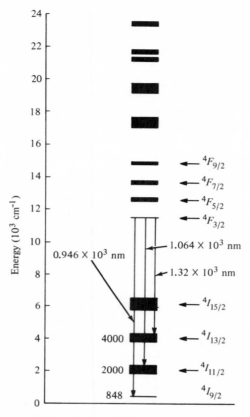

Figure 1-18   Energy levels and laser transition of neodymium ions in YAG.

on energy transfer between ions to bring the system into the upper laser level.

In addition to CW operation where powers of a few hundred watts can be achieved, it is also possible to repetitively Q-switch the YAG laser under continuous pumping conditions.[30,12] This possibility, which stems directly from the relatively long lifetime of the $^4F_{3/2}$ state, can normally achieve peak power of several kilowatts with pulse lengths of about 200 ns. The maximum repetition rate at or near maximum peak power will be limited to the inverse of the lifetime of the upper laser level and will approach 4000 Hz. Of course, Q-switched pulses at a higher repetition rate can be obtained, but only at the expense of peak power. It is also possible to operate the YAG laser in a pulsed mode with flash-lamp pumping, with the higher gain per pass leading to greater peak power, energies of a few joules per pulse, and repetition rates of greater than 40 pps.

Finally, we note that by a judicious selection of the feedback mirrors and operating temperatures, it is possible to suppress the normally preferential $^4F_{3/2}$ to $^4I_{11/2}$ laser transition and obtain oscillations at lower and higher wavelengths.

Since high-quality single crystals of YAG are hard to grow in diameters larger than a few millimeters, the total energy that can be obtained in a single pulse from such a laser will ultimately be limited by the size of the rod. However, good quality Nd^{3+} doped glass rods are available in larger sizes, and they have demonstrated the capability of producing high-energy and power pulsed laser action at 1.06×10^3 nm and several other wavelengths.[31]

The relevant energy levels in Nd doped glass are similar to those of Nd:YAG, and under a similar pumping scheme system, the laser operates as a four-level system. However, the glass host introduces substantial line broadening in comparison with ions in crystals, which plays a significant role in determining the suitability of the laser for a particular application. The larger line width increases the threshold, raises the amount of energy that can be stored in the material during the optical pumping operation, and therefore makes the glass laser a prime candidate for high-power Q-switched and mode-locked laser applications.

It is possible to obtain pulses in the 10^{-2} to 10^{-7} s range by either flash-lamp pulsing or spontaneous emission amplification.[32] Normal Q-switching techniques may be employed to produce pulses of from 10 to 120 ns. Simultaneous Q-switching and mode locking using saturable absorbers[33] may be used to generate pulses in the picosecond range, and to this end the very broad emission line of the glass laser (10 to 20 nm) is of immeasurable help. Very high peak powers can be obtained by releasing appreciable energy in a picosecond pulse.

As in the case of ruby, in applications requiring a particularly high level of energy and power per pulse, a combination oscillator-amplifier may be used to increase the output beyond its normal level obtained from an oscillator alone.

We have thus seen that the different properties of Nd doped YAG and glass lasers complement each other and make the YAG attractive for CW or high repetition rate operation, whereas the Nd doped glass is preferred for modest repetition rates (in the range of 1 pps), high-energy pulsing, Q-switching at high powers, and mode locking.

1·6·3   helium-neon laser

The HeNe laser was the first laser to employ a gaseous medium for the lasing action, and the first of any kind in which continuous laser action was demonstrated.[34] Its high temporal and spatial coherence and relative simplicity make it a highly suitable device for numerous measurement techniques and applications. A schematic representation of such a laser is given in Figure 1-19.

Since atomic resonance lines in gases are determined primarily by the Doppler width[4] and are relatively narrow, the most common pumping mechanism in a gas laser involves excitations through collision with electrons and other atoms in a gas discharge. In a HeNe laser, the discharge may be achieved in a tube by either passing a direct current through the gas mixture which typically contains 1 torr of He and 1 torr of Ne, or by applying a radio-frequency (RF) electric field to it. When the discharge occurs, some atoms are ionized, creating positive ions and free electrons. The free electrons are acted upon by the applied electric field which accelerates them and increases their energy. This is the initial step in the excitation process and, together with the aid of the important energy-level diagram of Figure 1-20, may be used to explain the attainment of population inversion between numerous electron energy levels of Ne in the HeNe laser.

When energetic electrons in the gas discharge strike He atoms, they efficiently excite these atoms, primarily into levels 2^1S and 2^3S. When these excited He atoms collide with unexcited Ne atoms, they may exchange energy raising the Ne atoms from the ground state into the $3s$ and $2s$ energy levels, respectively, while they drop back to their ground state. However, if this inelastic collision process is to take place with relatively high efficiency, the population of the excited He states has to be reasonably high, and the energy of the excited levels of He and Ne have to very nearly coincide. Fortunately, both conditions are readily satisfied in a mixture of He and Ne by virtue of the metastable nature of the 2^1S and 2^3S He levels, and the small energy difference between the excited states of He and Ne. This pumping mechanism will continuously act to populate the Ne $3s$ and $2s$ levels, and suggests the possibility of obtaining population inversion between these levels and lower Ne levels, which does happen in Ne since the relaxation times are favorable. The three most important HeNe laser lines are depicted in Figure 1-20 and involve the following transitions: $3s$ to $2p$ (red line at 632.8 nm),[35] $2s$ to $2p$ (1.15 $\times 10^3$ nm in the infrared),[34] and $3s$ to $3p$ (3.39 $\times 10^3$ nm in the infrared).[36]

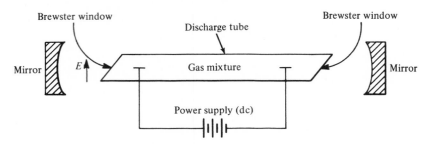

Figure 1-19 A schematic representation of a HeNe laser with Brewster windows using dc discharge.

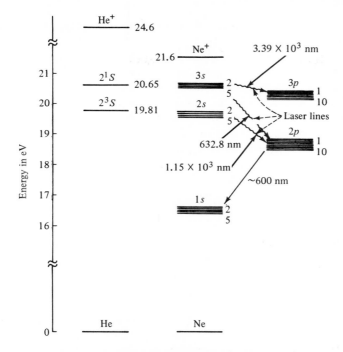

Figure 1-20 Energy-level diagram of helium and neon.

Even though the first HeNe laser ever built oscillated at 1.15×10^3 nm, the 3.39×10^3 nm line possesses the highest gain, whereas the 632.8 nm red line is the most widely used. Simultaneous oscillation in all of the above lines and at some other wavelengths is possible. If single-line oscillation such as the 632.8 nm line is desired, special measures have to be employed to suppress the lasing of the higher gain transitions. One such technique is illustrated in Figure 1-21. The Littrow* prism is designed

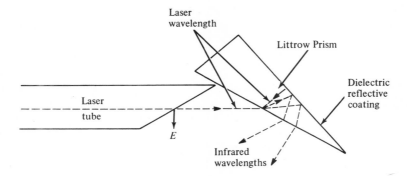

Figure 1-21 Prism separation of light wavelengths.

* See Glossary for a description of Littrow prism.

so that light at a wavelength at which oscillation is desired enters and leaves at Brewster's angle.   The undesired wavelengths are reflected at an angle which deflects them from the axis of the plasma tube.

A typical commercial HeNe laser has a plasma tube of from 10 cm to 1.8 m and can produce continuous power ranging from a fraction of a milliwatt to 80 mW.   The plasma tube usually has Brewster's angle end windows,* so that only light of the proper polarization is transmitted through the interface without suffering reflection, thus resulting in linearly polarized output light, usually in a TEM_{00} mode, as shown in Figure 1-6.

1·6·4   argon and other ion lasers

When high current densities are used to establish the discharge in a gas, it is possible while ionizing the gas to obtain population inversions between energy levels of the ions.   Lasers that employ ions as the active medium[37-39] have exhibited both pulsed and CW mode of operation, and have produced continuous high-power output in the visible part of the spectrum.[40]   The most important of these lasers is the argon-ion laser in which singly ionized argon acts as the lasing medium, which can have an output of several watts in either the blue (488.0 nm) or green (514.5 nm), or can operate in these and other lines in the blue-green region simultaneously.

The operation of the singly ionized argon laser (which does not require the introduction of any other gas into the discharge) may best be understood with the help of the energy-level diagram, Figure 1-22.   A dc or RF discharge is used to generate free electrons in the plasma with an average energy of 4–5 eV.   However, since the potential upper laser levels are approximately 20 eV above the ground state of the ion (1 eV = 8066 cm^{-1}), multiple collisions are required to raise the ions into levels that may serve as upper laser levels.   Once the ions are excited into these states, large population inversion may be achieved on either a momentary or continuous basis, depending on the relaxation rates.   Since the terminal laser levels are approximately 17 eV above the ion ground level, they have negligible thermal population even at the high plasma temperature.   The two sublevels of the $4s^2P$ state that serve as the lower laser level have very short lifetimes, quickly decay to the ion's ground level, and help maintain the population inversion during continuous pumping operation.

The large current density necessary for the pumping of ion levels requires high input power, expensive tubes (usually made of quartz, BeO, or ceramic) and water cooling to dissipate the large amount of heat generated in the process.

---

* See Glossary for a description of a Brewster window.

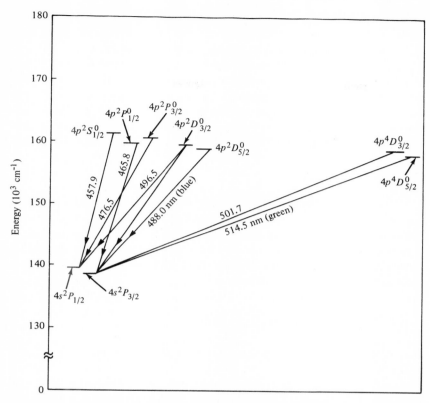

Figure 1-22   Argon-ion energy-level diagram and laser transitions.

The wavelength and power characteristics of a typical commerical argon-ion laser are given in Table 1-3.

If no dispersive element is introduced into the cavity, the laser will oscillate in most lines simultaneously. If a dispersive element such as a prism is introduced to deflect all lines except the desired one away from the tube axis, single-line operation is possible, but there is no increase in single-line power over the value obtained in multiline operation. Brewster's windows are used to linearly polarize the light, and the output is typically in a TEM_{00} mode. Commercial units that provide about 6 W of power in all lines, and approximately 2.5 W in either of the two stronger lines, are also available.

Lasing from numerous other ions such as krypton, neon, xenon, and many others have also been demonstrated,[39] but many of these will only operate on a pulsed basis. Lasers employing some of these ions are commercially available, and the most notable of these is the krypton-ion laser. This laser can emit CW light over a wide spectrum at the wavelengths of 647.1 nm (red), 568.2 nm (yellow), 520.8 nm (green), and

**TABLE 1-3   Typically Available Argon Lines
and Their Output Power**

Wavelength (nm)	Simultaneously (mW)	Singly, w/prism (mW)
514.5	700	700
501.7	150	150
496.5	150	150
488.0	700	700
476.5	250	250
472.7	—	30
465.8	—	30
457.9	50	50

476.2 nm (blue) simultaneously, or singly, with the use of a prism.   Typical power at the individual lines varies between a few tens of milliwatts to 200 mW (the 647.1 nm line being the strongest), and total power in all lines is about 300 or 400 mW.   Finally, it is worth noting that a mixture of two gases such as argon and krypton may be used to generate light at the wavelengths of both constituents.

1·6·5   carbon dioxide laser

Undoubtedly, the most important gas laser from both an industrial and scientific point of view is the CO_2 laser,[41,42] in which transitions between vibrational-rotational levels can provide large CW or pulsed power, with relatively high efficiency (up to 30 percent) at wavelengths approximating 10×10^3 nm.   These important characteristics stem directly from the fact that CO_2 is a member of a class of lasers called *molecular lasers*, which possess properties quite distinct from those in which atoms or ions act as the lasing medium.

In comparison with atoms and ions, the energy-level structure of molecules is more complicated and originates from three sources: electronic motions, vibrational motions, and rotational motions.   Just as in single atoms, electrons in molecules can be excited to higher energy levels, and transitions between these discrete levels normally correspond to frequencies in the visible and ultraviolet part of the spectrum.   Independent of the electronic energy state, the atomic nuclei, which are held together by molecular binding forces, will vibrate about their equilibrium position, giving rise to quantized vibrational energy levels.   The energy separation between vibrational levels of the same electronic energy state generally corresponds to frequency in the near and middle infrared range, and we thus see that each of the widely spaced electronic levels will be split into numerous vibrational sublevels.   Figure 1-23 indicates the three possible modes of vibration in the CO_2 molecule in the lowest electronic state: the symmetric, bending, and asymmetric vibrational

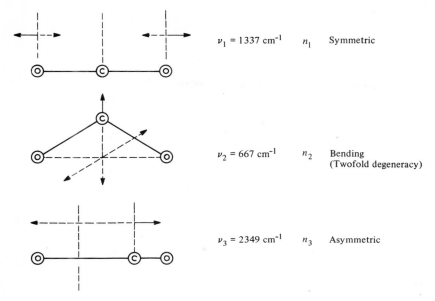

$\nu_1 = 1337$ cm^{-1} n_1 Symmetric

$\nu_2 = 667$ cm^{-1} n_2 Bending (Twofold degeneracy)

$\nu_3 = 2349$ cm^{-1} n_3 Asymmetric

Figure 1-23 *Vibrational motions of CO_2 molecule.*

motions. Each of the three modes is quantized, and their adjacent energy-level separations are approximately 1337 cm^{-1}, 667 cm^{-1}, and 2349 cm^{-1}, respectively. It should be noted that the bending motion is degenerate, reflecting the two possible directions of motion perpendicular to the molecular axis. Finally, a molecule in any electronic-vibrational level can undergo rotation about various axes in space. This rotational motion, due to the laws of quantum mechanics, will lead to closely spaced, discrete energy levels, and will further subdivide each vibrational level into a series of levels whose energy separations correspond to far infrared frequencies. Lasing transition occurs between a rotational sublevel of one vibrational level and another rotational sublevel of a lower vibrational level, where the quantized angular momentum numbers of the two rotational levels differ by unity.

The pertinent vibrational energy levels of the CO_2 laser in the electronic ground level are illustrated in Figure 1-24. When a gas discharge is established, CO_2 molecules are excited into higher electronic levels, from where they proceed to decay to the 00°1 level.* Favorable relaxation rates permit the establishment of population inversion between the 00°1 level and the 10°0 level, leading to lasing between numerous rotational levels around 10.6×10^3 nm, or between the 00°1 and 02°0 level resulting in possible oscillation around 9.6×10^3 nm. It has been found that the

* The notation $[n_1, n_2^l, n_3]$ is used to denote the degree of excitation of the symmetric, bending, and asymmetric vibrational modes, respectively.

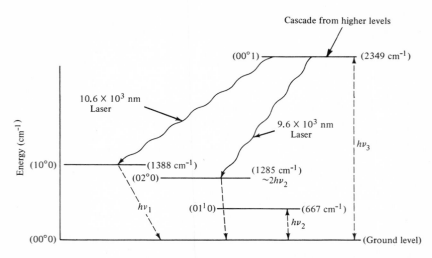

Figure 1-24   Some vibrational energy levels of the CO_2 molecule and laser transitions.

presence of various other gases in the discharge such as N_2 and He considerably increases the overall power and efficiency of the laser. The role of the N_2 molecules is to funnel the energy collected through collision with electrons into the upper laser level through a collision process with the CO_2 molecules. This collision process is highly efficient in transferring energy, primarily due to the long lifetime of the excited state of N_2, and the close energy coincidence between the two levels. The He is thought to increase the population of the $00°1$ state, and also to help empty the lower laser level.

Commercially available CO_2 lasers can supply several hundred watts of continuous power, or several kilowatts of peak power in a pulsed mode. Conventional cooling techniques relying on diffusion to the tube walls have limited continuous power output from the CO_2 laser to about 50 W/m. However, radically new designs, such as a gas transport laser for CW operation[43] in which the gas flows transversely to the cavity axes and is continuously recirculated, or a transversely excited atmospheric pressure (TEA) laser for high-energy pulsed operation,[44] may portend much higher than presently available powers and energies (more than 1000 W CW and kilojoules of energy in giant pulses several hundred nanoseconds long).

Finally, we note that the relatively long lifetime of the upper laser level permits Q-switching operation[45-47] in which peak power of the order of hundreds of kilowatts can be achieved. A rotating mirror may be employed in a Q-switching operation, whereas a saturable absorber such as SF_6 may be used to passively Q-switch[48] or mode lock[49] the laser. Even higher peak powers may be obtained from TEA lasers.

1·6·6   helium-cadmium laser

The HeCd laser[50-53] is a representative of a class of lasers where transitions between ionized levels of a metal vapor are used to obtain stimulated emission, and where a high ionization potential gas (usually He) is used as the buffer gas to pump the active ions through a collision process.   The significance of the HeCd laser lies in its continuous output at a wavelength of 325.0 nm in the ultraviolet[52,54] and its relative simplicity when compared to other ion lasers (e.g., Ar ion) which emit continuously in the blue region of the spectrum.

When a dc discharge is established in a binary gas mixture containing a high ionization potential gas such as helium and a low ionization potential metal vapor such as cadmium, a phenomenon termed cataphoresis takes place.[55]   Under this effect, the metal vapor is selectively transported toward the cathode end of the tube, thereby confining the corrosive metal vapors to a restricted section of tube, away from optical surfaces.   To obtain uniform distribution of metal vapor in the discharge, Cd atoms are continuously evaporated into the tube at a point close to the anode.   The atoms flow toward the cathode, only to condense on a cold surface before reaching the cathode.   The flow is thus restricted to a region between the heater-evaporator and the condenser, and never reaches the Brewster windows at the ends of the tube.

The relevant energy levels of a Cd ion are depicted in Figure 1-25 and may be used to explain the establishment of population inversion. The process starts with a collision in the discharge between electrons and He atoms which excites the atoms to a neutral metastable state.   The excited metastable He atoms then collide with neutral Cd atoms and ionize them.   This so-called Penning collision will result in an efficient transfer of energy even in the absence of coincidence in the two energy levels of He and Cd, since the excess energy can be taken by the electrons released in the process.   This collision results in the population of the $5s^2$ $^2D_{3/2}$ and $5s^2$ $^2D_{5/2}$ levels which serve as the upper laser levels for the 325.0 nm and 441.6 nm transitions, respectively.   The lower laser levels, which are the $5p$ $^2P_{3/2}$ for the 441.6 nm transitions, and the $5p$ $^2P_{1/2}$ for the 325.0 nm transition, are coupled to the ion ground level by a very fast transition, providing a favorable lifetime ratio and ensuring the possibility of population inversion.

Commercially available units can supply modest power (up to about 50 mW) at 441.6 nm, and about a tenth of this value at 325.0 nm.   The use of a single isotope of cadmium narrows the resonance line, increases the gain, and results in a threefold increase in power at the shorter wavelength.   The laser is, therefore, desirable for applications requiring modest continuous power in the shorter blue or near-ultraviolet wavelength, where its simple construction and operation without water cooling are advantageous.

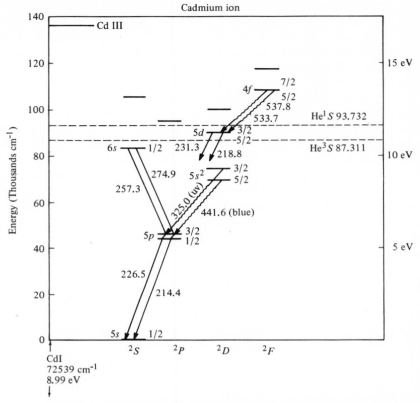

Figure 1-25   Energy-level diagram of cadmium ion. The wiggly lines are laser transitions (in nanometers.)[54] (With permission of Applied Physics Letters.)

Finally, we note that the type of process leading to laser action in cadmium is not unique to that metal, and similar laser transitions are attainable in other metals[52,56] (e.g., tin at $\lambda = 645.3$ nm, zinc at $\lambda = 747.9$ nm, and selenium at more than 20 different lines in the visible).

1·6·7 water-vapor laser

The spectral range between microwaves and infrared has long suffered from a lack of coherent energy sources.   With the discoveries of numerous laser lines in the submillimeter region in such molecules as H_2O[57] and HCN[58], the gap is rapidly being closed, and a new part of the spectrum is being opened for scientists and engineers.

The water-vapor laser[59] is perhaps the most common of the sub-millimeter wavelength lasers and has demonstrated lasing action at more

than one hundred pulsed lines and one dozen CW lines.   Peak power of up
to several hundred watts can be obtained in a pulsed mode of operation,
whereas typical power of a few milliwatts can be achieved on a CW basis,
all within the wavelength range of 7×10^3 to 220×10^3 nm.   The most
prominent CW lines are the 27.97×10^3 nm, and the 118.65×10^3 nm
lines.

Lasing in the water-vapor laser generally results from either a vibrational-rotational transition or a pure rotational transition in a particular
vibrational mode, and the establishment of population inversion in these
levels may be explained with the aid of the relevant energy levels displayed
in Figure 1-26.   The vibrational levels $v_1(100)$, $v_2(010)$, and $v_3(001)$ again
correspond to the symmetric, bending, and asymmetric motions of the
molecule, just as in the case of the CO_2 molecule.   For typical gas temperatures in the discharge, most molecules are in the vibrational ground state
of the electronic ground state.   From that state they are excited by

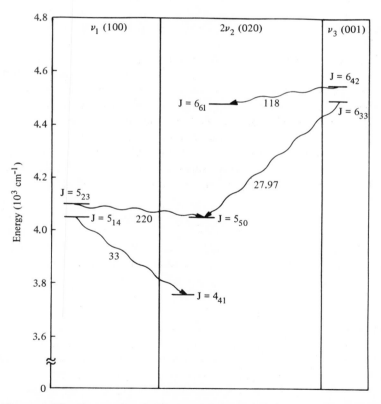

Figure 1-26   Energy-level diagram for H_2O showing several observed
laser transitions. Transitions are identified by the observed wavelength in
10^3 nm. For an explanation of notation and more complete diagram, see
Ref. 59.

electron impact to a higher electronic state and higher vibrational levels. The molecules then proceed to decay to the upper laser levels which are the rotational levels of the $v_1(100)$, $2v_2(020)$, and $v_3(001)$ vibrational levels of the electronic ground state. Even though transition probabilities between vibrational-rotational levels in H_2O do not have sufficient gain for laser action, perturbation mixing of vibrational levels increases the gain, and permits laser action when population inversion is achieved.

1·6·8   semiconductor lasers

Shortly after the observation of laser emission from active ions in solids and atoms in a gas mixture, the feasibility of obtaining lasing action in semiconductors was theoretically studied[60] and experimentally verified,[61-63] initially in GaAs and then in many other semiconductors. Despite the common thread of stimulated emission which characterizes all laser emission, semiconductor lasers are quite different from other types of lasers in both operating performance and pumping mechanism. Their distinctive features result from the fact that the electrons involved in a lasing transition are free to move in a large region of the semiconductor and are, thus, affected by the periodic potential in the lattice (see Section 2.3.6). In contrast with previously discussed solid-state and gas lasers where all individual atoms, ions, or molecules possessed identical energy levels whose distribution in thermal equilibrium obeyed Boltzmann statistics, the various energy levels in semiconductors can be occupied by at most two electrons in accordance with the Pauli exclusion principle, and the electrons obey Fermi-Dirac statistics.* Thus, the probability of an electronic state with energy E being occupied by an electron is given by

$$f_e(E) = \frac{1}{\exp[(E - E_f)/kT] + 1} \tag{1-41}$$

where E_f is the Fermi level,* and, similarly, the probability that a hole will occupy an energy state of level E is governed by the equation

$$f_h(E) = 1 - f_e(E) = \frac{1}{\exp[(E_f - E)/kT] + 1} \tag{1-42}$$

As with all lasers, lasing action proceeds after the establishment of population inversion inside the semiconductor. For population inversion to occur, the ratio of occupied states to unoccupied states near the bottom of the conduction band must exceed a similar ratio for states near the top of the valence band. This suggests the use of a degenerate semiconductor with a Fermi level in the conduction band for n-type material, and in the valence band for a p-type material. Radiative emission, which may be

* For a brief discussion of semiconductor theory, see Section 2.3.8.

either spontaneous or stimulated, depending on whether the rate of pumping is sufficiently high to establish population inversion, occurs when an electron in the conduction band recombines with a hole in the valence band, simultaneously emitting electromagnetic radiation at a frequency approximately corresponding to the band-gap energy. In addition to conservation of energy which determines the frequency of the emitted light in semiconductors, conservation of momentum also plays an important role in the recombination process. This conservation condition states that

$$\mathbf{k'} - \mathbf{k} = \mathbf{k}_{opt} \qquad (1\text{-}43)$$

where the wave vectors $\mathbf{k'}$ and $\mathbf{k}$ correspond to crystal momenta $\hbar\mathbf{k'}$ and $\hbar\mathbf{k}$, respectively, and $\mathbf{k}_{opt}$ is the propagation vector for the emitted radiation field. Since k_{opt} ($\sim 10^5$ cm^{-1}) is much smaller than either of the two crystal wave numbers k' or k ($\sim 10^8$ cm^{-1}), transition will occur only for the case in which $\mathbf{k'} \simeq \mathbf{k}$, a case that can be readily satisfied in direct gap semiconductors where the lowest minimum of the conduction band in k space is directly above the maximum of the valence band.

An important parameter for consideration in the evaluation of potential semiconductor laser material is the internal quantum efficiency, which is a measure of the efficiency with which electron excitation is internally converted into electromagnetic radiation and is defined by

$$\text{quantum efficiency} = \frac{\tau_{NR}}{\tau_R + \tau_{NR}} \qquad (1\text{-}44)$$

where τ_R is the radiative recombination lifetime, and τ_{NR} is the non-radiative recombination lifetime. In direct-gap semiconductors (e.g., Te, GaAs, CdS, PbS), $\tau_R \ll \tau_{NR}$ and the internal quantum efficiency approaches unity. In indirect-gap semiconductors (e.g., Si, Ge, GaP), $\tau_R \gg \tau_{NR}$ and the recombination process between electrons and holes is more likely to be accompanied by the excitation of lattice vibrations rather than the emission of electromagnetic radiation. In such semiconductors the quantum efficiency is below 10^{-4}, which weighs against the use of indirect-gap semiconductors for lasing materials. Indeed, most semiconductors that have demonstrated lasing action so far have been direct-gap materials. The overall laser efficiency of such materials at low temperatures may exceed 30 percent, which makes semiconductor lasers the most efficient lasers yet discovered.

The variety of laser wavelengths that may be obtained from semiconductors is illustrated in Figure 1-27, and is seen to span the part of the spectrum from the ultraviolet to the infrared.

Population inversion in semiconductors is normally achieved in one of three pumping methods. In homogeneous materials excitation is generally obtained either by electron beam bombardment or by optical pumping. In the first method a beam of high-energy electrons penetrates

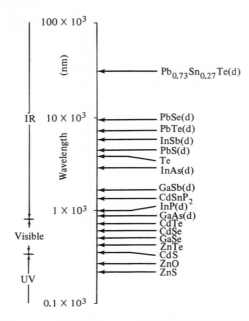

Figure 1-27   Some materials in which lasing has occurred.   Symbol "d" after a material indicates that diode lasers have been made of the material.

into the material and creates electron-hole pairs.   In the second case, electromagnetic radiation at a frequency slightly higher than the band-gap frequency is incident upon the material to generate the electron-hole pairs.   In this case, however, absorption of the incident radiation limits laser emission to a very small volume near the surface.   Consequently, the power that may be obtained from such optically pumped semiconductors is limited.   The third and most practical pumping scheme is applicable to *p-n* junctions and involves the injection of minority carriers into the *n* and *p* type regions by passing current through the diode.   The advantages of laser diodes (referred to as injection lasers) are quite obvious, the most important of which are small size, direct conversion of electrical energy into optical energy, and ease of modulating the output beam, which may be accomplished simply by modulating the diode current. Unfortunately, it is difficult to fabricate good *p-n* junctions of direct band-gap materials whose energy gap corresponds to frequencies in the ultraviolet and the blue or green regions of the visible part of the spectrum. For lasers emitting at these frequencies, electron beam or optical pumping must be employed.

The practical significance of injection lasers calls for a brief explanation of the operation of such devices.   The laser structure is schematically represented in Figure 1-28.   It consists of a planar *p-n* junction, with the

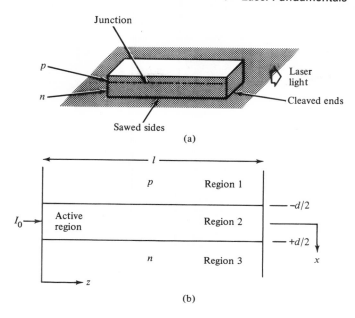

Figure 1-28 Diagrammatic sketch of injection laser. The light I_0 propagates in the z-direction. The pumping current is applied in the x direction.[64] **(With permission of IEEE, Inc.)**

two ends perpendicular to the plane of the junction cleaved to form parallel reflecting surfaces that create a dielectric cavity for the emitted radiation. Figure 1-29 depicts the space density of electrons in a region near a degenerate p-n junction in equilibrium and under forward-bias condition. In equilibrium when no voltage is applied (Figure 1-29a), the Fermi level has a constant value throughout the diode, and all energy levels below the Fermi level are essentially filled in both the n and p sides of the junction. When forward current flows through the diode, the density of electrons is altered and assumes the form depicted in Figure 1-29b. Here it is seen that, in the active region, electrons that moved in from the n side and holes that moved in from the p region are present, and it becomes possible for them to recombine while emitting electromagnetic radiation. This may lead to lasing action if all other conditions are favorable.

Just as in ordinary laser systems, the two opposite processes of absorption and emission of radiation will also be present in semiconductor lasers. If the fraction of occupied states with energy just below the top of the valence band is greater than that near the bottom of the conduction band, absorption will predominate over stimulated emission and no lasing action is possible. However, if the forward current is sufficiently high, the reverse is true, and a state of population inversion

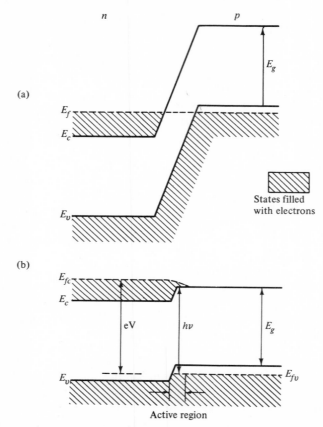

Figure 1-29   Density of electrons in the region of a degenerately doped p-n junction.   (a) With no applied voltage; and (b) with a forward-bias voltage.[64]   (With permission of IEEE, Inc.)

is established.   Lasing action will occur if the light wave suffers no net attenuation upon the completion of one round trip.   The gain necessary to satisfy the above requirement is provided, as in all lasers, by stimulated emission, whereas the losses sustained by the wave in the cavity are due primarily to reabsorption by the semiconductor itself and the radiation coupled out as emitted light.

The onset of laser oscillation is characterized by the narrowing of the emission spectrum, directionality of the radiation pattern, and a super-linear increase of output light with diode current.   Since threshold current density increases with temperature,[63] it is easier to obtain CW oscillation at low temperature (usually around 77°K), where power levels of a few watts are readily obtainable.   Under pulsed operation, peak powers of several watts can be obtained at room temperature and much higher powers at low temperatures. Typical pulse lengths under such mode of operation are several hundred nanoseconds, and shorter pulse lengths (several hundred picoseconds) may be obtained under Q-switched conditions.[65]

Recent advances in semiconductor laser technology have resulted in an appreciably reduced threshold current density and greatly increased efficiency, leading to CW operation at room temperature.[66] Current efforts at further reduction of threshold current density are continuing to center around novel heterostructures employing $Al_xGa_{1-x}As$ together with GaAs[67-70] and portend reliable compact injection lasers emitting CW radiation with high efficiency at room temperature in the near infrared.[71]

1·6·9 dye lasers

The great variety of lasers is further illustrated by a class of lasers utilizing organic dyes dissolved in various solvents (e.g., water, ethyl alcohol) as the active medium.[72] These dyes possess wide lasing lines which, together with their low cost, offer a relatively inexpensive tunable coherent source.

Lasing transitions in organic dyes occur between vibrational sub-levels associated with different electronic states of the molecules. The required population inversion is achieved by means of optical pumping either with flash lamps of fast rise time[73,74] or with pulsed,[75] Q-switched,[72] or CW[76] lasers. The absorption and emission spectra of a typical organic molecule are illustrated in Figure 1-30, where it is seen that the absorption spectrum is the approximate mirror image of the longer

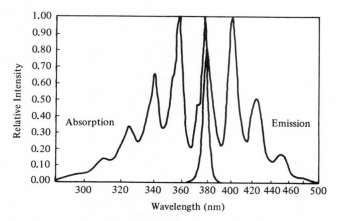

Figure 1-30 Absorption and fluorescence emission spectrum of a typical organic molecule.[77] **(With permission of Laser Focus.)**

wavelength emission spectrum.   To obtain emission at the high frequency end of the visible, it is necessary to pump the solution with ultraviolet radiation, which can be supplied by the 337.1 nm line of N_2 laser, the second harmonic of a Q-switched ruby laser at 347.1 nm, or a suitably chosen flash lamp.   For emission at longer wavelengths, laser pumps and flash-lamp pumps whose visible emission falls within the absorption range of the particular dye may also be employed.   Continuous lasing was difficult to achieve because of the accumulation of molecules in a particular state which readily absorbs the radiation at the laser wavelength.   This tends to increase the optical losses in the cavity and inhibits the lasing process. To obtain CW oscillation, special efforts must be taken to limit accumulation in that state, which explains the fact that lasing is more easily achieved on a pulsed basis, with typical pulse lengths of the order of several nanoseconds.   Repetition rates are usually limited by the pump to approximately 25 pps, although higher repetition rates may be achieved at some wavelengths with reduced output power.

Organic dyes usually have fluorescent emission spectra of several hundred angstroms[78] which endow this type of laser with its most distinctive feature—wide-range tunability.   Continuous tunability over the entire fluorescent emission band (which may range over a thousand angstroms)[79] can be achieved by substituting a diffraction grating for one of the mirrors in the cavity,[80] which results in the narrowing of output line widths to 1 Å, without loss in power.   Tunability over most of the visible part of the spectrum may be obtained by employing different dyes whose emission spectra span different, but preferably adjacent, parts of the desired wavelength range and thus "cover" the entire spectrum. Energy obtainable under pulsed operating conditions from commercially available units is generally below a millijoule for laser pumped systems, and a fraction of a joule for flash-lamp pumped system.   Peak output powers tend to depend on dye concentration and pulse rate and are usually of the order of several tens of kilowatts, for laser-pumped dye lasers, and even higher for flash-lamp pumped systems.   CW power is of the order of several tens of milliwatts and varies with wavelength.

Despite several distinct disadvantages such as tendency to decompose with increasing use, the dye laser, due to its unique feature of wide and yet simple tunability, may find extensive future use in applications requiring modest pulsed energies and CW powers while favoring frequency selectivity (e.g., spectroscopy, biological applications).

1·6·10   *brief survey of typical commercial lasers*

Table 1-4 summarizes the more important output characteristics of various types of typical commercially available laser systems.

TABLE 1-4 Typical Laser Systems

GAS LASERS

Type	Wavelength (s) (nm)	Beam Divergence (mrad)	Beam Diameter ($1/e^2$ pt., mm)	Operating Mode	Repetition Rate (pps)	Pulse Width (s)	Output Power (W) TEM_{00}	Output Power (W) Multimode
HeNe	632.8	0.8	1.4	CW			0.0006	
		1	1.1	CW			0.015	
Ar	451.9 to 514.5	0.8	1.4	CW			2	
	488.0 or 514.5	0.8	1.4	CW			0.7	
CO_2	10.6×10^3	2	10	CW			200	250
		2	10	Pulsed	1000	0.001		600
		2	10	Q-switched		0.5×10^{-6}		100000
			30	CW				1000
CO_2 (TEA)			0.25	Pulsed	400	0.4×10^{-6}		100000
HeCd	325.0	0.5	1.3	CW			0.005	

SOLID-STATE LASERS

Type	Wavelength (nm)	Beam Divergence (mrad)	Beam Diameter ($1/e^2$ pt., mm)	Operating Mode	Output Characteristics Max Pulse Energy (J)	Peak Power (W)	Pulse Width (μs)	Rep Rate (pps)
Cr^{3+}: Al_2O_3 (Ruby)	694.3	10	6	Pulsed	80	10^5	300–6000	1
		10	6	Q-switched	20	10^9	0.015	2 (ppm)

TABLE 1-4—continued

Type	Wavelength (nm)	Beam Divergence (mrad)	Beam Diameter (1/e² pt., mm)	Operating Mode	Output Characteristics			
					Max Pulse Energy (J)	Peak Power (W)	Pulse Width (μs)	Rep Rate (pps)
Nd³⁺:glass	1.06×10^3	10	6	Pulsed	125	10^6	500–10000	1
		10	6	Q-switched	30	10^9	0.015	2 (ppm)
Nd³⁺:YAG	1.064×10^3	3	4	Q-switched	0.005	5×10^3	0.1	50,000
		8	4	Pulsed	4			20
		3	4	CW	TEM$_{00}$—20W, Mult-mode—150W			

INJECTION LASERS

Type	Wavelength (nm)	Rep Rate (pps)	Pulse Width (μs)	Peak Power (W)	Diode or Array	Line Width (Å)	Energy per Pulse (mJ)	Current (A)		Operating Temperature (°C)
								Threshold	Peak	
GaAs	900.0	5000	0.2	8	diode	40		25	75	25
		5000	0.2	100	array	75		25	75	25

TUNABLE LASERS

Type	Tunable Spectral Range (nm)	Beam Divergence (mrad)	Beam Diameter (1/e² pt., mm)	Pulse Width (ns)	Energy per Pulse (mJ)	Rep Rate (ppm)	Avg. Power (mW)
Dye	360.0–650.0	3	5	2–8	0.02	25	<2.5
	560.0–640.0	2	3	CW			<50

References

1. T. H. Maiman, "Stimulated Optical Radiation in Ruby Masers," *Nature* **187**, 493 (1960).
2. A. Einstein, "Zur Quanten Theorie der Strahlung," *Phys. Zeit.* **18**, 121 (1917).
3. A. Yariv and J. P. Gordon, "The Laser," *Proc. IEEE* **51**, 4 (1963).
4. A. Yariv, *Quantum Electronics*, John Wiley and Sons, Inc., New York (1967).
5. S. Silver, *Microwave Antenna Theory and Design*, McGraw-Hill Book Co., New York (1949).
6. G. D. Boyd and J. P. Gordon, "Confocal Multimode Resonator for Millimeter Through Optical Wavelength Masers," *Bell System Tech. J.* **40**, 489 (1961).
7. G. D. Boyd and H. Kogelnik, "Generalized Confocal Resonator Theory," *Bell System Tech. J.* **41**, 1347 (1963).
8. H. Kogelnik and T. Li, "Laser Beams and Resonators," *Appl. Optics* **5**, 1550 (1966).
9. R. W. Hellwarth, *Advances in Quantum Electronics*, Columbia University Press, New York (1961).
10. F. J. McClung and R. W. Hellwarth, "Characteristics of Giant Optical Pulsations from Ruby," *Proc. IEEE* **51**, 46 (1963).
11. J. L. Helfrich, "Faraday Effect as a Q-Switch for Ruby Laser," *J. Appl. Phys.* **34**, 1000 (1963).
12. R. B. Chesler *et al.*, "An Experimental and Theoretical Study of High Repetition Rate Q-Switched Nd: YAG Lasers," *Proc. IEEE* **58**, 1899 (1970).
13. B. H. Soffer, "Giant Pulse Laser Operation by a Passive, Reversibly Bleachable Absorber," *J. Appl. Phys.* **35**, 2551 (1964).
14. P. Kafalas *et al.*, "Photosensitive Liquid Used as a Nondestructive Passive Q-Switch in a Ruby Laser," *J. Appl. Phys.* **35**, 2349 (1964).
15. L. E. Hargrove *et al.*, "Locking of He-Ne Laser Modes Induced by Synchronous Intracavity Modulation," *Appl. Phys. Lett.* **5**, 4 (1964).
16. S. E. Harris and R. Targ, "FM Oscillation of the He-Ne Laser," *Appl. Phys. Lett.* **5**, 202 (1964).
17. A. Papoulis, *The Fourier Integral and Its Applications*, McGraw-Hill Book Co., New York (1962).
18. H. W. Mocker and R. J. Collins, "Mode Competition and Self-Locking Effects in a Q-Switched Ruby Laser," *Appl. Phys. Lett.* **7**, 270 (1965).
19. C. C. Cutler, "The Regenerative Pulse Generator," *Proc. IRE* **43**, 140 (1955).
20. A. J. DeMaria *et al.*, "Picosecond Laser Pulses," *Proc. IEEE* **57**, 2 (1969).
21. A. W. Penney, Jr., and H. A. Heynau, "PTM Single-Pulse Selection from a Mode-Locked Nd^{3+}-Glass Laser Using a Bleachable Dye," *Appl. Phys. Lett.* **9**, 257 (1966).
22. A. A. Vuylsteke, "Theory of Laser Regeneration Switching," *J. Appl. Phys.* **34**, 1615 (1963).
23. E. B. Treacy, "Compression of Picosecond Light Pulses," *Phys. Lett.* **28A**, 34 (1968).
24. D. Maydan, "Fast Modulator for Extraction of Internal Laser Power," *J. Appl. Phys.* **41**, 1552 (1970).

25. D. Maydan and R. B. Chesler, "Q-Switching and Cavity Dumping of Nd : YAG Lasers," *J. Appl. Phys.* **42**, 1031 (1971).
26. W. S. C. Chang, *Principle of Quantum Electronics*, Addison-Wesley Publishing Co., Reading, Mass. (1969).
27. J. E. Geusic *et al.*, "Laser Oscillations in Nd-Doped Yttrium Aluminum, Yttrium Gallium, and Gadolinium Garnets," *Appl. Phys. Lett.* **4**, 182 (1964).
28. E. Snitzer, "Optical Maser Action of Nd^{+3} in a Barium Crown Glass," *Phys. Rev. Lett.* **7**, 444 (1961).
29. E. Snitzer, "Glass Lasers," *Proc. IEEE* **54**, 1249 (1966).
30. R. G. Smith and M. F. Galvin, "Operation of the Continuously Pumped, Repetitively Q-Switched YAG : Nd Laser," *IEEE J. of Quantum Electronics* **QE-3**, p. 406 (1967).
31. C. G. Young, "Glass Lasers," *Proc. IEEE* **57**, 1267 (1969).
32. C. G. Young *et al.*, "A High-Power Intermediate Pulse-Width Glass Laser," *IEEE J. of Quantum Electronics* **QE-3**, 238 (1967).
33. A. J. DeMaria *et al.*, "Self-Mode-Locking of Lasers with Saturable Absorbers," *Appl. Phys. Lett.* **8**, 174 (1966).
34. A. Javan *et al.*, "Population Inversion and Continuous Optical Maser Oscillation in a Gas Discharge Containing a He-Ne Mixture," *Phys. Rev. Lett.* **6**, 106 (1961).
35. A. D. White and J. D. Rigden, "Continuous Gas Maser Operation in the Visible," *Proc. IRE* **50**, 1697 (1962).
36. A. L. Bloom *et al.*, "Laser Operation at 3.39μ in a Helium-Neon Mixture," *Appl. Optics* **2**, 317 (1963).
37. W. B. Bridges, "Laser Oscillation in Singly Ionized Argon in the Visible Spectrum," *Appl. Phys. Lett.* **4**, 128 (1964).
38. W. B. Bridges, "Laser Action in Singly Ionized Krypton and Xenon," *Proc. IEEE* **52**, 843 (1964).
39. W. B. Bridges and A. N. Chester, "Visible and UV Laser Oscillation at 118 Wavelengths in Ionized Neon, Argon, Krypton, Xenon, Oxygen, and Other Gases," *Appl. Optics* **4**, 573 (1965).
40. E. I. Gordon *et al.*, "Continuous Visible Laser Action in Singly Ionized Argon, Krypton, and Xenon," *Appl. Phys. Lett.* **4**, 178 (1964).
41. C. K. N. Patel, "Interpretation of CO_2 Optical Maser Experiments," *Phys. Rev. Lett.* **12**, 588 (1964).
42. C. K. N. Patel, "Continuous-Wave Laser Action on Vibrational-Rotational Transitions of CO_2," *Phys. Rev.* **136**, A1187 (1964).
43. W. B. Tiffany *et al.*, "Kilowatt CO_2 Gas-Transport Laser," *Appl. Phys. Lett.* **15**, 91 (1969).
44. A. J. Beaulieu, "Transversely Excited Atmospheric Pressure CO_2 Lasers," *Appl. Phys. Lett.* **16**, 504 (1970).
45. M. A. Kovacs *et al.*, "Q-Switching of Molecular Laser Transitions," *Appl. Phys. Lett.* **8**, 62 (1966).
46. G. W. Flynn *et al.*, "Vibrational and Rotational Studies Using Q-Switching of Molecular Gas Lasers," *Appl. Phys. Lett.* **8**, 63 (1966).
47. C. K. N. Patel, *Symposium on Modern Optics*, March 1967, New York, p. 19, Polytechnic Press, New York (1968).
48. O. R. Wood and S. E. Schwarz, "Passive Q-Switching of a CO_2 Laser," *Appl. Phys. Lett.* **11**, 88 (1967).

49. O. R. Wood and S. E. Schwarz, "Passive Mode Locking of a CO_2 Laser," *Appl. Phys. Lett.* **12**, 263 (1968).
50. G. R. Fowles and B. D. Hopkins, "CW Laser Oscillation at 4416 Å in Cadmium," *IEEE J. of Quantum Electronics* **QE-3**, 419 (1967).
51. W. T. Silfvast, "Efficient CW Laser Oscillation at 4416 Å in Cd(II)," *Appl. Phys. Lett.* **13**, 169 (1968).
52. W. T. Silfvast, "New CW Metal-Vapor Laser Transitions in Cd, Sn, and Zn," *Appl. Phys. Lett.* **15**, 23 (1969).
53. J. P. Goldsborough, "Continuous Laser Oscillation at 3250 Å in Cadmium Ion," *IEEE J. of Quantum Electronics* **QE-5**, 133 (1969).
54. J. P. Goldsborough, "Stable, Long Life CW Excitation of Helium-Cadmium Lasers by dc Cataphoresis," *Appl. Phys. Lett.* **15**, 159 (1969).
55. T. P. Sosnowski, "Cataphoresis in the Helium-Cadmium Laser Discharge Tube," *J. Appl. Phys.* **40**, 5138 (1969).
56. W. T. Silfvast and M. B. Klein, "CW Laser Action on 24 Visible Wavelengths in Se II," *Appl. Phys. Lett.* **17**, 400 (1970).
57. A. Crocker *et al.*, "Stimulated Emission in the Far Infra-Red," *Nature* **201**, 250 (1964).
58. H. A. Gebbie *et al.*, "A Stimulated Emission Source at 0.34 Millimeter Wavelength," *Nature* **202**, 685 (1964).
59. W. S. Benedict *et al.*, "The Water-Vapor Laser," *IEEE J. of Quantum Electronics* **QE-5**, 108 (1969).
60. W. P. Dumke, "Interband Transitions and Maser Action," *Phys. Rev.* **127**, 1559 (1962).
61. R. N. Hall *et al.*, "Coherent Light Emission from GaAs Junctions," *Phys. Rev. Lett.* **9**, 366 (1962).
62. M. I. Nathan *et al.*, "Stimulated Emission of Radiation from GaAs *p-n* Junctions," *Appl. Phys. Lett.* **1**, 62 (1962).
63. T. M. Quist *et al.*, "Semiconductor Maser of GaAs," *Appl. Phys. Lett.* **1**, 91 (1962).
64. G. Burns and M. I. Nathan, "*P-N* Junction Lasers," *Proc. IEEE* **52**, 770 (1964).
65. J. E. Ripper and J. C. Dyment, "Internal *Q* Switching in GaAs Junction Lasers," *Appl. Phys. Lett.* **12**, 365 (1968).
66. I. Hayashi *et al.*, "Junction Lasers which Operate Continuously at Room Temperature," *Appl. Phys. Lett.* **17**, 109 (1970).
67. I. Hayashi *et al.*, "A Low-Threshold Room-Temperature Injection Laser," *IEEE J. of Quantum Electronics* **QE-5**, 211 (1969).
68. H. Kressel and H. Nelson, "Close-Confinement Gallium Arsenide *PN* Junction Lasers with Reduced Optical Loss at Room Temperature," *RCA Rev.* **30**, 106 (1969).
69. I. Hayashi and M. B. Panish, "GaAs-Ga$_x$Al$_{1-x}$As Heterostructure Injection Lasers which Exhibit Low Thresholds at Room Temperature," *J. Appl. Phys.* **41**, 150 (1970).
70. M. B. Panish *et al.*, "Double-Heterostructure Injection Lasers with Room-Temperature Thresholds as Low as 2300 A/cm^2," *Appl. Phys. Lett.* **16**, 326 (1970).
71. B. I. Miller *et al.*, "Semiconductor Lasers Operating Continuously in the 'Visible' at Room Temperature," *Appl. Phys. Lett.* **18**, 403 (1971).

72. P. P. Sorokin and J. R. Lankard, "Stimulated Emission Observed from an Organic Dye, Chloro-Aluminum Phthalocyanine," *IBM J. of Res. and Devel.* **10**, 162 (1966).
73. P. P. Sorokin *et al.*, "Flashlamp-Pumped Organic-Dye Lasers," *J. Chem. Phys.* **48**, 4726 (1968).
74. B. B. Snavely, "Flashlamp-Excited Organic Dye Lasers," *Proc. IEEE* **57**, 1374 (1969).
75. J. A. Myer *et al.*, "Dye Laser Stimulation with a Pulsed N_2 Laser Line at 3371 Å," *Appl. Phys. Lett.* **16**, 3 (1970).
76. O. G. Peterson *et al.*, "CW Operation of an Organic Dye Solution Laser," *Appl. Phys. Lett.* **17**, 245 (1970).
77. M. R. Kagan *et al.*, "Organic Dye Lasers," *Laser Focus* **4**, No. 17, 26 (September 1968).
78. I. B. Berlman, *Handbook of Fluorescence Spectra of Aromatic Molecules*, Academic Press Inc., New York (1965).
79. C. V. Shank *et al.*, "Near UV to Yellow Tunable Laser Emission from an Organic Dye," *Appl. Phys. Lett.* **16**, 405 (1970).
80. B. H. Soffer and B. B. McFarland, "Continuously Tunable, Narrow-Band Organic Dye Lasers," *Appl. Phys. Lett.* **10**, 266 (1967).

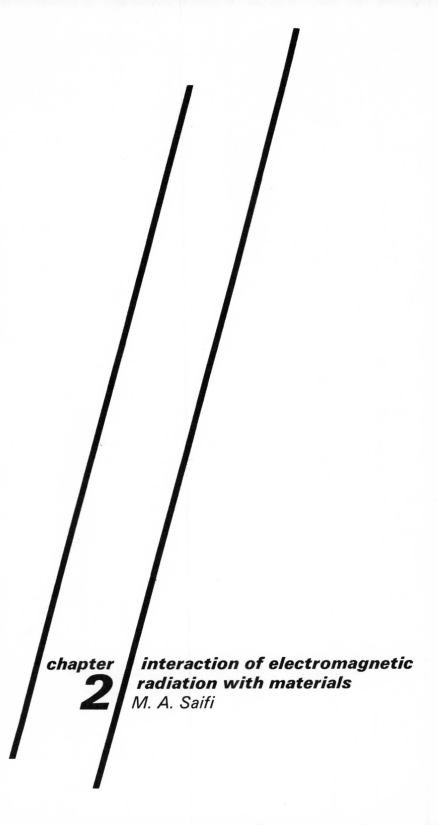

chapter
2
interaction of electromagnetic
radiation with materials
M. A. Saifi

2·0 introduction

Interaction of radiation with matter encompasses three subjects: first, electromagnetic radiation and its properties; second, material properties; and third, interaction phenomena. This chapter therefore is divided into these three categories.

In interaction of laser radiation with matter, often it is important to take into account the Gaussian distribution of the beam intensity. In this chapter, however, plane-wave concepts are used since they provide the necessary background to illustrate the fundamentals of interaction phenomena.

To describe the interaction phenomena, the optical properties, particularly the dispersion relations for dielectrics, metals, and doped semiconductors, are illustrated through simple classical models. This treatment it is hoped will be sufficient to stress the point that, in thermally induced processing with laser radiation, the main problem is coupling of the incident radiation to the material. Since the advent of lasers, apart from research in communications and nonlinear effects, industrial research has been concentrated in processing applications. As the number of applications increases, further research efforts will be devoted toward better understanding of reflection and absorption phenomenon under intense radiation. Present available literature offers few definitive views in this regard, and our treatment of this subject reflects it.

The nonlinear effects, such as Raman and Brillouin scattering and second harmonic generation, are also discussed, since it appears they will be increasingly used in many industrial applications.

It is apparent from the above that the chapter deals with many diverse topics. The reader should, therefore, be aware of the fact that this is only a brief review of those subjects which are of immediate import in obtaining some insight to the interaction of radiation with matter.

2·1 radiation field

The electromagnetic radiation consists of time varying electric and magnetic field components of a wave which propagates through a medium at a characteristic velocity. The propagation velocity in free space (vacuum) is about 3×10^8 m/s and is somewhat less in a material medium.

In this section we shall mainly discuss plane waves, i.e., electromagnetic waves in which the electric and magnetic field intensities, at any instant of time, vary only in the direction of its propagation. The basic features of an electromagnetic plane wave are shown in Figure 2-1. It consists of electric and magnetic fields which oscillate sinusoidally as a function of time and space. The electric field intensity E_x of the wave varies sinusoidally as a function of its spatial coordinate z and at any instant of time its amplitude is independent of x and y coordinates. The magnetic field associated with such a wave has only a y component, which also varies sinusoidally

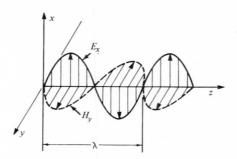

Figure 2-1 Electromagnetic plane wave. The electric and magnetic fields are in the x and y directions, respectively. The figure shows field intensities at a given time as a function of the z coordinate; the field intensities are independent of the x and y coordinates.

in the z direction. Apart from the spatial dependence, both the electric and magnetic fields oscillate (sinusoidally) as a function of time. The spatial distance within which the wave executes one complete oscillation is called the wavelength λ of the radiation, and the inverse of the temporal period of one complete oscillation gives its frequency v in cycles per second, usually denoted by hertz.

The fundamental equations which describe the electromagnetic behavior in any media are known as *Maxwell's equations*. The development of these equations from a few fundamental laws is discussed in several texts;[1,2,3] therefore, in the following we shall briefly outline its application to plane waves. The Maxwell equations (differential form) in mks units are listed below.*

$$\nabla \times \mathbf{E} = -\frac{\partial \mathbf{B}}{\partial t} \tag{2-1}$$

$$\nabla \times \mathbf{H} = \mathbf{J} + \frac{\partial \mathbf{D}}{\partial t} \tag{2-2}$$

$$\nabla \cdot \mathbf{D} = \rho \tag{2-3}$$

$$\nabla \cdot \mathbf{B} = 0 \tag{2-4}$$

The quantities appearing in the above equations and their mks units are given in Table 2-1.

* In Cartesian coordinates operator ∇ is given by $[\mathbf{a}_x(\partial/\partial x) + \mathbf{a}_y(\partial/\partial y) + \mathbf{a}_z(\partial/\partial z)]$. The dot and cross product of this with a vector is called divergence and curl. For reference, see S. A. Schelkunoff, "Applied Mathematics for Engineers and Scientists," Van Nostrand Reinhold Co., New York (1965).

TABLE 2-1 Quantities Appearing in Maxwell's Equations

Quantity	Description	mks Units
D	Electric flux density	coulomb/m^2
ρ	Electric charge density	coulomb/m^3
B	Magnetic flux density	weber/m^2
E	Electric field intensity	V/m
H	Magnetic field intensity	A-turn/m
J	Electric current density	A/m^2
ε	Permittivity	farads/m
μ	Permeability	henry/m

The first equation (Faraday's law of induction) states that a time varying magnetic flux density generates an electric field. The second equation states that the magnetic fields are generated either by conduction current **J** and/or displacement current $\partial \mathbf{D}/\partial t$. Maxwell's concept of displacement current $\partial \mathbf{D}/\partial t$ was a most important contribution, which helped explain the electromagnetic wave propagation. The generation of electric fields due to a time varying magnetic flux density is well known and is exploited in making devices such as transformers. However, how magnetic fields can be generated in free space (vacuum), where no conduction current is present, was not very clear prior to Maxwell's introduction of the concept of displacement current.

The third equation (Gauss's law) states that the charge density is a source or sink of electric flux lines. The charge density may be due to a free electronic charge (such as free electrons in a metal), or due to polarization produced by bound charges. This does not mean that the electric flux lines always originate and terminate on electrical charges. For example, in a charge free region where $\rho = 0$, the electric field intensity **E**, and hence the electric flux density **D**, may result from a time varying magnetic flux density **B** (Faraday's law) as stated earlier. Finally, the last equation states that the magnetic lines of flux must be continuous everywhere.

The quantities **D**, **E**, and **B**, **H** appearing in Maxwell's equations are related and are given by

$$\mathbf{D} = \varepsilon \mathbf{E} \tag{2-5}$$

and

$$\mathbf{B} = \mu \mathbf{H} \tag{2-6}$$

where ε is the permittivity of the medium and μ is its permeability.

The electric flux density **D** can also be written as

$$\mathbf{D} = \varepsilon \mathbf{E} = \varepsilon_0 \mathbf{E} + \mathbf{P} \tag{2-5a}$$

where **P** is polarization. The polarization arises because of charge separation induced by the electric field of the incident radiation.

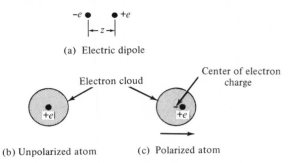

(a) Electric dipole

(b) Unpolarized atom   (c) Polarized atom

Figure 2-2   (a) Electric dipole.   (b) Unpolarized atom in which the center of charge of the electron cloud coincides with the positive nuclear charge.   (c) Polarized atom due to an applied electric field E.

If two equal but opposite charges e are separated by a distance z, they are said to form an electric dipole of dipole moment ez.   The dipoles give rise to electric fields which are of considerable importance in electromagnetic theory.   The dipole moment per unit volume is also called *polarization* per unit volume.   As an example, consider a neutral atom with spherical electron charge distribution as shown in Figure 2-2. In the unpolarized state the center of gravity of electron charge coincides with the positive charge of the nucleus.   Application of an electric field to such an atom causes the displacement of electron cloud with respect to the nucleus and develops polarization **P**.   It is this polarization with which we will be concerned in describing the optical properties of any material.

2·1·1   plane waves

For plane electromagnetic waves, electric and magnetic field intensities at any instant of time vary only in the direction of propagation and are constant in any plane perpendicular to the direction of propagation (see Figure 2-1).   In free space,

$$\rho = \mathbf{J} = 0$$

$$\mathbf{B} = \mu_0 \mathbf{H}$$

$$\mathbf{D} = \varepsilon_0 \mathbf{E}$$

where μ_0 and ε_0 are free space permeability ($\mu_0 = 4\pi \times 10^{-7}$ henry/m), and permittivity ($\varepsilon_0 = 8.8542 \times 10^{-12}$ farad/m), respectively.   Substituting the above in (2-1) to (2-4) gives

$$\varepsilon_0 \nabla \times \mathbf{E} = \mu_0 \nabla \times \mathbf{H} = 0 \tag{2-7}$$

$$\nabla \times \mathbf{E} = -\mu_0 \frac{\partial \mathbf{H}}{\partial t} \tag{2-8}$$

and

$$\nabla \times \mathbf{H} = \varepsilon_0 \frac{\partial \mathbf{E}}{\partial t} \tag{2-9}$$

These equations can be solved to obtain general expressions for $\mathbf{E}$ and $\mathbf{H}$ as a function of time and space coordinates. These equations are coupled in the sense that the electric and magnetic fields are interdependent. However, by manipulating these equations it is possible to obtain a simple second-order differential equation involving either $\mathbf{E}$ or $\mathbf{H}$ only. For the plane wave shown in Figure 2.1, $E_y = E_z = 0$. In this case the second-order differential equation comes out to be

$$\frac{\partial^2 E_x}{\partial z^2} = \mu_0 \varepsilon_0 \frac{\partial^2 E_x}{\partial t^2} \tag{2-10}$$

This is known as the wave equation, because a general solution shows that the electric field intensity oscillates both as a function of time t and space coordinate z, and propagates at a characteristic velocity, which are the properties of a wave. Assuming that the propagating wave is sinusoidal,* one possible solution of (2-10) is

$$\mathbf{E} = \mathbf{a}_x E_x \cos(\omega t - k_0 z), \qquad \omega = 2\pi v \tag{2-11}$$

where E_x is amplitude of the electric field intensity, v its temporal frequency (cycles per second), and k_0 the propagation constant. In the following it will be shown that k_0 determines the phase velocity of wave propagation and hence the term propagation constant. (The subscript zero is used to denote propagation in free space.)

Substituting (2-11) into (2-10) shows that k_0 and ω must satisfy the relation

$$k_0^2 = \omega^2 \mu_0 \varepsilon_0 \tag{2-12}$$

To illustrate the traveling wave nature of the expression (2-11), we show in Figure 2-3 one cycle of this wave plotted as a function of z, and for several different values of time. Some important features of the plane-wave propagation can be seen from this figure. For example, at a given instant of time, the electric field intensity varies sinusoidally as a function of z, and a complete cycle in space is given by λ_0, where

$$\lambda_0 = \frac{2\pi}{k_0} \tag{2-13}$$

This is known as the free space wavelength of the radiation. Also, if we consider a point of constant phase, for example, $\omega t - k_0 z = \pi/2$ (point

---

* For nonsinusoidal waves, Fourier components can be superposed; hence use of sinusoidal waves here is applicable to a general case.

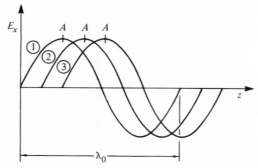

Figure 2-3 E_x *as a function of* z *at several values of time for a sinu-*
soidal propagating wave. **(1)** $\omega t = 0$, **(2)** $\omega t = \pi/4$, **(3)** $\omega t = \pi/2$. λ_0 *is the*
free space wavelength.

marked A in Figure 2-3), it appears to be traveling in the positive z direction. The velocity at which a point of constant phase travels can be
obtained by differentiating the phase expression with respect to time, i.e.,
obtaining dz/dt.

$$\omega t - k_0 z = \text{constant}$$

$$\omega - k_0 \frac{dz}{dt} = 0$$

$$v_0 = \frac{dz}{dt} = \frac{\omega}{k_0} \tag{2-14}$$

This is the velocity with which a point of constant phase travels in the
positive z direction. For a wave traveling in the negative z direction, the
argument of the cosine function will be $(\omega t + k_0 z)$. The velocity v_0 is
called the phase velocity of the wave and k_0 is generally referred to as
either the propagation constant or the wave vector. Substituting the
value of k_0 from (2-12) into (2-14) and using the numerical values of μ_0
and ε_0, we obtain

$$v_0 = \frac{1}{\sqrt{\mu_0 \varepsilon_0}} = 3 \times 10^8 \text{ m/s},$$

which is the velocity of wave propagation in free space. The above
expression shows that in free space the velocity v_0 is independent of the
frequency ω. In general, for a material medium $\mu > \mu_0$ and $\varepsilon > \varepsilon_0$ and
hence the velocity is always less than that in free space. Furthermore, in
a material medium μ and ε are functions of ω, and hence v in general will
be a function of frequency. The ratio of the velocity in free space to that

in the material is known as the *index of refraction*. The propagation constant k, for a material of permeability μ and permittivity ε is (see 2-12)

$$k = \omega\sqrt{\mu\varepsilon}$$

Hence, the phase velocity v in a material is given by

$$v = \frac{1}{\sqrt{\mu\varepsilon}}$$

This gives for the index of refraction

$$n = \sqrt{\frac{\mu\varepsilon}{\mu_0\,\varepsilon_0}} \tag{2-15}$$

Section 2.5.4 shows that for dielectric materials ε is in general frequency dependent, and $\mu \simeq \mu_0$. For such materials, then, n^2 is equal to its dielectric constant ε_r, where $\varepsilon_r = \varepsilon/\varepsilon_0$. If either μ or ε or both are complex, the index of refraction will be complex. A complex index of refraction, as will be shown later, implies absorption of energy from the propagating wave.

Finally, to complete the development of plane waves, we note that a propagating radiation wave consists of both the electric and magnetic fields. The magnetic field can be derived from (2-9) and (2-10). For the specific case of the plane wave shown in Figure 2-1, this comes out to be

$$H_y = \frac{k_0}{\omega\mu_0}\,E_x \cos(\omega t - k_0 z) \tag{2-16}$$

Note that for a plane wave, the vectors representing electric field intensity, the magnetic field intensity, and the propagation direction form a set of orthogonal vectors.

In the above, electric and magnetic field intensities were expressed as sinusoidal traveling waves. Exponential functions can also be used to express these quantities, provided either the real or the imaginary components of the exponential function is retained in the final expression. For example, (2-11) can also be written as

$$\mathbf{E} = \mathbf{a}_x\,E_x\,\mathrm{Re}\,\exp\,i(\omega t - k_0 z) \tag{2-11a}$$

where Re stands for the real part of the exponential function, which is $\cos(\omega t - k_0 z)$. Since it is generally understood that only the real or imaginary part of the exponential function is to be retained, the Re notation can be dropped. In the following sections the exponential notation will be often used, and it will be implicit that one consider only the real or imaginary part of the function.

2·1·2   intrinsic impedance and power

We shall now review the concepts of intrinsic impedance and energy flow associated with electromagnetic radiation.   In free space the electric and magnetic fields are in time phase, as shown by (2-11) and (2-16). In electrical circuit theory the circuit impedance is given by the ratio of voltage to current.   For the radiation field the ratio of electric field to magnetic field intensities is given by

$$\frac{E_x}{H_y} = \frac{k}{\omega\varepsilon} = \sqrt{\frac{\mu}{\varepsilon}} = \frac{V/m}{A/m} = \Omega \tag{2-17}$$

This quantity is known as the intrinsic impedance of the medium.   For free space both μ and ε are real, and therefore its intrinsic impedance is real and is equal to 377 ohms.   For material medium μ and ε may be real or complex.   If both μ and ε are real, the intrinsic impedance of the medium is real and the material will be lossless.   However, if either permeability (μ) and/or permittivity (ε) are complex, the intrinsic impedance will be complex and the material will be lossy (see Section 2.5.1).

To determine the power associated with the electromagnetic radiation, we note that the product of E and H gives

$$(E)(H) = \frac{V \times A}{m^2}$$

i.e., it gives power per unit surface area.   Using more elaborate arguments one could show that the instantaneous power density and its flow direction are given by the cross product of **E** and **H**, i.e.,

$$\mathbf{S} = \mathbf{E} \times \mathbf{H} \tag{2-18}$$

Since the cross product is a vector, the direction of **S** gives the direction in which power is flowing.   For the plane-wave case discussed earlier, **S** is given by

$$\mathbf{S} = \mathbf{a}_x E_x \times \mathbf{a}_y H_y = \mathbf{a}_z (E_x)(H_y)$$

This means that in this case power is flowing in the z direction, the direction of wave propagation.   Thus (2-18) not only gives power density associated with the radiation, but also specifies the direction of power flow.   The cross product **E** × **H** is known as the Poynting vector.   For a plane wave the power density can also be expressed in terms of the intrinsic impedance of the medium.   Using (2-17),

$$H_y = \frac{E_x}{Z} \left(Z = \frac{k}{\omega\varepsilon} = \text{intrinsic impedance} \right)$$

hence

$$S = E \times H$$

$$|S| = \left| \frac{E^2}{Z} \right| \qquad (2\text{-}19)$$

It is instructive to calculate the field intensities associated with Q-switched laser pulses. As was shown in Section 1.4.1, such lasers are capable of developing peak powers of 10^8 watts lasting for about 20 ns. By focusing the laser beam to a spot of about 0.1 mm in diameter, the laser produces peak power densities of the order of 10^{12} W/cm^2. The electric field associated with such power densities can be easily obtained using the relation

$$S = \frac{E^2}{Z}$$

which for free space gives

$$S = \frac{E^2}{377} \quad \text{W/m}^2$$

$$\therefore E \simeq 10^9 \ \text{V/m}$$

The interatomic electric fields in the material are of the order of 10^{10} to 10^{11} V/m. Thus we see that the fields produced by a laser beam can easily reach and even exceed interatomic fields either by using high power lasers or tighter focusing.

So far, plane waves, for which the instantaneous field intensities in a plane perpendicular to the propagation direction remain constant, have been discussed. This is not true for an actual laser beam wherein the field intensities for the lowest-order transverse mode follow a Gaussian pattern as shown in Section 1.3. However, the concepts of plane waves are sufficient to understand the optical properties of a material. In any laser beam induced process, thermal or nonthermal, the actual field distribution in the beam does play a significant role; such factors are discussed in the following chapters.

2·1·3   elliptically polarized wave

Direction of polarization is generally defined as the vibration direction of the electric field vector. The plane containing the vibration direction (i.e., electric field) and the propagation direction is called the *plane of polarization*, as shown in Figure 2-4. As an example, consider the plane wave discussed in the last section. For this wave the electric field

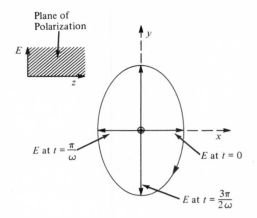

Figure 2-4   Rotation of E vector for elliptically polarized wave as seen by an observer at z = 0 plane.   The direction z is out of the paper plane.

is always in the x direction, and no other electric field components exist. Hence it is really a plane-polarized wave.   A more general type of polarization is elliptical polarization, and is so defined because the electric field vector in a plane perpendicular to the propagation direction traces out an ellipse in one cycle.   In this case, the electric field is composed of two components which are perpendicular to the propagation direction.

To illustrate the concept of elliptic polarization, consider two electromagnetic waves of the same frequency whose electric field intensities are given by

$$\mathbf{E}_x = \mathbf{a}_x E_1 \cos(\omega t - k_0 z) \tag{2-20}$$

and

$$\mathbf{E}_y = \mathbf{a}_y E_2 \cos(\omega t - k_0 z + \xi) \tag{2-21}$$

where E_1 and E_2 are electric field amplitudes, and $\mathbf{a}_x$, $\mathbf{a}_y$ are unit vectors in x and y direction, respectively.   Both the waves are traveling in the z direction except that these are polarized perpendicular to each other and have a phase difference of ξ.   The total electric field intensity at any point on the z axis is given by

$$\mathbf{E} = \mathbf{a}_x E_1 \cos(\omega t - k_0 z) + \mathbf{a}_y E_2 \cos(\omega t - k_0 z + \xi) \tag{2-22}$$

We first consider a special case for which $\xi = +\pi/2$, and in Figure 2-4 plot $\mathbf{E}$ as a function of time at $z = 0$ looking toward the incoming beam. In this case, expanding (2-22) gives

$$\mathbf{E} = \mathbf{a}_x E_1 \cos \omega t - \mathbf{a}_y E_2 \sin \omega t$$

For $E_1/E_2 < 1$, the resultant $\mathbf{E}$ vector traces out an ellipse with its major and minor axis coincident with the y and x axes.   To an observer looking into the incoming beam, this resultant vector rotates in the clockwise direction at an angular frequency of ω rad/s. This is called the right elliptically polarized wave. If we had taken the phase angle $\xi = -\pi/2$, Figure 2-4 would still describe the trace of the **E** vector at $z = 0$ plane, except that now the **E** vector will sweep in the counterclockwise direction. As before, we assume the observer to be looking into the oncoming beam. This type of wave is, therefore, known as left elliptically polarized.

Another special case one should consider is when $E_1 = E_2$. In this case the trace in the $z = 0$ plane will appear to be circular. Once again depending on the value of ξ, we obtain either a right or left circularly polarized wave.

The above treats two special types of elliptically polarized waves. In general $E_1 \neq E_2$ and ξ may assume values other than $\pi/2$. In such cases, the major and the minor axis of the ellipse do not coincide with the x and the y axis.[4]

An important application of the elliptically polarized wave is in determining the optical constants of a material and in the measurement of thin film thickness. The apparatus used for such measurements is called an ellipsometer and is discussed in Chapter 6.

2·2   *quantum aspects of the radiation field*

The theory outlined in the previous section describes electromagnetic radiation as a wave phenomena. We have shown that the electric and magnetic fields associated with radiation oscillate as a function of time and in the propagation direction. This is known as the classical description of electromagnetic fields, which can explain a great variety of phenomena such as diffraction, reflection, refraction and interference of electromagnetic waves. However, it does not explain results of many other experiments, the simplest being the photoelectric effect, which is discussed in Section 2.2.2. The development of quantum theory of radiation and matter has shown that, apart from its wave nature, electromagnetic radiation has certain particle characteristics and that one can also associate wave properties with particles such as electrons. The fundamental postulates of the quantum theory of radiation state that

i.   Electromagnetic radiation of frequency v consists of discrete bundles of energy hv, where h is a universal constant known as Planck's constant. This (light) quantum is called a *photon.*

ii.   The mass of the photon is zero and in free space its velocity is universally constant, i.e., 3×10^8 m/s.

iii. The momentum associated with the photon is equal to $\hbar k$, where k is magnitude of the wave vector ($\hbar = h/2\pi$).

Further clarification of the particle nature of light requires discussion of blackbody radiation, photoelectric effect, and radiation pressure.

2·2·1 blackbody radiation

It is well known that a hot body radiates electromagnetic radiation. Experiments have shown that the radiation emitted by such a body is continuous and covers a wide frequency range.   The emitted radiation is not uniformly distributed over the entire spectral range but shows maximum intensity at a wavelength which depends upon the temperature of the radiating body, as shown in Figure 2-5.   This wavelength at which the radiation intensity is a maximum, and below which the radiation intensity falls off, could not be explained on the basis of classical thermodynamic arguments.   The classical model[5] predicted the power I_λ radiated by a blackbody at a given wavelength λ to be proportional to $kT\lambda^{-4}$, where T is the body temperature and k is Boltzmann's constant.   It is apparent from Figure 2-5 that this law fails badly at shorter wavelengths and is reasonably accurate at longer wavelengths.

Max Planck's[6] theory of blackbody radiation in 1901 was the beginning of quantum theory.   Briefly, Planck's theory is as follows.   The radiation emitted by a blackbody is due to oscillating charges.   The oscillating charges, therefore, form a set of harmonic oscillators.   The key concept which Planck introduced was to assume that each oscillator of frequency v can have only discrete energy levels hv, $2hv$, etc.   The body as a whole consists of a set of harmonic oscillators with varying values of v. This idea that harmonic oscillators can take up energy values only hv at a time (i.e., their energy levels are quantized) is radically different from the classical concept in which, for each oscillator, allowed energy levels are continuous.

The intensity or the strength of each such oscillator can be described by a positive integer n, and its energy by nhv.   Note that if such oscillators

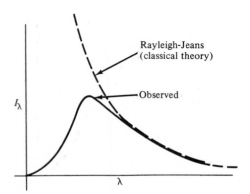

Figure 2-5 Blackbody radiation at temperature T. - - - - Classical theory. _____ Experimental.

radiate, their energy will diminish.   Since energy levels of each oscillator are quantized, this implies that energy exchange can occur either by absorption or radiation of a quantum of energy hv or some integral number of them.   Obviously an oscillator of high strength, i.e., large n, will radiate more, and those with low energy or small n will radiate less.   From statistical thermodynamics one could show that, for a system under thermal equilibrium, n is a function of v and for $hv \gg kT$, n falls off rapidly.   For a given temperature there is a characteristic value of v for which n is a maximum.   Therefore, oscillators for which $hv \gg kT$ are less intense. Planck's hypothesis, therefore, predicts blackbody radiation intensity to fall off at shorter wavelengths (large v), because all such oscillators are essentially in their lowest energy state.   In the region where $hv \ll kT$ (large λ) Planck's theory gives results very similar to the classical concept. The expression for I_λ from Planck's theory comes out to be

$$I_\lambda = \frac{2\pi c^2 h}{\lambda^5} \frac{1}{\exp(hc/\lambda kT) - 1} \tag{2-23}$$

where c = velocity of light in free space (3×10^8 m/s).

The total power radiated by a blackbody can be obtained by integrating the above equation over all wavelengths.   This gives

$$I = \int_0^\infty I_\lambda \, d\lambda = 5.67 \times 10^{-8} T^4 \qquad \text{W/m}^2 \tag{2-24}$$

This is known as the Stefan-Boltzmann law of radiation and has been experimentally verified.   The wavelength λ_m at which the radiation by a blackbody at temperature T is maximum can also be derived from (2-23). This is known as Wien's displacement law.

$$\lambda_m T = 2.884 \times 10^{-3} \text{ m}^\circ\text{K} \tag{2-25}$$

An interesting application of (2-25) has been in time resolved temperature measurement of a laser-heated surface[7], which showed that laser-heated metal surfaces can reach peak temperatures of the order of 10,000°K and that the temperature rise follows closely the laser pulse.

2.2.2   photoelectric effect

Photoelectric effect is the emission of electrons from a metal surface when irradiated with electromagnetic radiation.   In this section we shall outline the main features of the photoelectric effect and then show that the quantum nature of radiation satisfactorily explains this effect, whereas the classical concept fails.

Figure 2-6 shows energy levels of electrons in the conduction band of a metal. At room temperature the kinetic energy of these electrons is insufficient to overcome the potential barrier ϕ (volts) existing at the

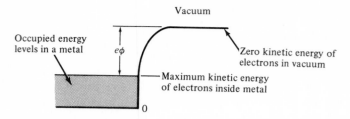

Figure 2-6   Occupied energy levels and work function of a metal surface.

metal surface.   The energy required to overcome the potential barrier ($e\phi$) is called the *work function*, where e is the electronic charge.   It is apparent that for electrons in the highest energy level of the conduction band, $e\phi$ is the energy that one must provide to overcome the potential barrier.   For electrons occupying lower energy levels, energy greater than $e\phi$ will have to be provided in order to cause emission.

In a photoelectric experiment one uses a metal plate as a cathode. Another plate is used as an anode (collector) and a potential is applied across the plates, which are kept in vacuum.   The arrangement is shown schematically in Figure 2-7.   When the cathode is illuminated with radiation of frequency v, and the potential across the plate is varied, the collector current as a function of applied voltage and light intensity is given by Figure 2-8.   The important feature to note is that for negative potentials there is a critical voltage V_c below which no electrons are emitted.   This is because the negative voltage acts as an additional potential barrier, which the electrons must overcome.   As the voltage is increased the anode current increases, and for $V \geq 0$ it reaches a saturation value I_s, which is linearly dependent on the intensity of the incident radiation. The interesting part of the experimental result is that V_c is independent of illumination intensity.

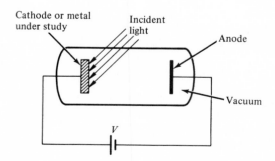

Figure 2-7   Schematic of photoelectric experiment.   The applied voltage V shown acts as a retarding potential on the emitted electrons.

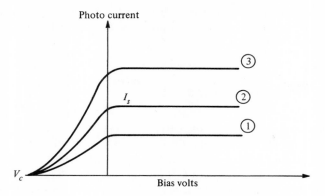

Figure 2-8 Photoelectrons as a function of light intensity and retarding potential V. Light intensity for $1 < 2 < 3$.

These experimental results cannot be explained by considering only the wave nature of radiation. For example, assume that electrons interact with the electric field of the incident radiation; then an increase in radiation intensity implies a higher electric field. Therefore, more energy is imparted to the electrons and hence these should be able to overcome V_c. On this basis one would expect V_c to be more negative for higher intensities. However, as mentioned previously, this is not the case. On the contrary, for a given frequency v, V_c is independent of radiation intensity.

On the basis of quantum theory of radiation, the photoelectric effect was first explained by Einstein. He assumed that monochromatic radiation of frequency v consists of photons of energy hv. In the interaction process the photon energy is absorbed by the electron. The emitted electrons have to overcome a potential barrier (work function) of energy $e\phi$; therefore, their maximum kinetic energy will be the difference between the photon energy and the work function, i.e.,

$$(\tfrac{1}{2}mv^2)_{max} = hv - e\phi \tag{2-26}$$

Since the application of an externally applied retarding potential adds to the work function, (2-26) gives

$$(\tfrac{1}{2}mv^2)_{max} = hv - e(\phi + V) \tag{2-26a}$$

As the retarding potential V is increased, there will be a critical value V_c at which $hv = e(\phi + V_c)$. Above this voltage, then, electrons will not be emitted. Furthermore, (2-26) and (2-26a) show that the maximum kinetic energy of the emitted electrons and the critical retarding potential V_c are linear functions of frequency v.

The above description of the photoelectric effect shows that the electron emission depends on the radiation frequency v and work function;

hence it should be possible to observe this effect at very low intensities. This effect is used in photon counting systems which are discussed in Chapter 9.

2·2·3   radiation pressure

Two important parameters of a dynamic system are its energy and momentum. We have shown that the energy of a photon is given by $h\nu$. The following qualitative arguments show that the momentum associated with photons is given by $\hbar\mathbf{k}$, where $\mathbf{k}$ is its wave vector.

It is known that a material particle of rest mass m and velocity v has a momentum mv in the direction of its velocity. Photons have zero mass and their velocity is fixed (see 2-18), i.e., the velocity of light in free space. To show that there is momentum associated with photons, Feynman[8] gives the following example. Let us assume that a plane wave is incident on a charged particle of charge e. The particle will oscillate in response to the electric field of the incident radiation, as shown in Figure 2-9. If the electric field of the incident radiation is in the x direction, the particle will acquire an oscillatory velocity in this direction. The magnetic field of the incident radiation is in the y direction, and the wave is propagating in the z direction. From electromagnetic theory we know that a charged particle moving in a magnetic field experiences a force

$$\mathbf{F} = e(\mathbf{v} \times \mathbf{B})$$

where $\mathbf{v}$ is particle velocity, and $\mathbf{B}$ is magnetic flux density of the incident radiation. Since e and $\mathbf{v}$ change sign simultaneously, then it can be seen that $e(\mathbf{v} \times \mathbf{B})$ is always in the direction of wave propagation. This force results in the radiation pressure. Thus using only classical physics it is shown that radiation pressure does exist. Feynman further shows that the momentum transferred by the radiation is given by

$$p = \frac{\text{energy absorbed}}{\text{velocity of light}}$$

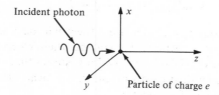

Figure 2-9   Charged particle interacting with a photon field. Light is polarized in the x direction and propagates in the z direction.

For a single photon the momentum magnitude is therefore given by

$$p = \frac{h\nu}{c}$$

which, using (2-14), gives

$$\mathbf{p} = \hbar\mathbf{k}_0 \tag{2-27}$$

Pressure due to transfer of momentum from photons to a material can be observed.   A recent study[9] has shown that laser beams can be used to observe radiation pressure without complications of the thermal effects. In this study micron size latex particles were suspended in water.   Water, as well as latex, is transparent to green ($\lambda = 514.5$ nm) light of an argon laser; hence thermal effects are not present.   Radiation, incident on the latex particles, exerts pressure which causes the particles to move in the direction of the propagating laser beam.   Such particles get trapped within the laser beam diameter at the container wall.   When the laser is shut off, the particles wander away due to random motion in the liquid.   This conclusively shows that the movement and trapping of the particles occurred due to the radiation pressure.   Possible applications of this effect in sorting of micron and submicron size particles have been discussed in Ref. 9.

In interaction processes, two conservation laws often most helpful in developing the mathematical formalism are conservation of energy and momentum.   The concept of momentum and its conservation will, therefore, be important when scattering of light is discussed.

2·3   theory of solids

Interaction of radiation with matter depends both on properties of the electromagnetic radiation, such as its frequency and intensity, and on the material properties.   In most cases interaction phenomenon can be illustrated with simple classical models.   However, there are certain aspects of the theory of solids, such as band theory of solids, quantization of the electronic energy levels, etc., that are best explained on the basis of quantum theory.   Therefore, in the following, Schrödinger's equation and band theory of solids are briefly reviewed.

2·3·1   Schrödinger's equation

In 1924, de Broglie[10] suggested that small particles of matter such as electrons have the property of also behaving like waves of wavelength

$$\lambda = \frac{h}{p}$$

where h is Planck's constant, and p is momentum of the particle.   In 1927, electron diffraction from a nickel crystal was observed[11] and analyzed analogously to the Laue[12] patterns of X-ray diffraction.   Diffraction (see Chapter 7) can be explained only on the basis of wave theory, thereby furnishing experimental confirmation of the de Broglie hypothesis.

During this same period, Bohr[13] developed the quantum theory of electrons in an atom.   According to this, electrons bound in an atom could occupy only discrete energy levels called the *stationary states*.   Bohr postulated that electrons are orbiting around the nucleus.   Radiation (photon) is emitted only when bound electrons move from a higher energy level (E_2) to a lower energy level (E_1), the photon energy being the difference between the two energy levels

$$E_2 - E_1 = h\nu$$

This means that the energy levels of a bound electron are quantized, much the same as Planck assumed the quantized energy levels of harmonic oscillators to explain blackbody radiation.

In 1926, Schrödinger[14] showed that a wave equation could be used to characterize bound electrons in agreement with Bohr's quantum theory. Schrödinger equation in Cartesian coordinates is

$$\frac{\hbar^2}{2m}\left(\frac{\partial^2}{\partial x^2} + \frac{\partial^2}{\partial y^2} + \frac{\partial^2}{\partial z^2}\right)\psi - V\psi = \frac{h}{i}\frac{\partial\psi}{\partial t} \qquad (2\text{-}28)$$

where m is mass of the particle, V is its potential energy, and $i = \sqrt{-1}$. The solution of Schrödinger's equation, ψ, is a function of space coordinates and time and is called the *wave function*.   According to quantum theory the wave function, ψ, contains all the relevant information about the behavior of the particle, such as its velocity, energy, position, etc.

It is not necessary for us to go into details of the possible solutions of (2-28) except to note that, if the potential energy function V is specified, then in principle it is possible to determine the wave function.   A special case occurs when potential V is independent of time as in, for example, a crystal (see Section 2.3.6).   In this case, ψ can be written as

$$\psi = \Phi(x, y, z)F(t)$$

where Φ is a function of space coordinates, and F is a function of time. Substituting this in Schrödinger's equation, one can show that [16]

$$F(t) = \exp\left(-i\frac{Et}{\hbar}\right)$$

where E is total energy of the electron.   The time independent part of Schrödinger's equation then becomes

$$\frac{\hbar^2}{2m}\left(\frac{\partial^2}{\partial x^2} + \frac{\partial^2}{\partial y^2} + \frac{\partial^2}{\partial z^2}\right)\Phi + (E - V)\Phi = 0 \qquad (2\text{-}29)$$

This is known as the time independent Schrödinger equation, which we shall use in reviewing the band theory of solids and energy levels of an electron in an isolated atom.

2·3·2   energy levels of an electron in an atom

The potential energy V of an electron of charge $-e$ at a distance r from a nucleus of charge Ze is given by

$$V = -Ze^2/4\pi\varepsilon_0 r$$

where

$$r = \sqrt{x^2 + y^2 + z^2}$$

This potential energy can be used in (2-29) to determine the wave function and energy levels of an electron in a hydrogen-like atom.   The solution[17] so obtained shows that the wave function can be described by three numbers n, ℓ, and m_ℓ.   These numbers, generally referred to as quantum numbers, can take only integer values (ℓ and m_ℓ could be zero) and essentially represent the quantization of energy levels and the angular momentum of the orbiting electron.   Table 2-2 gives the allowed values of these numbers and the associated quantities.

The quantum numbers n, ℓ, and m_ℓ describe the orbit of an electron around the nucleus.   Experimentally it is found that electrons also have an intrinsic spin angular momentum which can be either parallel or anti-parallel to its orbital angular momentum.   The spin states are assigned an additional quantum number called m_s, which is included in Table 2-2.

TABLE 2-2   Quantum Numbers of a Bound Electron Wave Function

Quantum Number and Its Allowed Values	Associated Quantity and Its Value
$n = 1, 2, \ldots$	Total energy[a] $$E_n = -\frac{1}{n^2}\frac{mZ^2e^4}{32\pi^2\varepsilon_0^2\hbar^2}$$
$\ell = 0, 1, 2, \ldots (n-1)$	Orbital angular momentum $L = \hbar\sqrt{\ell(\ell+1)}$
$m_\ell = -\ell, -\ell+1, \cdots 0 \cdots, \ell-1, \ell$	Component of orbital angular momentum
$m_s = +\frac{1}{2}, -\frac{1}{2}$	Component of spin angular momentum

[a] The negative energy implies the electron is *bounded*.

2·3·3   Pauli exclusion principle

When an atom containing more than one electron is treated quantum mechanically, a useful first approximation is to assume that the electrons do not exert forces on one another.   In this case the wave functions are specified by the four quantum numbers given above.   The Pauli[18] exclusion principle states that in a multielectron system no two electrons can have the same wave function.   In other words, a set of quantum numbers—n, ℓ, m_ℓ, and m_s—is assigned to each electron.   This principle applies equally well to electrons in a solid, except that in this case widely separated energy levels split into a band of allowed energy values.   It is important to note that even in a solid the allowed energy values are quantized, except that the adjacent values in a given band do not differ appreciably.

2·3·4   interatomic bond

Solid, liquid, and gaseous states of the same material (element or compound) occur at correspondingly higher temperatures, so the energy of solid is lower than the other two states.   As the interatomic spacing of free atoms is reduced, they combine to form molecules, which to a large extent retain their identity in liquid and solid states.   A molecule is defined as the smallest stable unit of more than one atom.   In general, the molecular state in a gas is more stable than widely separated individual atoms. It is for this reason that hydrogen is generally found in molecular state H_2.

Interatomic binding forces are due to the mutual attraction and repulsion of the electronic and nuclear charges of the constituent atoms.   The molecular binding forces can be understood from Figure 2-10.   When two atoms approach each other, the coulombic repulsion between the electronic clouds polarizes the atoms; i.e., the center of charge of the electron cloud does not coincide with the positive charge of its nucleus. Polarized (dipoles) atoms attract each other,[15] which causes interatomic distance to reduce further.   This increased reduction causes the positive nuclear charge of one atom to attract the negative electronic charge of the other atom.   This attraction still further reduces the interatomic spacing. Finally, a stable distance between the two atoms is maintained when the mutual repulsion between the respective nuclear charges and electronic charges just balances the attractive forces mentioned earlier.   All molecular binding forces are due to electrical charges; however, depending on the electronic configuration of the constituent atoms, these can be classified into four distinct types.

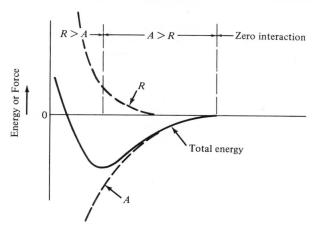

**Figure 2-10   Forces and molecular energy as a function of inter-
nuclear distance. A = attractive force; R = repulsive force.**

1. Van der Waals Bond: This type of bond develops if the atoms have
   closed shell electron configuration (closed shell means that all the
   electronic states corresponding to the quantum number, n, are occupied).
   The bonds attractive force is basically due to polarized atoms.   This is
   the weakest bond.
2. Ionic Bond: In this case, atoms exchange electrons to produce closed
   shell configuration.   The exchange of electrons produces positive and
   negative ions, and the resulting electrostatic attraction develops the
   ionic bond such as in a Na^+Cl^- molecule.
3. Covalent Bond: In covalent bonded molecules and crystals, the electrons
   are not exchanged but shared.   This means that the electron orbits are
   modified to encompass more than one atom as, for example, the H_2
   molecular bond.
4. Metallic Bond: This is a combination of van der Waals bond and
   covalent bond.   The valence electrons are shared not just by the
   adjacent atoms but by all atoms of the crystal.

   It should be emphasized that the above classification is merely a
convenient way of characterizing the bonds.   In a real crystal, more than
one type of bond is often present.   With this reservation in mind, one
would expect the properties of a crystalline solid to depend upon the nature
of the bond and its strength.   For example, if the binding forces are weak,
the crystal will be mechanically weak also and will melt at low temperatures
such as crystals in which van der Waals binding is predominant.   On the
other hand, ionic crystals have strong binding forces which are reflected in
their mechanical and thermal properties.   A broad outline of the physical
and structural properties associated with the four interatomic bonds is
given in Table 2-3.[19]

TABLE 2-3   Physical and Structural Properties Associated with the Four Interatomic Bonds[a]

Property	Ionic	Covalent	Metallic	Van der Waals
Structural	Nondirected, giving structures of high coordination.	Spatially directed and numerically limited, giving structures of low coordination and low density.	Nondirected, giving structures of very high coordination and high density.	Formally analogous to metallic bond.
Mechanical	Strong, giving hard crystals.	Strong, giving hard crystals.	Variable strength. Gliding common.	Weak, giving soft crystals.
Thermal	Fairly high M.P.[b] low coefficient of expansion. Ions in melt.	High M.P., low coefficient of expansion. Molecules in melt.	Variable M.P., long liquid interval.	Low M.P., large coefficient of expansion.
Electrical	Moderate insulators. Conduction by ion transport in melt. Sometimes soluble in liquids of high dielectric constant.	Insulators in solid and melt.	Conduction by electron transport.	Insulators.
Optical and magnetic	Absorption and other properties primarily those of the individual ions, and therefore similar in solution.	High refractive index. Absorption profoundly different in solution or gas.	Opaque. Properties similar in liquid.	Properties those of individual molecules and therefore similar in solution or gas.

[a] With permission of Cambridge University Press.
[b] Melting point.

2·3·5   space lattices and crystal classes

In solids, the molecules lose their individual identity and are bound together in a manner similar to that of interatomic binding. The difference between crystalline and noncrystalline materials is that, in the former, atomic array is periodic, whereas in the latter, the atomic groups are arrayed more randomly. Geometric configurations of three-dimensional periodic arrays are called *space lattices*; the study of their symmetry properties is called *crystallography*. The symmetry of the atomic groupings in a unit cell affects many of the optical, electrical, and mechanical properties of a crystalline solid.

A space lattice is defined by a network of straight lines in space so constructed that it divides space into equal volumes with no space

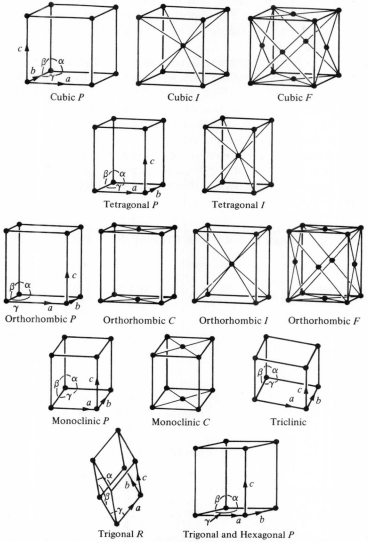

Figure 2-11   The fourteen Bravais or space lattices.   The cells shown are the conventional unit cells, which are not always the primitive cells. P = primitive unit cell, C = base centered, F = face centered, I = body centered, and R = rhombohedral.[25]   (Adapted with permission of John Wiley and Sons, Inc.)

excluded. At first it would appear that many such lattices could be constructed; however, Bravais in 1848 showed that there are only 14 possible distinct networks of lattice points. Unit cells of such lattices, known as *Bravais cells*, are shown in Figure 2-11. The unit cell is defined as one which, when translated along the axes of a lattice, gives rise to the lattice itself. It is important to note that the lattice points are not necessarily occupied by atoms. The important point is that atoms of a crystal are set in space either on the points of a Bravais lattice or in some fixed relation to those points.

Another important feature of Bravais lattices is that only seven sets of axes are needed to construct the 14 different space lattices. This leads to the classification of all crystalline solids as belonging to one of the seven crystal systems, where the term system refers to a set of axes. Table 2-4 (see also Figure 2-11) lists the seven crystal systems, their axes and the angular relationships between the axes.

Many crystalline solids have complex crystal structures, which can be derived from the seven crystal systems of Table 2-4, such as the diamond structure, hexagonal close-packed structures, etc. Table 2-5 gives crystal structures of some commonly known elements and chemical compounds.

TABLE 2-4   The Crystal Systems

Name	Axial Lengths	Axial Angles
Cubic	$a = b = c$	$\alpha = \beta = \gamma = 90°$
Tetragonal	$a = b \neq c$	$\alpha = \beta = \gamma = 90°$
Orthorhombic	$a \neq b \neq c$	$\alpha = \beta = \gamma = 90°$
Monoclinic	$a \neq b \neq c$	$\alpha = \beta = 90° \neq \gamma$
Triclinic	$a \neq b \neq c$	$\alpha \neq \beta \neq \gamma \neq 90°$
Rhombohedral (Trigonal R)	$a = b = c$	$\alpha = \beta = 90° \neq \gamma$
Hexagonal	$a = b \neq c$	$\alpha = \beta = 90° \neq \gamma = 120°$

TABLE 2-5   Bravais Unit Cells of some Elements and Compounds at Room Temperature

Unit Cell	Typical Crystalline Solids
Cubic	Al, Cu, Ag, Au, NaCl Alloys; CuNi and FeNi
Tetragonal	$BaTiO_3$, CdO, KDP
Orthorhombic	U, Nb_2O_5, $AgNO_3$
Monoclinic	V_3O_5, $ZnCl_2$, WO_3, ZrO_2, Se(red)
Triclinic	$NiWO_4$, $CoWO_4$
Rhombohedral	Bi, Sb
Hexagonal	La_2O_3, KO_3, Be, Co, Ti

2·3·6   band theory of solids

The most significant contribution of the quantum theory, as applied to solid-state physics, has been the emergence of a band theory of solids, which states: the energy levels that electrons can occupy in a solid are distributed over several energy bands; any two allowed energy bands are separated by a region of forbidden energy values which electrons cannot occupy.   Our main interest in this theory lies primarily in delineating the absorption processes in conductors, semiconductors, and insulators. Furthermore, knowledge of it is important in understanding the operation of semiconductor lasers.

About three quarters of all known elements are metallic and, therefore, in the early 1900's, solid-state theory was centered around explaining the properties of metals.   Drude[20] proposed that metals are composed of positive ions whose valence electrons are free to roam among the ionic array, with the only restriction that they are confined to remain within the boundaries of the metal crystal.   Lorentz[21] carried this model further by applying thermodynamic principles to the electron gas in a solid.   This theory was refined by Sommerfield,[22] who incorporated quantum concepts of discrete energy levels of the electrons and Pauli's exclusion principle. However, both Drude-Lorentz theory and Sommerfield quantum theory fail to explain why the electrical conductivity increases with temperature in semiconductors such as Si and CuO_2, whereas in such metals as Cu it decreases with temperature.   All the above theories assume a constant potential inside the crystal.   This assumption is not correct, because each atom contains at its center a small nucleus, in which all the positive charge resides.   The electric field in which the electrons move is stronger near the center of the atoms than at the point midway between atoms (Figure 2-12a); therefore, the electrostatic potential fluctuates from one atom to the next. The simplest model which takes into account the fluctuating potential is due to Kronig and Penney[23] as shown in Figure 2-12b.

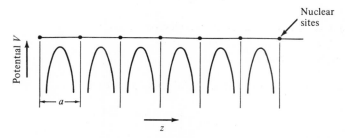

Figure 2-12a   *Periodic potential in a one-dimensional crystal.   Note that the potential is maximum at the nuclear sites and is minimum in between.*

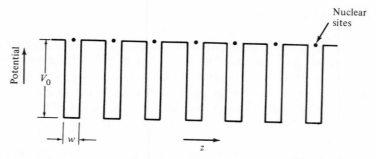

Figure 2-12b Kronig-Penney model. *(The limiting value P, see text, determines the width of the allowed energy bands. In general, the bands become broader as P decreases, and for P=0 we obtain the free electron case.*

To see qualitatively that the allowed energy levels form bands, we go back to the concept of a free atom. In Section 2.3.2 it was pointed out that the electrons in a free atom can occupy only certain discrete energy levels. However, as two atoms approach each other the electronic and nuclear (charge) interactions modify the potential function. In this approximation the discrete energy values split into two values differing slightly from each other. This process is continued when large aggregate of atoms combine to form the solid state. The process is schematically shown in Figure 2-13, where the allowed energy values are shown as a function of interatomic spacing.

We shall now briefly outline the solution of Schrödinger equation using the Kronig-Penney model. First, consider the Sommerfield model in which the periodic potential is replaced by a constant potential V inside the crystal. In this case the time independent Schrödinger equation, for a one-dimensional (z) crystal, is given by

$$\frac{d^2\phi}{dz^2} + \frac{2m}{\hbar^2}(E - V)\phi = 0 \qquad (2\text{-}30)$$

where ϕ = time independent free electron wave function,
E = total energy of the electron,
m = electron mass.

In exponential form the solution of this equation is

$$\phi = A \exp \pm \left[i \frac{\sqrt{2m(E - V)}}{\hbar} \right] z \qquad (2\text{-}31)$$

where A is a constant and the plus or minus sign in the exponent corresponds to electron motion in positive or negative z direction.

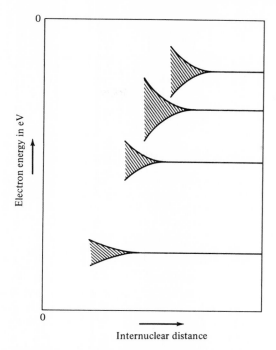

Figure 2-13   Electron energy levels as a function of internuclear distance.   Note that the energy levels of outer electrons (higher energy) split earlier and develop broader bands.

This may be compared with the time independent part of the electromagnetic plane-wave solution (2-11), which is

$$E = E_0 \exp[\pm ikz]$$

where k was defined as the propagation constant or wave vector.   Using the same notation for an electron wave vector, we obtain

$$k = \frac{1}{\hbar} \sqrt{2m(E - V)}$$

Squaring both sides gives

$$E - V = \frac{\hbar^2 k^2}{2m}$$

E is the total energy of the electron, and V is its potential energy; therefore, $(E - V)$ corresponds to kinetic energy of an electron in the one-dimensional crystal.   Kinetic energy of a particle in terms of its momentum is given by $p^2/2m$; therefore,

$$E - V = \frac{p^2}{2m} = \frac{\hbar^2 k^2}{2m}$$

or

$$p = \hbar k \qquad (2\text{-}32)$$

Thus the momentum of an electron is given by a relation similar to that of a photon (2-27). The wavelength of the electron from (2-13) is

$$\lambda = \frac{2\pi}{k} = \frac{h}{p}$$

which is also the de Broglie relation. The dependence of total energy E on wave vector k is depicted in Figure 2-14a. There are no restrictions placed either on the total energy E of the electron or the possible values which k can assume, because the electron has been assumed to move in a constant potential.

Now consider the consequences of making V a periodic function of z. In the Kronig-Penney model, Figure 2.12b, the potential V_0 is allowed to be infinitely large at the nuclear sites with the restriction that

$$\lim_{W \to 0} (V_0)(W) = P$$

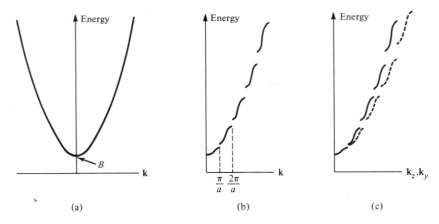

(a)   (b)   (c)

Figure 2-14   Electron energy as a function of wave vector k.

(a) *Sommerfield model, in this case E vs. k diagram is parabolic given by the equation*

$$E = \frac{\hbar^2 k^2}{2m} + B$$

(b) *Kronig-Penney model, the periodic nature of V creates energy gaps at*

$$k = +\frac{\ell\pi}{a}, \ell = 1, 2, \ldots$$

(c) *Overlapping bands due to anisotropy in V. Note that in one case the energy values not allowed in the z direction (solid curve) are allowed in the y direction (dotted curve).*

Replacing V by $V(z)$ in (2-30) we obtain

$$\frac{d^2\phi}{dz^2} + \frac{2m}{\hbar^2}[E - V(z)]\phi = 0 \qquad (2-33)$$

Since V now is a periodic function of z, one would expect the solution of (2-33) to be periodic in z. A detailed analysis shows that the periodic nature of $V(z)$ modifies the energy versus $\mathbf{k}$ (wave vector) diagram of Figure 2-14a in the following manner.

First, the energy is no longer a continuous function of wave vector $\mathbf{k}$, but shows discontinuities for values of wave vector $k = \pm(\pi/a)\ell$, where $\ell = 1, 2, \ldots$.

Second, the application of boundary conditions due to finite size of any crystal shows that the number of distinct electron wave functions which can be accommodated within a Brillouin* zone is $2N$, where N is the number of unit cells in the crystal. In other words, if there are $2N$ electrons in a given band, it is completely filled.

Third, the value of P determines the width of the allowed energy bands. In general, the bands become broader as P decreases, and for $P = 0$ we obtain the free electron case.

So far a one-dimensional crystal has been considered. In a real crystal the $E\text{-}k$ diagram of Figure 2-14b needs certain modifications. First, in any direction the maximum value of the wave vector $\mathbf{k}$, in any Brillouin zone, will depend upon the lattice spacing, a $(k = n\pi/a)$. Second, the energy values for a given k which are not allowed in one direction may be allowed in another direction, as depicted in Figure 2-14c. This turns out to be a significant factor which explains the conductivity of many divalent metals. According to the band theory (see Section 2.3.7), solids in which the highest lying energy band is completely filled should be either a semiconductor or an insulator. Since each band can accommodate at most $2N$ electrons, and there are two valence electrons per atom in a divalent metal, it would appear that the outermost band in this case is completely filled. Therefore, such metals should not be good electrical conductors. The fact that such metals are good electrical conductors is due to overlapping bands in different directions.

---

* A Brillouin zone encompasses a region in k-space given by

$$-\frac{m\pi}{a} \le k \le -\frac{(m-1)\pi}{a}, \quad \text{and} \quad \frac{(m-1)\pi}{a} \le k \le \frac{m\pi}{a}.$$

Thus, in one-dimensional model the first Brillouin zone covers the region $-\pi/a < k < \pi/a$, and the subsequent Brillouin zones have two intervals of half a period each as defined above. In the present context a Brillouin zone defines a region within which no energy gaps occur. For further reference, see R. M. Rose, L. A. Shepard, and J. Wulff, *The Structure and Properties of Materials*, Vol. IV, John Wiley and Sons, Inc., New York (1966).

2·3·7 conductors, semiconductors, and insulators

The band theory enables one to construct a rational explanation of electronic conduction in the solid state.   It is important to consider the magnitude of the energy gap between different bands and the relative fullness of the allowed energy bands with electronic states.   Since the inner core electrons are tightly bound (large P), the first few bands are narrow and always completely filled; we should therefore direct our attention to the last two bands as shown in Figure 2-15.   In Figure 2-15a the highest energy band, generally called the *conduction band*, is only partly filled.   This may well represent a monovalent (one valence electron) metal.   In the previous section it was pointed out that each band can accommodate $2N$ electrons.   Thus, for a monovalent metal, only half of the conduction band is occupied.   Figures 2-15b and 2-15c show the valence band completely filled but the conduction band empty.   These two examples differ in the sense that the band gap, E_g, is small in Figure 2-15b compared to that in Figure 2-15c.

In the following description, letters in parentheses refer to parts of Figure 2-15.

Now let us consider what happens when a constant electric field E is applied to the crystal (a).   The electrons experience a force and are accelerated.   This means they acquire additional energy and occupy available higher energy levels in the conduction band.   However, this process cannot continue indefinitely, since electrons go through several collision processes and lose their acquired energy.   The important fact is that the electrons acquire an average velocity in the direction of the electric field, and hence the crystal is a conductor.

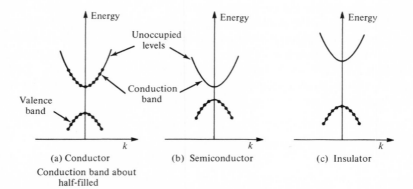

Figure 2-15   Energy band diagram for conductor, semiconductor, and insulator.   For semiconductors (b) at absolute zero, the conduction band is empty; however, at normal temperature, electrons from valence band are excited in the conduction band.

TABLE 2-6   Typical Values of Band Gaps in Semiconductors and Dielectrics

Semiconductor or Dielectric	Band Gap E_g (eV) at 300°K
Si	1.1
Ge	0.7
InSb	0.167
InAs	0.35
InP	1.26
GaSb	0.67
GaAs	1.35
GaP	2.24
Diamond	5.3
SrTiO$_3$	3.4

For the examples shown in (b) and (c), application of a static electric field (at $T = 0$) cannot cause electronic conduction because there are no allowed empty energy levels available. This does not mean that the electric field will have no effect on the crystal at all. In fact, we should expect a small distortion of the bands, which would give rise to polarization and, therefore, such material could be classified as dielectric. However, there is an important difference between (b) and (c); the band gap, E_g, for (b) is much smaller than that for (c). This means that if we provide thermal energy, i.e., increase the temperature, some of the valence band electrons of (b) will acquire sufficient energy to jump the band gap and occupy the empty levels in the conduction band. Thus, as the temperature increases, additional electrons are excited to the conduction band and the conductivity of such a material at first increases with temperature. This should be contrasted with the case of a metal, where the band gap and the unoccupied energy levels are such that thermally no additional electrons could be excited to the conduction band. Therefore, the conductivity of metals (due to higher scattering) decreases with increasing temperature.

Finally, for the crystal (c) the band gap, E_g, is so large that at normal temperatures only a few electrons can be thermally excited into the conduction band. Such a material will, therefore, be a dielectric. In dielectrics the band gap is generally of the order of 3 to 5 eV. Table 2-6 lists the band gap of some commonly used semiconductors and dielectrics.

2·3·8   Fermi level

In the previous discussion it has been implied that with increasing temperature the probability of occupying higher energy levels increases. That this is indeed the case can be shown by arguments of statistical mechanics. Without going into details of statistical mechanics, the following briefly outlines its main conclusion.

According to the Pauli exclusion principle, each quantum state can be occupied by no more than one electron of each spin. Therefore, at the absolute zero of temperature, the electrons occupy the lowest energy states in such a manner that the occupied states are just sufficient to account for the number of electrons in the system. At any finite temperature ($T \neq 0$), because of an overall increase in the system energy, it is apparent that some electrons will occupy higher energy levels. For electrons, since they obey the exclusion principle, Fermi-Dirac[24] statistics apply. The main conclusion of Fermi-Dirac statistics is that at a temperature T, the probability of finding an electron of any one spin in a given energy level E is given by

$$P(E) = \frac{1}{[\exp(E - E_f)/kT] + 1} \tag{2-34}$$

where E_f is the Fermi energy level.

The temperature dependence of the Fermi function is shown in Figure 2-16. From this we note that, for $T = 0$,

$$P(E) = 1 \quad \text{if } E < E_f$$

and

$$P(E) = 0 \quad \text{if } E > E_f$$

Therefore, in general, the energy value which divides the filled and vacant levels at absolute zero is the Fermi level. At a finite temperature if there happens to be an allowed level with $E = E_f$, it is equally likely to be occupied or empty, since $E_f = 1/2$ for $T \neq 0$. In the case of intrinsic semiconductors (undoped semiconductors), E_f lies very close to the center of the band gap; i.e., if the top of the valence band is designated as zero energy, then $E_f = E_g/2$. Figure 2-17 shows the Fermi level diagram for intrinsic and doped semiconductors. If the semiconductor is doped with

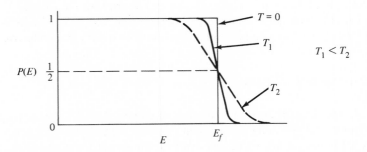

Figure 2-16 $P(E)$, *Fermi-Dirac probability distribution as a function of E for $T=0$ and two other temperatures.*

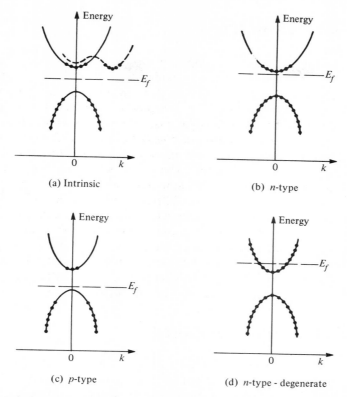

Figure 2-17 *Fermi level E_f in a semiconductor as a function of doping. Allowed energy values for the last two bands are shown as a function of wave vector* **k**. *If the minimum energy value in the conduction band and the maximum energy value in the valence band do not occur for same k (dotted curve (a)), the semiconductor is called indirect band gap; otherwise it is called direct band gap.*

impurities which provide additional electrons, i.e., n-type (donor) impurity, the additional electrons create new energy levels in the band gap.   Therefore, in this case, the Fermi level lies close to the conduction band as shown in Figure 2-17b.   If the impurity atoms have less valence electrons than the atoms of the parent material, some of the energy levels in the valence band remain unoccupied.   Such semiconductors are called p-type and, in this case, the Fermi level shifts toward the valence band as shown in Figure 2-17c.

A special case arises when the semiconductor is so heavily doped that even at $T = 0$, the allowed energy level falls within the conduction (n-type) band, which brings the Fermi level within the conduction band. Such semiconductors are called degenerate (Figure 2-17d) and are used in semiconductor lasers (see Section 1.6.8).

2·4 lattice vibrations

In previous discussions it was implicitly assumed that atoms (or ions) of a solid occupy fixed positions in a crystal lattice.   At any finite temperature, due to thermal energy, the atoms do not remain stationary but oscillate around their mean position.   The purpose of this section is to outline characteristic features of such vibrations.   If nearest neighbor atoms move in the same direction, they are called *acoustic modes of vibration*.   On the other hand, if neighboring atoms move in opposite directions, they are called *optic modes of vibration*.   The actual vibrations due to thermal energy are random, but these random oscillations could be thought of as due to superposition of many different harmonic oscillations.   The frequency spectrum is a characteristic feature of a particular crystal, because of its dependence on the atomic mass, crystal symmetry, and the nature and strength of the bonding forces.   Gaining some insight of the frequency spectrum of lattice vibrations is of primary interest because such vibrations give rise to scattering and absorption of radiation and play an important role in thermal and electrical conductivity.

2·4·1   acoustic vibrations

Consider a one-dimensional crystal of identical atoms of mass m connected through a massless spring of force constant f and unperturbed atomic spacing a.   For the moment the array will be considered infinitely long, and it will be assumed that there exists interaction between nearest neighbors only.   In equilibrium, the distance between neighboring particles is the lattice spacing, a, and due to vibrations, the deflection from the equilibrium position for the nth atom is identified by x_n.

In this model there are two forces acting on the nth atom.   First the force required to accelerate the nth particle.   Second the force due to compression or expansion of the springs connecting the nth atom to its two nearest neighbors, i.e., atoms at $(n-1)$ and $(n+1)$ lattice sites.   Therefore, from Figure 2-18, the equation of motion for the nth atom is given by

$$m\frac{d^2x_n}{dt^2} = -f(x_n - x_{n-1}) - f(x_n - x_{n+1})$$

$$= f(x_{n-1} + x_{n+1} - 2x_n) \tag{2-35}$$

Our interest is in those solutions of the equation in which the atomic displacement from their equilibrium position can be represented by a wave motion.   To illustrate this point further, Figure 2-19a shows atomic displacement x_n as a function of mean atomic position ξ for the linear chain model.   It is apparent that in this case 1st, 5th, and 9th atoms do not move from their equilibrium position, but the atoms in between are moved.   The interesting point is that the displacement of all the atoms together can be

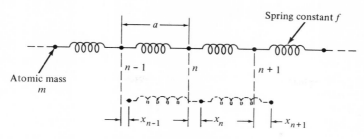

Figure 2-18   Linear chain model.

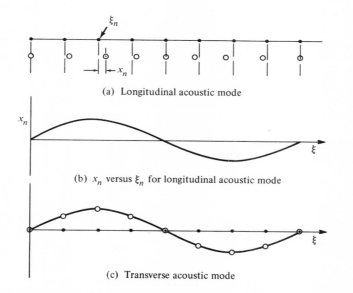

(a) Longitudinal acoustic mode

(b) x_n versus ξ_n for longitudinal acoustic mode

(c) Transverse acoustic mode

Figure 2-19   Atomic displacements for acoustic modes of a linear chain with two degrees of freedom where dots show mean atomic positions and circles give displaced positions.   (In (c) the displacement shown is in the transverse direction to the wave propagation.)

represented by a sinusoidal wave of Figure 2-19b.   As mentioned earlier, the actual atomic motion may be quite random, but such random motions can be constructed by superposing many sinusoidal oscillations of varying frequency and wavelengths.   Assuming a propagating wave-type solution for (2-35), displacement of the nth atom can be written as

$$x_n(t) = A \exp i(\omega t - qna) \qquad (2\text{-}36)$$

where $A =$ amplitude of oscillation,
  $\omega =$ oscillation frequency in rad/s,
  $na =$ equilibrium position of the nth atom, i.e., the spatial coordinate x,
  $q =$ propagation constant.

Substituting this in (2-35) gives

$$mw^2 = -f[\exp(-iqa) + \exp(iqa) - 2] = 4f\sin^2\frac{qa}{2} \qquad (2\text{-}37)$$

The maximum value of ω therefore is given by

$$\omega_{max} = 2\sqrt{\frac{f}{m}}$$

and, in general, from (2-37)

$$\omega = \omega_{max}\sin\frac{qa}{2} \qquad (2\text{-}38)$$

This expression gives the frequency of the wave in terms of its wave vector q, i.e., in terms of the wavelength since wavelength $\lambda = 2\pi/q$.   Each wave vector q has a corresponding frequency ω.   If we plot ω versus q, the frequency spectrum as shown in Figure 2-20 is obtained.   This is known as the *dispersion relation*.

The above derivation has been based on an infinitely long chain. However, if the chain is of finite dimension and consists of say $(N + 1)$ atoms, then we need to apply two boundary conditions, i.e.,

$$x_0(t) = 0 \quad \text{and} \quad x_N(t) = 0$$

These boundary conditions specify that atoms at the two ends of the chain remain fixed.   The occurrence of the boundary means that a certain number of interatomic forces are set equal to zero.   This gives rise to so-called "surface modes of vibrations," which we shall not be concerned with.

The application of these boundary conditions shows that the relationship between ω and q is not basically altered from (2-38) but that now q can

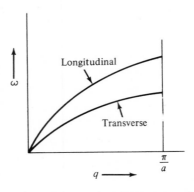

Figure 2-20   Typical dispersion curve for longitudinal and transverse acoustic vibrations.

assume only certain discrete values given by[25]

$$q = \frac{\pi}{Na} j \qquad (2\text{-}39)$$

where $j = 1, 2, \ldots, N - 1$. In the present linear chain model, the atomic movement and the wave propagation occurs in the same direction. Such vibrations are called *longitudinal acoustic*. In a real crystal the atomic motion could be perpendicular to the direction of wave propagation. If the neighboring atoms move in the same direction, but perpendicular to the direction of wave propagation (see Figure 2-19c) the vibrations are called *transverse acoustic*.

2·4·2 optic vibrations

In acoustic vibrations the adjacent atoms move in the same direction. It is also possible to have vibrations in which the adjacent atoms move in opposite directions, as shown in Figure 2-21. These are known as *optic vibrations*[26] for the simple reason that some of these vibrations can be excited by electromagnetic radiation. In analogy to acoustic vibrations, two types of optic vibrations are possible. If the atomic motion and wave propagation occur in the same direction, the vibrations are called *longitudinal optic*. In the *transverse optic* branch* the atomic vibration and wave propagation occur perpendicular to each other.

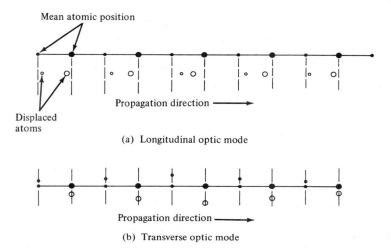

Mean atomic position

Displaced atoms

Propagation direction ⟶

(a) Longitudinal optic mode

Propagation direction ⟶

(b) Transverse optic mode

Figure 2-21 Atomic displacements in longitudinal and transverse optic modes of vibration of a diatomic linear chain and with two degrees of freedom.

* The ω-q dispersion curve for a particular mode of vibrations is also called a *branch*.

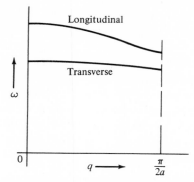

Figure 2-22   Typical dispersion curves for longitudinal and transverse optic vibrations.

Calculations of the dispersion relation for optic modes of vibration proceeds in a manner similar to that given in the previous section. However, if the adjacent atoms are not the same, e.g., as in a NaCl crystal, then due to their different masses, one needs to solve two equations of motion— one for each type of atom. A typical dispersion curve for optic modes of vibrations is shown in Figure 2-22. The interesting feature is that, for optic vibrations, ω does not vary as much with q as in the case of acoustic vibrations. Furthermore, for the acoustic branch, $\omega \to 0$ as $q \to 0$, but this is not the case for the optic branch.

In summary, lattice vibrations of a crystal consist of four distinct types of vibrations: longitudinal acoustic, transverse acoustic, longitudinal optic, and transverse optic. There may be several such branches in a crystal; the exact number depends upon the number of atoms per unit cell and the symmetry of the crystal.

2·4·3 phonons

The theory of lattice modes of vibrations briefly outlined above forms a very important part of the theory of solid-state physics. The thermal energy of a solid is basically the excitation of lattice vibrations. The thermal conductivity, specific heat, and many of the electrical, optical, and mechanical properties of a solid are greatly affected by lattice vibrations. For example, the electrical conductivity of a metal decreases with increasing temperature because of increased scattering from lattice vibrations at high temperatures. In Section 2.2, it was shown that an electromagnetic field has both a particle and wave nature. Particle characteristics of zero mass, energy $h\nu$, and wave vector $\mathbf{k}$ were attributed to photons. Similarly, particles corresponding to lattice modes of vibrations are called *phonons*, which are also assumed to have zero mass. The energy of a phonon is given by hv, where v is the phonon frequency and its momentum is given by $\hbar\mathbf{q}$, where $\mathbf{q}$ is the phonon wave vector. In interaction processes involving photons (electromagnetic field), phonons (lattice vibrations), and electrons, it is always required that the total energy and momentum of the system be conserved. These concepts are used in discussing scattering processes.

2·5   dispersion in solids

The concepts of electromagnetic radiation and the properties of solids outlined in the last few sections will now be applied to illustrate wave propagation in materials and the microscopic aspects of the interaction of radiation with matter. Whenever electromagnetic radiation encounters a boundary surface between two materials of different indices of refraction, reflection occurs; therefore, boundary conditions and expressions relating reflection and refraction (or transmission) phenomena to the indices of refraction will be given. Finally, simple models will be used to show the microscopic origins of the indices of refraction and their frequency dependence.

2·5·1   wave propagation in materials

Maxwell's equations are applicable to electromagnetic wave propagation in materials as well as in free space. The material properties are introduced by suitable choice of ε, μ, and σ which represent permittivity, permeability, and electrical conductivity, respectively.

Each of these parameters could be real or complex. For the present it will be assumed that all are real, which is equivalent to saying that the losses in the medium are essentially due to conduction currents (ohmic). In a linear medium ε, μ, and σ are independent of the field intensities. However, if one or all of these parameters are field dependent, the medium is called nonlinear. For a linear medium, (2-1) and (2-2) give

$$\nabla \times \mathbf{E} = -\mu \frac{\partial \mathbf{H}}{\partial t}$$

and

$$\nabla \times \mathbf{H} = \sigma \mathbf{E} + \varepsilon \frac{\partial \mathbf{E}}{\partial t} \tag{2-40}$$

where $\mathbf{J}$ has been replaced by $\sigma\mathbf{E}$, $\mathbf{D}$ by $\varepsilon\mathbf{E}$ and $\mathbf{B}$ by $\mu\mathbf{H}$. Following a procedure similar to that used for deriving (2-10), we obtain

$$\nabla^2\mathbf{E} = \mu\varepsilon\frac{\partial^2\mathbf{E}}{\partial t^2} + \sigma\mu\frac{\partial\mathbf{E}}{\partial t} \tag{2-41}$$

We are interested in plane-wave type solutions to the above equation. Since the conductivity term introduces ohmic losses, it is expected that the field intensities will reduce as the wave propagates through the medium. For a plane wave polarized in the x direction and propagating in the z direction the electric field is given by

$$E_x = E \exp i[\omega t - (\beta_1 - i\beta_2)z]$$

$$= E \exp(-\beta_2 z) \exp i(\omega t - \beta_1 z) \tag{2-42}$$

The term $(\beta_1 - i\beta_2)$ is called the *complex propagation constant* and will be denoted by γ. The values of β_1 and β_2 in terms of material constants ε μ, and σ can be determined by substituting (2-42) into (2-41). which gives

$$\gamma^2 = (\beta_1 - i\beta_2)^2 = \omega^2\varepsilon\mu - i\omega\sigma\mu \tag{2-43}$$

The above derivation shows that, for a lossy medium, the propagation constant γ is given by a complex number. The other quantities of interest, such as index of refraction, intrinsic impedance, and magnetic field intensity, can be derived by following procedures similar to those outlined in Section 2.1. Therefore, the use of a complex index of refraction will be illustrated and only the final expressions for intrinsic impedance and magnetic field intensity will be given.

The complex index of refraction is defined as

$$n^* = \frac{\text{propagation constant for the material}}{\text{propagation constant for free space}}$$

$$= \frac{\gamma}{k_0} = n - i\kappa \tag{2-44}$$

where n determines the phase velocity of the wave and κ the field attenuation, which is also called the extinction coefficient. The field intensities for a plane wave in terms of complex index of refraction using (2-11) and (2-16) can be written as

$$E_x = E \exp i[\omega t - k_0(n - i\kappa)z] \tag{2-45}$$

and

$$H_y = E\frac{\gamma}{\omega\mu} \exp i[\omega t - k_0(n - i\kappa)z] \tag{2-46}$$

The absorption coefficient α of a material gives the power density attenuation per unit length, and therefore it will be proportional to the attenuation coefficient of E^2.   Thus, from (2-42) and (2-45),

$$\alpha = 2\beta_2 = 2k_0\kappa$$

Since $k_0 = 2\pi/\lambda_0$ (see 2-13), where λ_0 is the free space wavelength

$$\alpha = \frac{4\pi\kappa}{\lambda_0} \qquad (2\text{-}47)$$

Figure 2-23 shows power density associated with a plane wave propagating in a lossy medium.   Absorption W per unit area in a length z of the material is equal to that lost by the propagating wave, which from Figure 2-23 is given by

$$W = I_0[1 - \exp(-\alpha z)] \qquad (2\text{-}48)$$

where I_0 is the power density at $z = 0$.   The length within which the power density drops down to $1/e$ of its initial value is called the *depth of penetration* δ.

From (2-48) and Figure 2-23, we obtain

$$\delta = \frac{\lambda_0}{4\pi\kappa} \qquad (2\text{-}49)$$

For most metals at optical and infrared frequencies, the depth of penetration is of the order of few tens or hundreds of nanometers.

In the above derivations, the losses of the medium were introduced through the conductivity term.   However, the loss term can also be introduced by suitable choice of permittivity or permeability.   For example, in the neighborhood of an optic mode frequency, the losses occur due to damping of resonant modes excited by the incident radiation.   In this case, the permittivity is given by a complex number.

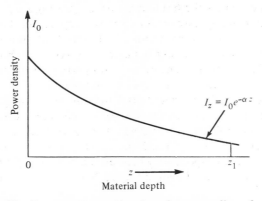

Figure 2-23   Power attenuation in a lossy medium for a plane wave propagating in the z direction.

Absorption in a lossy dielectric probably is one reason why the CO_2 laser ($\lambda = 10.6 \times 10^3$nm) has been so effectively used in hole drilling and scribing on ceramics. Therefore, the use of complex permittivity in Maxwell's equations is illustrated. Let

$$\varepsilon = \varepsilon_1 - i\varepsilon_2 \qquad (2\text{-}50)$$

where ε_2, the imaginary part of the dielectric constant, represents the loss term. Substituting $\sigma = 0$ and $\varepsilon = \varepsilon_1 - i\varepsilon_2$ in (2-40), and following a procedure similar to that used in obtaining relations (2-43), we obtain

$$(\beta_1 - i\beta_2)^2 = \omega^2\mu(\varepsilon_1 - i\varepsilon_2) \qquad (2\text{-}51)$$

The difference between the loss term introduced through finite conductivity of the medium and complex permittivity is important. The conductivity term introduces losses due to absorption of radiation by conduction electrons and their subsequent scattering by phonons, ionized impurities, grain boundaries, etc. The absorption, therefore, is spread out over a very broad frequency range. Losses due to complex permittivity arise due to excitation of lattice vibrations and their subsequent damping by crystal imperfections, etc. For example, it has been observed that NaCl crystals crack[27] at [100] planes under intense radiation, which has been attributed to stimulated Brillouin scattering. The absorption in dielectrics therefore may be very high in narrow frequency ranges.

2·5·2   *boundary conditions*

Whenever an electromagnetic wave encounters a boundary separating two media whose optical properties are different, a fraction of the incident energy is reflected and the remaining energy is transmitted across the boundary. Since across the boundary surface (see Figure 2-24) the parameters ε, μ, and σ change discontinuously, we may expect the field vectors to exhibit corresponding discontinuities. Figure 2-24 shows two homogeneous, isotropic media having a plane S as common boundary, and otherwise infinite in extent. The material properties for the two media are specified by ε_1, μ_1, σ_1, and ε_2, μ_2, and σ_2, respectively. A plane wave is incident at the boundary, where its direction of propagation makes an angle θ_i with the normal to the surface. The angles which the propagation direction of reflected and transmitted waves make with the surface normal are given by $\theta_r(\theta_r = \theta_i)$ and θ_t. Field vectors in the two media can be resolved into components which are parallel and perpendicular to the plane of incidence,* as shown in Figure 2-24. Boundary conditions,[28]

---

* The plane containing the electromagnetic wave propagation direction vector and normal to the surface *s* is called the *plane of incidence*.

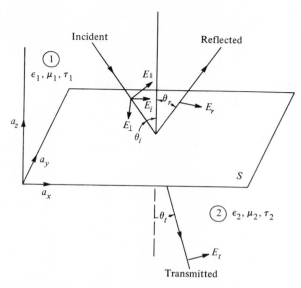

Figure 2-24   Reflection from an interface.   Parallel and perpendicular components of E_i are shown.   Similarly, E_r and E_t can be decomposed into parallel and perpendicular components.

which the field vectors must satisfy, can be derived from Maxwell's equations and are

$$E_{1t} = E_{2t} = 0 \qquad (2\text{-}52)$$

$$H_{1t} - H_{2t} = J_s \qquad (2\text{-}53)$$

$$B_{1n} - B_{2n} = 0 \qquad (2\text{-}54)$$

$$D_{1n} - D_{2n} = \rho_s \qquad (2\text{-}55)$$

where the subscripts 1 and 2 stand for the medium and t and n for the tangential and normal components; J_s and ρ_s are the surface current density and externally introduced surface charge density, respectively.

True surface current density J_s is present only in material for which the electrical conductivity σ is infinite.   Since the conductivity for most materials of interest is finite, J_s in (2-53) will be taken as zero.

Conditions (2-52) and (2-54) state that the tangential components of the electric field and the normal component of the magnetic flux density should be continuous across the boundary.   On the other hand, the normal component of the electric flux density and the tangential component of the magnetic field could vary discontinuously across the boundary. Applications of these conditions to the general case illustrated in Figure

2-24 involve rather complex mathematical expressions, and the results obtained are known as Fresnel equations (see Section 6.1). Therefore, only the special case when the incident reflected and transmitted waves propagate perpendicular to the surface will be considered.

2·5·3   reflection and transmission

The case of normal incidence is shown in Figure 2-25. Let the subscripts i, r, and t represent the incident, reflected, and transmitted waves and γ_1, γ_2 the propagation constants of the media 1 and 2, respectively. The propagation constants γ_1 and γ_2 may be real or complex and are in general given by (2-43). Electric fields in the two media are then given by

$$E_1 = E_i \exp i(\omega t - \gamma_1 z) + E_r \exp i(\omega t + \gamma_1 z) \qquad (2\text{-}56)$$

and $E_2 = E_t \exp i(\omega t - \gamma_2 z)$. The corresponding magnetic fields are obtained using the relation (2-51) which gives

$$H_1 = \frac{\gamma_1}{\omega\mu_1} E_i \exp i(\omega t - \gamma_1 z) - \frac{\gamma_1}{\omega\mu_1} E_r \exp i(\omega t - \gamma_1 z) \qquad (2\text{-}57)$$

and

$$H_2 = \frac{\gamma_2}{\omega\mu_2} E_t \exp i(\omega t - \gamma_2 z)$$

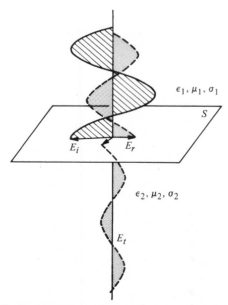

Figure 2-25   Reflection and transmission at normal incidence.   Note: The case shown assumes $\sigma_1 = 0$ and $\sigma_2 \neq 0$.

For most materials of interest, $\mu_1 = \mu_2 \simeq \mu_0$ and $J_s = 0$. Therefore, the application of boundary conditions (2-52) and (2-53) at the surface S ($z = 0$) gives

$$E_i + E_r = E_t$$

and

$$\frac{\gamma_1}{\omega\mu_0} E_i - \frac{\gamma_1}{\omega\mu_0} E_r = \frac{\gamma_2}{\omega\mu_0} E_t \tag{2-58}$$

From the above two equations we obtain

$$\frac{E_r}{E_i} = r = \text{amplitude reflection coefficient}$$

$$= \frac{\gamma_1 - \gamma_2}{\gamma_1 + \gamma_2}$$

In terms of index of refraction, $\gamma_1 = k_0(n_1 - i\kappa_1)$ and $\gamma_2 = k_0(n_2 - i\kappa_2)$,

$$\frac{E_r}{E_i} = r = \frac{(n_1 - n_2) - i(\kappa_1 - \kappa_2)}{(n_1 + n_2) - i(\kappa_1 + \kappa_2)} \tag{2-59}$$

The power reflection coefficient R is given by

$$R = \left|\frac{E_r}{E_i}\right|^2 = \frac{(n_1 - n_2)^2 + (\kappa_1 - \kappa_2)^2}{(n_1 + n_2)^2 + (\kappa_1 + \kappa_2)^2}$$

In most laser applications, medium 1 is normal atmosphere, hence $n_1 \simeq 1$ and $\kappa_1 = 0$, which gives

$$R = \frac{(1 - n_2)^2 + \kappa_2^2}{(1 + n_2)^2 + \kappa_2^2} \tag{2-60}$$

The power transmission coefficient (T) in the material can be obtained from

$$T = 1 - R = \frac{4n_2}{(1 + n_2)^2 + \kappa_2^2} \tag{2-61}$$

2.5.4   dispersion and absorption in dielectrics

Now consider the microscopic aspects of electromagnetic wave propagation through dielectric solids. In the previous section it was assumed that material properties, such as conductivity, permeability, and permittivity, were known. In this section a simple model will be used to illustrate the frequency dependence of permittivity, i.e., the dielectric constant. Equation 2-15 (Section 2.1.1) shows that the dielectric constant determines the index of refraction provided $\mu \simeq \mu_0$. (For a dielectric material,

$\sigma = 0$.) For most common materials, $\mu \simeq \mu_0$ and remains practically constant; therefore, the optical properties are essentially dependent upon their dielectric behavior.

Application of electric fields to any material causes either the displacement of the electronic cloud bound to an atom or ion, or the displacement of ions, or both. If the applied electric field is oscillating at a frequency ω, the electronic and ionic displacements will also oscillate at a frequency ω, unless the frequency is so high that the electrons and/or ions cannot follow such rapid oscillations. The displacement of ions and bound electrons from their equilibrium position develops polarization P. However, such oscillations also experience damping due to interaction with adjacent ions or due to lattice vibrations, as discussed in Section 2.4. The damping or the loss term, as will be shown below, causes P and ε to assume complex values.

The simplest model (Drude-Lorentz)[29] which shows the microscopic aspects of the frequency dependence of the dielectric constant assumes the electronic cloud bound to the nucleus through a spring. A similar model can be used to account for binding between two adjacent atoms or ions. In such a model, Figure 2-26, the equation of motion for a bound charge is given by

$$m\frac{d^2x}{dt^2} + \eta\frac{dx}{dt} + fx = eE\exp(i\omega t) \qquad (2\text{-}62)$$

where x = displacement of electron cloud,
       m = mass of the electron,
       η = damping constant,
       e = charge of an electron,
       E = electric field intensity of the incident radiation,
       ω = frequency of the incident radiation.

The steady-state solution of (2-62) is

$$x = \frac{eE}{m}\frac{1}{\omega_0^2 - \omega^2 + i\Gamma\omega}\exp(i\omega t) \qquad (2\text{-}63)$$

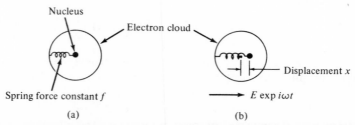

Figure 2-26   Model used to calculate dispersion in dielectrics. Damped oscillations are excited in response to the electric field of the incident radiation.

where $\omega_0^2 = f/m$, the natural frequency of oscillation and $\Gamma = \eta/m$, the scattering or damping frequency. The polarizability per unit volume is defined by

$$\zeta = \frac{Nex}{E}$$

where x is the complex amplitude of the displacement, and N is the number of charged particles per unit volume. The polarization P is given by

$$P = \zeta E$$

In general, the electric flux density D and the electric field intensity E are related by

$$D = \varepsilon E = \varepsilon_0 E + P$$

therefore,

$$\varepsilon = \varepsilon_0 + \frac{P}{E} = \varepsilon_0 + \zeta \tag{2-64}$$

Since $P = \zeta E$, from (2-63) and (2-64), note that, for a lossy dielectric, P will be complex and, hence, the permittivity ε will also be complex. Therefore, the complex index of refraction (see 2-19) and dielectric constant are given by

$$\varepsilon_r = \frac{\varepsilon}{\varepsilon_0} = 1 + \frac{P}{\varepsilon_0 E} = (n - i\kappa)^2 \tag{2-65}$$

Substituting the value of P and using relations (2-63) and (2-64)

$$\varepsilon_r = (n - ik)^2 = 1 + \frac{Ne^2}{\varepsilon_0 m} \frac{1}{\omega_0^2 - \omega^2 + i\Gamma\omega} \tag{2-66}$$

For bound electrons, the resonant frequency ω_0 generally lies in the ultraviolet region. An estimate of this frequency can be made from a knowledge of the static ($\omega = 0$) dielectric constant of a gas. For most gases at atmospheric pressure, the static dielectric constant is close to unity, $(1 + 250 \times 10^{-6})$. Therefore, from (2-66)

$$n^2 = \varepsilon_r = 1 + \frac{Ne^2}{\varepsilon_0 m} \frac{1}{\omega_0^2} \tag{2-66a}$$

Substituting the value of N (about 10^{24} atoms/m^3) and other constants,

$$\omega_0 \simeq 6 \times 10^{15} \text{ rad/s}$$

Thus, for bound electrons the resonant frequency is much higher than optical frequencies ($\omega \simeq 6 \times 10^{14}$ rad/s). Therefore, the index of refraction for most gases at optical and lower frequencies is close to unity.

Equation (2-63) and subsequent derivations are equally valid for ionic motion as well, provided proper mass and electronic charge values are used. Since ionic mass is three orders of magnitude higher than the electronic mass, the resonant frequency ω_0 for ionic oscillations is much lower and falls in the far-infrared region. It is for this reason that, at optical frequencies, the ionic contribution to the dielectric constant is small, whereas at infrared and lower frequencies it is quite important.

The derivation of (2-66) has assumed that there is only one kind of oscillator. However, atomic systems are complex and have more than one resonant frequency, depending upon the configuration of their electronic cloud. To take this into account (2-66) can be modified by replacing ω_0 by ω_j and summing on all the different resonant frequencies, corresponding to both electronic and ionic oscillations. With these modifications, (2-66) becomes

$$(n - i\kappa)^2 = 1 + \sum_j \frac{N_j e^2 f_j}{\varepsilon_0 m_j} \frac{1}{\omega_j^2 - \omega^2 + i\Gamma_j \omega} \tag{2-67}$$

where the subscript j stands for the jth oscillator (electron or ion) and f_j for the oscillator strength.

Finally, in the case of a solid, the local field correction (also known as Lorentz-Lorenz[30] correction) modifies the resonant frequency ω_0 as given by

$$\omega_j^2 = \omega_{0j}^2 - \frac{e^2}{3m} \frac{N_j}{\varepsilon_0}$$

This correction arises due to the fact that the electric field at the ionic site is, in general, different from the applied field due to polarization fields produced by other charges. It is apparent that this modification shifts the resonant frequency toward lower values.

Figure 2-27 shows the reflectivity and optical constants of quartz[31] in the wavelength region of 5×10^3 to 35×10^3 nm. It is interesting to note that at the frequencies where the extinction coefficient is high (large κ), the reflectivity is also high, as can be seen from relation (2-56).

To see the effect of resonant frequency on the optical constants, consider the simple case of a single oscillator with no damping ($\Gamma = 0$) for which (2-66) applies. In this case the square of the index of refraction is given by

$$n^2 = 1 + \frac{Ne^2}{\varepsilon_0 m} \frac{1}{\omega_0^2 - \omega^2} \tag{2-68}$$

The frequency dependence of n^2 based on (2-68) is shown in Figure 2-28a; $n^2 \simeq 1$ for $\omega \ll \omega_0$ or $\omega \gg \omega_0$. However, when $\omega \sim \omega_0$, n^2 is very large and either positive or negative. In this region, (2-56) shows that the material will be highly reflecting.

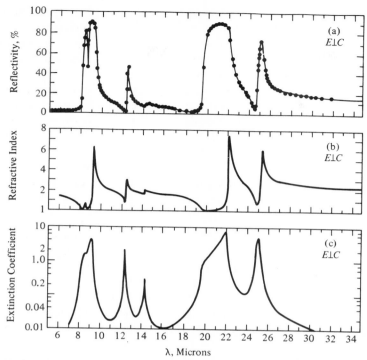

Figure 2-27   Reflectivity, refractive index, and extinction coefficient of quartz for the ordinary way.   (a) Theoretical curve for reflectivity (solid trace) is adjusted by variation of dispersion parameters until satisfactory fit with measured values (points) is obtained; (b) and (c) traces for n and κ, respectively, as computed from the adjusted dispersion parameters. Four major and several minor resonances are seen to coincide in the three curves.   (Data are taken from the work of W. G. Spitzer and D. A. Kleinmann, Phys. Rev. 121, 1324 (1961).)   (Published with permission of Academic Press, Inc.)

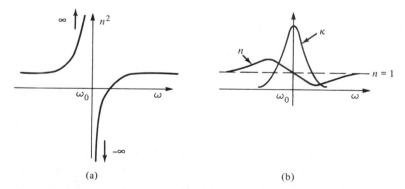

Figure 2-28   (a) n^2 as a function of incident radiation frequency for a lossless oscillator model.   (b) Extinction coefficient κ and index of refraction n as a function of frequency for a simple oscillator model.

Next, consider the effect of restoring the damping term $i\Gamma\omega$. For values of ω far away from ω_0, it can be shown that the extinction coefficient $\kappa \to 0$ and $n \to 1$. However, for values of $\omega \simeq \omega_0$, the extinction coefficient assumes high values. Physically this is expected, because a large extinction coefficient implies large damping losses, which can occur only if the oscillations are strong. It is well known that strong oscillations can be excited near a resonance frequency. This is also evident in Figure 2-27, in which regions of high reflectivity and κ correspond to resonant frequencies.

2·5·5   dispersion and absorption due to free electrons

In dielectrics, the interaction takes place with bound charges. However, in metals and heavily doped semiconductors strong interaction will occur with free electrons. The free electrons can be treated as contributing either to conductivity or to a dielectric constant. For handling optical properties it is more natural to treat them as if they contributed to a dielectric constant. Under applied electromagnetic fields, the equations of motion for free electrons are exactly the same as those for the bound electrons discussed in the previous section, except that the spring constant f in this case is zero. However, the oscillating electrons will experience scattering due to electron–electron collision, collisions with phonons, ionized impurities, and crystal defects. Thus, there will be a damping constant involved which may be vastly different from that obtained through static conductivity measurements. From (2-63), we obtain the free electron displacement by substituting $\omega_0 = 0$:

$$x = \frac{eE}{\varepsilon_0 m} \frac{1}{-\omega^2 + i\Gamma\omega}$$

If the crystal contains N free electrons per unit volume, the polarization due to free electrons is given by

$$Nex = \frac{Ne^2 E}{\varepsilon_0 m} \frac{1}{-\omega^2 + i\Gamma\omega}$$

The complex permittivity, due to free electrons and the lattice, is given by

$$\varepsilon_r = \varepsilon_\infty + \frac{Ne^2}{\varepsilon_0 m} \frac{1}{-\omega^2 + i\Gamma\omega} \tag{2-69}$$

where ε_∞ is the contribution from bound electrons discussed in the previous section. Experimentally, it has been found that for most metals the above expressions have to be modified.[33,34] These modifications generally involve change in the number of free electrons (N), the effective electron mass (m), and/or additional terms involving more than one damping frequency (Γ). The term $\sqrt{Ne^2/\varepsilon_0 m}$ has the units of s^{-1} and is defined as the plasma frequency of the free electrons. In the absence of damping, reflectivity is minimum[35] at the plasma frequency and occurs due to collective motion of free electrons. For most metals the plasma frequency generally lies in the ultraviolet region.

The index of refraction (assuming $\mu = \mu_0$) is given by

$$(n - i\kappa)^2 = \varepsilon_\infty + \frac{Ne^2}{\varepsilon_0 m} \frac{1}{-\omega^2 + i\Gamma\omega}$$

Equating the real and imaginary parts gives

$$n^2 - \kappa^2 = \varepsilon_\infty + \frac{Ne^2}{\varepsilon_0 m} \frac{1}{\omega^2 + \Gamma^2} \tag{2-70}$$

and

$$2n\kappa = \frac{\Gamma}{\omega} \frac{Ne^2}{\varepsilon_0 m} \frac{1}{\omega^2 + \Gamma^2} \tag{2-71}$$

Table 2-7 gives the reflectivity and the indices of refraction for several metals calculated from experimental data of thin film reflectance.

TABLE 2-7 Optical Indices and Reflectivity of Some Metals[32]

Element	$\lambda_0 \times 10^3$ nm	n	κ	R
Al	0.3	0.25	3.33	92.1
	0.546	0.82	5.99	91.6
	0.7	1.55	7.00	88.8
	0.95	1.75	8.5	91.2
	10.0	26.0	67.3	98.0
Ag	0.302	1.2	0.8	12.4
	0.55	0.055	3.32	98.2
	0.70	0.075	4.62	98.7
	1.0	0.129	6.83	98.9
	10.0	10.69	69.0	99.1
Au	0.2	1.24	0.92	15.4
	0.55	0.331	2.324	81.5
	0.7	0.131	3.842	96.7
	1.0	0.179	6.04	98.1
	9.9	25.2	55.9	97.4
Cu	0.45	0.87	2.2	58.3
	0.55	0.756	2.462	66.9
	0.70	0.15	4.049	96.6
	1.0	0.197	6.272	98.1
	10.8	12.6	64.3	98.8

In thermal processing of materials, such as welding, drilling, and scribing of metals, it is believed that such processes work better with short wavelength lasers, such as YAG ($\lambda = 1060$ nm) or ruby ($\lambda = 694.3$ nm), than with the CO_2 ($\lambda = 10,600$ nm). From (2-70) and (2-71), we can easily see why this is the case. In metals, the free electron density (N) is about 10^{28}/m³, and the scattering frequency (Γ) is about 10^{16} s⁻¹. Substituting these in (2-70) and (2-71), with values of e, m, and ε, $n^2 - \kappa^2$ comes out to be about -10 at 1060 nm and -1000 at 10,600 nm. Thus at all of the above wavelengths n is less than κ. Moreover, the values of n and κ at 694.3 nm and 1060 nm are smaller than their values at 10,600 nm. Therefore the reflection losses at the CO_2 wavelength are higher as compared to those at YAG and ruby wavelengths (see Table 2-7).

The reflectance values given in Table 2-7 were measured at room temperature. However, in thermal processing with lasers, the power intensity used is so high that, during a very short initial portion of the laser pulse, the surface temperature of the material under process rises rather rapidly. This increase in temperature reduces the scattering time τ, and, since the scattering frequency $\Gamma = 2\pi/\tau$, Γ increases with temperature. Once again (2-70) and (2-71) show that the values of both n and κ decrease as Γ increases. This in turn implies that the reflection losses decrease with increasing temperature.

Thus for metals, short wavelength lasers are more efficient for welding and drilling. However, even for CO_2 laser the reflection losses are reduced at high temperatures, and because of their high overall efficiency (14 percent for CO_2 as compared to <2 percent for YAG and ruby), the CO_2 lasers are increasingly used in thermal processing applications.

2·5·6 optical properties of semiconductors

The band gap in semiconductors is generally of the order of 1 eV, and their conductivity can be controlled by proper doping. This small band gap, as compared to that for insulators, means that intrinsic absorption due to band-to-band transitions occurs primarily in the visible and infrared regions. This absorption could be thought of as due to an internal photoelectric effect,[37] in which absorption of a photon causes electrons from the valence band to be excited to the conduction band as shown in Figure 2-29. For doped semiconductors, the conduction electrons (or holes in the valence band) behave as free charge carriers and give rise to absorption of the type discussed in the previous section. Therefore, the optical properties of semiconductors in the infrared region depend largely upon doping. In general, the extinction coefficient increases with wavelength as λ^p, where p depends upon the band structure.[38,39] The absorption coefficient as a function of wavelength for a semiconductor is depicted in Figure 2-30.

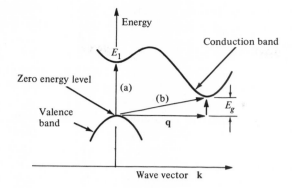

Figure 2-29 Direct and indirect band-to-band transition in semiconductors.

(a) Electrons from valence band are excited to conduction band by direct absorption of a photon of energy $\geq E_1$.

(b) Phonon assisted indirect band-to-band transition with photons of energy $\simeq E_g$; q is the phonon wave vector required for momentum conservation.

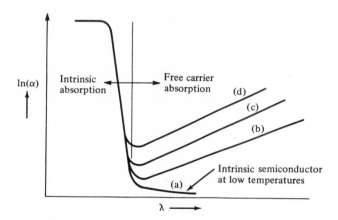

Figure 2-30 Absorption in semiconductors as a function of doping and wavelength.

(a) Intrinsic at low temperatures with no thermally excited carriers.
(b), (c), (d) Doped semiconductor. (b) has lowest doping.

2·6 nonlinear interactions

In Section 2.5.1 it was pointed out that if permittivity (ε) or conductivity (σ) depend upon the intensity of incident fields, the medium is called *nonlinear*. While propagating through such a medium, a fraction of the incident radiation experiences frequency shifts.   Three such processes are known as Raman scattering, Brillouin scattering, and second harmonic generation.

2·6·1   Raman scattering

Scattering of electromagnetic radiation due to excitations in matter which give rise to a frequency shift of the incident radiation is called Raman scattering.   The term excitations is used in a broad sense and includes such phenomena as molecular vibrations, lattice vibrations in solids, electron plasma oscillations, etc.   Scattering generally implies collisions of two or more particles in which energy and momentum are exchanged between the interacting particles.   The frequency shift of the incident radiation corresponds to energy exchange, and the direction of the scattered radiation is determined by momentum exchange.   The quantum mechanical description of Raman scattering is rather simple.   For a quantum mechanical discussion of the conservation of energy, consider the energy diagram of Figure 2-31 which represents the energy levels of a molecule and a photon. In Figure 2-31a the molecule is unexcited initially.   An incident photon of frequency v_1 is absorbed, while *simultaneously* a photon at frequency $v_3 = v_1 - v_2$ is emitted.   To conserve energy, the molecule is excited to the vibrational level of energy hv_2.   It is important to note that absorption and emission of photons occurs simultaneously and the excited vibration, hv_2, corresponds to one of the modes of molecular vibrations.   If the molecule is initially at the energy level hv_2, then the simultaneous absorp-

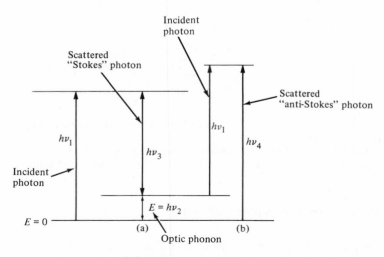

Figure 2-31   Energy conservation diagram for "Stokes" and "anti-Stokes" Raman scattering.

tion and emission of photons give out scattered radiation at the frequency v_4, as shown in Figure 2-31b. In this case energy conservation requires $v_4 = v_2 + v_1$. It is apparent that in the first process molecular vibrations at frequency v_2 were created, whereas in the second process such vibrations were annihilated. When, as in the first process, the scattering causes a downward shift in frequency, the emitted photon is called a *Stokes photon*. In the second case, scattering causes an upward shift in the frequency and this photon is called an *anti-Stokes* photon.

So far we have considered only the conservation of energy. Momentum conservation in Raman scattering gives the direction of the scattered photon. From (2-27), the momentum of a photon or phonon is given by $\mathbf{p} = \hbar \mathbf{k}$ where $\mathbf{k}$ is the wave vector in the direction of propagation. For a Stokes line we therefore obtain

$$\hbar \mathbf{k}_1 = \hbar \mathbf{k}_3 + \hbar \mathbf{q}_2$$

or

$$\mathbf{k}_1 = \mathbf{k}_3 + \mathbf{q}_2 \qquad (2\text{-}72)$$

Similarly, for the anti-Stokes scattering

$$\mathbf{k}_4 = \mathbf{k}_1 + \mathbf{q}_2$$

where $\mathbf{k}$ and $\mathbf{q}$ are the wave vectors for photons and phonons, respectively, and the subscripts correspond to the frequency of the incident and scattered photons. In general, $k_1 \simeq k_3 \simeq k_4$; therefore, q is comparable in value to k. Since k is small, this means that scattering generally occurs only from long wavelength phonons ($\lambda = 2\pi/q$). Furthermore, the frequency shift is a direct measure of the vibrational or rotational frequency of the molecule; these frequencies typically lie in the infrared to far-infrared regions; as a result, the wavelength of the scattered radiation is shifted from that of the incident radiation by about 10 nm.

An important fact to note is that the frequency or the wavelength shift due to Raman scattering is independent of the frequency of the incident radiation and depends only on the frequency of the phonon. Thus, one could work with lasers operating in the visible region of the spectrum (provided the material is transparent to the laser radiation), where low-noise, highly sensitive detectors are readily available.

Since the frequency shifts are characteristics of the molecule or crystal, Raman scattering is an important tool for studying the material properties, and the method is known as Raman spectroscopy. In practice, it is finding increasing applications in material characterization and in air pollution studies. Such applications are discussed in Chapter 6.

The above discussion does not explicitly elucidate the basic features of the interaction phenomenon which gives rise to Raman scattering. In Section 2.5.4 on the optical properties of a material, it was pointed out that the dielectric constant or the index of refraction is mainly a function of electronic and ionic polarizabilities. It turns out that the electronic and ionic polarizabilities in some cases are a function of nuclear position. This means that as the ions vibrate around their mean position, the electronic and ionic polarizabilities also continuously oscillate around a mean value. Mathematically this is expressed by stating that the polarizability ζ is given by

$$\zeta = \zeta(y)$$

where y is the interionic distance.

In general, for small nuclear displacements, $\zeta(y)$ can be expanded in a Taylor series. Retaining only the first two terms, we obtain

$$\zeta = \zeta_0 + y\left(\frac{\partial \zeta}{\partial y}\right)\bigg|_{y=0} = \zeta_0 + Ry$$

where $y = 0$ is the mean nuclear position, and R is called the differential polarizability $\partial\zeta/\partial y$. If there are N ions per unit volume, the permittivity ε is given by

$$\varepsilon = \varepsilon_0 + \zeta = \varepsilon_0 + N\zeta_0 + NRy \tag{2-73}$$

It can be shown[40] that only those optic vibrations for which the differential polarizability is nonzero give Raman scattering. The effect of differential polarizability on the incident radiation can be seen by using (2-73) to calculate the electric flux density.[41] Let ω_2 denote the molecular vibration frequency. Then the molecular position y can be written as

$$y(t) = y \cos \omega_2 t$$

Therefore, from (2-73) and (2-5),

$$D = \varepsilon E = \zeta_0 (E \cos \omega_1 t)(\varepsilon_0 + N\zeta_0 + NRy \cos \omega_2 t)$$

$$= \zeta_0 (\varepsilon_0 + N\zeta_0) E \cos \omega_1 t$$

$$+ \tfrac{1}{2}\zeta_0 NRyE[\cos(\omega_1 - \omega_2)t + \cos(\omega_1 + \omega_2)t] \tag{2-74}$$

In the above $(\omega_1 - \omega_2)$ is the Stokes photon frequency and $(\omega_1 + \omega_2)$ is the anti-Stokes photon frequency. This derivation shows that the scattered radiation consists of both Stokes and anti-Stokes photons of equal intensity, which is not correct. The reason is that it is a purely classical derivation and does not take into account the fact that for anti-Stokes photons it is necessary that, even in the absence of incident radiation, the molecule be oscillating at the frequency ω_2. At normal temperatures the probability that such vibrations exist is considerably small; therefore, the intensity of anti-Stokes frequency component is much less than the Stokes component. The intensity of the Stokes component is about 10^{-6} of the incident radiation intensity. Therefore, in Raman spectroscopy it is desirable to use an intense monochromatic source of radiation, and lasers meet these requirements.

2·6·2 *Brillouin scattering*

Scattering of electromagnetic radiation from acoustic modes is known as Brillouin scattering. In describing it, a simple classical model will be presented which will show the mechanism responsible for Brillouin scattering.

Acoustic waves could be thought of as elastic waves traveling through a crystal. The material has regions in which atoms come closer to each other corresponding to compression where the material density increases; and in the dilated volume it decreases. Note from (2-66) that the dielectric constant depends on the volume density, N. In the regions where the acoustic wave increases the volume density, ε will increase and vice versa in the regions where the density is reduced. From this point of view, consider a fixed distribution of high and low dielectric constant regions as shown in Figure 2-32. Assuming no change in permeability μ, the index of refraction can be obtained from

$$n = \varepsilon^{1/2}$$

Let n_1 and n_2 be the index of refraction of the two regions, and $\Delta\varepsilon$ change in the dielectric constant due to the density variations, as shown in Figure 2-32

$$n_1 = (\varepsilon - \Delta\varepsilon)^{1/2} \simeq \sqrt{\varepsilon}\left(1 - \frac{1}{2}\frac{\Delta\varepsilon}{\varepsilon}\right) \qquad \text{for} \quad \Delta\varepsilon \ll \varepsilon$$

and

$$n_2 = (\varepsilon + \Delta\varepsilon)^{1/2} \simeq \sqrt{\varepsilon}\left(1 + \frac{1}{2}\frac{\Delta\varepsilon}{\varepsilon}\right)$$

Electromagnetic radiation incident perpendicular to such regions will

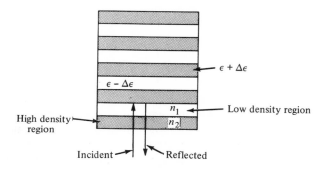

Figure 2-32 Incident and reflected radiation from regions of high and low density set up by an acoustic wave.

be weakly reflected from each interface, the reflectivity of each interface being (see 2-59)

$$R = \left(\frac{n_1 - n_2}{n_1 + n_2}\right)^2 = \left(\frac{\Delta\varepsilon}{2\varepsilon}\right)^2$$

The density variation, therefore, gives weak reflection from the interface. So far it has been assumed that such regions are stationary and have a fixed dielectric constant.   Both of these assumptions are not true for a traveling acoustic wave.   First, if the interface were moving in the same direction as the incident radiation, then the frequency of the reflected radiation would shift due to the Doppler effect (see Section 6.2.3).   The following discussion shows this frequency shift by assuming a traveling density wave in which the dielectric constant varies with density.

The density variation due to a traveling acoustic wave can be written as

$$\rho = \rho_0 + \Delta\rho \cos(\omega_s t - q_s z)$$

where ρ_0 = average material density,
ω_s = acoustic (or density) wave frequency,
q_s = acoustic wave vector magnitude.

Assuming permittivity to be a linear function of density gives

$$\varepsilon = A[\rho_0 + \Delta\rho \cos(\omega_s t - q_s z)] \qquad (2\text{-}75)$$

where A is a proportionality constant relating permittivity to the material density.   The electric flux density D for incident radiation of frequency ω_1 and propagation constant k_1 is, therefore,

$$D = \varepsilon E_1 \cos(\omega_1 t - k_1 z)$$

$$= A[\rho_0 + \Delta\rho \cos(\omega_s t - q_s z)]E_1 \cos(\omega_1 t - k_1 z)$$

Following a procedure similar to that in deriving (2-74), we obtain

$$D = A\rho_0 E_1 \cos(\omega_1 t - k_1 z) + \frac{E_1}{2} A \Delta\rho \cos[(\omega_1 - \omega_s)t - (k_1 - q_s)z]$$

$$+ \frac{E_1}{2} A \Delta\rho \cos[(\omega_1 + \omega_s)t - (k_1 + q_s)z] \quad (2\text{-}76)$$

Note that due to a traveling acoustic wave the scattered radiation consists of frequencies equal to $(\omega_1 - \omega_s)$ and $(\omega_1 + \omega_s)$.   The intensity of the Brillouin scattered radiation is about 10^{-6} of the incident radiation. Furthermore, the acoustic mode frequencies (about 10^{10} Hz) are much smaller than the optic mode frequencies (about 10^{12} Hz); therefore, the frequency and wavelength shifts (about 10^{-2} to 10^{-3} nm) involved in Brillouin scattering are small compared to those in Raman scattering.

The above model and calculations are used only to illustrate the mechanism of Brillouin scattering.   To be completely correct, one should couple the acoustic wave solution into Maxwell's equations, the mathematics of which soon become unwieldy.[42,43]   Another important assumption has been that the acoustic wave and incident radiation propagate in the same direction.   Since the scattered Stokes photon ($\omega = \omega_1 - \omega_s$) is traveling in the opposite direction, and its wave vector is approximately the same as k_1, momentum conservation requires that

$$k_1 - q_s = -k_1$$

$$q_s = 2k_1$$

or

$$\lambda_s = \tfrac{1}{2}\lambda_1$$

This, therefore, is a very special case in which the photon and phonon wave vectors are collinear.   If they are not collinear, the scattered radiation shows angular dependence, which is discussed in Section 6.2.4.

Quantum mechanically, scattering from acoustic modes can be considered in the same manner as Raman scattering.   However, Raman scattering arises from nonzero differential polarizability, whereas Brillouin scattering arises from density variation caused by the acoustic vibrations. Since density variations are associated with every acoustic mode, all acoustic modes are "Brillouin active," but not all optic modes are Raman active.

2·6·3   second harmonic generation

In this section the effect of large electric fields on the electronic polarizability shall be discussed.   In particular, it will be shown that the electric field dependence of the electronic polarizability can be used to generate radiation at a frequency twice that of the incident radiation.[44]   This is known as second harmonic generation.

Electric flux density and induced polarization are related by

$$D = \varepsilon_0 E + P$$

in which P itself is a function of the applied electric field since the displacement (see 2-63) and polarizability are field dependent.   In general, when the applied field is weak, P and E are linearly related.   Therefore,

$$D = \varepsilon_0 E + P = \varepsilon_0 E + \eta_1 E$$

and

$$\varepsilon = \varepsilon_0 \left(1 + \frac{\eta_1}{\varepsilon_0}\right) \tag{2-77}$$

where η_1 is known as dielectric susceptibility, and ε is independent of E. Under high fields, P and E do not follow the linear relationship given above, and exhibit P versus E characteristic as shown in Figure 2-33b. It is apparent that the induced polarization P follows E linearly up to E_A, and for $E > E_A$ it shows saturation or nonlinear effects.

In general, then P can be described by

$$P = \eta_1 E + \eta_2 E^2 + \eta_3 E^3 \cdots \tag{2-78}$$

where coefficients η_1, η_2, etc., can assume positive or negative values.

Substituting the above in (2-5a)

$$D = \varepsilon_0 E\left(1 + \frac{\eta_1}{\varepsilon_0} + \frac{\eta_2}{\varepsilon_0} E + \frac{\eta_3}{\varepsilon_0} E^2 + \cdots\right) \tag{2-79}$$

If the applied electric field is reversed (in the absence of nonlinear effect, i.e., $\eta_2 = \eta_3 = \cdots 0$), D also changes sign and its magnitude remains the same. However, this is not generally the case with nonlinear materials, as can be seen from (2-79), if E is replaced by $-E$

$$D_- = -\varepsilon_0 E\left(1 + \frac{\eta_1}{\varepsilon_0}\right) + \frac{\eta_2}{\varepsilon_0} E^2 - \frac{\eta_3}{\varepsilon_0} E^3 + \cdots$$

D_- is the electric flux density for negative values of E. Thus, unless $\eta_2 = \eta_4 = \eta_6$ are all zero, the P versus E curve will be as shown in Figure 2-33b. For crystal structures such that the unit cell has a center of symmetry, P reverses sign with E. This means that for such materials the coefficients of even-order terms (in 2-78) are all zero. However, if the crystal structure does not possess a center of symmetry,[45] then η_2, η_4, etc., are generally nonzero. Crystals of this type can be used for second harmonic generation.

Consider an x-polarized plane wave of frequency ω incident on a nonlinear crystal, which is transparent at frequencies ω and 2ω. If the

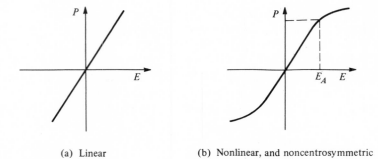

(a) Linear   (b) Nonlinear, and noncentrosymmetric

Figure 2-33   Polarization P versus electric field for linear and non-linear crystals.

nonlinear coefficient η_3 is much less than η_2, retaining only the first two terms in (2-78) gives

$$P = \eta_1 E_x \cos(\omega t - k_1 z) + \eta_2 E_x^2 \cos^2(\omega t - k_1 z)$$

This expression can also be written as

$$P = \eta_1 E_x \cos(\omega t - k_1 z) + \frac{\eta_2 E_x^2}{2}[1 + \cos(2\omega t - 2k_1 z)] \qquad (2\text{-}80)$$

This shows that the nonlinearity in P gives rise to both a second harmonic wave in P as well as a constant term. Therefore, $P(2\omega)$ is given by

$$P(2\omega) = \frac{\eta_2 E_x^2}{2} \cos(2\omega t - 2k_1 z) \qquad (2\text{-}81)$$

This wave is also referred to as the "forced" wave, and its phase velocity from (2-81) is given by

$$v_1 = \frac{2\omega}{2k_1} = \frac{\omega}{k_1}$$

which is the same as that of the incident wave. The polarization wave $P(2\omega)$ generates electromagnetic radiation at frequency 2ω. This radiation whose electric field intensity we denote by $E(2\omega)$ will be proportional to $P(2\omega)$. The $E(2\omega)$ wave is referred to as "free wave." Once the free wave is generated it will travel through the crystal at its phase velocity given by

$$v_2 = \frac{2\omega}{k_2}$$

where k_2 is the propagation constant at frequency 2ω.

In the discussion of dispersion in dielectric media, it was pointed out that generally k is a function of frequency. If $k_2 \neq 2k_1$, then the forced and free waves travel through the crystal at different velocities. This difference in velocity is of crucial importance in second harmonic generation because, if the forced and free waves do not remain in phase, the interference effect markedly reduces the available second harmonic power.

Calculations show that the second harmonic power density is given by[46]

$$I(2\omega) \propto E^4 (\omega) \frac{\sin^2 \dfrac{\ell \omega}{c}(n_1 - n_2)}{n_1 - n_2} \qquad (2.82)$$

where n_1 and n_2 are index of refraction at frequencies ω and 2ω, respectively, c is velocity of light in free space, and ℓ is length of the crystal.

Therefore, $I(2\omega)$ is a maximum when $n_1 = n_2$. If $n_1 \neq n_2$, then $I(2\omega)$ depends on the length of the crystal and has a maximum when

$$\frac{\ell\omega}{c}(n_1 - n_2) = \frac{\pi}{2}$$

or

$$\ell = \frac{\lambda_0}{4(n_1 - n_2)} \tag{2-83}$$

where λ_0 is the free space wavelength at the fundamental frequency. The thickness ℓ given by (2-83) is called the *coherence length* for second harmonic generation.

Equation (2-82) shows that maximum power at second harmonic frequency can be obtained if $n_1 = n_2$. It turns out that this condition can be satisfied in certain birefringent crystals by suitable choice of propagation direction and polarization of the incident radiation[47,48] and has been successfully used in efficient second harmonic generation.

According to (2-82), $I(2\omega) \propto E^4(\omega)$; therefore, second harmonic intensity can be increased by increasing the intensity of the incident radiation. Since the fundamental field intensity is several orders of magnitude greater inside a laser cavity than outside, enhanced second harmonic generation can be achieved if the nonlinear crystal is placed inside the cavity. This scheme was developed by Geusic[49] *et al.*, and has been used for generating the second harmonic in Nd:YAG lasers, i.e., for conversion from 1060 nm to 530 nm radiation.

2.6.4 absorption under intense radiation

The application of lasers in welding, scribing, and other thermally induced material processing exposes the material to highly intense electromagnetic radiation. In all such applications the laser radiation is first absorbed either by free electrons, bound electrons, or lattice vibrations and then converted to heat by collision processes. This section outlines the probable effects of high radiation intensity on the absorptivity of the material.

Absorptivity of a material is defined as

$$A = 1 - R$$

where A is absorptivity and R is reflectivity. This definition assumes that the absorption coefficient of the material is sufficiently large so that, except for reflection, no energy is transmitted out of the system. In models describing thermally induced processes with laser radiation, it is assumed that most of the incident radiation is absorbed by the material (i.e., $R \simeq 0$ and $A \simeq 1$).

For example, the depth of holes drilled in various materials using a YAG laser is given in Table 3-5, Chapter 3. The model discussed assumes absorption of all the incident energy. Agreement between the calculated and experimental results is rather good, despite the fact that the normal reflectivity of copper is 98 percent and that of silicon 30 percent. Similar results have been obtained by other investigators.[50]   This shows that when the incident intensity is high, absorptivity of the material becomes large.

Although this phenomenon is very interesting, little progress has been made in explaining it in a detailed and definitive way.   One reason probably is that several mechanisms simultaneously play a role in enhancing the absorptivity.   This makes it difficult to explain the results of any experiment.   In the following we shall discuss only those effects which probably play a significant role in enhancing the absorptivity.

1.   Temperature Effects   As the name "thermal processing" indicates, a large increase in temperature occurs under intense $[I > 10^4$ W/ cm$^2]$ radiation.   It is therefore reasonable to ask how this increase in temperature, which may occur during the initial duration of a laser pulse, affects its absorption properties.

In case of metals, which are usually highly reflecting, an increase in absorptivity implies a decrease in reflectivity.   It is well known that the electrical resistivity of a metal increases with temperature due to an increase in the scattering frequency, Γ.   In Section 2.5.5 it was pointed out that this reduces the reflectivity of a metal.   This effect, although important, can explain changes in reflectivity of only a few percent.

In the case of semiconductors, temperature plays a dual role.   An increase in temperature not only increases the scattering frequency, but also generates free carriers either by band-to-band transitions or thermal excitations.[51]   As discussed in Section 2.5.6, both of these effects enhance the absorptivity of a semiconductor.

2.   Effects of Defects   Most materials at elevated temperature have defect structures such as ion vacancies, which become efficient scattering centers for conduction electrons.   In laser-induced thermal processes, only a very small portion of a material is exposed to intense radiation.   It is, therefore, apparent that the mechanical boundary conditions of the radiation-affected area are fixed.   These boundary conditions cause high stresses and strains, which in turn may develop defect structures such as dislocations and even mechanical breakdown of the heat affected zone. Due to the increased surface area in such a mechanically damaged surface, intrinsic absorptivity will increase.   Moreover, the formation of even a small crater increases absorption due to multiple reflection within the crater.[50]

3. Effect of Vaporized Material   Vaporization of very small amounts of material during the initial portion of a laser pulse could drastically affect its optical properties.   If the vaporized material consists essentially of neutral particles (Section 2.7), it may act as a thin surface layer of lower index of refraction and high transparency.   A thin surface layer of this kind could act as an antireflection coating on a normally reflecting substrate.   On the other hand, if the vaporized material consists of charged particles, radiation will be more efficiently absorbed by it and then transferred to the underlying substrate by thermal conductivity.   The second process becomes important only when $I > 10^6$ W/cm^2.[52]   The effect of a dense vaporized material has been used to explain high absorptivity exhibited by many materials under ultra-short ($\sim 10^{-11}$ s duration) high-intensity radiation.[53]

2·7   particle emission

Another class of phenomenon which could be considered in the interaction processes is that of particle emission from the laser irradiated surface. The emitted particles generally consist of electrons, ions, vaporized material, or plasma (ionized gas), and their study has helped elucidate many aspects of the interaction process.   Essentially, the particle emission can involve three phenomena.

1. Thermionic emission of electrons and/or ions, i.e., charged particles.
2. Emission of vaporized material, consisting mostly of neutral but highly energetic particles.
3. Plasma formation.

Starting from thermionic emission they require successively higher intensities of the incident radiation.   Therefore, depending upon the radiation intensity and its duration, one or all of these may be present in a laser-induced thermal process.   The rate of material removal in micromachining and hole drilling is affected by the presence of a surface layer of charged or neutral particles and, therefore, should be considered in a thermodynamic model of the process.

2·7·1   electron and ion emission

In Section 2.2.2 it was pointed out that electrons are emitted from a metal surface if they acquire sufficient energy to overcome the work function. From the Fermi-Dirac (see Section 2.3.8) distribution function, note that the probability of finding such electrons increases with temperature. The relation between thermionic current density j, the surface temperature

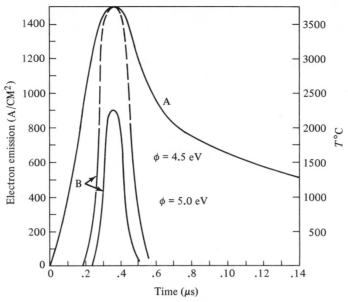

Figure 2-34   Curve A is the calculated plot of surface temperature as a function of time for the application of a single neodymium laser pulse. Curve B is the calculated plot of thermionic electron emission as a function of time for the temperatures indicated in curve A and for surfaces of work function 4.5 eV and 5.0 eV.[55]

(T), and the metal work function (ϕ) is given by Richardson's[54] equation

$$j = AT^2 \exp(-\phi/kT)$$

where A is a constant and is generally equal to $60.2 \text{ A cm}^{-2}\,{}^{\circ}\text{K}^{-2}$ for many metals.

Experimentally it is observed that the thermionic emission from a laser-irradiated metal surface closely follows the laser pulse, indicating a rapid rise of the surface temperature.[55,56,57]   Calculated values of metal surface temperatures agree well with the observed thermionic currents and Richardson's equation, as shown in Figure 2-34.

Positive ion emission from laser-irradiated surfaces has also been observed.[58]   Their origin again appears to be thermionic.

2·7·2   neutral particle emission

In addition to the emission of charged particles, evaporated material consisting of neutral atoms and/or molecules is emitted from a laser-irradiated surface.   For example, in one experiment a thin coating of aluminum on a glass substrate was vaporized (incident power density $\simeq 10^9 \text{ W/cm}^2$) without any damage to the glass, and it was found that charged particles constituted only 1 percent of the evaporated material.[59] Such emitted material is fairly transparent to laser radiation.

An interesting aspect of such experiments is that some emitted particles have energy of the order of 100 eV. It is highly unlikely that this is thermal energy, since the temperature and energy involved (about 10^5 degrees) are sufficiently high to dissociate the molecules. One interpretation is that thermally emitted electrons and ions first absorb the laser energy and then transfer it to neutral particles by collision.[60]

When a metal surface is irradiated with a high intensity (about 10^{10} W/cm^2), short duration laser pulse (about 50 ns), it has been observed that the vaporized material is emitted after the laser beam declines from its peak value. It is proposed that in this case absorption occurs so rapidly that material at some depth below the surface reaches its vaporization temperature before the material at the surface has time to absorb its latent heat of vaporization. This leads to development of high pressure and subsequent superheating of the underlying material until the temperature rises above the critical point, at which instant the delayed (relative to laser peak) ejection of the material proceeds like a thermal explosion.[61] Such a model will also explain existence of high-energy particles in the plume of ejected material. Validity of this model has been questioned by some investigators.[62]

2·7·3 plasma production

Plasma production using a laser is of great interest because of its possible application in producing a high-density, high-temperature plasma in which thermonuclear reactions could occur.[63,64] Plasma with density close to that of a solid (about 10^{28} atoms/m^3) and temperatures as high as $10^{6\circ}$K has been obtained with laser irradiation of solid particles. Several models have been proposed to explain the plasma generation and subsequent absorption of radiation by it. Since our main interest is to emphasize those aspects which affect micromachining and hole drilling by a laser beam, we shall outline the relevant conclusions only.

Briefly, it appears that the blow-off material (consisting of ions, electrons, and neutral molecules discussed in the previous section) is removed early in the laser pulse. Later, a portion of the incident radiation energy is absorbed in the plume by several processes, particularly by interaction with the charged particles. This causes rapid ionization of the plume which thus forms a plasma. Further absorption of the energy by the plasma rapidly increases its temperature, wherein it begins to undergo a rapid expansion. The reduction in plasma density so obtained reduces radiation absorption and once again the plume becomes transparent.

In attempting to relate the mechanisms just described to the practical situation of material removal, particularly for the case when high-intensity

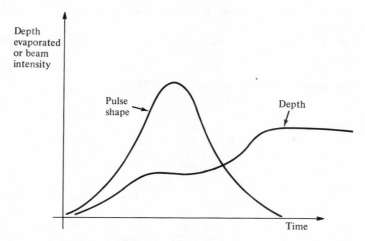

Figure 2-35   Proposed time dependence of the depth to which material is evaporated with respect to the incident laser pulse.

Q-switched pulses are employed, the following qualitative model can be used.   Material evaporation is assumed to begin early in the pulse.   At some short time later, the material in front of the surface becomes opaque (absorbing plasma) and essentially shuts off or isolates the surface from the incoming radiation.   Later in the pulse, or even after its termination when this blow-off material has become very hot, reradiation from the hot plasma reaches the sample surface and cause still further evaporation. Thus, the time dependence of the depth to which material is evaporated with respect to the incident laser pulse may appear as in Figure 2-35.

The incident laser energy does not go effectively into supplying the latent heat of vaporization of the solid material but rather into raising the temperature of a small amount of material evaporated fairly early.[65] Although detailed experimental evidence is not yet available to confirm this, it appears that optimum peak power and pulse widths exist for a given material above which proportionate increases in the amount of material removed will not be seen.

References

1. H. H. Skilling, *Fundamentals of Electric Waves*, John Wiley and Sons, Inc., New York (1948).
2. A. Hoyt, *Engineering Electromagnetics*, McGraw-Hill Book Co., New York (1962).
3. J. A. Stratton, *Electromagnetic Theory*, McGraw-Hill Book Co., New York (1941).

4. F. A. Jenkins and H. E. White, *Fundamentals of Optics*, 3rd Ed., McGraw-Hill Book Co., New York (1957).

5. M. R. Wehr and J. A. Richards, Jr., *Physics of the Atom*, Addison-Wesley Publishing Co., Reading, Mass. (1967).

6. F. K. Richtmyer, E. H. Kennard, and T. Lauritsen, *Introduction to Modern Physics*, McGraw-Hill Book Co., New York (1955).

7. F. A. Richards and D. Walsh, "Time-Resolved Temperature Measurement of a Laser-Heated Surface," *Brit. J. Appl. Phys.* Series 2, **2**, 663 (1969).

8. R. P. Feynman, R. B. Leighton, and M. Sands, *The Feynman Lectures on Physics*, Vol. I, Addison-Wesley Publishing Co., Reading, Mass. (1965).

9. A. Ashkin, "Acceleration and Trapping of Particles by Radiation Pressure," *Phys. Rev. Lett.* **24**, 156 (1970).

10. deBroglie, *Compt. Rend.* **177**, 107, 148 (1923). Also see P. L. Bergmann, *Introduction to the Theory of Relativity*, Prentice-Hall, Inc., Englewood Cliffs, N.J. (1942).

11. C. Davisson and L. H. Germer, "Scattering of Electrons by a Single Crystal of Nickel," *Phys. Rev.* **30**, 705 (1927). Also see F. Seitz, *Modern Theory of Solids*, McGraw-Hill Book Co., New York (1940).

12. B. D. Cullity, *Elements of X-ray Diffraction*, Addison-Wesley Publishing Co., Reading, Mass. (1956). Also see E. A. Wood, *Crystals and Light*, D. Van Nostrand Co. Inc., Princeton, N.J. (1964).

13. N. Bohr, "The Constitution of Atoms and Molecules," *Philosophical Magazine* **26**, 1, 476, 875 (1913).

14. R. L. Sproull, *Modern Physics*, John Wiley and Sons, Inc., New York (1963).

15. M. Born, *Atomic Physics*, Blackie & Sons, Ltd., London (1951).

16. R. L. Sproull, *Modern Physics*, p. 142, John Wiley and Sons, Inc., New York (1963).

17. C. L. Hemenway, R. W. Henry, and M. Coulton, *Physical Electronics*, John Wiley and Sons, Inc., New York (1962).

18. R. L. Sproull, *Modern Physics*, pp. 195–197, John Wiley and Sons, Inc., New York (1963).

19. R. C. Evans, *An Introduction to Crystal Chemistry*, Cambridge University Press (1964).

20. J. C. Slater, *Quantum Theory of Molecules and Solids*, Vol. 3, McGraw-Hill Book Co., New York (1967). Also see P. Drude, *Ann. Physik* **1**, 566; and **3**, 369 (1900).

21. H. A. Lorentz, *The Theory of Electrons*, G. P. Stechert and Co., New York (1923); also see J. C. Slater, *Quantum Theory of Molecules and Solids*, Vol. 3, p. 4, McGraw-Hill Book Co., New York (1967).

22. A. Sommerfield, "An Electronic Theory of Metals Based on Fermi's Statistics," *Z. Physik* **47**, 1, 43 (1928).

23. R. de L. Kronig and W. A. Penney, "Quantum Mechanics of Electrons in Crystal Lattices," *Proc. Roy. Soc.* **A130**, 499 (1931). Also see R. L. Sproull, *Modern Physics*, John Wiley and Sons, Inc., New York (1963).

24. C. L. Hemenway *et al.*, *Physical Electronics*, p. 45, John Wiley and Sons, Inc., New York (1962).

25. C. Kittel, *Introduction to Solid State Physics*, 3rd Ed., John Wiley and Sons, Inc., New York (1966).

26. C. Kittel, *Introduction to Solid State Physics*, 3rd Ed., p. 109, John Wiley and Sons, Inc., New York (1966).

27. M. P. Lisitsa and I. V. Fekeshgazi, "Time and Spectral Characteristics of Emission Accompanying Damages of Rock Salt and Glan by a Laser Beam," *Ukrayin Fiz. Zh.* (U.S.S.R.), Vol. 12, 1701–1713 (1968). Also see R. Y. Chiao, C. H. Townes, and B. P. Stoicheff, "Stimulated Brillouin Scattering and Coherent Generation of Intense Hypersonic Waves," *Phys. Rev. Lett.* **12**, 592 (1964).

28. J. A. Stratton, *Electromagnetic Theory*, p. 34, McGraw-Hill Book Co., New York (1941).

29. J. C. Slater, *Quantum Theory of Molecules and Solids*, Vol. 3, p. 97, McGraw-Hill Book Co., New York (1967).

30. J. C. Slater, *Quantum Theory of Molecules and Solids*, Vol. 3, p. 115, McGraw-Hill Book Co., New York (1967).

31. M. Grarbuny, *Optical Physics*, Academic Press Inc., New York (1965).

32. *American Institute of Physics, Handbook*, pp. 6–112, McGraw-Hill Book Co., New York (1967).

33. S. Roberts, "Optical Properties of Copper," *Phys. Rev.* **118**, 1509 (1960).

34. F. Abeles, Ed., *Optical Properties and Electronic Structure of Metals and Alloys*, John Wiley and Sons, Inc., New York (1966).

35. J. C. Slater, *Quantum Theory of Molecules and Solids*, Vol. 3, p. 155, McGraw-Hill Book Co., New York (1967).

36. M. N. Libenson, G. S. Romanov, and Y. A. Imas, "A Calculation on the Influence of the Temperature Dependence of the Optical Constants of a Metal on the Nature of Its Heating by Laser Radiation," *Soviet Phys.: Technical Phys.* **13**, 925 (1969).

37. T. S. Moss, *Optical Properties of Semiconductors*, Academic Press Inc., New York (1959).

38. O. Madelung, *Physics of III-V Compounds*, John Wiley and Sons, Inc., New York (1964).

39. W. Spitzer and H. Y. Fan, "Infrared Absorption in *n*-type Silicon," *Phys. Rev.* **108**, 268 (1957).

40. A. Yariv, *Quantum Electronics*, John Wiley and Sons, Inc., New York (1967).

41. F. O. Rice and E. Teller, *The Structure of Matter*, Science Editions, Inc., New York (1961).

42. A. Yariv, *Quantum Electronics*, pp. 433–435, John Wiley and Sons, Inc., New York (1967).

43. C. Kittel, *Introduction to Solid State Physics*, 3rd Ed., John Wiley and Sons, Inc., New York (1966).

44. P. A. Franken and J. F. Ward, "Optical Harmonics and Nonlinear Phenomena," *Rev. Mod. Phys.* **35**, 23 (1963).

45. J. C. Burfoot, *Ferroelectrics*, Van Nostrand Reinhold Co., New York (1967).

46. P. A. Franken and J. F. Ward, "Optical Harmonics and Nonlinear Phenomena," *Rev. Mod. Phys.* **35**, 23 (1963).

47. J. A. Giordmaine, "Mixing of Light Beams in Crystals," *Phys. Rev. Lett.* **8**, 19 (1962).

48. P. D. Maker *et al.*, "Effects of Dispersion and Focusing on the Production of Optical Harmonics," *Phys. Rev. Lett.* **8**, 21 (1962).

49. J. E. Geusic *et al.*, "Continuous 0.532μ Solid State Source Using $Ba_2NaNb_5O_{15}$," *Appl. Phys. Lett.* **12**, 306 (1968).

50. M. K. Chun and K. Rose, "Pulse Output and the Ejection of a Mass of Metal under the Action of a Giant Laser Pulse," *J. Appl. Phys.* **41**, 614 (1970). Also see A. M. Bonch-Bruevich, *Soviet Phys: Technical Phys.* **13**, 640 (1968).

51. W. B. Gauster and J. Bushnell, "Laser-Induced Infrared Absorption in Silicon," *J. Appl. Phys.* **41**, 3850 (1970).

52. S. I. Anisimov *et al.*, "The Action of Powerful Light Fluxes on Metals," *Soviet Phys.: Technical Phys.* **11**, 945 (1967).

53. A. Caruso and R. Gratton, "Interaction of Short Laser Pulses with Solid Materials," *Plasma Phys.* **11**, 839 (1969).

54. C. L. Hemenway *et al.*, *Physical Electronics*, p. 60, John Wiley and Sons, Inc., New York (1962).

55. D. Litchman and J. F. Ready, "Laser Beam Induced Electron Emission," *Phys. Rev. Lett.* **10**, 342 (1963).

56. F. Gioni, L. A. Mackenzie, and E. J. McKinney, "Laser-Induced Thermionic Emission," *App. Phys. Lett.* **3**, 25 (1963).

57. C. M. Verber and A. H. Adelman, "Laser Induced Thermionic Emission," *Appl. Phys. Lett.* **2**, 220 (1963).

58. J. K. Cobb and J. J. Murray, "Laser Beam-Induced Electron and Ion Emission from Metal Foils," *Brit. J. Appl. Phys.* **16**, 271 (1965). Also see S. Namba *et al.*, "Propagation of Ruby Laser Beam in Air," *Scientific Papers I.P. CR.* **60**, 101 (1966).

59. J. F. Ready, *Effects of High Power Laser Radiation*, John Wiley and Sons, Inc., New York (1971).

60. L. P. Levine, J. F. Ready, and E. Bernal, "Production of High-Energy Neutral Molecules in the Laser-Surface Interaction," *IEEE J. of Quantum Electronics* **QE4**, 18 (1968).

61. J. F. Ready, "Development of Plume of Material Vaporized by Giant-Pulse Laser," *Appl. Phys. Lett.* **3**, 11 (1963).

62. H. Weichel and P. V. Avizonin, "Expansion Rates of the Luminous Front of a Laser-Produced Plasma," *Appl. Phys. Lett.* **9**, 334 (1966).

63. N. A. Basov *et al.*, "Heating and Disintegration of a Plasma Produced by a Laser Giant Pulse Focused on a Solid Target," *Soviet Phys.: Technical Phys.* **24**, 659 (1967).

64. A. F. Haught and D. Polk, "High-Temperature Plasmas Produced by Laser Beam Irradiation of Single Solid Particles," *Phys. Fluids* **9**, 2047 (1966).

65. E. Archbold, D. W. Harper, and T. P. Hughes, "Time-Resolved Spectroscopy of Laser-Generated Microplasmas," *Brit. J. Appl. Phys.* **15**, 1321 (1964).

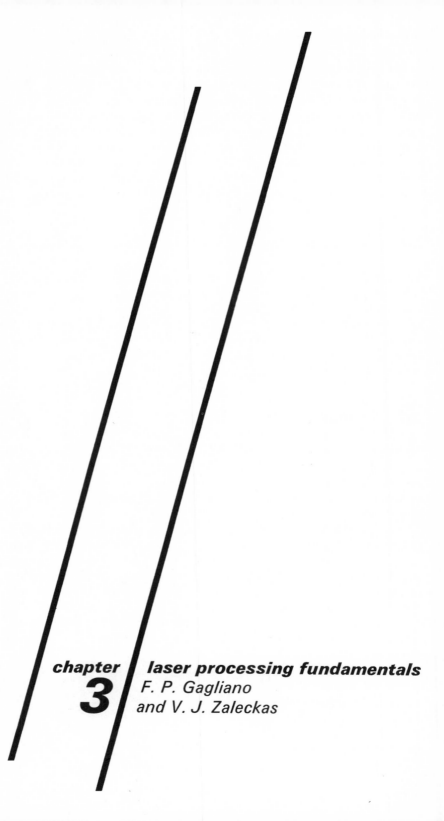

chapter
3

laser processing fundamentals
F. P. Gagliano
and V. J. Zaleckas

3·0 introduction

In the processing of materials, applications such as welding, drilling, and the various forms of micromachining are generally considered. Such processes are fully appreciated only when one has an understanding of the various technical disciplines encompassed by each. A general model depicting a laser processing application would include the following: the laser and its output characteristics, optics to direct and focus (if necessary) the raw beam onto the sample being worked, and the material itself. Chapter 1 dealt with the laser and its output characteristics. This chapter is arranged to treat the remaining elements of this model in some detail.

3·1 optics considerations for material processing

The unfocused, "raw" output of the laser generally does not provide sufficient power density to raise the temperature of most materials above their melting or boiling points. Also, the diameter of the raw beam, typically being at least a few millimeters, is too large for those applications requiring that heat affected zones be confined. For these reasons, focusing or concentrating the output beam of the laser is required for the majority of material working applications.

3·1·1 fundamental relations

This section reviews those relations and concepts considered necessary for a general understanding of laser beam focusing by an ideal lens. Based on some initial assumptions, a relation for spot size is developed and its meaning is discussed as related to various optical variables which can be controlled.

A rather complete description of Gaussian beam propagation has been developed.[1,2,3] If the assumption is made that the coherent beam from the laser possesses a Gaussian intensity profile in the transverse dimension, then the above referenced theory can be applied to predict the propagation characteristics of such radiation in free space and also its interaction behavior with various optical elements.

Near the optic axis, the Gaussian beam is regarded as a TEM wave with a spherical phase front and transverse field distribution as depicted in Figure 3-1.[2]

The field amplitude is E, and the beam radius w is defined as that transverse distance at which E has fallen to $1/e$ times its value on axis (or equivalently, the distance at which the intensity has fallen to $1/e^2$ its on-axis value).

The two parameters of most interest in describing the propagation characteristics of such a beam are the beam radius, $w(z)$, at any axial

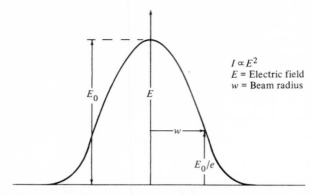

*Figure 3-1   Variation of transverse field amplitude E with radial
position for a Gaussian beam.*

position, z, and the phase front radius $R(z)$, given below and illustrated
graphically in Figure 3-2.

$$w^2(z) = w_0^2\left[1 + \left(\frac{\lambda z}{\pi w_0^2}\right)^2\right]$$ (3-1)

$$R(z) = z\left[1 + \left(\frac{\pi w_0^2}{\lambda z}\right)^2\right]$$ (3-2)

where λ is the radiation wavelength.

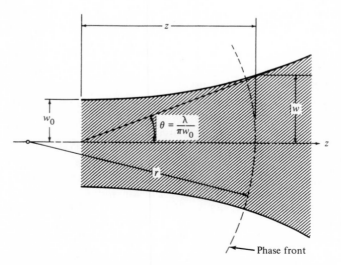

Figure 3-2   Gaussian beam propagation[2] starting from a waist w_0.

The beam expands as it propagates through space. The intensity distribution remains Gaussian in every beam cross section, with the width of that Gaussian profile changing along the axis. At the beam waist where the phase front becomes plane, the beam contracts to a minimum diameter $2w_0$ ($z = 0$, $R = \infty$). For most practical lasers, the location of the beam waist generally lies within the cavity itself, as seen in Chapter 1.

From (3-1), it can be seen that for large z the beam expands linearly, with a far-field divergence angle given by (assuming θ is small)

$$\theta = \lim_{z \to \infty} \frac{dw}{dz} = \frac{\lambda}{\pi w_0} \qquad (3\text{-}3)$$

In general, when a Gaussian beam passes through an ideal lens (i.e., one that leaves the transverse field distribution unchanged), a new beam waist is formed and the parameters in the expansion laws (Equations 3-1 and 3-2) are changed. These effects are illustrated in Figure 3-3 where the most general situation is shown.

Before passing through the lens, beam waist of radius w_1 is located at distance d_1 to the left of the lens whose focal length* is f. The lens produces another beam waist at a distance d_2 (to the right of the lens) with a radius w_2. The transformed waist and its position can be found from the following relations:

$$\frac{1}{w_2^2} = \frac{1}{w_1^2}\left(1 - \frac{d_1}{f}\right)^2 + \frac{1}{f^2}\left(\frac{\pi w_1}{\lambda}\right)^2 = \frac{1}{w_1^2}\left(1 - \frac{d_1}{f}\right)^2 + \left(\frac{1}{f\theta_1}\right)^2 \qquad (3\text{-}4)$$

$$d_2 - f = \frac{(d_1 - f)f^2}{(d_1 - f)^2 + (\pi w_1^2/\lambda)^2} \qquad (3\text{-}5)$$

Note that for the general case being considered, the minimum spot radius w_2 does not occur at the lens focal plane f. From (3-4), it can be seen that

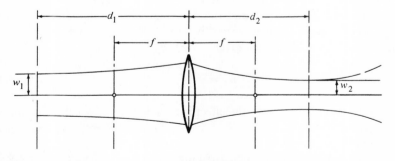

Figure 3-3 Effect of a lens on the propagation of a Gaussian beam.[2]

* Defined in the Glossary.

the minimum spot radius varies directly with the lens focal length and inversely with distance d_1.

At this point, several simplifying assumptions can be made, the justification of which will become clear later when numerical examples are cited. The first is that the far-field divergence angle, θ_1, is small and the beam radius upon entering the lens can be assumed equal to the untransformed waist radius w_1. The second is that the term $1/w_1^2[1 - (d_1/f)]^2$ in (3-4) contributes little to the value of w_2^2. Note that these approximations also imply that $d_2 - f$ is small and, hence, the focused spot occurs at the lens focal plane.

For the transformed beam waist, and hence the focused spot radius, (3-4) then becomes

$$w_2 = f\theta_1 = \frac{f\lambda}{\pi w_1} \qquad (3\text{-}6)$$

From this approximation the following can be noted:

1. The focused spot radius is directly proportional to the lens focal length and the radiation wavelength λ and inversely proportional to the untransformed waist w_1 (and thus, in light of the approximation just made, inversely proportional to the diameter of the beam entering the lens).
2. For radiation at a given wavelength λ, the focused spot radius is thus minimized by minimizing the ratio f/w, which can be taken as the working f/number* of the lens.
3. The entrance aperture of the lens fixes an upper limit on the value of w_1.

In practice, one has little control over the beam waist, w_1, which is formed primarily as a consequence of laser cavity geometry. However, before entering the "focusing" lens, a beam expander can be used to increase w_1 before focusing, thus decreasing the size of the focused spot. The effects of a beam expander are illustrated in Figure 3-4.

The initial waist is w_1 and the distance between the lenses is made equal to the sum of their respective focal lengths. In this case, the transformed waist w_2 is then given simply by

$$w_2 = w_1\left(\frac{f_2}{f_1}\right) \qquad (3\text{-}7)$$

Thus, assuming $f_2 > f_1$, the effect is to increase w_1, which can equivalently be considered as a decrease in the far field divergence angle (see Equation 3-3).

From a practical material working standpoint, the depth of focus achieved when focusing the laser output is also of importance. In this

* See Glossary.

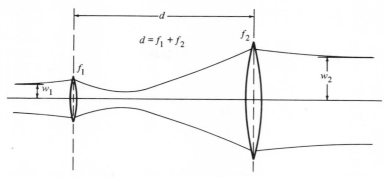

Figure 3-4   Effects of a beam expander on the propagation of a Gaussian beam.[2]

context, depth of focus can be considered as that distance over which the minimum beam waist does not vary enough to effect the results of material working applications due to variations in the position of the workpiece. Specifically, it can be defined as that axial position at which the intensity has fallen off to some percentage of its maximum value achieved at the waist.

Qualitatively, (3-2) for the wavefront radius can be used to show the relation between depth of focus and other parameters.   In the near field, (i.e., for small z) the depth of focus varies directly with the wavefront radius $R(z)$, and increases in depth of focus are achieved only at the expense of an increase in the size of the focused spot.   Similar conclusions can be drawn by noting that the depth of focus is inversely related to the far-field divergence angle θ.

If specific limits are imposed on the variation of w_2, the focused spot size, with z, exact relations for the depth of focus can be obtained from (3-1).   Specifically, if the depth of focus z is arbitrarily defined as that point at which w_2 has increased by 5 percent, then

$$z = \pm \frac{0.32\pi w_2^2}{\lambda} \tag{3-8}$$

Table 3-1 lists values of z for various values of w_2, the spot radius, assuming a radiation wavelength λ of 1060 nm.

TABLE 3-1

w_2 (μm)	z (μm)
1	± 0.95
5	± 23.7
10	± 95
20	± 380
50	± 2370

3·1·2   spot size—power density

From the relations presented in Section 3.1.1, estimates can be made for the focused beam size. In addition to knowing the focal length of the focusing lens, the untransformed beam size must also be known. Several methods exist for experimentally measuring this quantity. One is to measure the transverse distribution of the beam intensity by incrementally scanning a small pinhole across the beam and measuring the intensity at each point. From the intensity distribution data so obtained, the beam radius can be determined.

Another method[4] employs a calibrated iris placed in the beam path and a means for measurement of the relative power transmitted through the iris. A round iris of radius a will intercept (i.e., block) an amount of power, P_{iris}, given by

$$P_{iris} = P_{incid} \times e^{-2[a/w]^2} \tag{3-9}$$

where P_{incid} is the incident power and w is the beam radius. If $a = w$, then 13.5 percent of the incident power is intercepted. A power meter is used to measure the beam power passing through the iris, and w is determined by means of the following procedure:

(a) The iris is opened wide and P_{incid} is measured.
(b) The iris is then closed down until the transmitted power measures $0.865 P_{incid}$. The radius of the iris at this point then equals the beam radius.

The following numerical example illustrates the use of the relations given in Section 3.1.1. Consider a Nd : YAG laser operating at a wavelength of 1060 nm producing 1 W CW power in the fundamental (Gaussian) TEM mode with a beam waist ($2w$) equal to 1 mm. These conditions are easily achieved by using internal apertures, for example.

Assume the focusing lens parameters to be

$$f = 2 \text{ cm}$$

$$\text{aperture (lens diameter)} = 1 \text{ cm}$$

$$d_1 \text{ (distance from lens to waist)} = 10 \text{ cm}$$

In order to achieve the minimum possible spot radius, a 10× ($f_2/f_1 = 10$) beam expander is used to expand the untransformed waist to the size of the lens aperture. Using (3-4),

$$\frac{1}{w_2^2} = \frac{1}{(5 \times 10^{-3})^2}(1 - 5)^2 + \frac{1}{(20 \times 10^{-3})^2(0.672/10 \times 10^{-3})^2}$$

$$= 0.64 \times 10^6 + 0.55 \times 10^{12}$$

(The insignificance of the term $1/w_1^2(1 - d_1/f)^2$ can be clearly seen in this example.)

$$w_2 = 1.34 \ \mu m$$

A focused spot diameter of 2.68 μm would therefore be expected for a perfect lens.

The peak power density, or peak intensity I_0, obtained within the focused spot is found from the total power P_0 as follows.

$$P_0 = \int_0^\infty I(r) 2\pi r \, dr = \int_0^\infty I_0 e^{-2r^2/w_2^2} 2\pi r \, dr = I_0 \frac{\pi w_2^2}{2} \qquad (3\text{-}10)$$

Hence

$$I_0 = \frac{2P_0}{\pi w_2^2} \qquad (3\text{-}11)$$

Thus, for the specific example cited above, the peak power density I_0 is found to be

$$I_0 = \frac{2(1 \ \text{W})}{\pi(1.34 \times 10^{-4} \ \text{cm})^2} = 3.56 \times 10^7 \ \text{W/cm}^2$$

3·1·3   effective spot diameter

Due to the relatively high power densities and small size, direct measurements of the focused optical spot diameter are difficult to obtain. An "effective" spot diameter, defined by the resultant heat affected zone within the material, can be determined by metallurgical cross sectioning. This heat-affected zone primarily depends on the focused power from the laser, the total energy absorbed, and the thermal properties of the material. Therefore, its measurements may differ appreciably from optical spot size calculations.

3·1·4   material surfaces

The purpose of beam focusing and optics in general, as related to laser processing, is to direct and/or concentrate the beam from the laser onto the surface of the material being worked. The coupling or transfer of this energy into the material depends, to a large extent, on the material surface itself. This section briefly considers material surfaces from a qualitative viewpoint.   The discussion that follows applies specifically to the surfaces of metals and most semiconductors, but the treatment can also apply, in principle, to nonmetals.

The surfaces of most materials are different from any similar plane of atoms in the subsurface or interior of the materials.   (We are not referring to atomic binding and nearest neighbor theory.)   For example, even for the "inert" or noble metals like gold and platinum, there can be (and usually are) surface films of greases and other predominately organic contaminants, as well as adsorbed gases.   The more reactive metals will always have an oxide and/or other inorganic films, such as chlorides, sulfides, and nitrides.   The presence of these films and metal compounds will have an influence on the interaction of laser energy with the surface.

The topography of a material surface generally consists of a number of high and low spots, normally in a (repetitive or uniform) pattern derived from the method of preparation.   These spots or asperities are sometimes visible to the unaided eye.   The vertical distance between these high and low spots is often referred to as surface roughness, roughness height, waviness, or lay.   These measurements are normally specified in reference to a nominal surface using appropriate instrumentation, such as a profilometer.   The measurement is expressed as the mean deviation from this nominal surface or profile in microinches (μin.).   The surfaces that one may encounter in laser processing can range in roughness from 2–8 μin. for a superpolished finish to the standard tool machined surfaces of 16–200 μin., and to 100–1000 μin. for casting and cutting operations.

The interaction of electromagnetic energy with materials was covered in Chapter 2.   Some discussion on the reflectivity of material surfaces (from a less theoretical position) is included here for metallic surfaces. Most metals reflect a large portion of a laser beam; therefore correspondingly higher power beams are required for most transformation processes. However, the surfaces of most materials reflect light during only a small portion of the laser pulse.   As the temperature of the surface increases, reflectivity often decreases with a corresponding increase in absorptivity. The absorptivity of liquid Al and Cu for ruby light is given as:[5] Al $= 0.20$, Cu $= 0.15$.   The corresponding room temperature values are approximately 0.11 for Al and 0.04 for Cu.

The reflectance of most metals increases with wavelength; hence more power will be required from a laser with a long wavelength than from one with a short wavelength.   For example, as the wavelength increases from 690 nm to about 1000 nm, an order of magnitude increase in power is required in order to melt some materials.   Figure 3-5 gives the percent reflectance or transmittance versus wavelength for some materials.   The data are for normally incident light on specular surfaces at room temperature.   When a low power laser beam is incident on a polished metal specimen, there is no melting because the light is largely reflected.   To produce surface melting and/or vaporization, the power must be increased.

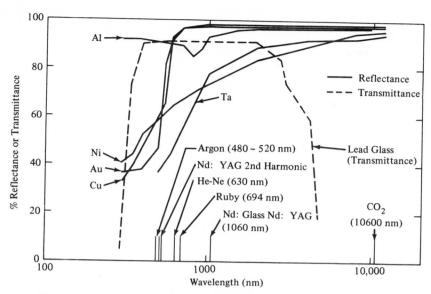

Figure 3-5 *Room temperature reflectance (or transmittance) versus wavelength for the materials shown.*

However, a sudden increase in the absorption of light makes it difficult to control the welding of some materials.   For example, when thin ribbons of a highly reflective metal, such as gold, are welded, the intensity and duration of the laser beam must be adjusted carefully to prevent the ribbon from vaporizing.[6] This could happen because the laser beam intensity required to break down the surface reflectivity is greater than that required for stable propagation of the fusion front once the surface has melted.[13]   One possible way of overcoming the problem is to decrease the beam power after applying a short breakdown pulse. A simpler approach, and often quite effective, is to coat intentionally or change the material surfaces so that they become good absorbers. For the case of bright copper sheet, its reflectance to 694.3 nm was reduced from approximately 95 percent to less than 20 percent by oxidizing the surface to a CuO/Cu_2O film approximately 1000 to 1500 nm thick.

When the size of surface asperities are of the order of the wavelength of the laser light, the effect of reflectivity is clearly demonstrated. Figure 3-6 shows the depth of penetration of the melt puddle in pieces of copper exposed to ruby radiation. The copper was prepared with surface finishes in the range of 0.025 to 100 μm; it appears that above about 2 μm the absorption process is independent of surface finish. Figure 3-7 shows the appearance of the exposed copper surface for several degrees of roughness.

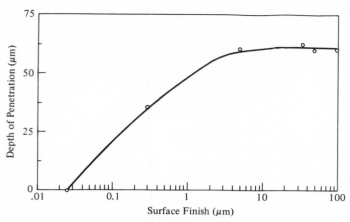

Figure 3-6 Depth of melting versus surface finish for copper. Focused power density was approximately 3×10^6 W/cm$^{2.14}$ (With permission of Academic Press Inc.)

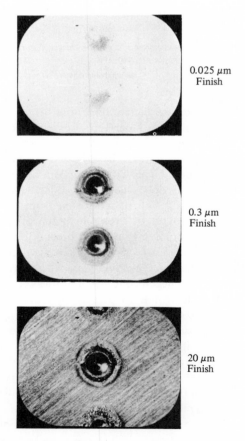

0.025 μm
Finish

0.3 μm
Finish

20 μm
Finish

Figure 3-7 Appearance of the exposed copper surface for the finish indicated.[14] (With permission of Academic Press Inc.)

3·1·5   other considerations

This section reviews some considerations relating to the effects when nonideal lenses are used, as well as laser outputs which do not conform to the assumptions of Gaussian beam theory.

Most high-powered lasers used in manufacturing applications, particularly the solid-state pulsed lasers, do not oscillate in the fundamental transverse mode (TEM_{00}) and, hence, do not conform to the assumption previously made of a Gaussian intensity profile across the beam. Such lasers generally oscillate in higher-order transverse modes, resulting in greater output power but only at a sacrifice in modal purity. The far-field divergence angle of higher-order transverse mode beams is also larger than for a fundamental mode beam, assuming that the waist is the same in each case. The use of relations, such as (3-6), to determine focused spot radius under such circumstances is, of course, no longer strictly correct. However, to a first approximation, (3-6) can be used to estimate the focused spot size if the actual far-field divergence angle of the beam in question is used. The same lens parameters, beam expansion, etc., as they relate to spot size would still apply in this case. Thus, normally the higher the transverse mode the larger will be the focused spot size.

As an illustration of these concepts, again consider the CW Nd : YAG laser. Typical multimode output characteristics for this laser might be the following (without the use of internal apertures):

$$CW \text{ power} = 15 \text{ W}$$

$$\text{Beam diameter} = 3 \text{ mm}$$

$$\text{Beam divergence} = 2.5 \text{ mrad } (\tfrac{1}{2} \text{ angle})$$

Using a lens with the same parameters as that used in the example of Section 3.1.2, the achievement of the minimum focused spot size in this case requires the use of a 3.33 × (10/3) beam expander. The resultant beam divergence is thus reduced to

$$\frac{2.5 \text{ mrad}}{3.33} = 0.75 \text{ mrad}$$

The focused spot radius is found using (3-6).

$$w_2 = f\theta_1$$

$$w_2 = (20 \times 10^{-3} \text{ m})(0.75 \times 10^{-3} \text{ rad})$$

$$= 15 \text{ } \mu m$$

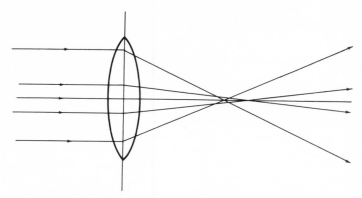

Figure 3-8   Geometrical illustration of spherical aberration.

The peak focused power density or intensity I_0 in this case is thus

$$I_0 = \frac{2 \times 15 \text{ W}}{\pi(15 \times 10^{-4} \text{ cm})^2} = 4.24 \times 10^6 \text{ W/cm}^2$$

which is seen to be approximately an order of magnitude less than the power density calculated for the "single mode" case.

The significance of this example lies in the fact that even though higher powers can be achieved through multimode operation, the resultant focused power density obtained will normally be less than for a laser operating in the fundamental mode.

In all discussions up to now, the lens was assumed to be ideal. In practice, all optical systems are subject to aberrations. For the focusing and collimating optics used in laser applications, many aberrations become unimportant and performance is limited mainly by spherical aberration where the image of the point source is spread out into a blurred spot. (This type of aberration is a symmetrical defect of optical systems in which rays from an on-axis point source which enter the optical system at different distances from the optical axis do not come to a common focus.) Figure 3-8 geometrically illustrates the situation where it is seen that rays nearest the optical axis will focus at one point, while those rays further from the axis focus at a point nearer the lens. The result is to cause an increase in the size of the focused spot over what is predicted by the relations so far presented.[7]

3.2   materials and their properties

A general review of materials and their properties as related to thermally induced changes is given in this section. Basic thermodynamic relations are defined and the general concepts of thermally induced phase changes are discussed.

3·2·1   thermodynamic considerations

For an isolated system which undergoes a change in state,

$$\Delta E = q + w = q + PdV \qquad (3\text{-}12)$$

where E = internal stored energy,
q = net amount of heat added,
w = net external work done on the system.

Equation (3-12) is a statement of the first law of thermodynamics, namely that energy in a system is conserved.

A basic quantity useful not only in itself, but in defining other quantities, is that of enthalpy (H) and is defined as the sum of internal stored energy and the pressure-volume product as

$$H \equiv E + PV \qquad (3\text{-}13)$$

For a system change occurring at constant pressure, it can be shown that

$$\Delta H = q \qquad (13\text{-}14)$$

and hence, at constant pressure, the change in enthalpy is equal to the heat input.

A change in state caused by a rise in temperature (T) can be characterized by a quantity known as heat capacity, C, where

$$C \equiv \frac{dq}{dT} \qquad (3\text{-}15)$$

In general, there are a number of heat capacities, but the two most commonly used are those at constant pressure, C_p, and constant volume, C_v, defined as follows:

$$C_p = \left(\frac{dq}{dT}\right)_p = \left(\frac{\partial H}{\partial T}\right)_p \qquad (3\text{-}16)$$

and

$$C_v = \left(\frac{dq}{dT}\right)_v = \left(\frac{\partial E}{\partial T}\right)_v \qquad (3\text{-}17)$$

3·2·2   phase transformations

The term phase can be defined as any homogeneous part of a system which is physically distinct and separated from other parts of the system by definite bounding surfaces. For example, water can exist in a solid phase as ice, in a liquid phase as water, or in a gaseous phase as vapor. A pure substance is defined as one which is chemically homogeneous and fixed in chemical composition.[8]   The state of a pure substance, when it exists as a single phase, can be completely specified by the values of two independent properties, namely pressure and temperature, provided electric, magnetic, and surface tension effects do not exist.   If, for example, in the case of a gas, the pressure and temperature were specified, then density, internal energy, viscosity, etc., are fixed.   The pressure and temperature of any one phase of a substance can be varied independently over wide ranges.   When two phases of a pure substance coexist in equilibrium, there is a fixed relationship between pressure and temperature. These values of pressure and temperature are generally called the saturation pressure for a given temperature and the saturation temperature for a given pressure, and the corresponding phase of the pure substance existing under such conditions is called a saturated phase.   A fixed relationship between saturation pressures and temperatures is characteristic of all pure substances.   For example, the pressure versus temperature phase diagram for copper would appear as shown in Figure 3-9.

Consider the processing of copper along the path of the dashed line in Figure 3-9.   Changes in state within a single phase and changes in the transformation reactions between phases are assumed to occur at constant pressure, namely atmospheric.   Therefore $\Delta H = q$.   Assume the copper sample is heated from room temperature (25°C) to 2595°C, the point of vaporization, at a relatively slow rate so that incremental temperature

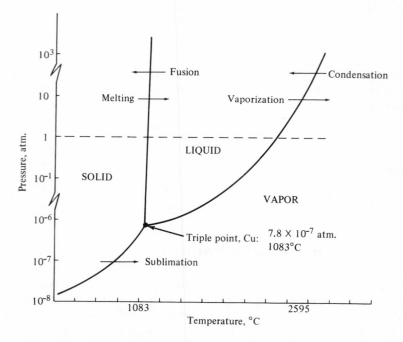

Figure 3-9   Pressure-temperature phase diagram for copper.

measurements can be made.   A typical temperature versus time plot for the data would appear as shown in Figure 3-10.   From both the pressure-temperature and temperature-time diagrams, the following can be noted:

A. Solid Phase   Assuming the pressure is constant, the amount of heat required to raise the temperature from 25°C to 1083°C (i.e., to the melting point, but just before melting commences) is given by (3-14).   If the heat capacity, C_p, is assumed to be independent of temperature, this quantity of heat is given as

$$\Delta H = q = C_p \, \Delta T \qquad \text{(J/g)} \tag{3-18}$$

For a given volume, V, of material, and assuming it remains constant with increasing temperature

$$q = \rho V C_p \, \Delta T \qquad \text{(J)} \tag{3-19}$$

where ρ is the density.

B. Transformation Reaction, Solid to Liquid   In the transformation reaction, a finite time is required for complete liquefaction.   During this time heat is added to the system with no increase in temperature. This "isothermal" heat goes into destroying the crystalline structure of the material, i.e., it overcomes the bond energies of the solid phase, resulting in a far less ordered array of the atomic structure, namely a liquid.

This quantity of heat absorbed at the isotherm is called the *latent heat of fusion*, ΔH_f, often seen as L_f.   [Note: ΔH_f and L_f are used interchangeably throughout the text.]   At the 1083°C isotherm, a mixture

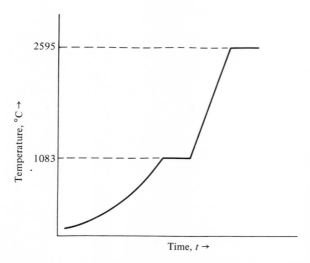

Figure 3-10   Temperature-time diagram, representative for copper.

of solid and liquid exists and if this mixture is kept stable—i.e., at thermo-dynamic equilibrium—then for a further increase in pressure there will be a corresponding increase in temperature to maintain the sample on the uni-variant curve, i.e., the saturation equilibrium line between solid and liquid.

Mathematically, this univariant curve is described by the Clapeyron equation:

$$\frac{dP}{dT} = \frac{\Delta H_f}{T \, \Delta V_f} \tag{3-20}$$

or equivalently as

$$\frac{\Delta P}{\Delta T} = \frac{\Delta H_f}{T_e(V_2 - V_1)} \tag{3-21}$$

where $\Delta P/\Delta T$ is the slope of the univariant line between solid and liquid,

T_e is the equilibrium temperature normally taken as the melting point, and

V_2 and V_1 are the volumes of the liquid and solid, respectively.

C. Liquid Phase   Upon restoring atmospheric pressure, the copper sample will spontaneously go to complete liquefaction. The material (liquid) now has a different heat capacity, larger than the corresponding value for the solid.

If it is again assumed that ρ, C_p, and V are not significantly different from their room temperature values,

$$q = \rho V(Cp \, \Delta T + \Delta H_f) \tag{3-22}$$

This equation describes the energy change for temperatures up to but below that required for vaporization.

D. Transformation Reaction, Liquid to Vapor   This reaction can be described in a manner similar to the solid–liquid transformation. Using the same basic assumptions for constancy of property values, the total energy change for the system in going from room temperature to complete vaporization is given as

$$q = \rho V(C_p \, \Delta T + \Delta H_f + \Delta H_v) \tag{3-23}$$

where $\Delta H_v(L_v)$ is the latent heat of vaporization.

3·2·3   thermal diffusivity

Since most material working with lasers is effected with a high-temperature, short-time-duration function, problems associated with the flow of heat in laser-treated materials are of the transient type. This means that the temperature at any point in the material is variable with time, so that steady-state temperature profiles are normally not established for the total time of the reaction.   In the steady-state case, thermal equilibrium is normally established.   In this case heat flow problems are solved by the determination of the rate of conduction of heat through the material. For the transient state, the emphasis is on the rate of change of temperature within the material—such as in determining the depth of heat penetration from the interaction of a laser beam with the surface.

The rate of change of temperature is dependent on the rate of heat flow in a material.   These factors are related by the thermal conductivity, K.   But thermal conductivity is not the only factor that influences the heat flow, since the rate of change in temperature also depends on the specific heat, c, of the material concerned.   In fact, it is inversely proportional to the volumetric specific heat, ρc.   We can state the relationship of these factors as

$$\frac{K}{c/\text{unit vol.} \times \text{mass}} = \frac{K}{c \times \text{density}} = \frac{K}{c \times \rho} \tag{3-24}$$

The expression in (3-24) has the dimensions of $1^2\,t^{-1}$, characteristic of a diffusion coefficient and has, therefore, been given the descriptive term thermal or heat diffusivity (to recognize the fact that it represents the diffusion coefficient of temperature or, more properly, heat).

For all unsteady-state heat-flow problems the term $K/\rho c = \kappa$ is involved (see Section 3.3).   The significance of this term is that it determines how rapidly a material will accept and conduct thermal energy. Thus, for the case of welding, high thermal diffusivity will normally allow larger fusion penetration with no thermal shock cracking.   Table 3-2 lists the thermal diffusivity of several metals and alloys.

Many materials have relatively low thermal diffusivities which may limit their laser weldability.   The stainless steels and the heat-resistant alloys, such as René 41,[9] experience rather shallow fusion depths.   These metals are relatively easy to vaporize so that hole drilling processes can be effected (see Section 4.2).   On the other hand, the evaporation of a material having higher diffusivity values, such as silicon, in some cases results in a small amount of the condensed liquid phase being retained.

Thermal diffusivity is largely determined by the value of the thermal conductivity, since the product ρc does not vary to any great extent for many materials.   Table 3-3 shows that ρc, the volume specific heat, varies by less than 2.5 : 1, whereas the thermal conductivity varies by about 7 : 1 and the specific heat per unit mass at constant pressure, properly called the heat capacity, C_p (i.e., $c = C_p$), varies by approximately 10 : 1. This helps explain, for example, why metals with high C_p, such as aluminum and magnesium, have no marked advantage over the other metals when considering heat flow problems.   However, when ρc is considered, it is obvious why nickel and high-nickel alloys are good candidates for

TABLE 3-2

Material	*Thermal Diffusivity κ^a* ($\times 10^{-4} m^2/s$)
Metals (commercially pure)	
Aluminum	0.91
Beryllium	0.42
Chromium	0.20
Copper	1.14
Gold	1.18
Iron	0.21
Molybdenum	0.51
Nickel	0.24
Palladium	0.24
Platinum	0.24
Silicon	0.53
Silver	1.71
Tantalum	0.23
Tin	0.38
Titanium[b]	0.082
Tungsten	0.62
Zinc	0.41
Alloys	
Brass (70:30)	0.38
Phosphor bronze (5% Sn)	0.21
Cupro nickel (30% Ni)	0.087
Beryllium copper (2% Be, γ phase)	0.29
Inconel (76% Ni, 16% Cr, 8% Fe)	0.039
6061, 0 temper aluminum alloy (1% Mg, 0.6% Si, 0.25% Cu, 0.25% Cr)	0.64
304 type stainless steel (19% Cr, 10% Ni)[c]	0.041

[a] Calculated from the data of physical properties contained in Ref. 10.
[b] Values for thermal conductivity and specific heat are the average of the spread for several alloys of 99.0 percent commerically pure grades at 93°C (200°F).
[c] Wrought stainless steel in the annealed condition.   Values of thermal conductivity and specific heat apply at 100°C.

laser welding.   Nickel retains its absorbed energy for a longer time than most other metals because of its large heat capacity per unit volume. Furthermore, it requires more energy per unit volume to raise nickel to a given temperature than for another material with a lower ρc product. Hence, one can appreciate why the depth of fusion penetration for nickel is comparable to other metals even though its thermal diffusivity value is less than most of these metals.   Figure 3-11 shows unusually large grains in the microstructure of a laser melted nichrome (a high-nickel-content alloy) specimen where the surface was exposed to a 2.5 ms pulse of ruby radiation.   The large grain structure is evidence that a time-temperature relation necessary for recrystallization has occurred.

TABLE 3-3

Metal	K $(cal/s/cm/^\circ C)$	C_p $(cal/g\,^\circ C)$	ρc (cal/cm^3)
Aluminum	0.53	0.215	0.58
Beryllium	0.35	0.45	0.84
Chromium	0.16	0.11	0.79
Copper	0.94	0.092	0.82
Gold	0.71	0.031	0.60
Iron	0.18	0.11	0.87
Molybdenum	0.34	0.066	0.68
Nickel	0.22	0.105	0.94
Palladium	0.17	0.058	0.70
Platinum	0.16	0.031	0.67
Silicon	0.20	0.162	0.38
Silver	1.0	0 056	0.59
Tantalum	0.13	0.034	0.56
Tin	0.15	0.054	0.40
Tungsten	0.40	0.033	0.64
Zinc	0.27	0.092	0.66

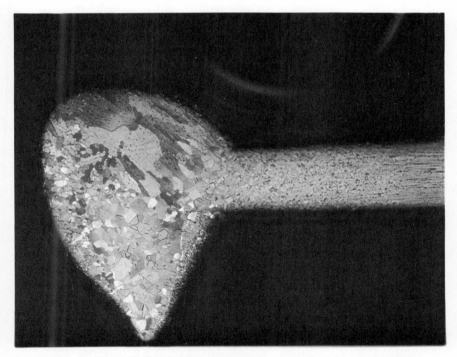

Figure 3-11   Microstructure of a laser melted nichrome specimen which was exposed to a 2.5 ms pulse of ruby radiation.

Variation of diffusivity with variables such as temperature is similar to the variations found with thermal conductivity. The variation with temperature is normally neglected and/or an average value is chosen for the temperature range of interest.

3·3   thermal processing models

When laser light is focused onto the surface of a material, a certain percentage of the light may be absorbed and converted to thermal energy. When sufficient energy is absorbed, phase changes, in the form of melting and vaporization, can occur. In this section, analytical methods and models applicable to material working applications, such as welding, drilling, and micromachining using both pulsed and Q-switched lasers are presented.

3·3·1   assumptions

The following basic assumptions and considerations generally apply to the discussions of this section.

1. As was indicated in Chapter 2, light is absorbed in materials due to an interaction with both bound and free electrons, the electrons being raised to higher energy states upon absorption of optical energy. The conversion of light energy to heat is governed by some type of collision process in which excited electrons give up their energy by means of collisions with lattice phonons and with other electrons, ionized impurities, and defect structures. The mean free collision time is typically of the order of 10^{-12} to 10^{-14} s.[11] In the time duration of the shortest laser pulse to be considered, typically no less than 10^{-9} s, the absorbing electrons will have had time to make many collisions. Thus, the first assumption made is that the laser energy is instantaneously converted to heat at the point at which the light was absorbed. The establishment of a local equilibrium during the pulse duration is assumed and the usual concept of temperature is taken to be valid, thereby allowing the use of conventional heat flow analysis.[11]

2. Several properties of the absorbing materials, such as thermal conductivity, specific heat, and density, are taken to be independent of temperature, i.e., they are assumed to remain constant during the heating process. Optical properties, such as absorption coefficient, reflectivity, etc., will be dealt with where appropriate in each area discussed.

3. Heat losses due to reradiation from the material are considered negligible. For the laser intensities or flux densities under consideration, typically 10^6 to 10^9 W/cm^2, thermal radiation from the material surface will proceed at rates three to four orders of magnitude less than that of the laser pulse intensity.[11]

3.3.2   solid phase—temperature profiles

Fundamental conditions for heat transfer by conduction within a solid body require that:

1. A temperature gradient exist.
2. The resulting heat flow be in a direction of decreasing temperature.

The basic law which defines heat conduction in one dimension can be stated, with reference to Figure 3-12, as follows. The quantity of heat per unit area, q, conducted in the x direction of a homogeneous solid can be written as the product of the temperature gradient along the path, dT/dx, and the thermal conductivity K, as

$$q = -K\frac{dT(x)}{dx} \tag{3-25}$$

In the one-dimensional case, the temperature is assumed constant in the y and z directions.

For transient heat conduction, where the temperature T is a function of both position x and time t, the quantity of heat entering and leaving a volume element of the body is not the same at any given instant. From energy balance, this results in a change in the internal energy of the element. With reference to (3-19), this can be expressed as

$$dq = \rho C_p V \frac{\partial T(x, t)}{\partial t} dt \tag{3-26}$$

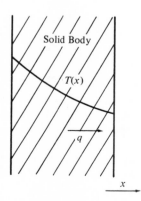

Solid Body

$T(x)$

q

x

Figure 3-12   Linear one-dimensional heat conduction in a solid.

From (3-25) and (3-26), the unsteady one-dimensional heat conduction equation is seen to be the following:

$$\frac{\partial T(x, t)}{\partial t} = \frac{K}{\rho C_p} \frac{\partial^2 T(x, t)}{\partial x^2} \tag{3-27}$$

The general partial differential equation (satisfied by the transient temperature field) in a three-dimensional body can be easily derived in an analogous manner. For the most general case where heat is produced in the solid at a point (x, y, z) and supplied at the rate $A(x, y, z, t)$ per unit volume per unit time, the equation is given as:

$$\frac{\partial^2 T}{\partial x^2} + \frac{\partial^2 T}{\partial y^2} + \frac{\partial^2 T}{\partial z^2} - \frac{1}{\kappa} \frac{\partial T}{\partial t} = -\frac{A}{K}(x, y, z, t) \tag{3-28}$$

where T = temperature at point (x, y, z) and time t; i.e., $T = T(x, y, z, t)$,
  K = thermal conductivity,
  κ = thermal diffusivity.

For the case when the system or body under consideration does not contain heat sources or sinks, T must satisfy

$$\frac{\partial^2 T}{\partial x^2} + \frac{\partial^2 T}{\partial y^2} + \frac{\partial^2 T}{\partial z^2} = \frac{1}{\kappa} \frac{\partial T}{\partial t} \tag{3-29}$$

and for steady-state conduction where T is independent of time,

$$\frac{\partial^2 T}{\partial x^2} + \frac{\partial^2 T}{\partial y^2} + \frac{\partial^2 T}{\partial z^2} = 0 \tag{3-30}$$

must be satisfied.

The first of several examples considers solutions to (3-28) when the maximum temperature is below the melting point; i.e., the material remains in its solid phase. Temperature profiles, i.e., temperature as a function of both position and time, will be found for appropriate values of A, which are chosen so that the source of heat is representative of that generated by laser radiation.

If the transverse dimensions of the laser beam are large, then uniform temperatures in the xy plane can be assumed, and the problem can be considered one dimensional with dependence only on z. Equation (3-28) then becomes

$$\frac{\partial^2 T(z, t)}{\partial z^2} - \frac{1}{\kappa} \frac{\partial T(z, t)}{\partial t} = -\frac{A(z, t)}{K} \tag{3-31}$$

For radiation at the surface, a particular form for the function $A(z, t)$ must be chosen and the heat flow equation (3-31) solved. First, consider a rather simple case where there is no internal source of heat present. For a semi-infinite solid, i.e., one bounded by the plane $z = 0$

and extending to infinity in the positive z direction, let the following initial and boundary conditions apply:

$$T(0, t) = T_s, \text{ a constant for } t > 0$$

$$T(x, 0) = 0$$

The surface ($z = 0$) is kept at a constant temperature T_s and the initial temperature is zero. The solution to the heat flow equation (3-31) under these conditions with $A(z, t) = 0$ is[12]

$$T(z, t) = T_s\left(1 - \text{erf}\frac{z}{2\sqrt{\kappa t}}\right) = T_s \,\text{erfc}\,\frac{z}{2\sqrt{\kappa t}} \tag{3-32}$$

where

$$\text{erf}\,x = \frac{2}{\sqrt{\pi}}\int_0^x e^{-\zeta^2}\,d\zeta \tag{3-33}$$

Equation (3-32), plotted in Figure 3-13, is introduced to show the dependence that heat flow within a material has on the material's properties. From (3-32) it can be seen that the time required for a point in the material to attain a given temperature varies inversely as the diffusivity. Thus materials with high heat diffusivity ($K/\rho C_p$) accept and conduct thermal energy very quickly. Also, the time for any point to reach a given temperature is proportional to the square of its distance from the surface under the specified assumptions and boundary conditions.

The absorption of radiation by materials can be adequately described by the equation:

$$I(z, t) = I(0, t)e^{-bz} \tag{3-34}$$

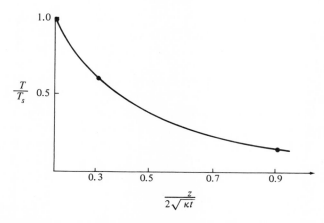

Figure 3-13   *Plot of (3-32) showing variation of* $T(z, t)/T_s$ *with the parameter* $Z/2\sqrt{\kappa t}$.

where $I(0, t)$ describes the temporal shape of the incident radiation absorbed at the material surface $z = 0$, $I(z, t)$ is the intensity within the material, and b is the optical absorption coefficient (see Chapters 2 and 6 for further discussion). As was initially stated, it is assumed that all the light energy absorbed goes into heating the material. Further, if it is assumed that the spatial pulse shape is uniform with an infinite extent in the xy plane, then

$$A(z, t) = bI(z, t) = bI(0, t)e^{-bz} \qquad (3\text{-}35)$$

If the further assumption that $I(0, t) = I_0$ (a constant) is made, straightforward solutions to the one-dimensional heat-flow equation can be obtained for the following two cases:

1. The optical absorption coefficient is large, corresponding to the case in which the absorption of incident radiation and hence heat generation takes place only in the surface plane of the material. For this special case, the solution to the heat-flow equation is given as[12]

$$T(z, t) = \frac{2I_0}{K} \left[\left(\frac{\kappa t}{\pi} \right)^{1/2} e^{-z^2/4\kappa t} - \frac{z}{2} \operatorname{erfc} \frac{z}{2\sqrt{\kappa t}} \right] \qquad (3\text{-}36)$$

which, at the surface of the material, reduces to

$$T(0, t) = \frac{2I_0}{K} \left(\frac{\kappa t}{\pi} \right)^{1/2} \qquad (3\text{-}37)$$

2. When the absorption coefficient is not large, corresponding now to the case when heat is generated within the material assumed to be a semi-infinite solid, the solution is

$$T(z, t) = \frac{2I_0}{Kb} (bt)^{1/2} \operatorname{ierfc} \frac{z}{2(\kappa t)^{1/2}}$$

$$+ \frac{I_0}{2Kb^2} e^{(b^2\kappa t + bz)} \operatorname{erfc}\left[b(\kappa t)^{1/2} - \frac{z}{2(\kappa t)^{1/2}} \right]$$

$$+ \frac{I_0}{2Kb^2} e^{(b^2 t + bz)} \operatorname{erfc}\left[b(\kappa t)^{1/2} + \frac{z}{2(\kappa t)^{1/2}} \right] \qquad (3\text{-}38)$$

The solution given by (3-38) can be extended to include the case in which the rate of heat production; i.e., $A(z, t)$, is a function of time through the use of Duhamel's theorem. The solution can be given in the form:[11]

$$T(z, t) = \int_z^\infty \int_0^t \frac{I(\tau)}{I_0} \frac{\partial}{\partial t} \frac{\partial T'(z', t - \tau)}{\partial z'} \, dz' \, d\tau \qquad (3\text{-}39)$$

where T' represents the solution given by (3-38). The results of numerical integration of (3-39) for tungsten and copper samples initially at 0°C and exposed to a Q-switched laser pulse of the assumed shape and duration shown in Figure 3-14 are given in Figures 3-15 and 3-16.

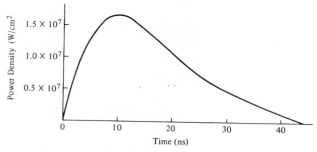

Figure 3-14   Laser pulse shape used in obtaining the results shown in Figures 3-15 and 3-16.[11]   (With permission of American Institute of Physics.)

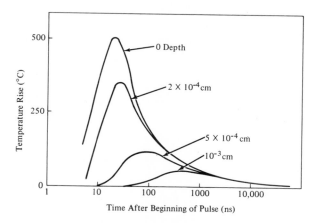

Figure 3-15   Calculated temperature rise as a function of time, with depth as a parameter, in a tungsten sample initially at $0°C$ when a laser pulse of the shape and intensity shown in Figure 3-14 is absorbed at the surface.[11]   (With permission of American Institute of Physics.)

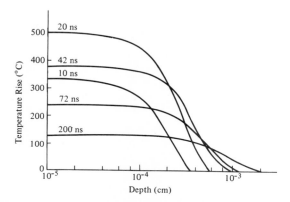

Figure 3-16   Calculated temperature as a function of depth with time as a parameter in a copper sample initially at $0°C$ when a laser pulse of the shape and intensity shown in Figure 3-14 is absorbed at the surface.[11] (With permission of American Institute of Physics.)

Although the results given are valid only for the case of a uniform spatial intensity distribution, they do illustrate important points which will now be discussed and which are generally applicable in all cases.

An important result is the extremely large rates of change of temperature and temperature gradients that are predicted. Gradients as high as 10^6 deg/cm and rates of increase of 10^{10} deg/s are expected. Also, the rate of temperature decrease after the duration of the laser pulse is rapid, indicating rather small thermal time constants.

One can also qualitatively deduce the effects of varying the laser pulse shape. A shorter, higher power density pulse leads to considerably higher peak surface temperatures than does a longer, lower power density pulse containing the same total energy. It would also produce a more uniform temperature distribution and a greater depth of penetration of the heat at the end of the laser pulse.[11] It is precisely for this reason that the use of short-duration, Q-switched pulses in thin-film material removal applications offers an advantage over conventional pulsed or CW outputs, especially where penetration beyond a certain depth may result in undesirable thermal damage. However, the physical properties of the material must also be considered. For example, for lower thermal conductivities the peak surface temperature increases and the penetration depth of thermal energy at a given time decreases.

3.3.3 melting

Melting is considered here as it applies to the process of laser welding. A complete treatment of the melting problem involves the analysis of a boundary separating the liquid and solid phases moving into the material.[13] The assumptions to be made are the following:

1. The thermal properties of the liquid and solid regions are taken to be equal and constant.
2. The depth of penetration of the heat-affected zone is taken to be small relative to the diameter of the impinging laser radiation, thus restricting the problem to the one-dimensional case.
3. The heat input is considered uniform, both in its spatial and temporal extent.

The geometry and coordinate system used in the heat-transfer analysis is given in Figure 3-17.

In general, separate heat-conduction problems exist in the liquid and solid regions, the exact positions of which are unknown since the position of the moving interface $s = s(t)$ is unknown and is one of the quantities to be determined. The general one-dimensional heat flow equation

$$\frac{\partial T_i}{\partial t} - \kappa_i \frac{\partial^2 T_i}{\partial z^2} = 0, \qquad i = 1\ 2 \text{ (liquid, solid)} \qquad (3\text{-}40)$$

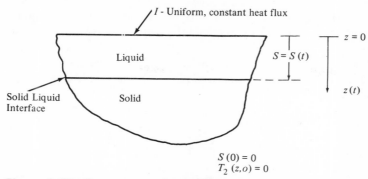

Figure 3-17   Geometry and coordinate systems used in the heat-transfer analysis discussed in text for a melting solid.[13]

applies in each region.   A boundary condition that must be satisfied at the interface between liquid and solid is that the temperature in both regions equal the melting temperature T_m; i.e.,

$$T_1 = T_2 = T_m \quad \text{at} \quad z = S, \qquad t > 0 \tag{3-41}$$

where T_1 is the temperature of the liquid, and T_2 the temperature of the solid.   Conservation of energy at the interface requires that the net heat flux between liquid and solid regions must equal the rate at which heat is absorbed per unit area during the phase change; i.e.,

$$K_2 \frac{\partial T_2}{\partial z} - K_1 \frac{\partial T_1}{\partial z} = \rho L_f \frac{\partial S}{\partial t}, \qquad z = S \tag{3-42}$$

where L_f is the latent heat of fusion.
The following is an expression of the conservation of energy at the surface, namely

$$I = -K_1 \frac{\partial T_1}{\partial t} \qquad \text{for } z = 0, \quad t > 0 \tag{3-43}$$

and states that the net flux of heat at the surface or the rate at which heat is transferred across the surface per unit area per unit time is equal to the input heat flux.   Implied in this assumption is the fact that there are no reflection losses and that the absorption coefficient is infinite.   The following boundary conditions result from restricting the problem to a semi-infinite body.

$$\lim_{z \to \infty} T_2(z, t) = T_\infty \qquad \text{(taken to be zero)} \tag{3-44}$$

$$\lim_{z \to \infty} \frac{\partial T_2}{\partial z} \to 0 \tag{3-45}$$

A generalized solution to the above nonlinear problem has been obtained using an analog computer.[13]   The results are summarized in Figure 3-18, which gives the depth of melting and the surface temperatures as functions of time.

The time t_m at which the surface $z = S = 0$ begins to melt can be found from (3-37), which applies to this problem up to the point at which melting starts.

$$T(0, t_m) = T_m = \frac{2I_0}{K}\left(\frac{\kappa t_m}{\pi}\right)^{1/2} \tag{3-46}$$

$$\therefore \qquad t_m = \frac{\pi}{\kappa}\left(\frac{KT_m}{2I_0}\right)^2$$

The curves of Figure 3-18 are used to calculate the theoretical depth melted as follows.   First, the parameter $Y = L_f/T_m C_2$ (where C_2 equals the heat capacity of the solid), and t_m are calculated for the material being considered.   Then from the curves in the upper portion of the figure, the time t_v to reach vaporization at the surface $z = 0$ is found from a knowledge of T_v, the vaporization temperature.   The depth melted for times $t_m < t < t_v$ can be found from the lower curves.

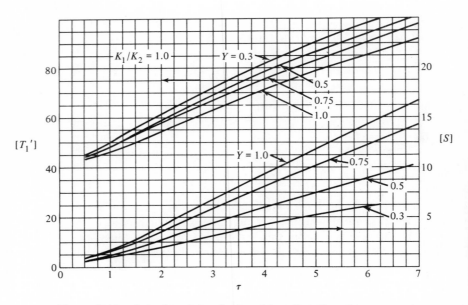

Figure 3-18   Calculated depth of melting, S, and surface temperature, T_1'**, as functions of time,** t**.**
$[S] = (8.33\rho L_f S/It_m)$, $[T_1'] = 40T_1'/T_m$, $\tau = t/t_m$, $Y = L_f/C_2 T_m$. **Temperature in** °F, L_f = **latent heat of fusion.**[14]   **(With permission of Academic Press Inc.)**

Taking a value for Y of 0.45^{14}, which is typical of many metals, S_{max}, the melting depth occurring during vaporization limited melting, is given by

$$S_{max} = \frac{0.16I}{\rho L_f}(t_v - t_m) \tag{3-47}$$

3.3.4 vaporization

Vaporization is important because of its role in material removal processes, such as hole drilling, thin-film micromachining, etc. Many models of varying degrees of complexity can be formulated and applied to this problem, depending on the initial assumptions, imposed boundary conditions, etc. In the majority of work to date, the presence of a liquid state is neglected. In general, the analysis describes the inward propagation of a moving boundary, in this case between the solid and vapor. Exact solutions involve initial transients as well as the steady-state propagation of the boundary. In the most general case of a finite optical absorption coefficient, internal heat generation within the material must be accounted for by selection of an appropriate function for the term $A(x, y, z, t)$ in the heat-conduction equation (3-28). In what follows, a solution is presented which considers all the above.[15] In addition to the more exact solution presented, the limiting case of an infinite absorption coefficient (i.e., a totally absorbing surface, common to many metals) under steady-state conditions is discussed and experimental results presented.

In any treatment of this problem, a knowledge of the temperature distribution within the solid as a function of both position and time is desired. Specifically, solutions should yield the velocity with which material can be removed from the solid surface, i.e., how fast the drilling process is, and the temperature profile within the solid.

As in the previous cases considered, solutions to the heat-conduction equation under the assumptions and initial boundary conditions imposed on the problem are required. The following assumptions, not previously made (in Section 3.3.2 or 3.3.3), are imposed on this problem:

1. The laser beam intensity, I, is of sufficient magnitude to cause vaporization of the material.
2. The gas that is created due to vaporization of the material is transparent to the incident laser energy.
3. The effects of radial heat conduction and the liquid phase are ignored.

Penetration of the laser light into the material results in a physical model representing the laser drilling process consisting of a distributed heat source coupled to a moving boundary (solid–vapor interface). Figure 3-19 represents the geometry and coordinate system used.

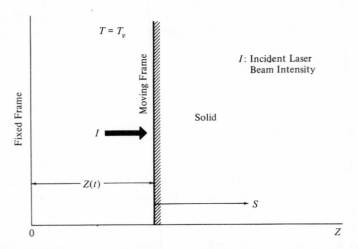

Figure 3-19 **Geometry and coordinate system for thermal model applicable to material removal.**[15]

The velocity of the moving interface separating solid and vapor, $\dot{Z}(t)$, as well as the temperature $T(s, t)$ within the solid are to be found. The one-dimensional heat flow equation, written to include a distributed laser-heat source moving with the front surface, is

$$\frac{\partial^2 T}{\partial z^2} - \frac{1}{\kappa}\frac{\partial T}{\partial t} = -\frac{I}{K} b e^{-b(z-Z)}, \qquad z > Z \qquad (3\text{-}48)$$

where the quantity $A(z, t)$ in (3-28) has been replaced by

$$A(z, t) = bI e^{-b(z-Z)}, \qquad z > Z \qquad (3\text{-}49)$$

Conservation of energy at the moving interface requires that the energy given to the vaporized material equal the energy conducted from the solid. Thus

$$\rho L_v \dot{Z} = K \frac{\partial T}{\partial z}\bigg|_{z=Z} \qquad (3\text{-}50)$$

Solutions of (3-48) and (3-50) will yield the desired temperature and velocity.

Boundary conditions imposed on the model are the following:

$$T = T_v \quad \text{at} \quad z = Z \qquad (3\text{-}51)$$

$$T = 0 \quad \text{at} \quad z = \infty \qquad (3\text{-}52)$$

Before (3-48) and (3-50) can be solved, two independent initial conditions are required. The first,

$$Z = 0 \quad \text{at} \quad t = 0 \qquad (3\text{-}53)$$

assumes that at time $t = 0$ the drilling process begins. The second initial condition regarding temperature depends upon how the material is heated, i.e., what the temperature profile is before the onset of drilling. From solutions to this "preheating" problem, some of which were discussed in Section 3.3.2, an approximation to the exact initial temperature profile is made and given as

$$T = T_v(1 + qz)e^{-qz} \quad \text{at} \quad t = 0 \tag{3-54}$$

The parameter q is chosen such that (3-54) most closely matches the exact initial profile.

The method of solution consists of calculating the temperature and velocity by perturbing the temperature profile around the initial and steady-state front surface velocities. The results of this iterative procedure are inner and outer solutions, neither of which are exactly correct for all time t; the inner solution being a good approximation for values of time t near zero and the outer solution correct for large values of time ($t \to \infty$). The outer solution also approaches the exact solution as t approaches zero.

Equations (3-48) and (3-50) are transformed into a moving dimensionless reference frame and written as follows:

$$\frac{\partial \theta}{\partial \tau} - u \frac{\partial \theta}{\partial s} - \frac{\partial^2 \theta}{\partial s^2} = \frac{B}{\lambda} e^{-Bs} \tag{3-55}$$

$$u = \lambda \frac{\partial \theta}{\partial s}\Big|_{s=0} \tag{3-56}$$

where $\theta = T/T_v$

$$s = \frac{IC_p}{KL_v}(z - Z)$$

$$u = \frac{\rho L_v}{I}\dot{Z}$$

$$\tau = \frac{I^2 C_p}{\rho K L_v^2}t$$

A heating parameter λ, absorption parameter B, and a normalized initial parameter Q are defined, where

$$\lambda = \frac{C_p T_v}{L_v}$$

$$B = \frac{KL_v}{IC_p}b$$

$$Q = \frac{KL_v}{IC_p}q$$

In this new system, (3-54) becomes

$$\theta = (1 + Qs)e^{-Qs}, \qquad \tau = 0 \qquad\qquad (3\text{-}57)$$

Figures 3-20 and 3-21 show typical variations of θ versus distance and u versus time, respectively, for a chosen set of parameters B, Q, and λ. For simplicity, only the outer solutions are plotted, they being more closely representative of the exact solution.

The curves shown in Figure 3-20 predict temperatures inside the material which are greater than the surface temperature T_v. This arises from absorption of the laser pulse within the material (finite absorption coefficient) resulting in a distributed internal heat source. Vaporization of the front surface acts as a cooling mechanism, removing energy from regions near the front surface. If sufficient heat generation within the

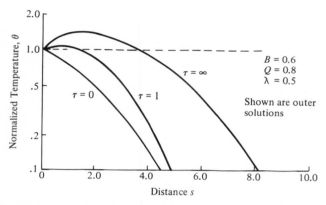

Figure 3-20 **Normalized temperature θ versus distance s with normalized time τ as a parameter.**[15]

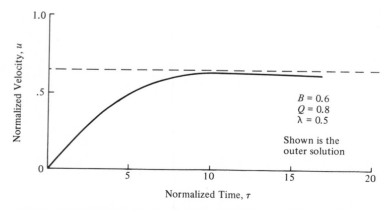

Figure 3-21 **Normalized velocity u versus normalized time τ.**[15]

solid occurs, removal of energy by vaporization of the front surface may not be sufficiently rapid to prevent the inner portion of the material from reaching temperatures that are higher than the subsurface vaporization temperature.

An important physical consequence of this is that, if the subsurface temperature is sufficient to cause vaporization of the material at depths below the surface, the resulting internal pressure caused by the vaporized material *may* be sufficient to fracture and hence cause "explosive" removal of the intervening solid material.   If such a mechanism did exist in laser drilling, it could result in a process more efficient than the processes that rely on complete vaporization of all material to be removed.   Experimental confirmation of this has appeared in the literature.[16]   Table 3-4 summarizes results obtained on various materials.   The second and third columns of the table compare, respectively, the actual absorbed laser energy and the amount of energy calculated (from thermodynamic energy balance) for removal of the amounts of material observed in the experiment.   A more efficient drilling process is clearly indicated for the materials listed in the lower portion of the table.

A possible explanation for this is the explosive removal mechanism just discussed.   Obviously, the greater the maximum subsurface temperature is, the more possible it is for an explosion to occur; and it can be shown that the smaller the absorption parameter B, the higher will be the maximum temperature.   In the limit, as $B \to 0$, the maximum subsurface temperature T_{max} is reached and given by

$$T_{max} = T_v \left(\frac{1 + \lambda}{\lambda} \right) \tag{3-58}$$

Calculated values for B and T_{max}/T_v are listed in columns 4 and 5 of Table 3-4.   Of particular significance is a comparison of silver versus bismuth and iron versus cadmium, where the values of T_{max}/T_v are approximately the same.   Here it is seen qualitatively how the value of B can be

TABLE 3-4

Element	Absorbed Energy (J)	Vaporization Energy (J)	B^a	T_{max}/T_v
Ag	0.82	0.47	8.4	1.34
Cu	0.87	0.43	8.3	1.45
Fe	1.16	1.03	9.3	1.50
Cd	1.16	1.28	1.1	1.50
Bi	1.29	1.76	0.16	1.37
Pb	1.30	1.80	0.48	1.26

^{a} B is calculated for $I = 3.25 \times 10^8$ W/cm^2.[15]

used to predict when subsurface explosions during laser drilling might occur. Materials that had more material removed than predicted by straightforward energy balance (Cd, Bi, Pb) had substantially lower values of B than those materials (Ag, Cu, Fe) that had less material removed. It might at first be expected that in the limit of very small values of B, which can be achieved in practice by increasing I, the drilling process would be most efficient. This is not necessarily so because, as B decreases by increasing the laser intensity, the position of the temperature peak within the solid shifts toward the surface and, hence, although an explosion might be more likely to occur, less material would be removed.

In the steady state, the temperature is given by

$$\theta_{ss} = e^{-vs} - \frac{1}{\lambda(B-v)}(e^{-Bs} - e^{-vs}) \tag{3-59}$$

and the normalized steady-state velocity by

$$v = u_{ss} = \frac{1}{1+\lambda} \tag{3-60}$$

In terms of the original variables, (3-60) becomes

$$\dot{Z}_{ss} = \frac{I}{\rho(L_v + C_p T_v)} \tag{3-61}$$

which could also be derived from energy balance. Under the following conditions, (3-61) can be used to estimate the depth to which material is drilled:

1. The time t_v to reach the vaporization temperature at the front surface is small with respect to the laser pulse length t_p.
2. Subsurface explosions do not occur, i.e., B is large and T_{max}/T_v is small.
3. The time to reach steady state, t_{ss}, is small with respect to t_p.

Under these conditions, the depth to which material is removed is given as

$$d = \dot{Z}_{ss} \times t_p \tag{3-62}$$

If, when the intensity I varies as a function of time, it is assumed that the speed of the moving boundary adjusts itself at any instant of time to the steady-state speed associated with the flux at that time, the depth vaporized can be given as[11]

$$d = \int_0^{t_p} \dot{Z}(t)\, dt = \frac{1}{\rho(L_v + C_p T_v)} \int_0^{t_p} I(t)\, dt \tag{3-63}$$

The three conditions listed above can be satisfied in practice in the limit of a totally absorbing surface, i.e., $b \to \infty$, and intensities of sufficient magnitude to ensure that t_v and t_{ss} are much less than t_p.

TABLE 3-5

Element	t_v (ns)	t_v (ns) $I = const^a$	d_{obs} (μm)	d_{calc} (μm)
Cu	7.75	0.129	16	21.4
Al	5.77	0.054	20	31.2
W	8.05	0.179	10	12.4
Pt	3.98	0.044	9	16.9
Ni	5.47	0.046	14	16.0
Si	4.94	0.033	26	37.4

[a] $I = 7.4 \times 10^8$ W/cm².

Table 3-5 summarizes the results obtained using the steady-state approximations for incident Q-switched laser pulses on several metals, where for most metals, b exceeds 10^6 cm^{-1} and particularly for the case of Q-switched laser pulses, intensities greater than 10^8 W/cm² are easily achieved. The exact temporal shape of the pulse along with a trapezoidal approximation is shown in Figure 3-22. The linear approximation is used in the following discussion.

For a totally absorbing surface, the time for the surface to reach the vaporization temperature T_v for an applied heat flux increasing linearly with time is given as[17]

$$t_v = \left[\frac{T_v}{\frac{4}{3}\left(\frac{\kappa^{1/2}}{K\sqrt{\pi}} \frac{I_0}{c}\right)} \right]^{2/3} \tag{3-64}$$

where c is defined in Figure 3-22.

Calculated values of t_v are listed in Table 3-5. For a constant heat flux, (3-37) is used to determine t_v, i.e.,

$$t_v \bigg|_{I=const} = \frac{\pi}{\kappa}\left(\frac{KT_v}{2I_0}\right)^2 \tag{3-65}$$

This is also listed in Table 3-5. From $t_v \big|_{I=const}$ estimates can be made for the time t_{ss} required to achieve steady-state conditions, i.e., the propagation inward of a fixed temperature distribution at constant velocity.[17a] Specifically,

$$t_{ss} = 25 t_v \bigg|_{I=const} \tag{3-66}$$

which is seen to give values of t_{ss} ranging from 1 ns to 5 ns. This time can be considered as analogous to a time constant with respect to approach to the steady-state velocity. When the heat flux rises linearly to I_0 in the time shown in Figure 3-22, namely 40 ns, the assumption can be made that steady state is achieved concurrent with the onset of vaporization at the surface, i.e., at time $t = t_v$. Since t_v is short compared to t_p, the total laser pulse length, the process is assumed to start at $t = 0$.

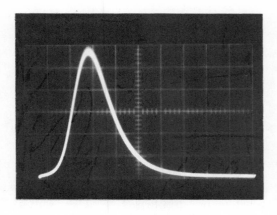

$I_0 = 7.4 \times 10^8$ W/cm^2

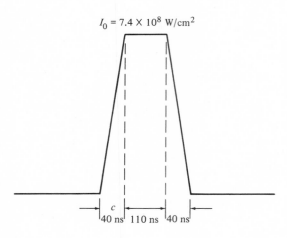

c
40 ns | 110 ns | 40 ns

Figure 3-22   Oscilloscope trace showing actual temporal shape of Q-switched pulse along with the corresponding trapezoidal approximation.

Consider copper as a specific example.   From (3-63) and using the linear approximation shown in Figure 3-22,

$$d = \frac{1}{\rho(L_v + C_p T_v)}$$

$$\times \left[\int_0^{40\text{ ns}} \frac{I_0}{40} t \, dt + \int_{40\text{ ns}}^{150\text{ ns}} I_0 \, dt + \int_{150\text{ ns}}^{190\text{ ns}} I_0 \left(1 - \frac{t - 150}{40} \right) dt \right] \quad (3\text{-}67)$$

Substituting values for the physical constants of copper

$$d = 19.5 \; \mu\text{m}$$

Columns 4 and 5 of Table 3-5 summarize the results obtained on the various materials chosen, listing both calculated and experimentally observed depths. These results were obtained using a Q-switched Nd : YAG laser operating in the fundamental TEM_{00} mode at 1060 nm.

The model considered above treated temperature variation only in one dimension—namely, the drilling direction z. As shown, temperature variations within the solid can be predicted, and in certain cases the depth drilled can be obtained. In many drilling processes using the laser, another important consideration is the temperature variations which exist in the radial direction. Knowing this temperature profile, the distribution of thermal stresses and the shape of the drilled hole can be obtained.[18]

Analytically, there are two significant differences between the model to be presented below and the one just discussed. First, since it is based on a moving source technique, the velocity of vaporization must be known in order to calculate the temperature field. This is done either through experimentation or through use of the first model discussed in this section. Second, possible finite absorption of the laser beam within the material is neglected. The absorption, and hence heating due to the laser, is assumed to occur entirely in the surface plane of the material. All other assumptions previously made apply here.

Figure 3-23 represents the geometry and coordinate system used. The laser beam impinges on the circular area of diameter $2a$, initially in the plane $z = 0$, with its center located at the origin O. As the drilling process proceeds, the front of the laser beam, i.e., the surface heat source, moves down along the z axis from the origin at a rate previously determined.

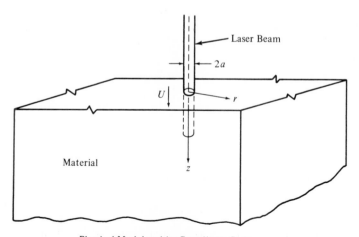

Physical Model and its Coordinate System

Figure 3-23   Geometry and coordinate system for two-dimensional thermal model.[18]

Since finite absorption of the laser pulse (and hence internal heat generation) is neglected, the unsteady heat-flow equation in Cartesian coordinates (3-29) is the following

$$\nabla^2 T = \frac{1}{\kappa} \frac{\partial T}{\partial t} \qquad (3\text{-}68)$$

The solution to (3-68) for an instantaneous point source located at the point x', y', z' can be written as

$$T(x, y, z, t) = \frac{Q(x', y', z')}{8(\pi\kappa t)^{3/2}} \exp\left[-\frac{(x - x')^2 + (y - y')^2 + (z - z')^2}{4\kappa t} \right]$$

$$(3\text{-}69)$$

where Q is defined as the strength of the point source located at (x', y', z') which instantaneously liberates an amount of heat $Q\rho C_p$.

Equation (3-68) is linear in temperature and hence the superposition principle may be applied to the solution describing the temperature rise produced by point sources in a solid. Thus, by integrating the solution for an instantaneous point source (3-69), with regard to appropriate space and time variables, one can obtain solutions for heat sources of any temporal and spatial configuration. Specifically, it is desired to obtain the solution for a continuous heat source distributed over the laser spot and moving in the z direction.

Equation 3-68 is first transformed into polar coordinates, where the instantaneous point source is then considered as being distributed into a ring around the origin with radius r' in the plane $z' = 0$ and having strength $Qr'\,d\theta'$ for the angle $d\theta'$. Integration of the resulting solution with respect to both $r(0 \to a)$ and $\theta(0 \to 2\pi)$ yields the temperature distribution due to an instantaneous source distributed over the laser spot. Integration with respect to time t then results in the continuous source solution and is given as

$$T(r, z, t) = \int_0^a \int_0^t \frac{q(r', t')r'}{4\sqrt{\pi[\kappa(t - t')]^{3/2}}} \left[\exp\left\{ -\frac{r^2 + r'^2 + z^2}{4\kappa(t - t')} \right\} \right]$$

$$\times I_0\left(\frac{rr'}{2\kappa(t - t')} \right) dt'\, dr' \quad (3\text{-}70)$$

where I_0 is the modified Bessel function of the first kind and zeroth order and

$$Q(r') = q(r')dr'$$

The actual solution of interest is the temperature distribution due to a disc source moving in the z direction from $z' = 0$ and varying in location as $z' = f(t')$. Equation (3-70) can be easily modified to describe this case by replacing z with $[z - f(t')]$.

$$T(r, z, t) = \int_0^a \int_0^t \frac{q(r', t')r'}{4\sqrt{\pi(\kappa(t - t'))^{3/2}}} \left[\exp\left\{ -\frac{r^2 + r'^2 + (z - f(t'))^2}{4\kappa(t - t')} \right\} \right]$$

$$\times I_0\left(\frac{rr'}{2\kappa(t - t')}\right) dt' dr' \quad (3\text{-}71)$$

The results obtained when (3-71) is applied to the specific applications of laser drilling in Al_2O_3 and Si, with appropriate boundary conditions, are presented and discussed in Chapter 4.

3.4   metallurgical considerations—introduction

In many cases, the interaction of high-intensity laser light with metals has produced unusually fine-grained or dendritic microstructures within the laser-affected zone. Metallographic inspection of these heat affected zones (e.g., laser welds) often reveals unusually complex microstructures which are difficult to identify (Figure 3-24). This is not to imply, however, that the basic metallurgy of alloy systems is different when one metal reacts with another upon absorption of laser energy. What is suggested is that, because of the high temperatures that can be achieved in a very short cycle time, new structures are evidenced which could not have been retained with lesser values of dT/dt.

Indeed, recent studies[19] of rapidly quenched metals have identified new structures and established the presence of significant deviations from normally existing phase relationships, such as the extension of solid solubility limits. Specifically, it was found that a rapidly quenched liquid specimen of the Ag-Cu eutectic alloy produced a single-phase structure.[20] This was direct evidence that the Hume-Rothery rules* for solid solution of binary alloy systems do apply to the Ag-Cu system, though under equilibrium conditions a eutectic system was always found. This would lead one to conclude that because of the quench-like cooling, an alloy weld of silver and copper made by laser energy could have higher ductility and overall improved properties as opposed to a conventional brazed

---

* Hume-Rothery found that the extent of primary solid solution is seriously constrained whenever the difference in atomic radii exceeds 15 percent. Silver and copper have a difference of 11.5 percent. He also states the dependence of solid solution on two additional rules: (1) the *electrochemical factor*, which states that the more electropositive the one component and the more electronegative the other component, the greater is the tendency to form intermetallic compounds; and (2) the *relative valency effect*, which postulates that a metal of lower valency, i.e., number of valence electrons, is more likely to dissolve one of high valency than the other way around. This last rule would not apply to the Ag-Cu system since both have one valence electron in the neutral atom state. The electrochemical factor, however, applies well to this system, since both silver and copper are very strongly electropositive. The reader is referred to any one of a number of excellent texts on physical metallurgy for a more detailed treatment of the subject. For example, see Darken and Gurry.[21]

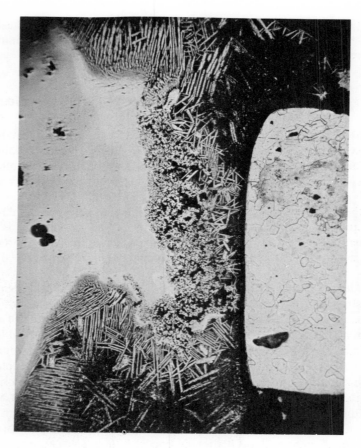

Figure 3-24   Example of a complex weld structure between tantalum (on the left) and nickel wires.   Electron microprobe analysis along the weld zone revealed indeterminant compounds of Ta_xNi_y.   Mag. approximately 200X.

joint, which may suffer from a brittle condition. The fact that laser welds have been made with dissimilar metal systems is no guarantee that they will stand up to a designed function, especially if subjected to high stresses.

For the process of laser welding, the extremely fast temperature rise and almost equally fast cooling cause a nonequilibrium type of solidification.   Figure 3-25 shows a fine dendritic structure fairly common for laser welds of many metal combinations. (This type of structure is similar to that found for cast metals.)   For certain metal combinations it may be necessary to perform a subsequent stress relief or annealing operation on the weld joint.   On the other hand, the swirl-like pattern (Figure 3-26) resulting from the short-time, high-temperature reaction produces a mechanical intermixing of the metal constituents, with some amount of elemental diffusion across the interfaces.   This usually contributes to the strength of the weld structure, provided the thermal expansion coefficients and other properties are compatible.

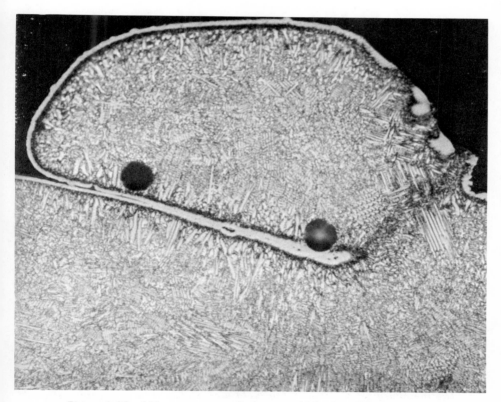

Figure 3-25   Microstructure of a laser weld for beryllium copper wire. Dendritic and acicular-type structures are commonly found for many metal alloys.   Mag. approximately 382 X.

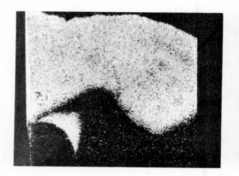

(a) Copper Constituent.

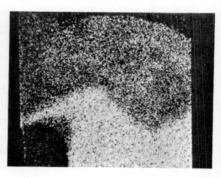

(b) Palladium Constituent.

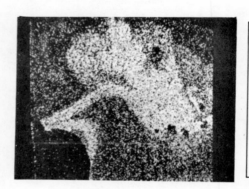

(c) Chromium Decorating.

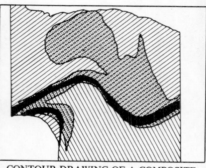

CONTOUR DRAWING OF A COMPOSITE
SYNTHESIS OF FIGURES

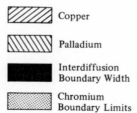

Copper

Palladium

Interdiffusion
Boundary Width

Chromium
Boundary Limits

*Figure 3-26   Electron microscopy analysis of a Be-2%, Cu to Pd weld.
The metallurgical section of the weld was etched with a chromic acid
solution.   Mag. 130X.*

3·4·1   solidification and microstructure

The solidification sequence in a given volume of molten material depends on several factors.   These factors are best considered in terms of the bulk properties of materials, such as temperature, latent heat, composition, thermal conductivity, density, and surface-free energy.

Discussion of the solid–liquid phase transformation stated the acceptability of applying the condition of equilibrium to a laser melted metal in contact with the solid phase.   The Clapeyron equation, representing the univariant curve of the pressure-temperature relationship, is used to describe small detectable changes from equilibrium values of T and P.

$$\frac{\Delta T}{\Delta P} = \frac{T_e(V_2 - V_1)}{\Delta H_f} \qquad (3\text{-}72)$$

The terms V_2 and V_1 are the volumes of the liquid and solid, respectively, and are essentially constant for both, although not the same.

A plausible model for the solidification of a small volume (0.01 to 0.05 mm^3) of a pure metal is illustrated in Figure 3-27.   It might be representative of the dynamic condition of a molten puddle as effected by a laser pulse focused to give a power density of approximately 3.5 kW/mm^2. At the moment of laser shutoff (time $t = 0$), the temperature, T_m, of the molten volume can be considered to be uniform throughout the volume of the melt.   This assumption is quite reasonable since the temperature is very high, and the temperature gradient between the surface and the bottom of the melt puddle is relatively small.

Since the surface area to volume ratio of the melt is appreciably large, i.e., greater than 10, solidification or fusion is primarily governed by conduction of heat into the large heat sink of the solid phase, which is at ambient temperature.   The large interfacial area between liquid and solid affords an efficient and rapid means of cooling.   It is to be expected, then,

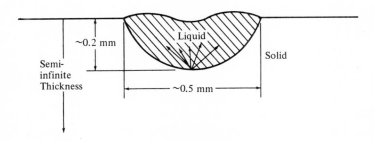

Figure 3-27   Model depicting the solidification of a pure metal.

that the first liquid to solidify will be that along the liquid–solid interface, with preference given at the deepest penetration of the melt. This is indicated by the directions and magnitude of the arrows in the figure. It is further to be expected that the microstructure formed will be fine grained (or of a very close dendritic spacing)[22,23] in the area of initial solidification and somewhat larger in the region of final solidification. Also, the very last element to solidify will be in the depressed region of the surface in contact with the air or atmosphere above the melt.

The mechanism of solidification can be best understood by taking an atomistic approach. The initiation of solidification occurs at locations of minimum energy content, e.g., at the surface of a "seed" crystal or a cluster of "cold" atoms that have deviated from equilibrium to a sufficient degree to form an embryo temporarily possessing a lattice structure. Since the solid state is thermodynamically a more stable state than the corresponding liquid state, nucleation of solid particles will initiate at sites along the liquid–solid interface where the highest probability of nucleating sites occurs. However, the primary force for initiation of solidification is the large temperature gradient existing at the liquid–solid interface, thereby setting the condition for excellent conduction cooling. Solidification will then propagate into the liquid at some decreasing rate.

The principle of conduction cooling was well applied to the study of retained high-temperature phases. Pol Duwez,[19] in his 1967 Campbell Memorial lecture, reviewed the results of quenching from the liquid state. He stated that conduction cooling is best realized when the following conditions are satisfied: (1) A very good thermal contact exists between the liquid and the substrate, i.e., the parent solid phase; (2) the liquid layer is relatively thin; and (3) the time between initial contact of liquid with the substrate and the end of solidification is as short as possible. Obviously, with the laser, the liquid is always in contact with the solid phase, so that the time from laser shutoff to the end of solidification should be as short as those found for the fast quenching experiments.

One of the techniques developed for the liquid quenching approach is the Gun technique, in which a liquid globule is accelerated to a high speed and then spread on a heat-conductive substrate under centrifugal force, a type of "splat cooling." Cooling rates for liquid iron on a copper substrate were computed from a theoretical analysis[24] which showed that, for a 100 μm liquid spread thickness, the cooling rates in °C/s for heat transfer coefficients of infinity, 100, and 1, were 8×10^5, 7×10^5, and 6×10^4, respectively. A cooling rate of 3×10^5 °C/s was approximated based on high-speed camera analysis of a laser affected melt puddle of beryllium copper on palladium. The camera frame rate was 8500 frames/s, and the final solidified bead measured 0.35 mm in diameter and was approximately 50 μm thick. Figure 3-28 shows the transverse section of such a weld bead, typical of the one used in the high-speed photography study.

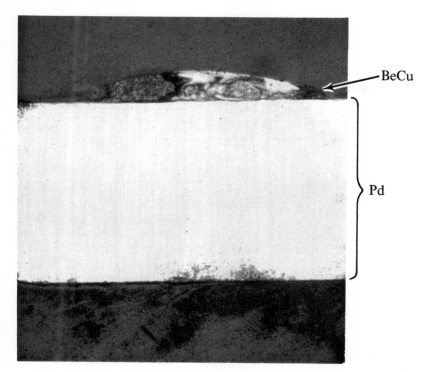

Figure 3-28   A 50 μm thick beryllium-copper solidified melt spread on palladium.   Mag. 200X.

Since it can be concluded that the rapid cooling of a laser-melted volume of metal in contact with its solid phase is essentially by conduction, then one can look more closely at the heterogeneous nucleation from the solid surface into the liquid phase.   Heterogeneous nucleation is defined[25] as the formation of a nucleus of a certain critical size by the catalytic action from a suitable surface in contact with the liquid.   (Although the discussion is restricted to a single-component metal, the principles apply equally to binary systems.)   Nucleation initiates at low energy sites at the liquid–solid interface, as illustrated in Figure 3-29.

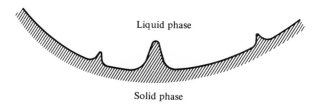

Figure 3-29   Protuberances at the liquid-solid interface.

Supercooling Before proceeding further with nucleation, a look at the solid–liquid phase change by considering the cooling rate curve for a pure metal would be helpful. Figure 3-30 shows the temperature-time plot for a single component system.

The difference $(T_0 - T_1)$ represents the degree of undercooling or supercooling of the liquid before solidification starts. In practice, many metals undergo appreciable supercooling before solidification; for example, molten platinum can be supercooled by as much as 370° below its equilibrium temperature (T_e or T_0 from Figure 3-30).[26]

A condition that must be satisfied to undercool or supercool a liquid is that *none* of the solid phase be present.[27] There must be a real distinction between the liquid and the solid for the nucleation time period which is related to the metastability of the supercooled liquid. In order to understand the metastability of a supercooled liquid it is necessary to consider the mechanism involved in the formation of a nucleating crystal. This would require a treatment on the thermodynamics of solidification,[27] which is not given here. However, from free-energy concepts, it can be shown that at the solid–liquid interface, the free energy of the solid which is at a temperature below the equilibrium temperature (i.e., the fusion temperature) is less than that of the liquid phase. This is a consequence of the thermodynamic definition of equilibrium. Thus, the solid is the more stable phase, and the transformation of liquid to solid would always proceed spontaneously.

Nucleation from the Liquid Phase If one considers the initial conditions for the start of nucleation, i.e., the stability of a geometrical particle or crystal under equilibrium conditions, it will be seen that very small particles have a larger surface area-to-volume ratio than larger particles. Their stability will differ appreciably since equilibrium between

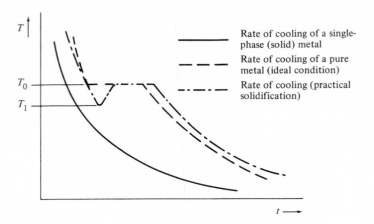

Figure 3-30 *Typical temperature-time plot for a single component system.*

solid and liquid across a curved interface differs from that across a planar interface.   The smaller particles will tend to redissolve and the larger ones will tend to grow.   Consider the generally convex surface of a small particle.   The individual atoms that go to make up the potential nucleating particle are, on the average, less tightly bound in a convex surface than those of a flat surface (i.e., they have, on the average, a poor fit into the lattice structure so that few of them are in equilibrium with their nearest neighbors).   As the radius of curvature increases, more atoms are available at the surface and more atoms, statistically, will be situated in stable lattice sites.   Then the total free energy of the particle will be negative and the reaction (solidification) will go to completion.   There is, in fact, a critical size at which the free energy of the particle is a maximum before decreasing. The process of redissolving or growing is, of course, temperature dependent. The critical radius is defined in Ref. 27 as that existing at any temperature below T_0, (i.e., a temperature necessary for an embryonic particle to form), for which the rate of dissolution of the particle back into the liquid state equals the rate of growth in the solid state.   Thus a large degree of supercooling can be effected which would in turn generally favor a rapid solidification, provided the latent heat can be removed quickly enough.

The above considerations show that solidification of laser-melted metals can be treated from the heterogeneous nucleation theory because of a large degree of supercooling.   The theory is found to help explain the microstructures seen in laser fusion welding and similar melt reactions. In addition, it provides some basis for the observed relationship between dendrite spacing and degree of supercooling.[28]

One additional cause of supercooling in alloy systems is the rejection of solute by the freezing solid and the consequent enrichment of the liquid near the growing interface, i.e., the protuberance.   The enriched liquid then has a lower freezing temperature.[29]   Therefore, if solidification is to continue, the temperature of the liquid in contact with the solid must be low enough to maintain the necessary amount of supercooling.   Since the freezing temperature of the liquid rises with increasing distance from the surface of the solid, it is possible for the amount of supercooling to increase for a distance into the liquid before decreasing to zero.   If the thickness of supercooled liquid is large, then the growth extensions of the protuberances can proceed well in advance of the completely solidified portions, and, as noted, a dendritic pattern of growth is obtained.   Under the conditions previously discussed, the growth of a dendrite consists of not only the main axis of growth but also of secondary and higher-order axes that branch off the existing axes.

3.4.2   grain growth

For pure metals, dendritic structures are not seen, but instead columnar grains are found, quite similar in orientation to ingot castings taken from a mold.   When a melt puddle is made in a pure metal, by laser-energy absorption, the liquid at the solid–liquid interface is quickly cooled to the equilibrium melting temperature T_0 and stable nuclei are formed on the protuberances along the interface.   These nuclei grow rapidly into grains of roughly spherical shape, liberating a large latent heat of fusion.   This heat plus the superheat of the liquid metal must be dissipated through the interface and the layer of solidified metal.   Therefore, the rate of growth of the crystals soon becomes limited by the rate of heat removal rather than by the inherent growth velocity (the latter is extremely large).   The temperature distribution in the solidifying metal at this stage has a relatively shallow gradient.   The small amount of supercooling in advance of the growing grains does not permit nucleation of new grains, and many of the grains in the solidifying layer give way to more favorably oriented grains, which, in many cases, are the parent grains originating in the solid phase. These two factors give rise to the columnar structure.   The columnar grains tend to have a characteristic crystal direction as their axis, and they advance uniformly into the liquid.   In pure metals, this type of solidification continues to the upper center of the melt puddle (Figure 3-27). Figure 3-31 is a very good example of this type of grain growth, as experienced with a laser melted puddle.

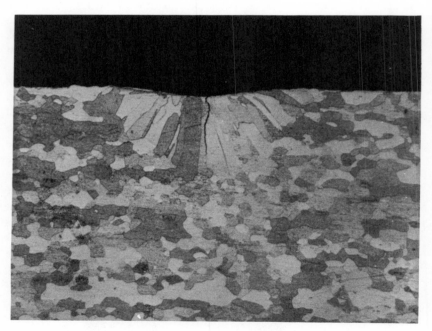

Figure 3-31 Laser-melted arc-cast molybdenum demonstrating columnar grain growth into the fusion zone.   Note the outline shape of fused zone as compared to the sketch of Figure 3-12.[14]   (With permission of Academic Press Inc.)

References

1. G. Gaubau, "Optical Relations for Coherent Wave Beams," *Electromagnetic Theory and Antennas*, E. C. Jordan, Ed., p. 907, Pergamon Press, New York (1963).
2. H. Kogelnik, "Imaging of Optical Modes—Resonators with Internal Lenses," *Bell System Tech. J.* **44**, 455–494 (March 1965).
3. H. Kogelnik and T. Li, "Laser Beams and Resonators," *Appl. Optics* **5**, No. 10, 1550–1567 (October 1966).
4. R. L. Fork, D. Herriott, and H. Kogelnik, "A Scanning Spherical Mirror Interferometer for Spectral Analysis of Laser Radiation," *Appl. Optics* **3**, No. 12, 1471 (December 1964).
5. J. E. Anderson and J. E. Jackson, "An Evaluation of Pulsed Laser Welding," *Proc. Electron and Laser Beam Symposium* (sponsored by Pennsylvania State University and Alloyd General Corporation), A. B. ElKareh, Ed., pp. 17–50 (1965).
6. M. I. Cohen, "Laser Beams and Integrated Circuits," *Bell Labs Record* **45**, 247–251 (September 1967).
7. D. K. Wilson, "Design of Best-Form Lenses for Laser Application," *Optical Spectra*, p. 52 (March/April, 1968).
8. J. B. Jones and G. A. Hawkins, *Engineering Thermodynamics*, John Wiley and Sons, Inc., New York (1963).
9. H. S. McCracken, "Parameters Effecting Laser Welding," 1967 Materials Engineering Exposition and Congress, Cleveland, Ohio, *ASM Tech. Report C7-19.1*.
10. K. K. Kelly, Contributions to the Data on Theoretical Metallurgy, U.S. Department of the Interior, *Bureau of Mines Bulletin No. 584*.
11. J. F. Ready, "Effects Due to Absorption of Laser Radiation," *J. Appl. Phys.* **36**, 462 (1965).
12. H. S. Carslaw and J. C. Jaeger, *Conduction of Heat in Solids*, Oxford University Press, New York (1959).
13. M. I. Cohen, "Melting of a Half-Space Subjected to a Constant Heat Input," *J. Franklin Inst.* **283**, 271–285 (April 1967).
14. M. I. Cohen and J. Epperson, "Applications of Lasers to Microelectronic Fabrication," *Electron Beam and Laser Beam Technology*, Academic Press Inc., New York (1968).
15. F. W. Dabby and U. C. Paek, "High Intensity Laser Induced Vaporization and Explosion of Solid Material," *IEEE J. Quantum Electronics* **QE-8**, 106–111 (1972).
16. H. Klocke, "Untersuch Ungen Zum Materialabbau Durch Laserstrahlung," *Spectrochimica Acta* **243**, 263 (1969).
17. M. I. Cohen, private communication.
17a. H. G. Landau, "Heat Conduction in a Melting Solid," *Quart. Appl. Math.* **8**, 81 (1950).
18. U. C. Paek and F. P. Gagliano, "Thermal Analysis of Laser Drilling Processes," *IEEE J. Quantum Electronics* **QE-8**, 112–119 (1972).
19. P. Duwez, "Structure and Properties of Alloys Rapidly Quenched from the Liquid State," *Trans. Am. Soc. Metals* **60**, 607 (1967).

20. R. K. Linde, "Kinetics of Transformation of Metastable Silver-Copper Solid Solutions," Ph.D. Thesis, California Institute of Technology, Pasadena, Calif. (1964).
21. L. S. Darken and R. W. Gurry, *Physical Chemistry of Metals*, McGraw-Hill Book Co., New York (1953).
22. H. Matyja, B. C. Giessen, and N. J. Grant, "The Effect of Cooling Rate on the Dendrite Spacing in Splat-Cooled Aluminum Alloys," *J. Inst. Metals* **60**, 30 (1968).
23. R. H. Willens and B. C. Giessen, "Rapidly Quenched (Splat Cooled) Metastable Phases; Their Phase Diagram Representation, Preparation Methods, Occurrence and Properties," in *The Use of Phase Diagrams in Ceramics, Glass, and Metal Technology*, A. M. Alper, Ed., Academic Press Inc. (1970).
24. R. C. Ruhl, "Cooling Rates in Splat Cooling," *Materials Sci. Eng.* **1**, 313 (1967).
25. D. Turnbull, "Kinetics of Solidification of Supercooled Liquid Mercury Droplets," *J. Chem. Phys.* **20**, 411 (1952).
26. D. Turnbull, "Formation of Crystal Nuclei in Liquid Metal," *J. Appl. Phys.* **21**, 1022 (1950).
27. B. Chalmers, *Principles of Solidification*, p. 62, John Wiley and Sons, Inc., New York (1964).
28. N. H. Fletcher, "Size Effect in Heterogeneous Nucleation," *J. Chem. Phys.* **29**, No. 3, 572–576 (1958).
29. A. G. Guy, *Elements of Physical Metallurgy*, 2nd Ed., p. 156, Addison-Wesley Publishing Co., Reading, Mass. (1959).

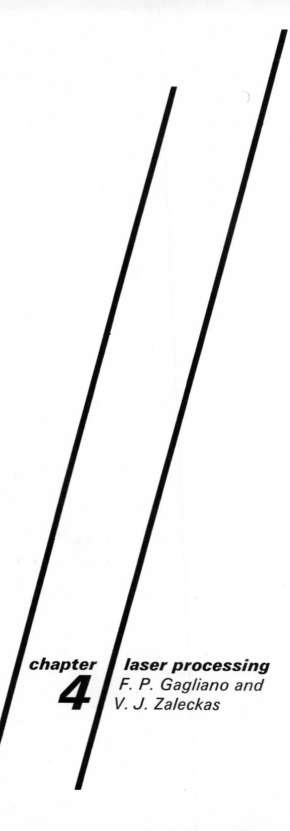

chapter
4

laser processing
F. P. Gagliano and
V. J. Zaleckas

4·0   introduction

The purpose of this chapter is to review examples of laser processing, primarily those in the general categories of welding, drilling, and micro-machining.   Each category is illustrated by general principles and a review of pertinent laser applications.   Then, by the review of a production application, the analytical and practical aspects of applying the laser are illustrated.   The examples chosen also demonstrate the need for a variety of lasers by emphasizing the required operating characteristics.

4·1   welding

Fusion welding is one major fabrication process where the laser has found a relatively active although not a large field of applications.   The cross-sectional thickness of the weld design is often the limiting factor which accounts for the dearth of welding applications.   The unidirectional thermal penetration of the absorbed laser intensity is limited to a relatively shallow depth of fused material.   It would seem then that electronic and microelectronic interconnections of cross-sectional thicknesses less than 0.5 mm are the prime areas for an increasing use of laser welders.[1] (charshan 1982)

Metals are the predominant materials that have been joined by laser welding.   Some thermoplastics, however, can be heat sealed or welded, since the absorption by organic polymers of infrared radiation is generally very good.   This fact coupled to the relatively low melting and softening temperatures of plastics makes this type of application very attractive to the packaging industry.   Other nonmetallics, such as quartz, have also been joined.[2] (charshan.

4·1·1   fusion depth and weld geometry

The physical size and geometry of the component parts of a weldment are presently restricted to the small-scale category, from the microminiature, e.g., integrated circuit (IC) technology and thin films, to an upper limit related to the fusion depth.   Normally, the maximum thickness of metal that can be welded where full weld penetration is desired, as in a butt joint, is approximately 1 mm.[3]   Up to about twice this thickness can be welded with complete fusion penetration if some material depletion[4,5] is acceptable.   However, recent investigations[6,7] with a CO_2 convection laser have shown that deep penetration welds can be made using multi-kilowatt CW outputs.   Figure 4-1 shows a longitudinal section of a butt weld with complete fusion penetration made in 302-type stainless steel 6.35 mm thick.

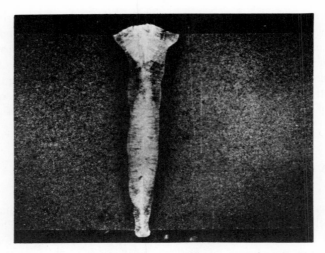

Figure 4-1.   Butt weld of 0.25 in. (6.35 mm) thick 302-type stainless steel using a CO_2 laser operated as an amplifier unit giving an output of 3.5 kW.   The material was moved under a 25 cm focal-length mirror at a speed of 2 cm/s.[6]   (With permission of United Aircraft Research Laboratories.)

For a pulsed laser-welder, the duration of the light energy is short, nominally 2–10 ms so that the generated depth of the fusion front in the material is limited.   This limit is dependent on the thermal properties of the materials, as was shown in Chapter 3.

In any laser-induced transformation on a material, whether it be welding, drilling, or evaporation, the first objective is to deliver sufficient beam intensity to the surface of the material to compensate for surface reflectivity losses.   Upon sacrificing some of the energy because of the surface reflectance, which may be as high as 95 percent of the incident intensity, the remainder is then efficiently absorbed to some depth (see Section 2.5.3).

At this step of the laser light-material interaction, some form of heat transfer mechanics takes over, so that the extent of penetration of the fusion front or volume of material vaporized can be related to the laser parameters.   Some idea of the energy needed can be obtained from the data of Table 4-1.   In addition to the more common metals, the table lists many other materials with their enthalpy values at a given temperature. The last column gives the amount of energy required to be absorbed by a unit mass of material to have its temperature increased from "room temperature" to the value given in the second column.   The values are calculated from the general heat content equation (see Section 3.2)

$$H_T - H_{298.16} = aT + bT^2 + cT^{-1} + d \qquad (4\text{-}1)$$

TABLE 4-1 Enthalpy Values (ΔH_{T-298})

Material	$T(°K)^a$	Kcal/Mole	$J/\mu g$ ($\times 10^{-3}$)
Aluminum	1900	13.63	2.11
Beryllium	2700	19.30	8.95
Carbon (graphite)	4000^b	21.31	7.42
Chromium	2600	25.33	2.04
Copper	2370	16.48	1.08
Gold	2400	17.33	0.37
Gold	3264^c	135.24	2.87
Iron	2800	28.26	2.11
Molybdenum	4300	41.04	1.79
Nickel	2700	24.51	1.74
Palladium	2300	19.24	0.76
Platinum	3700	31.18	0.67
Silicon	2300	24.43	3.64
Silver	1900	14.03	0.54
Tantalum	3270	20.78	0.48
Tin	1900	13.34	0.47
Titanium	3000	25.84	2.25
Tungsten	3700^d	22.16	0.50
Zinc	1000	6.65	0.42

[a] The temperature is selected at a value 2/3 the interval between the melting and boiling points.
[b] Sublimation.
[c] Boiling point—gas.
[d] Melting point—liquid.

where $a + 2bT - cT^{-2} = C_p$ (the heat capacity), $a, b, c,$ and d are constants determined from experimental data, and T is the temperature in degrees Kelvin.[8]

The data in Table 4-1 apply only to an isolated mass of material, thermally insulated and under constant pressure. Although these conditions do not exist in practice, the calculated data can provide a good working guideline in setting initial laser parameters.

For the general case, maximum penetration occurs when the surface temperature has reached the boiling point. Materials differ widely in their maximum achievable melt depths, primarily due to differences in thermal properties. Magnesium and similar low-temperature melting alloys tend to have excessive material depleted surfaces, particularly if their thermal diffusivity is low. Metals with high vapor pressure have a greater tendency to vaporize when irradiated with a focused laser beam. Alloys with an appreciable zinc content tend to "overmelt" in attempts to weld them. Large aggregates of zinc atoms can boil out of the melt, producing uneven melting and often with a resultant porous weld structure.[9]

An example of a weld where complete fusion penetration is required for maximum weld strength is shown in Figure 4-2. The material is

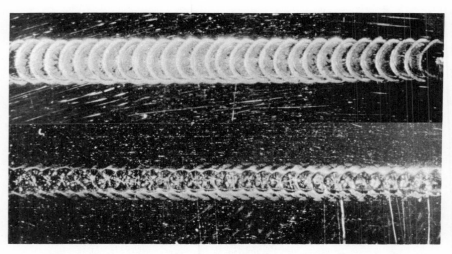

Figure 4-2   Butt welding relatively thin materials.   The photograph shows the front side to the laser beam (top), and the back of 7 mil (0.18 mm) thick stainless steel (bottom).

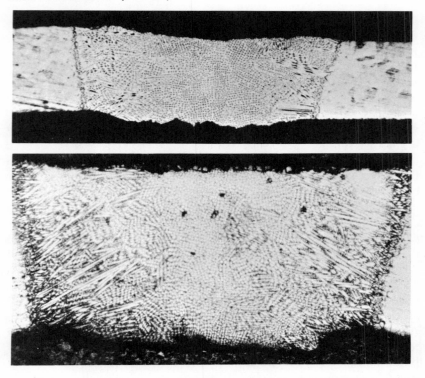

Figure 4-3   Seam weld of 0.046 cm thick (top) and 0.068 cm thick (bottom) alloy steel (AMS 5544).[10]   *Mag. 35X.   (With permission of the* **Welding Journal.)**

0.18 mm thick 402-type stainless band steel.   The weld was made using overlapping spots with a ruby laser.   The beam energy was 12 J and the pulse length was 5.5 ms pulsed at a rate of 20/min.   The effective spot diameter was approximately 1 mm and the power density on the weld area was 6×10^5 W/cm^2 (a 67 mm focal length lens defocused into the steel by 3.8 mm).

A CW or a high repetition rate (more than 30 pulses per second (pps)) laser would, of course, be a better choice for seam welding.   Figure 4-3 shows some results for alloy steels using the CO_2 laser.[10]   The samples were welded with a beam output of 195 W, CW.   The beam was focused with an $f/1$ Irtran II lens* to a spot size of about 1.2 mm in diameter and which gave a power density of approximately 15 kW/cm^2 on the surface. The welding speed was 0.5 cm/s.

However, with the multi-kilowatt CO_2 lasers, seam welding of thicker materials at greater speeds is feasible.   For example, the weld shown in Figure 4-1 was made with a focused power density of approximately 10^6 W/cm^2.   It is theorized that at this intensity a void is established, i.e., a drilled hole, allowing energy to be absorbed in the body of the material. If the material is moved at some threshold rate related to the time required for expulsion of material, then the void becomes stable and translates with the movement with subsequent filling and solidification occurring behind it.   Although the fusion depth reported in Refs. 6 and 7 is about three to four times deeper than any other known laser weld, the proposed mechanism of the weld formation implies that thermal penetration by conduction in the solid and/or liquid state has not been extended beyond about 1 mm because of the multi-kilowatt CW power outputs.

Joint geometry also influences the thickness that can be welded. Since there is little time for material flow and a relatively small amount of molten material, the process will most always require close fitting joints. In practice, there are many joint designs that do not require full fusion penetration.   Indeed, full fusion penetration may be quite impractical or unnecessary to the design function.   Figure 4-4 illustrates several common types of joint geometries that are applicable to laser welding.[12] One good example of joint geometry and need of good fitting between the component parts is shown in Figure 4-5.

---

* Eastman Kodak Company zinc sulfide material.   The Irtran lenses have a transmittance of about 85-90 percent to 10.6×10^3 nm radiation but have a relatively low damage threshold level.   Coated germanium lenses are 95 percent transmittive and are considered to be quite stable to ambient conditions normally found in the laboratory or manufacturing shop floor.   The salt (KCl and NaCl) lenses though possessing the highest damage threshold levels may be difficult to keep free of adsorbed moisture and other vapors which makes them rather impractical to use in a manufacturing environment.   The salt lenses happen to be the least expensive.   Gallium arsenide lens material has been found to take a high-quality permanent optical finish and is considered to be the best of the semiconductor materials possessing a high (100 W/cm^2) damage threshold, but is much more expensive than any of the other lenses.[11]

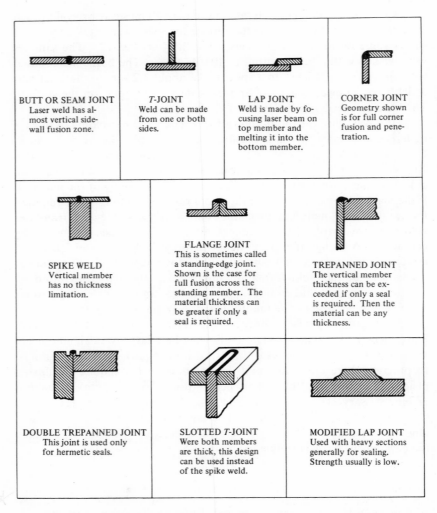

BUTT OR SEAM JOINT
Laser weld has almost vertical sidewall fusion zone.

T-JOINT
Weld can be made from one or both sides.

LAP JOINT
Weld is made by focusing laser beam on top member and melting it into the bottom member.

CORNER JOINT
Geometry shown is for full corner fusion and penetration.

SPIKE WELD
Vertical member has no thickness limitation.

FLANGE JOINT
This is sometimes called a standing-edge joint. Shown is the case for full fusion across the standing member. The material thickness can be greater if only a seal is required.

TREPANNED JOINT
The vertical member thickness can be exceeded if only a seal is required. Then the material can be any thickness.

DOUBLE TREPANNED JOINT
This joint is used only for hermetic seals.

SLOTTED T-JOINT
Were both members are thick, this design can be used instead of the spike weld.

MODIFIED LAP JOINT
Used with heavy sections generally for sealing. Strength usually is low.

Figure 4-4   Some joint designs for laser welding.[12]   (*With permission of* **Machine Design.**)

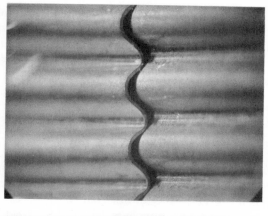

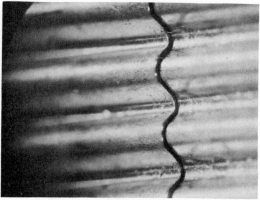

Figure 4-5   Examples of poor fitting (top) and good fitting (bottom) for seam welding of corrugated sheet steel.

4·1·2   welding speeds

In continuous welding, the speed is limited by several factors. It is primarily a function of the power density on the material and the time for fusion penetration to some depth. These factors hold for both the CW and the pulsed lasers. However, for pulsed lasers, the pulse repetition rate is also a major factor. A rate of 1 pps is commonplace today, and at an appreciably high energy level (>10 J). Although present laser welding equipment requires a relatively long delay between one weld spot and the next, a change in length of this delay does not affect the weld quality.

Pulsed laser welding is a relatively slow process when compared to other welding techniques, averaging between 0.5 and 5 cm/min for over-lapping spots with a pulsing rate of 1 pps. However, high repetition rate

(>30 pps), high-energy ($\sim 1 - 40$ J/pulse) pulsed lasers are now available. This would then increase the speeds to about 5 to 50 cm/min. On the other hand, welding with a high power CO_2 laser pulsed at 100 to 1000 Hz would give speeds of 12 to 60 cm/min. With higher power CO_2 and YAG systems, welding speeds as high as 125 cm/min can be expected.[13]

4·1·3   laser systems and their operating parameters

In considering laser systems for welding applications, one major factor that must first be determined is the output of the system in power and energy. When operating lasers in the pulsed mode, the duration of the lasing action is important. For characterizing laser welding, these parameters and others may be separated into two groups—a primary group of two and a secondary group of four.

Energy and Power   The output energy for solid-state pulsed systems, commonly measured in joules, is a function of a charging voltage obtained from the power supply, on a bank of capacitors designated the energy storage unit. The stored energy is discharged in a high intensity flash lamp which excites the laser rod for stimulated emission.

Ruby and neodymium: glass are the two lasing materials used in most commercial pulsed welding systems. Also, large Nd: YAG crystals are now available which can produce high energies from standard flash pumped cavity designs. Ruby is generally more rugged and can be pumped harder to produce higher energies. Nd: glass has a lower lasing threshold, and while operating over a wider temperature range (up to 85°F) can, in general, give higher slope efficiencies, i.e., the calculated slope of the output against the input energies. Its lower thermal conductivity and susceptibility to damage under higher pumping levels limits its ability to achieve high average output power. However, there are indications that some of these shortcomings have been overcome.[14] One approach uses a disc or segmented design which allows for increased cooling efficiency with subsequent higher output energies.

The Nd: YAG crystal not only has a low threshold energy but also a low thermal time constant, lower than either the ruby or Nd: glass. Consequently, commercially available Nd: YAG systems have a higher average power capability than the ruby or the Nd: glass lasers. Figures 4-6, 4-7, and 4-8 show typical energy output plots for high-energy ruby, Nd: glass, and Nd: YAG commercial systems, respectively. (The volume of laser crystal is essentially the same for the ruby and Nd: YAG, whereas the Nd: glass rod is more than twice the volume of the ruby and YAG rods.) The energy readings for all cases were obtained at a pulsing rate of not more than 1 pps.

CW gas lasers, specifically the CO_2 laser, operate by simple discharge of a direct current into the gas (CO_2-N_2-He mixture). Efficiencies of 15 percent to 20 percent of the input power are obtainable in presently available systems. Commercial systems are now available with CW power outputs of up to 1 kW, which appreciably extend their welding capability. Outputs of tens of kilowatts have been reported for the electric-discharge convection laser (EDCL) type.[15] The transverse excited atmospheric (TEA) type laser has shown the capability of producing peak powers in excess of 20 MW when operated in the pulsed excitation mode.[16] Figure 4-9 gives the CW power output for a commercial 250 W rated unit as a function of the discharge current for constant gas pressures.

CW operation with powers higher than 300 W can also be obtained with continuous lamp discharge pumping of Nd:YAG crystals. Krypton and tungsten-halogen (iodine or bromine) lamps have been successfully used in single and double ellipse cavities with lamp lives of a few hours to several hundred hours depending on the operating power level. Efficiencies of these high-power CW YAG systems are nominally rated at 2 percent with krypton pumping and about 0.5 percent with tungsten-iodine pumping. Higher powers (up to 1200 W CW) can be obtained using several YAG crystals in series.[17]

Pulse Length The following discussion is applicable to pulsed operation of the solid-state lasers.

Pulse length is effectively controlled by the amount of capacitance (actually capacitance-inductance groups) in the excitation circuit. The proper matching of the flash lamp to the electronics and the optical coupling geometry in the laser head assembly both greatly aid in optimizing the laser pulse characteristics for effective welding. In general, the longer the pulse length, the more the workpiece or weldment will react along the fusion mechanism of energy absorption, heat transfer, melting, intermixing of constituents, and subsequent solidification. With good control of the laser beam, vaporization and particle expulsion can be minimized.

Present commercial systems can achieve pulse lengths up to about 12 ms. With respect to temporal pulse shape, studies have shown that, in general, an exponentially decaying pulse shape is favored for welding work as opposed to a square wave shape. For example, consider gold, which has a high reflectivity (see Section 3.1.4) at the wavelength of ruby, yet very good thermal properties, such as high diffusivity. It would be desirable to have the first part of the laser pulse overcome the initial high reflectivity of the solid surface, then continue at lower intensity to minimize vaporization, yet effect sufficient heat transfer for melting. Figure 4-10 shows an oscilloscope trace showing the time variation of the power in a typical pulse from a ruby laser.

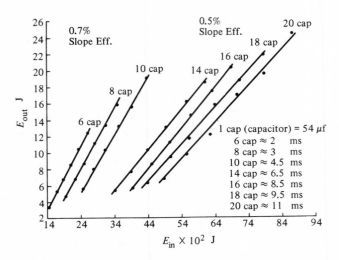

Figure 4-6   Energy output characteristics of a ruby laser.   (Data for the laser system shown in Figure 4-34.)

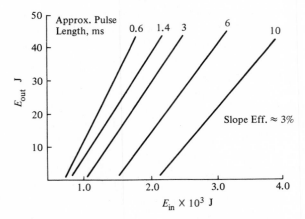

Figure 4-7   Energy output characteristics of a typical Nd:glass laser. (From American Optical Corporation data.)

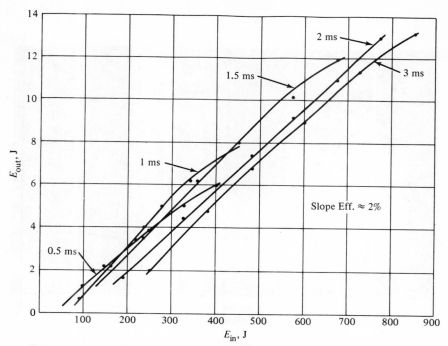

Figure 4-8   Energy output characteristics of a Nd:YAG pulsed laser.

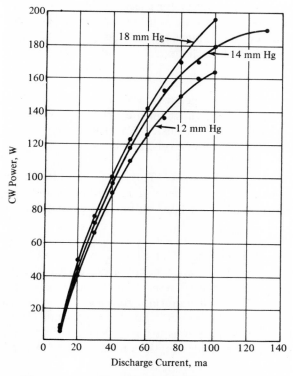

Figure 4-9   CW power output of a CO_2 laser.

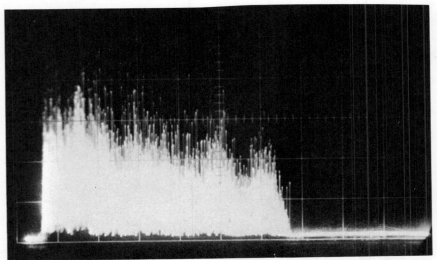

Figure 4-10   Typical long pulse shape from a ruby laser.   High LC value gives a generally decaying shape.   Note the highly spiked nature of the pulse.

The best possible condition for energy input to a weldment is to have the energy delivered at constant surface temperatures as opposed to input at a temporally constant intensity.[4]   Although this is highly desirable, it is not known whether such control is readily adaptable to commercial systems.

Wavelength   The characteristic wavelength for each lasing material determines to a large degree how much of the beam focused on a material is absorbed and converted into heat.   Wavelength changes can be effected by use of devices like harmonic generators.

Power Density or Intensity   This is a dependent variable.   It is commonly expressed in watts per square centimeter and is the result of concentrating the unfocused laser output power, normally by a simple lens.

Focusing and Spot Size   This plays a major role in providing a wide latitude in determining the amount of power density a given material sees.   For high-energy pulsed laser systems the beam intensity at the focal plane generally is not uniform across the focal spot because of the spatial distribution of the output.   For focused beams (Section 3.1), the optical spot diameter is given as a function of the beam divergence and the focal length of the condensing lens used ($2w = f\theta$; where θ is the full angle divergence).

Defocusing techniques (adjusting the workpiece surface at a plane other than the focal plane of the beam focusing lens) provide added control on the amount of heat generated in the weld area.   Simple experiments on bulk material (greater than 250 μm thick) have generated data of the kind shown in Figure 4-11.   The data illustrate the effect of the laser beam—material interaction by the variations in the effective spot size generated in the material.   The increase in the effective spot diameter as the average power per pulse is increased is due in part to the increased energy per pulse and also to an increase in the beam divergence.   Engineering working curves can be constructed from effective spot size measurements as shown in Figure 4-12.   (This particular plot was developed for the welding application shown subsequently in Figure 4-18.)

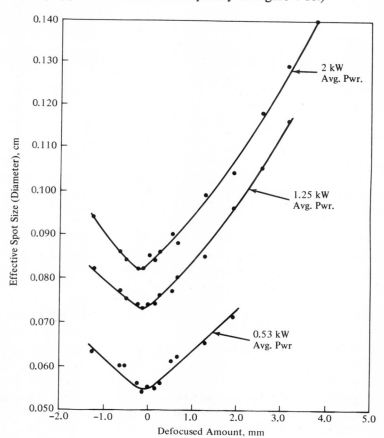

Figure 4-11   Effective spot size on Ni-Co-Fe (low expansion) alloy.

    Ruby laser: **0.6943 × 10³ nm output**

    Beam size: **3/8 in. dia.**

    Lens: **15 mm dia.–25 mm focal length**

Note: Average power is defined as the average power per pulse.

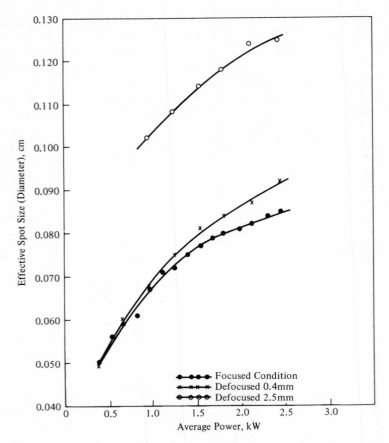

Figure 4-12   *Effective spot size on Ni-Co-Fe (low expansion) alloy.*
Ruby laser: 0.6943 × 10³ nm output
Beam size: 3/8 in. dia.
Lens: 15 mm dia.–25 mm focal length
Note: Average power is defined as the average power per pulse.

Other Factors   The joint design and the welding speed, discussed previously, are also factors that affect laser welding production capability. Their importance is illustrated by a recent study for the laser welding of a reed type relay which has two different diameter wires for the switch actuating coil windings. The wire coil leads and the reed switch leads are joined to 0.38 mm thick tin-coated brass terminals. Figure 4-13 shows the relay with laser welded connections. Three connections are seen at one end. The other end has the same three connections except that the coil wires (which are polyurethane coated) are 0.075 mm in diameter instead of 0.15 mm in diameter (the primary winding). The relay switch leads are 0.55 mm in diameter.

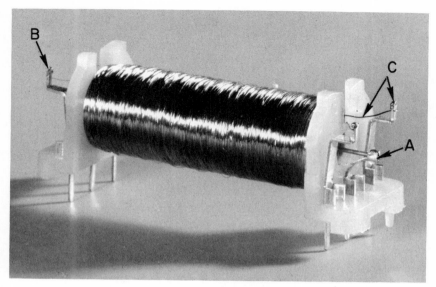

Figure 4-13   Terminal welding (arrows A, B, and C) of a dual wire-wound reed-type relay.

Initial attempts at effecting the welds showed that the switch lead-to-terminal connection could be routinely made by focusing the beam at the interface between one side of the wire and the " U " bend terminal (arrow A in Figure 4-13).   The coil wire-to-terminal connection presented some difficulties because of a large difference in their relative mass, especially for the smaller gauge wire.   For the case of the smaller (0.075 mm diameter) size wire, the relative mass of the tab to $1\frac{1}{2}$ turns of the wire is $22:1$ (arrow B).   With two turns of the larger (0.15 mm diameter) size wire, the ratio is $4:1$ (arrow C).

A design change of the terminal tab (see Figure 4-14) gave a mass ratio of $3:1$ for three turns of the 0.075 mm diameter wire and $1.5:1$ for two turns of the 0.15 mm diameter wire.   Consistent and uniform welds were then obtained (Figure 4-15).   All connections were welded with the same energy, 4.8 J focused through a 35 mm focal-length lens.   The pulse length was 3.7 ms.   (The problems of relative mass of the weld components   and   the   joint   design   have   been   investigated   quite thoroughly.[1,18,19])

It was also required that the six welds for each relay be welded within 4 s in order to make the application economical.   A Nd:YAG laser flash pumped at 3 pps could weld fifty relays in less than $2\frac{1}{2}$ min.   This kind of engineering analysis will very often provide the necessary guidelines for a potential application to become a manufacturing reality.

Altering the laser beam by means of *filters*, *apertures*, *masks*, and *beam-shaping optics* must also be considered.   Filters are rarely used,

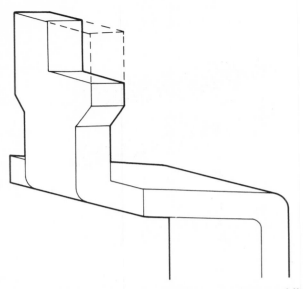

Figure 4-14   Suggested terminal design for laser welding.

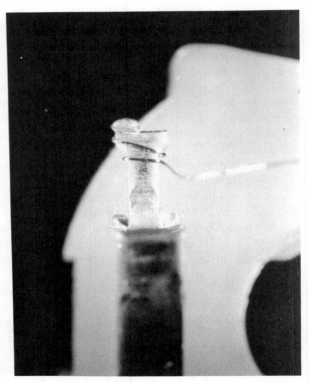

Figure 4-15   Enlargement of a wire-terminal weld showing the weld bead and geometry.

but apertures and masks are frequently used in hole drilling and thin-film machining. Beam-shaping optics have been used in a relatively large number of applications of the laser: the fabrication of microminiature devices,[20] thin-film circuitry, and metal lead frames.[21]

As an example of beam shaping, a method for noncontact welding of beam lead integrated circuit devices to thin films on alumina substrates using a pulsed laser is described.[22]   A beam lead is a gold electrical contact that extends out from the silicon chip typically 0.22 mm. It was shown that simultaneous welding of multiple beam leads (16—four on each side of silicon chips ranging in size from 0.75 mm to 1.8 mm square) could be accomplished with one pulse from a ruby laser using optics to generate a four-line square pattern.[23]   However, applying this pattern to integrated circuit connections introduced several problems. The mass of the beam leads was much less than the mass of pieces involved in previous work done with a laser; and, because of the size of the chips, special hold-down techniques were required. *Intimate contact* between the beam leads, which are typically 0.012 mm thick by 0.11 mm wide, and the substrate is necessary. A satisfactory technique was developed[24] which consisted of placing a Teflon® film over the chip and substrate and using a vacuum chuck to draw the film down tightly over the two. No damage occurs to the Teflon during welding.

Although the analyzed results indicated that the technique was basically sound and individual welds, shown in cross section in Figure 4-16, were of good quality, the energy distribution along each line and

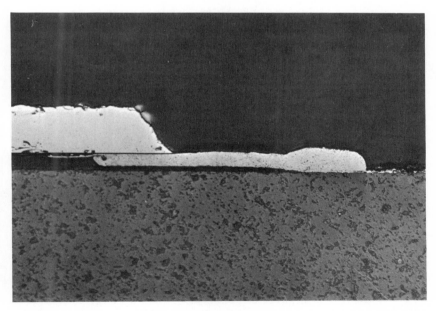

Figure 4-16   Longitudinal section of weld between a gold beam lead and a gold-titanium thin film.   Mag. 200X.

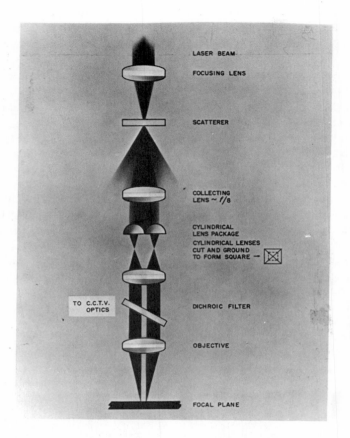

LASER BEAM

FOCUSING LENS

SCATTERER

COLLECTING
LENS ~ f/8

CYLINDRICAL
LENS PACKAGE
CYLINDRICAL LENSES
CUT AND GROUND
TO FORM SQUARE —

TO C.C.T.V.
OPTICS

DICHROIC FILTER

OBJECTIVE

FOCAL PLANE

Figure 4-17 Optical system for beam-lead integrated circuit welding to thin-film conductors.

from one line to another was not consistent.   This could be traced directly to nonuniformity in the spatial distribution of the laser output.   Subsequently, a relatively simple scattering technique, as shown in Figure 4-17, was developed[23] that supplies a reliable, repeatable output.[25]   The scatterer, or diffuser, placed in the path of the beam results in a more uniform intensity at the focal plane.

4·1·4   advantages of laser welding

Justifying the use of the laser for welding applications requires a knowledge of existing welding techniques and an awareness of the areas where improvements can be technically effected and economically realized.   Among the more obvious are production rate and yield.   The least obvious areas can be listed as advantages for the use of the laser as a welding tool.

1. Because of the short time factor associated with this source of heat, welds adjacent to heat-sensitive elements can be effected./ For example, Figure 4-18 shows the laser weld of a transistor element to a nickel alloy part used in the manufacture of transistor devices.[26]   Tweezer welds of the Ni tab (attached to the semiconductor material) to the Kovar post could not meet the vibration test requirements of 15,000 g's minimum. Centrifuge tests of laser welded samples showed bending of the tab members between 20,000 g's and 25,000 g's but no failure of the weld joints.

A cross section of a weld of one of the tabs to the post is shown in Figure 4-19.   The tab is approximately 0.13 mm thick and the post about 0.45 mm in diameter.   A laser beam having an energy of 7.5 J and a 3 ms pulse length was focused with a 25 mm focal-length lens onto the edge of the post in line with its longitudinal axis.   At this point, the beam was defocused with respect to the nickel tab by approximately 0.4 mm.   The weld area, with this defocusing approach, covers more than 180° around the periphery of the post.   With these conditions and neglecting losses, the power density was estimated as 6×10^5 W/cm^2 using the data of Figure 4-12.

2. The short time factor also allows heat-treated and magnetic materials to retain their properties just outside a very small and limited heat affected zone as shown in Figure 4-20.

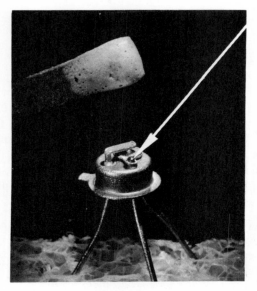

Figure 4-18   A transistor unit showing the laser weld (arrow) of the nickel tab containing the semiconductor material to the nickel alloy post.[26]

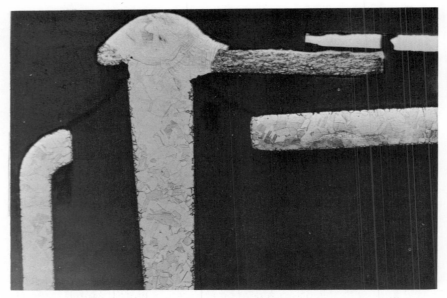

Figure 4-19   Cross section representing a typical transistor unit weld. Note the proximity of the weld to the glass filler, yet no thermal cracking of the glass is evident.

3. Welding in otherwise inaccessible areas is realized with the laser beam. Problems associated with making physical contact of welding electrodes are nonexistent with a light beam.

4. Laser welding, as shown in Figure 4-21, can be performed in many environments, through transparent enclosures and external fields.

5. Materials difficult to weld by the more conventional techniques are sometimes quite easily and reliably joined using the laser. Section 4.1.5 gives a detailed treatment of a manufacturing application for the welding of a multi-element precious metal alloy wire of high electrical resistivity to a phosphor bronze spring. A wide range of materials can be laser welded and general discussions along these lines can be found in the literature.[27,28] Table 4-2 gives a compatibility listing of metals based on the formation of binary systems. Some estimates can be made for alloys consisting of three metal elements.

6. Distortion and shrinkage of the weldment are negligible.

7. Most insulated wires can be effectively welded without prior removal of the insulation (Figure 4-13).

Figure 4-21   The weld repair of vacuum tube leads inside the glass envelope.   The top wire, 3 mm distant from the bottom wire, was initially bent by using the laser at a little less energy than required for the weld.[27] (With permission of Pennsylvania State University.)   →

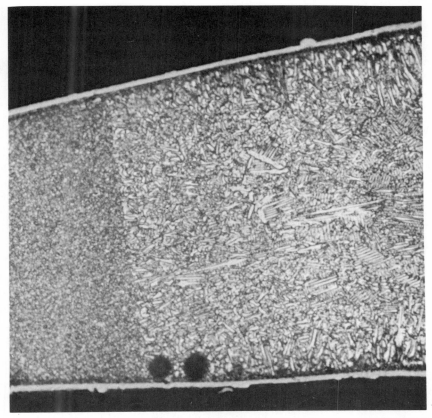

Figure 4-20   Laser welding of 125 μm (5 mils) diameter heat treated beryllium copper wire (Figure 3-25) showing the extent of the heat-affected zone.   The weld would lie to the right of this photograph.   The section is along the wire.   (Difficulties in sectioning produced the taper shown.) To the left of the very pronounced transition line is the microstructure of the original heat-treated condition.   The light envelope about the sample is a 5 μm thick Permalloy electroplate.   Mag. approximately 585X.

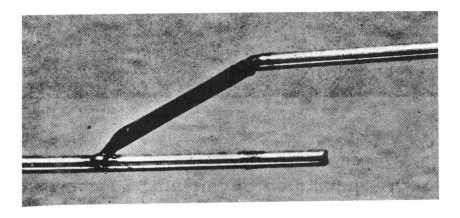

TABLE 4-2 Weldability of Binary Metal Combinations

Legend:
E = Excellent
G = Good
F = Fair
P = Poor
— = No data available

	W	Ta	Mo	Cr	Co	Ti	Be	Fe	Pt	Ni	Pd	Cu	Au	Ag	Mg	Al	Zn	Cd	Pb	Sn
W																				
Ta	E																			
Mo	E	E																		
Cr	E	P	E																	
Co	F	P	F	G																
Ti	F	E	E	G	F															
Be	P	P	P	P	F	P														
Fe	F	F	G	E	E	F	F													
Pt	G	F	G	G	E	F	P	G												
Ni	F	G	F	G	E	F	F	G	E											
Pd	F	G	G	G	E	F	F	G	E	E										
Cu	P	P	P	P	F	F	F	F	E	E	E									
Au	—	—	P	F	P	F	F	F	E	E	E	E								
Ag	P	P	P	P	P	P	F	P	F	E	E	F	E							
Mg	P	—	P	P	P	F	P	P	P	F	P	F	F	F						
Al	P	P	P	P	F	P	P	F	P	F	P	F	F	F	F					
Zn	P	—	P	P	F	P	P	F	P	F	F	G	F	G	P	F				
Cd	—	—	—	P	P	P	—	P	F	P	F	P	F	G	E	P	P			
Pb	P	—	P	P	P	P	—	P	P	P	P	P	P	P	P	P	P	P		
Sn	P	P	P	P	P	P	P	P	F	P	F	P	F	F	P	P	P	P	F	

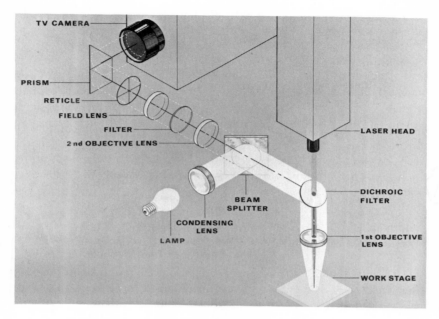

Figure 4-22a Work stage viewing by closed-circuit TV

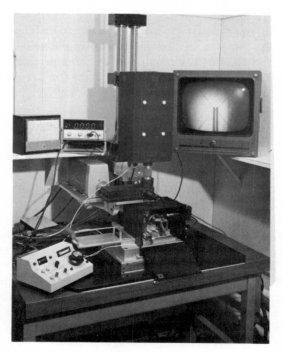

Figure 4-22b Ruby laser system with closed-circuit optics.

8. Conventional tooling and fixturing are easily adaptable to production procedures.

9. Laser beam optics can be readily adaptable to closed-circuit TV viewing, thus providing magnified on-the-spot "inspection" of the processed object. Figures 4-22a and 4-22b illustrate schematically and pictorially how this is done.

Welding techniques can be used for other than making joints and interconnections. For example, selective alloying can be accomplished to join diodes and similar devices. It has been demonstrated that the laser can form silicon diodes by alloying aluminum to a depth of about 1 μm in n-type silicon.[29] Alloy junctions using phosphorus instead of aluminum have also been reported.[30]

4.1.5   analyzing and solving a welding problem

Many electrical and electromechanical connections are made in the electronic industry. These connections are designed to function in service for extended periods of time. Those that are repetitive or cyclic in operation, such as make and break of relay contacts, require mechanical strength and endurance (high fatigue strength) in addition to long-term electrical reliability and stability. One other major requirement for switches is that wear resistance must be high and/or constant at some acceptable value, thus the need for noncorrosive and nonoxidative material. These conditions are commonly met by using precious metal alloys. The mechanical requirements of repetitive operation are usually met by the use of spring temper materials of good electrical conductivity, such as beryllium copper or phosphor bronze.

To achieve all the combined properties described above, the practice is to join relatively small masses of precious metal contacts to a mechanically supportive member of the assembly. The joint or connection then becomes an important consideration in the fabrication of relays and similar components. It must have and retain an adequate degree of the properties of both members of the connection unit.

Soldering, brazing, and fusion welding are the processes used in making electrical and electromechanical connections. Soldering is not normally used for making connections that will undergo dynamic operation, and brazing techniques are usually too involved and expensive for large production runs. Brazed joints are also prone to fatigue cracking, depending upon the component material composition. Resistance welding is the more common joining technique for applications of the type discussed.

This section details a feasibility study of using the laser to effect a fusion weld between a multicomponent precious metal alloy contact material and a phosphor bronze spring leaf member.[31]   The connection had been previously made using resistance welding.   However, the I^2R type of heating gave limited fusion penetration in the weld zone resulting in weak and nonuniform welds.   This was caused by the relatively large difference in electrical resistivity between the two materials: 33.4×10^{-6} ohm-cm[32] for the Paliney® 7 precious metal alloy and 11×10^{-6} ohm-cm[33] for the phosphor bronze.   With I^2R heating, the precious metal wire contacts shown in Figures 4-23 and 4-24 are preferentially heated and melted so that for the normal duration of the current pulse, little melting of the phosphor bronze takes place.   This results in a very shallow fusion region in the phosphor bronze spring.   Increasing the current and/or the electrode pressure or extending the time period invariably produces an excessive liquid metal flow of the contact wire, consequently weakening the joint at the wire-fusion zone.   With the laser as the source of energy into the weldment, electrical properties of the materials are usually not a determining factor for the weldability of a weld system and its subsequent quality.

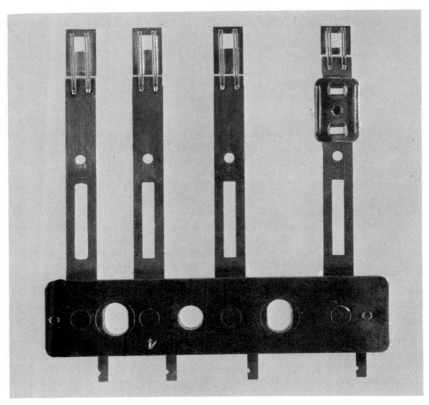

Figure 4-23   Laser welded spring wire contact assembly.   Mag 2.5X.

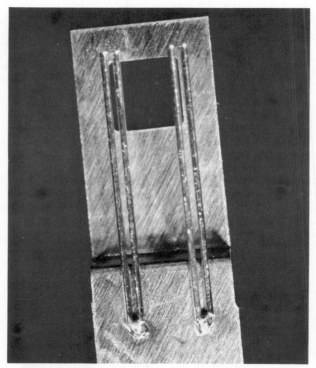

Figure 4-24   Enlarged spring unit.   Mag. 12X.

The Paliney 7-Phosphor Bronze Weld System: Basic Properties
Table 4-3 gives some physical properties of the phosphor bronze and
Paliney 7 alloys.   Although both alloys and especially the Paliney material
are complex with respect to their chemical composition, the physical
properties of importance for a fusion joint show that the combination
is really quite compatible.

TABLE 4-3 Some Physical Properties of Phosphor Bronze and Paliney® 7 [a]

	Paliney 7 [a]	Phosphor Bronze [b]
Crystal structure	FCC	FCC
Lattice constant, Å	—	3.705
Melting point, °C	1085	950
Coef. thermal exp., linear, μ in./in/°C	15×10^{-6}	17.8×10^{-6}
Thermal diffusivity, cm²/s	$(0.1)^{c}$	0.21

[a] Commercial designation of a precious metal alloy of composition: 35% Pd, 30% Ag, 14% Cu, 10% Pt, 10% Au, and 1% Zn.
[b] 5% Sn alloy A.
[c] Estimated.

System Metallurgy Since copper, palladium, and silver are the major constituents of the weld, a look at their equilibrium phase diagrams would help in understanding the metallurgy of the system and the expected integrity of the weld. Figures 4-25 through 4-27 show the phase diagrams of the possible systems, except for the Pd-Cu system, which is a solid solubility type similar to the Ag-Pd binary system.

Figure 4-25 shows a eutectic diagram for the Ag-Cu system where, except for limited solubility at either end of the composition range, nearly all the alloy combinations are mixtures of phases. When silver is alloyed with palladium, there is solid solubility for all compositions (Figure 4-26). This type of combination of one metal with another is highly desirable for a weld joint in most joining applications.

When one looks at the ternary system for Ag-Cu-Pd, the presence of the Ag-Cu phase can influence the integrity of the weld joint. Its presence may be noticed in the weld microstructure as colonies of the eutectic or near eutectic composition precipitating in alternating layers of the α and β phases.[34] However, if we assume the welded material to have the composition of 55 percent Cu, 25 percent Pd, and 20 percent Ag, then looking at the eutectic isotherm of the ternary at approximately

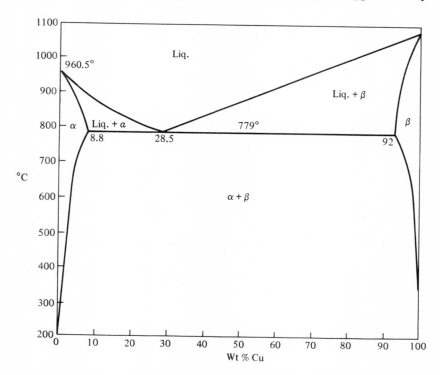

Figure 4-25. Ag-Cu system.[35] *(**With permission of Butterworth-Newness-Shiffe Group.**)*

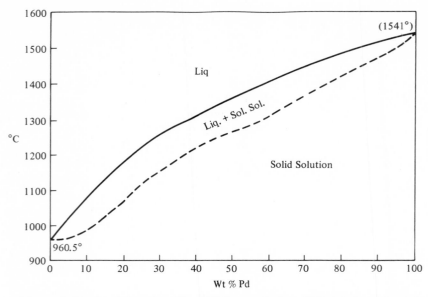

Figure 4-26   Ag-Pd system.[36]   (*With permission of* Metals Handbook.)

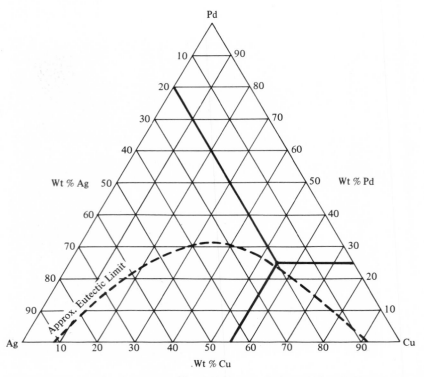

Figure 4-27   Ag-Cu-Pd system.[36]   (*With permission of* Metals Handbook.)

1010°C, Figure 4-27, it is seen that our assumed composition lies just outside the eutectic limit. This assumption is based on the fact that platinum forms a solid solution with palladium and gold a solid solution with silver, so that for the purpose of our assumption we can identify the Pt with the Pd and the Au with the Ag. The tin constituent can be considered to be dissolved in the copper, since it was in that state in the phosphor bronze.

There is some support to the above argument. It was found[36] that Pd increases the mutual solubility of Ag and Cu for each other. The first addition of Pd increases the temperature of the Ag-Cu eutectic; with further addition the eutectic reaction is eliminated; thus, complete solid solubility can be achieved. At high temperatures, most of the alloys of the ternary are single-phase solid solutions. Attainment of high temperatures over 1200°C with a laser is easy; therefore complete solid solubility can be achieved, thereby resulting in a quality weld.

The Laser Welding System   Figure 4-22b shows an experimental contact welding system setup. The TV monitor shows a pair of the contact wires positioned onto the phosphor bronze within a work chamber containing a welding fixture located below the vertically mounted laser head assembly. Figure 4-28 shows a closeup of the prototype welding fixture. The wires are fed from the left through a cutter mechanism up

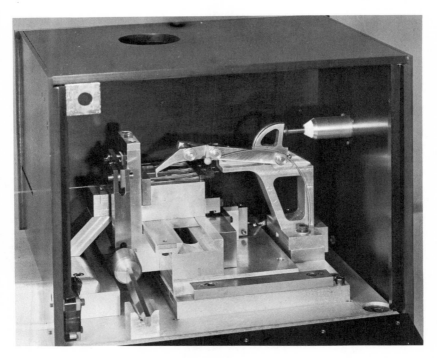

Figure 4-28   Prototype wire feeder and welding fixture.

against a stop. The welding fixture is indexed over eight positions to complete the welding of a relay assembly.

Estimates of Laser Output Requirements   In this section, a model (presented in Section 3.3.3) for laser welding is used to estimate the laser output parameters required for this application. Knowing the required depth of melting, both the absorbed heat flux and its time of application to achieve the required melting depth are calculated. The laser output power is then found from the absorbed heat flux.

Figure 4-29 illustrates schematically the geometry of the wire-spring leaf assembly. In order to apply the "melting" model, several simplifying assumptions must be made concerning both the geometry and physical properties of the spring assembly.

The physical properties of both Paliney 7 and phosphor bronze are very similar (see Table 4-3). Therefore, in order to simplify the use of the model, the Paliney contact wires will be neglected. The problem then is to determine the laser parameters required to melt, without vaporization, phosphor bronze to the thickness of the leaf spring (0.023 cm). Because of the boundary conditions imposed on the model, the overall

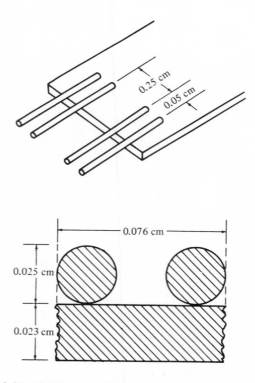

Figure 4-29   Schematic of the wire-spring leaf assembly.

thickness of the phosphor bronze is assumed large compared to the required melt depth. The model discussed in Section 3.3.3 assumes one-dimensional heat flow in the direction normal to the surface (Figure 3-17). In addition, the model assumes constant incident intensity I_0 fully absorbed at the sample surface. These assumed conditions are not satisfied in this problem, and hence will affect the accuracy of the final result. The significance of these assumptions will be discussed after application of the model.

The required melt depth, 0.023 cm, along with the physical properties of phosphor bronze (see Table 4-4) are the known parameters for this problem. From Figure 3-18, the nondimensional depth of melting [S] is given as

$$[S] = \frac{8.33\rho L_f S}{I_0 t_m} \tag{4-2}$$

where S = melt depth equal to 0.023 cm
$\quad I_0$ = absorbed incident intensity,
$\quad \rho$ = density,
$\quad L_f$ = heat of fusion.

$$t_m = \frac{\pi}{\kappa}\left[\frac{K^2 T_m^2}{4I_0^2}\right], \text{ the time for the onset of surface melting} \tag{4-3}$$

where K = thermal conductivity,
$\quad T_m$ = melting point,
$\quad \kappa$ = thermal diffusivity

Substituting for t_m in (4-2) and solving for I_0,

$$I_0 = \frac{[S]}{8.33\rho L_f S}\frac{\pi K^2 T_m^2}{4\kappa} \tag{4-4}$$

The nondimensional parameters $[T_1']$ (related to the surface temperature) and Y (see Section 3.3.3) are found using the properties of phosphor bronze listed in Table 4-4.

$$[T_1'] = \frac{40 T_1'}{T_m} = \frac{40 T_v}{T_m} = 72$$

$$Y = \frac{L_f}{T_m C_p} = 0.53$$

where the surface temperature (T_1') at maximum melt penetration is assumed equal to the vaporization temperature. This implies that the depth S, equal to 0.023 cm, is then the vaporization limited fusion depth as defined in Section 3.3.3. From the above values for $[T_1']$ and Y,

TABLE 4-4   Some Properties of Phosphor Bronze

Density, ρ, g/cm^3	8.86
Melting point, °C	950
Boiling point, °C	1700
Thermal conductivity, K, cal/s/cm/°C	0.17
Heat capacity, C_p, cal/g°C	0.09
Heat of fusion, L_f, cal/g	45 (estimated)

Figure 3-18 is then used to determine the nondimensional parameter $[S]$ which is found to be

$$[S] = 5.20$$

Equation 4-4 can now be used to find the input heat flux required to satisfy the above. Substituting the appropriate values,

$$I_0 = 2.77 \times 10^4 \text{ W/cm}^2$$

and from Equation 4-3, $t_m = 2.20$ ms.

Again referring to Figure 3-18, the nondimensional parameter τ (related to surface heating times) can be found. Specifically

$$\tau = \frac{t_v}{t_m} = 3.35$$

where t_v is the time required to reach the vaporization limited melt depth or equivalently the laser pulse length.

$$\therefore \quad t_v = \tau \times t_m = 7.4 \text{ ms}$$

Several factors must now be considered in order to make a realistic estimate of the required laser output power. These include:

1. The required optical spot size
2. Transmission losses through the optical system
3. Surface reflectivity of phosphor bronze
4. The effect of the Paliney wires

1. The optical spot size is assumed to be equal to the average cross-sectional measurement of the effective spot diameter (see Section 3.1.3)—equal to ~0.08 cm for this example.
2 and 3. The optical transmission losses are easily found and for a typical system would be approximately 20 percent. The surface reflectivity of phosphor bronze is estimated to be 60 percent. Therefore, 40 percent of the incident intensity is coupled into the material and available for heating.
4. The volume of wire that is melted must be accounted for. From geometric considerations (Figure 4-29), a volume of 4×10^{-5} cm^3, which is equal to 1/3 of the melt volume of phosphor bronze, is used.

By taking the above factors into account, the power output from the laser can now be calculated. Specifically, from the assumed focused spot diameter, the power is calculated as follows (the intensity is assumed uniform across the focused spot).

$$P = I_0(\pi w^2) = 139 \text{ W}$$

where w is the optical spot radius, 0.08/2 cm.

Including the losses discussed in 2, 3, and 4, the actual power from the laser is corrected to be

$$P = 139 \text{ W} \left(\frac{1}{0.8}\right)\left(\frac{1}{0.4}\right)(1.33) = 578$$

<u>Summary</u>   From the above calculations, the required laser output is then estimated to be the following:

Power	578 W
Pulse length	7.4 ms
Energy/pulse	4.3 J

The above results can serve only as initial guides because of the many simplifying assumptions made. Hence the exact welding parameters required for the application must be optimized through experimentation.

In the system illustrated subsequently in Figure 4-34, the following parameters were actually used.

Power	2000 W
Pulse length	3 ms
Energy/pulse	6 J

A 43-mm lens, defocused approximately 1.2 mm from the surface, was used to obtain the required focused power density.

<u>Results and Analysis</u>   Figure 4-30 is an action-stopped photograph showing the welding of a wire pair to the phosphor bronze spring. The spring assembly is held in the experimental welding fixture so that the mating of the wires against the spring is under a slight contact pressure. The brass barrel piece at the top holds the objective lens which converges the ruby radiation at the weld joint.

Figure 4-31 is a transverse section of a typical wire pair welded to the phosphor bronze spring material showing full penetration of the fusion front. Note the large degree of intermixing of the materials as evidenced by the swirl-like pattern seen in the micrograph; the dark bands are copper rich areas primarily due to the phosphor bronze. The diameter of the weld bead at the top surface of the phosphor bronze measures approximately 0.85 mm, and the thickness of the heat affected zone within the phosphor bronze measures approximately 0.05 mm, insignificant in terms of altering the spring temper condition of the phosphor bronze. The number of voids (dark spots) is decreased significantly when similar samples of material are carefully cleaned. The strength and bend properties of the weld joint do not appear to be appreciably influenced by the presence of voids.[31]   Pull tests show that the average breaking strength

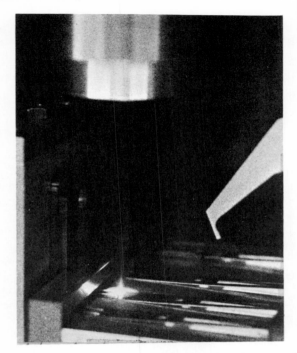

Figure 4-30   Action-stopped photograph showing actual laser weld taking place.

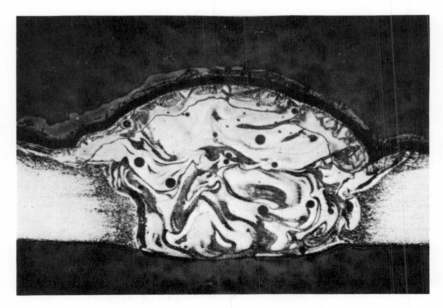

Figure 4-31   Transverse section of a welded wire pair.   Mag. 70X.

of welded samples is equal to 84 percent of the breaking strength of the Paliney 7 wire.

Electron microprobe analysis was performed on the sample of Figure 4-31. Figures 4-32 and 4-33 are probe displays of an area in the center of the weld. Note the heavier concentrations of copper corresponding to the dark swirl-like pattern seen in the electron backscatter picture. But of more significance is the strong indication that there has been an appreciable amount of elemental distribution throughout the weld fusion zone.

The production laser system for this application is shown in Figure 4-34. The ruby laser has the capability of being pulsed at a repetition rate of 1 pps with a beam energy output of 20 J per pulse and pulse lengths of from 0.5 to 6 ms. Wire is fed from two spools into the work enclosure and then onto a weld fixture similar to the prototype unit of Figure 4-28. The production rate is three switch assemblies (Figure 4-23) per minute.

The ruby laser cavity is set horizontally in the head assembly and the beam is deflected down by a mirror through the objective lens onto the weld area. A TV camera is mounted above the head assembly and the closed-circuit TV (CCTV) monitor is seen at the left. On the right is the power supply and pulse forming network. The table pedestals, which house the electronics and circuitry for automatic operation, have push-

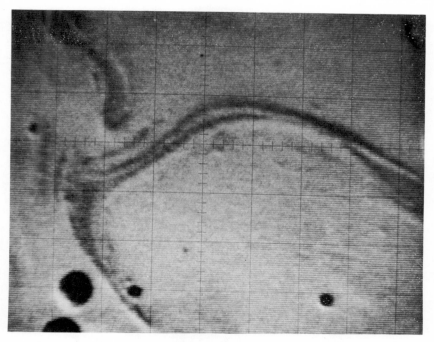

Figure 4-32 Electron probe backscatter image of the center area of the specimen of Figure 4-31. Mag. 800X.

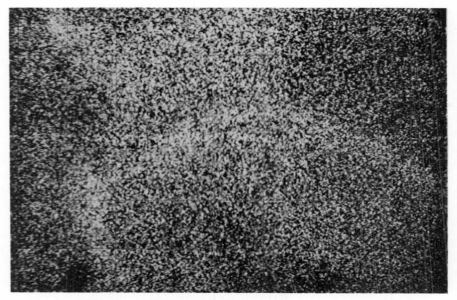

Figure 4-33   Electron probe X-ray pickup from the copper constituent. Mag. 800X.

button operator control for starting a completely automated wire feeding, welding, cutting, and indexing cycle; and, in addition, controls are provided for ON-OFF, manual, fire, test, and safety features.

This specific example illustrates a high-power pulsed laser system effectively used as a production welder. The example described has shown that metal combinations, which are difficult to weld by conventional methods, can be effectively joined using the laser.

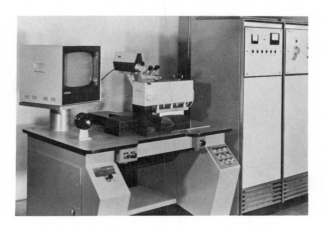

Figure 4-34   Production laser welding system.

4.2   drilling—introduction

Bulk removal of materials was one of the first demonstrated uses of the power of a laser.   One simple technique for classifying the power of a focused beam from ruby lasers during the early 1960's was according to the number of stacked razor blades that could be pierced.   It was not too surprising, therefore, that the first efforts in laser processing of materials was in the general area of hole drilling.[37,38,39]   Some of these efforts led to the first major industrial application of the laser: the drilling of diamond dies.[40,41]

The dies are used in drawing intermediate 15 gauge (American Wire Gauge) (1.44 mm diameter) copper wire to standard diameters, from about 19 gauge to 30 gauge, for use in telephone communications cable.[41] Figure 4-35 (top) shows the internal profile of a die as drilled and rough

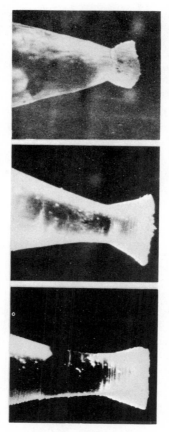

Figure 4-35   Laser drilling of a diamond wire drawing die; as drilled (top), mechanically lapped and sized (center), finished die after polishing (bottom).   The drilling operation (for a 100 point stone) required 250 pulses on the front side, which is seen at the left of the photograph, and 300 pulses for the back.   Beam energy was 2-3 J and pulse length was 0.6 ms.   Repetition rate was at 1 pps.

shaped by a commercial ruby laser system. Note that the cone sides are smooth, and that the front and back cones are concentric. The size of the minimum opening is 0.46 mm. The center figure shows a typical die as mechanically lapped and sized, and the bottom figure shows a typical die as finished.

The Swiss watch industry in Europe has been routinely using flash pumped Nd:YAG systems operating at approximately 20 pps with a pulse width of about 100 μs and an energy of approximately 150 mJ/pulse to drill ruby stones used in timepiece movements.[42,43] Figure 4-36 shows relatively long, narrow holes in 0.25 mm thick ruby gem stones. The hole diameter is about 30 μm and requires from 3 to 6 pulses for

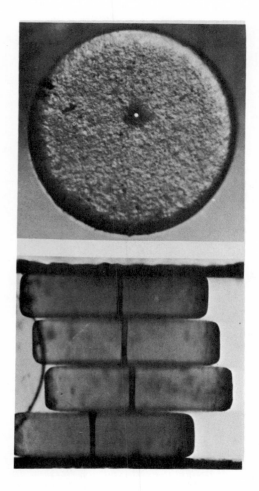

Figure 4-36. Laser drilled ruby gem stones.[43] Mag. 48X. (With permission of Raytheon Company.)

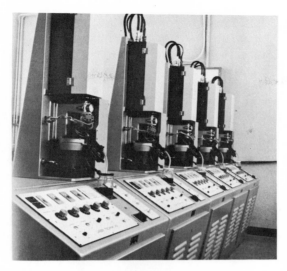

Figure 4-37   Nd:YAG production drilling system.[43]   (*With permission of Raytheon Company.*)

complete penetration. Figure 4-37 shows a production line setup of five systems.

One can readily appreciate the advantages of using laser energy for hole piercing by considering the following factors:

1. Because there is no physical contact between the hole-forming tool and the material, problems such as drill-bit breakage and wear are nonexistent.
2. Precise hole location is simplified because the optics used to focus the laser beam can also be used to align and locate.
3. Large aspect ratios (hole depth to hole diameter) can be achieved.

4·2·1   beam characteristics

Control of beam parameters becomes exceedingly important when concerned with the precision and geometric uniformity of drilled holes for production applications.

Laser hole drilling of materials is most effectively performed using the pulsed mode of operation. The solid-state ruby, Nd:glass and, recently, the high repetition rate Nd:YAG as well as the CO_2 gas laser systems have shown the greatest potential for hole drilling applications. The gas laser has an appreciably more uniform output beam profile than the solid-state lasers, therefore giving it an advantage for drilling holes of more circular uniformity. Although the high-energy pulsed solid-state laser outputs have a nonuniform, complex, high-order mode structure,[44] reproducible holes can be obtained.   There are several techniques employed, of which an aperture placed in the path of the output beam is the simplest and often the most effective means.   In addition, an internal aperture within the cavity will force the laser to operate in lower-order modes, thereby improving the hole geometry.

It was shown (Section 3.1) that beam expanders can be used to illuminate fully the diameter of the focusing lens (lens aperture) and to reduce the divergence angle, therefore achieving a smaller optical spot size.   For a given lens system, the position of the minimum diameter of the transformed beam can be calculated (3-5) and, in practice, the material to be drilled should be kept at this position in order to use the maximum power density available for maximum penetration.   The size of the focal spot and therefore the diameter of the drilled hole can be changed by simply changing the focal length or by changing the size of the aperture.

Short focal-length lenses are often used for hole drilling; and, since the working distance is also short, these lenses can be easily damaged from workpiece debris.   Subsequent laser pulses result in increased energy absorption by the lens because of the debris material coating the lens and, ultimately, the lens cracks.   A replaceable or moving transparent medium may be used to protect the lens.   Glass, Mylar, or Teflon films have been used with ruby wavelengths.   An alternative is to use reflecting objectives which have short focal lengths but relatively long working distances (see Glossary).

4.2.2   material considerations

The number of mechanisms that have been proposed for material removal in hole drilling reveal the limited amount of systematic work performed in this area.   Some investigators[45,46] have suggested the generation of a type of shock wave which propagates into the material in a unidirectional manner to produce deep holes.   The arguments were based on the following:[46]

1. Vaporizing the desired hole would require much more *energy* than was contained in the single pulse.
2. The *time* required for heat to be conducted through the full thickness of the material is much longer than the laser pulse duration.
3. The *heat* would tend to diffuse uniformly in all directions from the irradiated spot rather than being confined to the cylindrical volume of the hole which was effected.

Other studies[47,48] have indicated that coupled energy, from generation of shock waves, is not a major factor in hole drilling but that the

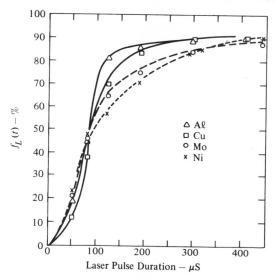

Figure 4-38 Fraction of material removed in liquid state. These measurements are the average ratio of molten material removed to the total material removed from three specimens subjected to an average power of 30 kW but different time durations.[48] *(With permission of M. K. Chun.)*

bulk of material removal is by liquid ejection. Figure 4-38 shows the fraction of material removed in the liquid state for several metals as a function of pulse duration for the same average power input using a pulsed Nd:glass laser. Of interest is the rapid incremental increase of the liquid fraction for pulses between 50 μs and 100 μs in duration, where the power density is least likely to be attenuated by subsequent plume and ejected material. A recent theoretical study[49] presents a model which allows for transmission of laser energy past the front surface. The analysis shows that subsurface temperatures will exceed the surface temperature leading to the possibility of explosive removal of material as the governing mechanism.

Rarely is hole drilling performed with a pulse length in excess of 1.5 ms; most materials undergo vaporization of sufficient volume for

TABLE 4-5[a]   **Depth of Material Removed**[50]

	10^7 W/cm^2 600 μs Laser Pulse (μm)	10^9 W/cm^2 44 ns Q-switched Pulse (μm)
Aluminum	780	3.6
Copper	900	2.2
Nickel	580	1.2
Brass	780	2.5
Stainless steel	610	1.1

[a] With permission of J. F. Ready.

practical material removal using pulse lengths of 100 to 700 μs. Q-switched pulse lengths (5–250 ns) normally produce vaporization to a much shallower depth—usually not exceeding a few micrometers. Table 4-5 gives the depth of removal of material for both 600 μs and 44 ns pulse lengths in several metals.[50]

4.2.3   hole geometry and beam parameters

It has been shown that when holes are drilled in a material, the depth of the hole increases with the power delivered by the laser (Figure 4-39). There appears to be an upper limit, however, to the depth achievable in a single laser pulse.   This upper limit may result from the fact that the laser plume becomes more opaque as it becomes large and more highly excited (Figure 4-40).   The latter portions of the laser pulse must pass through the plume of vaporized material, and therefore additional energy is absorbed by the plume rather than by the workpiece.   However, for materials (e.g., brass) that contain a large percentage of high vapor-pressure elements, this upper limit is greatly extended.   In drilling, this condition becomes an advantage for certain applications.   The tempera-ture required to just melt the brass alloy is sufficiently great to generate localized pockets of exceedingly high pressures so that, for a drilling process, conglomerates of zinc atoms greatly enhance the vaporization mechanism.

Figure 4-41 shows a 1.0 mm entrance and 0.5 mm exit hole in 2.4 mm thick 70:30 brass.   One pulse from a ruby laser of approximately 75 J energy and 5 ms pulse length was used in producing the hole.   A 43 mm focal-length lens concentrated the energy to a power density of 10 MW/ cm^2.   These results essentially agree with other findings.[48]

In drilling fired high-purity alumina ceramic, bulk material removal is primarily effected by particulate (essentially liquid droplets solidifying in transit) expulsion from the formed crater or hole.   The relative amount of liquid expulsion to the total mass of material removed per pulse of laser energy appears to be a function of the total energy content of the pulse.[51]   These observations have been noted for both the solid-state and the CO_2 lasers.   For example, Figure 4-42 relates the penetration depth in fused silica as a function of drilling time using a CO_2 laser.[52]

Similar results have been obtained using the ruby laser on relatively thick alumina ceramic material.   Figure 4-43 is a plot of penetration depth versus pulse length for 3.2 mm thick 99.5 percent Al_2O_3 hard ceramic.   The dashed part of the curves are uncertain because of a lack of data for the short pulse lengths (<300 μs); however, the form could comply with a proposed mechanism of hole drilling (discussed in Section 4.2.4).   Figure 4-44 indicates the strong dependence of hole geometry on the time duration of the laser pulse as well as its power, i.e., the energy content of the pulse.

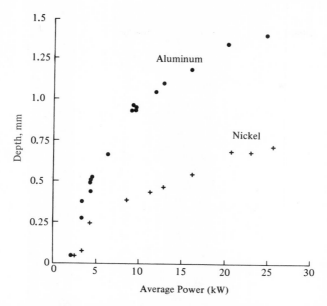

Figure 4-39 Hole depth as a function of delivered power for aluminum and nickel. Each point plotted is the average depth of several holes, using one pulse per hole. Pulse length was 0.8 ms. (With permission of M. I. Cohen.)

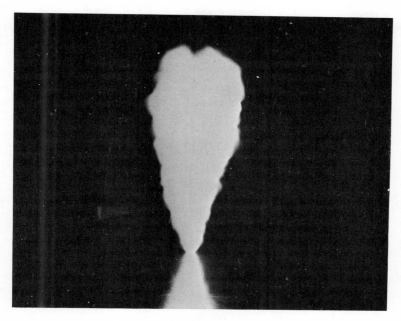

Figure 4-40 Laser plume developed in a hole drilling experiment.

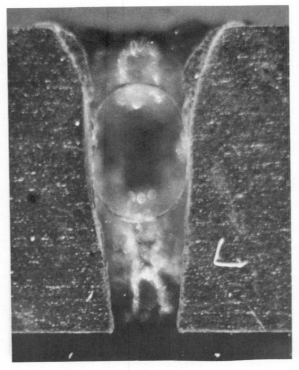

Figure 4-41   A hole made in 2.4 mm thick 70:30 brass.   One pulse of 75 J from a ruby laser produced the hole seen in cross section.   Mag. approximately 20X.

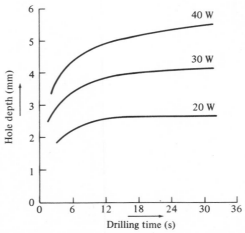

Figure 4-42   Dependence of hole depth on drilling time in fused silica using CO_2 radiation.

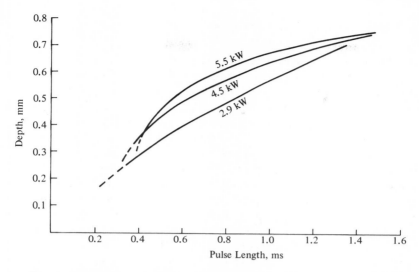

Figure 4-43   Hole depth in Al₂O₃ ceramic as a function of pulse length for ruby radiation.   A 15 mm focal-length lens was used.   The beam was apertured down to 5.5 mm so that an effective f/number of 2.7 was used to produce approximately 0.25 mm diameter holes.

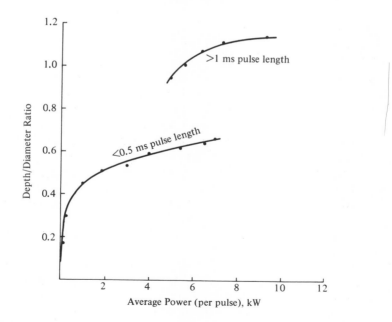

Figure 4-44   Aspect ratio as a function of average power per single pulse in a polycrystalline Al₂O₃ ceramic.

4·2·4 high-speed photography

In order to offer some explanation of the drilling mechanism and to study the degree of resolidification, high-speed movies of the drilling reaction from a ruby laser focused on an alumina substrate were taken. The intensity of the focused radiation was determined to be 4×10^7 W/cm^2. The sequence of eight photographs in Figure 4-45 which was printed from the high-speed film, shows the more dramatic and technically significant frames of the total film coverage photographed at a speed of 11,000 frames/s. This is equivalent to a time interval between frames of 91 μs. Frames 2 through 6 cover a total lapsed time of approximately 1.3 ms, quite close to the oscilloscope measured pulse width (see Figure 4-46) of 1.48 ms. Frame 1 is probably flash-lamp light transmitted through the ruby rod before laser threshold was reached. The spoke-like images seen at the bottom left of the photographs and emanating from the cross hairs are reflections off the gold thin-film pattern on the ceramic sample. The conclusions drawn from the high-speed study essentially agree with the analysis[48] of mass of material removed in percentage of liquid to the total amount. It is estimated that approximately 60 percent of the volume of removed material is by explosive expulsion of hot solid and liquid particulate matter. This percentage was arrived at by counting the number of discernible particles from all the frames and using a corrected size factor. The reader is referred to Ref. 51 for a thorough treatment of the analysis.

A description for the mechanism of laser hole drilling is offered as follows.

A. Initial penetration (absorption) into the surface, greatly increasing the vibrational and electronic energy content of the Al_2O_3 molecular structure much beyond their equilibrium values.
B. Subsurface (~ 5 nm to 50 nm) vaporization of localized areas.
C. Explosive expansion of these areas with subsequent removal of particulate matter. (Referring back to Chapter 3, in the discussion on vaporization, this explosive expansion step would suggest a value of less than 1 for the nondimensional parameter B.)
D. Rapid rise of temperature with heating to melting and vaporization of adjacent areas within the focused beam spot.
E. Steps B, C, and D may be repeated several times for the duration of the laser pulse.

Material in and near the surface is explosively removed as the leading portion of the laser pulse is absorbed by the ceramic providing more than enough energy to break the molecular and atomic bonds of the alumina structure. Large groups or clusters of molecules, as well as other particles (i.e., ionized species and quite probably electrons), are expelled from the surface in all three (plus plasma) states of matter.

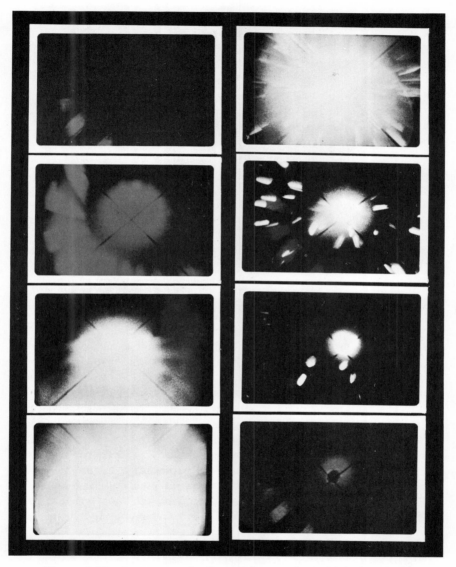

Figure 4-45   Sequence of selected frames from high-speed photo-graphy of ruby laser drilling in polycrystalline alumina.   See frontispiece for color rendition.

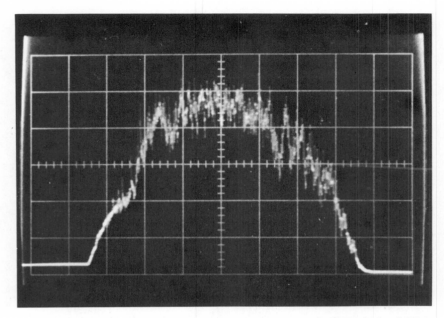

Figure 4-46   Ruby pulse shape for alumina substrate hole drilling (1 cm per major division, 0.2 ms/cm).

Radiation from the latter part of the laser pulse is absorbed by the remaining material which rapidly begins to melt.   The bulk of this molten mass is then evaporated by additional absorption and/or the rapid excursion of temperature.   At the end of the lasing action, a certain amount of molten ceramic resolidifies on the boundaries of the hole.

The high-speed photography analysis has presented some physical evidence of the forces which a high-intensity pulse of laser light can produce in the process of hole drilling.   The apparent mechanism that is suggested would indeed be extremely difficult to describe completely mathematically.   The literature shows that a few theories have been proposed, of which Refs. 45, 49, and 53 are notable.   The essentials of Refs. 45 and 49 are presented in Chapter 3 of this book.   Reference 49 is a significant extension of Ref. 53.

4·2·5   some practical considerations and applications

In practice, relatively large hole diameters (greater than 0.25 mm) and depths (greater than 1 mm) are obtained by using repetitive laser pulses at lower power levels.   Such holes have less taper and better definition than those drilled with higher-energy pulses.

An example of drilling through relatively thick materials is shown in Figure 4-47.   The sample is 3.2 mm thick polycrystalline, high-density alumina, and the objective was to provide precisely located patterns of holes of 0.25 mm to 0.30 mm diameter in 6.4 mm diameter discs.   The holes were drilled with a beam energy of 1.4 J, focused through a 25-mm focal-length lens onto the surface of the disc.   An average of 40 pulses at a repetition rate of 1 pulse every 5 s was used to drill a hole; each pulse had a time duration of 0.5 ms.   A 4.75-mm aperture was inserted in the path of the laser beam.   The power density at the focal spot at the surface of the ceramic disc was approximately 4 MW/cm^2 for the above-stated parameters.

Figure 4-48 shows a representative longitudinal section of a laser drilled hole.   This hole was made without the use of an aperture and at a higher energy level, 1.8 J, thus giving the larger entrance diameter, which measures 0.50 mm, compared to the exit hole diameter, which measures 0.09 mm.   The hole was made using multiple shots, adjusting for the increasing hole depth by refocusing after every third shot.   This was done in an attempt to locate the focal plane of the lens at the bottom of the (blind) hole.   Note that the profile of the exit hole is quite square, as is characteristic.   The entrance hole usually has some degree of taper, with tapers of approximately 1° to 10° typical.   Aspect ratios of 25 to 1, as determined by using the half-depth diameter for longitudinal sections

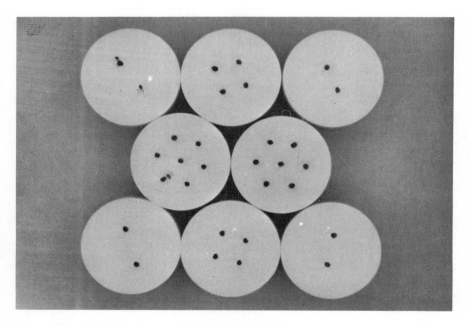

Figure 4-47   Laser drilling through high density polycrystalline alumina ceramic.   Mag. approximately 3X.

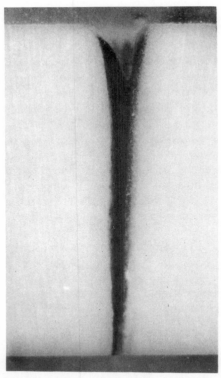

Figure 4-48   Longitudinal section of a typically drilled hole in a 3.2 mm thick alumina ceramic using pulsed ruby radiation.   Mag. 32X.

or the average diameter of the entrance and exit holes, have been demonstrated.[38,54]

Aperturing the emitted beam before lens convergence has a refining effect on hole formation.   The results of a simple experiment are summarized in Figure 4-49.   Note the very pronounced change in slope at a point corresponding to an aperture size of 2.8 mm, which is close to the 3.2 mm experimental aperture.   Assuming a Gaussian distribution of the beam intensity emitted from the face of the laser rod, which was 9.5 mm in diameter, then the 3.2 mm aperture transmits 90.5 percent of the total energy of the beam.   This would explain the relatively small increase in drilled hole size with increasing aperture opening beyond the 3.2 mm size.

Other studies[38,55] state that deep hole drilling using relatively short focal-length lenses could be explained by internal multiple reflections of the incident energy as the hole formation progressed.   This apparent "light pipe" effect is illustrated in Figure 4-50, which shows the effect of refocusing versus no refocusing for multiple-shot hole drilling in relatively

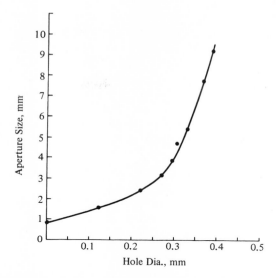

Figure 4-49 *The effect of using differing aperture sizes placed external to the cavity, but before beam convergence on alumina ceramic. Parameters are 1.53 J beam energy and 0.5 ms pulse length, 25 mm focal-length lens.*

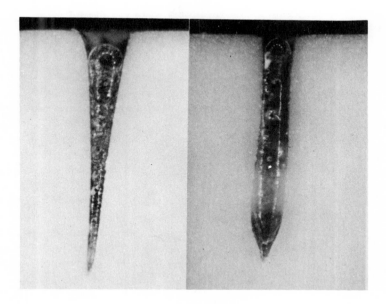

Figure 4-50   *The effect of refocusing versus no refocusing for multiple-shot hole drilling.   Mag. approximately 16X.*

thick alumina.   The longitudinal section on the left shows the hole profile made by refocusing to the extent of 0.2 mm/pulse.   The one on the right shows the profile with only initial focusing on the surface and no refocusing.   The same parameters were used in making both holes (3.1 J beam energy, 0.5 ms pulse length, 15 repetitive shots focused with a 39 mm focal-length lens, no aperture).   No refocusing apparently yields straight wall holes.   On the other hand, controllable refocusing can effect holes of almost any taper because the entrance hole diameter acts as an aperture to the converging beam, and less energy is transmitted to the bottom of the hole for each refocusing step.

Drilling in ceramic and other nonmetallic materials (up to about 0.75 mm in thickness) has almost exclusively been performed in the pulsed mode of operation for both the solid state and gas (CO_2) lasers. Both through holes and blind holes have been drilled in IC processed silicon wafers for alignment and registration purposes.   Figure 4-51

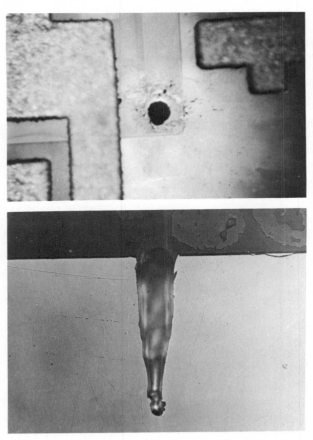

Figure 4-51   Registration holes in a silicon wafer (top), and a longitudinal section through a typical hole (bottom).

shows a 0.025 mm hole in 0.175 mm thick Si wafer using 350 μs pulses from a ruby laser and a beam energy of approximately 300 mJ.

Deep hole metal drilling has been investigated[38,56] for aircraft and consumer products applications; these investigations confirm the general remarks made earlier with respect to maximum hole depths achievable with the laser.   For example, single-pulse depths for ferrous materials, such as sheet steels, high-carbon steels, stainless, and other alloy steels, reach a maximum at about 1 mm.   About half this depth is achieved for nonferrous metals, except as was noted for brass and similar alloys. With good control of the beam parameters and well-designed optics, hole taper can be essentially eliminated and recast layers of metal greatly reduced.   Figure 4-52 illustrates these conditions for an alloy steel.

Resolidified or recast material about the periphery of the hole can be minimized to an appreciable degree by several techniques.[38,57]   These techniques take advantage of the fact that the removed material spews out much like a volcanic eruption (see Sections 4.2.2 and 4.2.3).   Masking or coating with paraffin wax and silicone grease has been used.[57]   The surfaces of the metal to be drilled will provide for the expelled material to be cast onto the coating which can then be removed by standard degreasing and cleaning operations.   Drilling two thicknesses of metals in tandem, so that the first acts as a mask for the underlying one, has produced essentially lip-free holes.[38]

Some uniformity of hole diameter is generally lost when attempting to drill small holes in sheet stock of less than 0.5 mm.   Holes of 0.01 mm to about 0.2 mm in diameter can be made in common metals of 0.5 mm and less in thickness, using relatively low powers in three pulses or less.

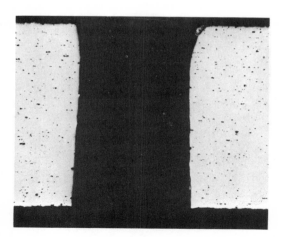

Figure 4-52   A single pulse of 15 J and 1 ms from a ruby laser produced a 0.75 mm diameter hole (seen in longitudinal section) in 1 mm thick René 41 alloy.[56]   (With permission of G. Bellows.)

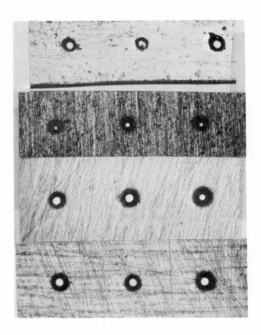

Figure 4-53   Hole piercing through thin materials (top to bottom)
0.125 mm thick section of aluminum, copper, nickel-iron alloy, and steel.
The holes are entrance holes and measure, on the average, 60 μm for Al,
35 μm for Cu, and 70 μm for both the NiFe and steel materials.   The same
laser parameters were used for all four samples.   The materials were
rough polished with 600 grit size cloth to approximate equal surface
topography.   Copper is one of the more difficult materials to laser
machine, and the evidence seen here appears to bear this out.   Mag.
approximately 30X.

Figure 4-53 shows ruby laser-drilled holes measuring 0.025 to 0.08 mm
in diameter in 0.125 mm thick aluminum, copper, nickel-iron alloy, and
low-alloy steel.   One application of small hole drilling in thin materials
is in the fabrication of the electron gun section of the camera tube used in
Picturephone® equipment.[58]   Figure 4-54 shows a sketch of a cross
section of the apertures in the gun.   The objective was to drill a 0.05 mm
diameter hole in 0.05 mm thick nickel foil.   The tolerance on the hole
size, which must be centrally located within a 0.025-mm radius with
respect to the center of the other apertures, is ± 0.005 mm.   Figure 4-55
shows a laser-drilled hole and, for comparison, one fabricated by the
electroforming method.   (The photographs represent the best of a group.)
The laser drilling parameters are 3 J beam energy from a Nd: glass laser,
a pulse of approximately 0.6 ms, through a 1.25 mm diameter aperture,
and focused by a 10 X objective lens.

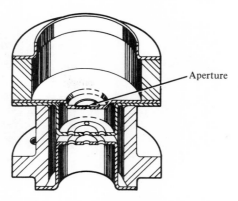

Figure 4-54   Sketch of aperture assembly in electron gun section.

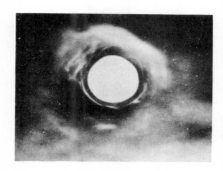

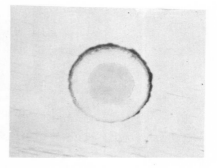

LASER DRILLED
50 µm thick nickel

ELECTROFORMED
25 µm thick nickel

Figure 4-55   Comparison of a laser-drilled hole and an electroformed hole in the same material.   Note the large difference in damaged material even though the electroforming technique had the thinner cross section. Mag. 450X.

In attempting to enhance the hole geometry and impróve on the precision of maintaining the hole diameter within the specified tolerance, various techniques were investigated.   In one series of experiments, high-pressure air was directed on the laser exit side of the nickel foil.   As seen in Figure 4-56, it is quite evident that the rush of air through the pierced holes was very effective in purging the holes of molten metal, which ordinarily resolidifies in an irregular pattern due to uneven surface-tension forces existing in the liquid state.   In another series of experiments, an epoxy compound was coated on the exit side of the foil.   As expected, a large volume of gas was provided by the thermal decomposition which kept most of the holes quite clean.   The result is shown in Figure 4-56.

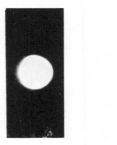

40 psig air pressure

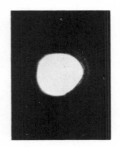

Epoxy coated

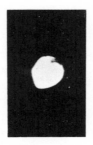

No pressure
differential

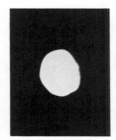

Uncoated

Figure 4-56   Enhancement of hole geometry.   Mag. approximately 400X.

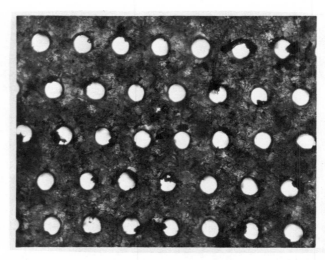

Figure 4-57 CO_2 laser pierced holes in 0.15 mm thick natural gum rubber.   The holes measure 0.09 mm in diameter and are spaced 0.25 mm between centers.   Approximately 1 kW peak power was incident on the rubber which was fixtured to an x-y table traveling at 38 cm/min.   The laser was pulsed at 25 Hz with a pulse duration of 60 μs.

246

Drilling of shallow holes in bulk material has practical application in the dynamic balancing of gyro and other rotating components.[59,60] Balancing is accomplished in much the same way as in conventional techniques, i.e., by locating the point or area of imbalance by strobe light and then trimming with the laser, using shallow hole drilling parameters. The laser pulse is triggered in phase with the point of imbalance at a pulse rate related to the rotating speed; material removal of milligrams per pulse is achieved.

Hole drilling in other materials has also been investigated. Non-metallics such as rubber, glass, plastics, and ferrites have been drilled using the CO_2 laser.[61,62,63,64] Figure 4-57 shows CO_2 laser pierced holes in natural gum rubber.[62]

4·2·6   the study of drilling ceramic material

Laser drilling in hard, high-temperature fired alumina ceramic is attractive because drilling ceramics by conventional means is not a simple task; it usually requires diamond-tipped, hardened-steel drill bits. Small-size holes, less than 0.25 mm in diameter, are extremely difficult for current tool technology. Breakage of the drill often results when the thickness of the ceramic is appreciably greater than the diameter of the hole to be drilled. Aspect ratios for holes in hard brittle materials are nominally 2 to 1 for conventional drilling and about 4 to 1 for ultrasonic drilling. Although holes can easily be put in alumina in the "green" state (aspect ratio for punching techniques is approximately 3 to 1), precision of hole location is lost because of the nonisotropic and inconsistent shrinkage behavior during the firing stage. The example discussed below is an application of several kinds of lasers for drilling 0.25 mm diameter holes in 0.7 mm thick alumina ceramic.

Material Description   The alumina material is specified commercial grade 99.5 percent minimum Al_2O_3 with a small percentage (<0.5 percent) MgO and usually containing some trace elements as impurities. The shape is in sheet form normally prepared by "doctor blade" or isostatic pressing. The dimensions of the "fired" parts are normally 9.5 cm by 11.4 cm by 0.07 cm thick. They may have a waviness across the surface of as much as ± 0.03 cm. The surface is normally smooth and somewhat specular but can have a dull or matt-like finish if a grinding operation is performed.

Requirements   The sheets are used as substrates for thin metal film deposition, and require a pattern of 61 holes (see Figure 4-58).

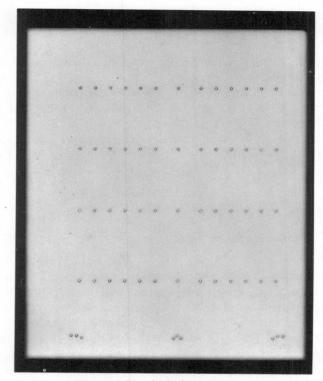

Figure 4-58   61 hole pattern.

The applicable dimensions of the holes are:

Diameter	0.25 mm nominal
Tolerance (for a specified diameter)	±0.025 mm
Taper	0–5 degrees
Spacing	1.64 mm (minimum) ±0.025 mm noncumulative 76.00 mm (maximum—linear) ±0.40 mm cumulative

The requirement is millions of drilled holes per year; therefore, the need for rapid, long-term operation from a laser system is paramount.

Laser Systems   Several laser systems were considered and used in the study, as listed in Table 4-6.

Since speed of hole drilling (elapsed time per substrate) is a major consideration for production purposes, all except the pulsed Nd:YAG laser were operated with numerically controlled (N/C) $x - y$ table movement of the substrate under the beam.   Table 4-7 gives the data for N/C operation.

TABLE 4-6   Laser Systems and their Basic Capabilities for Substrate Alumina Ceramic Hole Drilling

Laser System	Energy (J)	Max. Peak Power (kW)	Pulse Length (ms)	Repetition Rate[a] (pps)
CO_2 (conventional gated)	0.5–250 (CW)	1	0.06–CW	1–100 (2 J)
CO_2 (transient pulsed)	0.1–75 (CW)	50	0.01–0.15	100 (0.25 J)
Ruby	0.5–80	50	0.4–6	1 (20 J)
Nd: glass	0.5–80	50	0.4–10	1 (15 J)
Nd: YAG (pulsed)	0.5–25	30	0.1–5	10 (8 J)

[a] The repetition rate holds for the indicated energy level.

TABLE 4-7   N/C Laser Drilling System Parameters (61 Hole Pattern)[a]

Laser System	Peak Power (kW)	Pulse Length (ms)	Rep. Rate (pps)	Drilling Time/Hole (ms)	Time/Substrate[b] Total
CO_2 (conventional gated)	0.28	7.5	—[c]	7.5	1.05
CO_2 (transient pulsed)	3.0	0.1	70	130.0	1.19
Ruby	2.6	1.5	1	1.5	2.35
Nd: glass	3.3	2.2	1	2.2	2.35
Nd: YAG (pulsed)	2.8	0.3	40	100.0	1.14

[a] See Figure 4-58.
[b] Normalized to the same table speed of 2 in./s free running and 0.5 s stop-start time per hole.
[c] N/C table speed limited (~ 500 ms between holes).

Experimental Data   The information presented here is that obtained with the standard gated CO_2 gas laser and the pulsed ruby laser. Data obtained with the other lasers listed in Table 4-6 indicate that the results are similar for similar lasers (i.e., the characteristics of the holes are similar for those made with the CO_2 lasers and correspondingly similar for those made by the solid-state lasers). However, there are subtle differences within each group, and there definitely are distinct differences between the two types of lasers, i.e., the gas and the solid-state lasers. Some initial results with both CO_2 lasers showed an excess amount of resolidified material in the holes, often closing the holes.

There are two factors that contribute to a large amount of resolidified material and both have an effect on the material properties. One factor is the absorption by the alumina of the frequency of the laser radiation. The 10.6×10^3 nm radiation of the CO_2 laser is quite readily absorbed by alumina. Once the surface of the material has been broken down, there is essentially 100 percent absorption of the CO_2 energy. If the laser-on time or pulse duration is relatively long, then there will be a significant temperature rise outside the effective spot diameter. This can be readily seen since, among nonmetallics, alumina has a rather high thermal conductivity (0.011 cal/cm/°C/s at room temperature and 0.037 cal/cm/°C/s at its melting temperature).[65] The other factor is the peak power per pulse available from the lasers. Table 4-7 shows a large difference in the peak powers between the gated CO_2 and the other lasers.

The problem of undesired resolidified material is greatly eliminated by reducing the pulse duration and by cooling techniques engineered into the work chamber. One technique "assists" the laser pulse by flushing the melted material through the hole as it is drilled. The combination of a vacuum at the bottom of the substrate and a blast of gas (air jet) at the top of the substrate prevents the excess buildup on the walls of the hole. This concept is illustrated schematically in Figure 4-59. This approach, with the aid of a good heat sink in the form of a copper vacuum holding fixture, effectively cools the substrate and physically removes the large fraction of melted material.

The optimized operating parameters are shown in Table 4-8. As illustrated in Figure 4-60, the amount of resolidified material on the walls of the hole and about the periphery of the entrance was substantially reduced. For the case of the transient pulsed CO_2 laser, increasing the energy per pulse to about 0.3 J, reducing the number of pulses to about 10 per hole, and keeping the duty cycle at a minimum resulted in similar improvements.[66]

The holes, shown in Figure 4-61, which were produced with the solid-state lasers (ruby, Nd:glass, and the high-energy pulsed Nd:YAG)

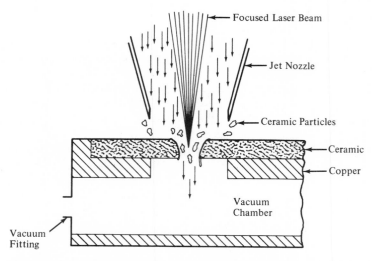

Figure 4-59 Schematic illustration of actions effected by a focused CO_2 laser beam with air-jet and vacuum assisted features during laser drilling of substrate.

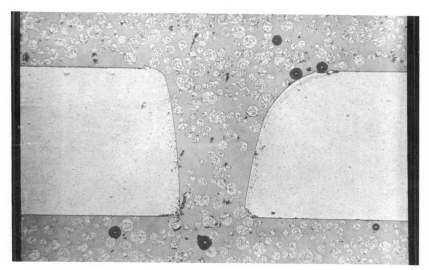

Figure 4-60   Longitudinal section of a typical hole drilled in 0.07 cm thick alumina substrate with a single laser pulse from a CO_2 laser.

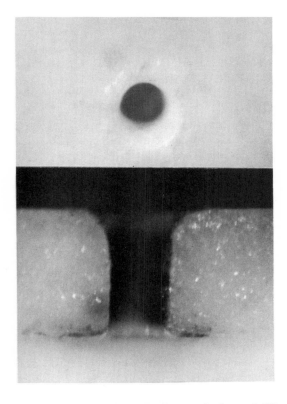

Figure 4-61   Hole geometry from ruby laser drilling.

TABLE 4-8   Jet Assisted CO_2 Laser Drilling Parameters

61-Hole Substrate

Air Pressure, psig	50
Jet nozzle diameter, mm	1
Lens focal length, cm	12.7
Number of pulses	one/hole
Pulse duration, ms	7.5
Energy per pulse, J	~2
Entrance hole diameter, mm	~0.28
Exit hole diameter, mm	~0.20
Total elapsed time for drilling (speed limited by N/C table)	1 min 56 s

appear to have less taper and about the same amount of resolidified material, although there is no gas jet assist nor heat sink required. The drilling parameters used for the solid-state lasers are listed in Table 4-9

TABLE 4-9   Pulsed Laser Alumina Hole Drilling Parameters

Laser	Beam Energy (J)	Aperture Diameter Size (mm)	Apertured Beam Energy (J)	Pulse Length (ms)	Lens Focal Length (mm)
Ruby	25.0	5.5	4	1.48	15
Nd : glass	32.0	5.5	5	2.20	15
Nd : YAG	3.5	—	—	1.20	32

and show that the basic parameters of pulse length and energy per pulse are not too different for these lasers, as might be expected. However, the higher repetition rate for the Nd:YAG plus its ability to drill a hole in 1.2 ms makes this laser a contender for this application.

The simple heat balance equation, $q = \rho V[C_p \Delta T + L_f + L_v]$ (see Section 3.2.2, Equation 3-23) was used to estimate that 2.34 J was required to drill each hole. Reasonable agreement is evident. The calculation was based on the following values for alumina:

$\rho = 3.98$ g/cm^3

$C_p = 0.37$ cal/g °C

$\Delta T = T_v = 3500$°C

$L_f = 260$ cal/g (extrapolated from Ref. 6 data)

$L_v = 2.6 \times 10^3$ cal/g (estimated $10 \times L_f$)

$K = 0.011$ cal/cm/°C/s

<u>Thermal and Stress Analysis</u>   As indicated previously in the high-speed photographic analysis, the absorption of high-intensity radiation in alumina material gave evidence of large thermal forces acting in the formation of a laser-drilled hole. Under certain conditions, radial cracks

would occur at the hole which could propagate to an adjacent hole or another high-stress location, such as the edge of the ceramic material. A model was developed[67] to describe the temperature profile and the associated thermal stress distributions for the laser drilled holes. The model is given in Chapter 3 (Section 3.3.4, Figure 3-23). Its application to alumina ceramic hole drilling is given here for the case of ruby radiation only.

Consider the energy of 4 J in a pulse length of 1.5 ms (Table 4-9). This gives a power density of 1.67×10^8 W/cm² for a beam divergence of 3 mrad. Drilling in a relatively thick specimen (3.2 mm) can be analytically treated with the model for a semi-infinite body, using the assumptions stated in the model. Specifically, (3-71) will be solved with the following conditions imposed on the problem.

1. A semi-infinite body is assumed. Thus $T \to 0$ as $Z \to \infty$; and $\partial T/\partial Z = 0$ at $Z = 0$.
2. The intensity distribution is uniform across the focused spot, with $I_0 = 1.67 \times 10^8$ W/cm².
3. The focused spot diameter is approximately 0.50 mm.

The calculation of the temperature distribution in the material is dependent on the velocity of sublimation (i.e., vaporization). This is found experimentally by measuring the hole penetration depth, $f(Z)$, as a function of time. Figure 4-62 shows the hole depth as a function of pulse

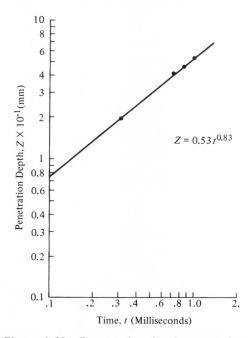

$$Z = 0.53 t^{0.83}$$

Time, t (Milliseconds)

Figure 4-62   Penetration depth versus time.

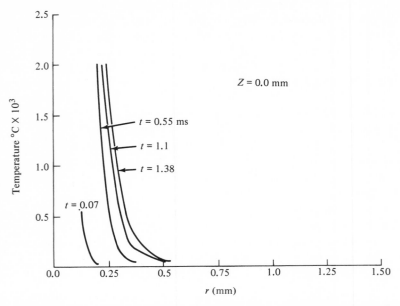

Figure 4-63   Radial temperature distribution at the surface for various times.

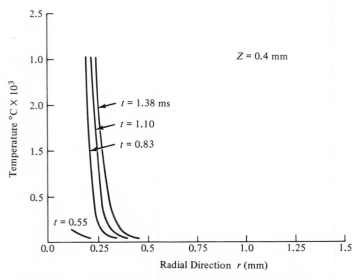

Figure 4-64   Radial temperature distribution at a heat source location of 0.4 mm from the surface and for various times.

length, t. The velocity of sublimation can readily be obtained by differentiating $f(Z)$ with respect to t. On a log–log plot, the relationship takes the form of

$$\log Z = \log k + a \log t \qquad (4\text{-}5)$$

where Z = hole depth,

$\qquad k$ = a constant, numerically equal to the hole depth scale intercept,

$\qquad a$ = the slope of the line plot.

Equation (3-71) (Section 3.3.4) is used in a computer program to generate the temperature distributions shown in Figures 4-63 and 4-64. The data are for various pulse lengths of approximately the same beam energy incident on the alumina surface.

Figure 4-65 gives the tangential stress distribution as well as its radial propagation at a heat source location $Z = 0.25$ mm from the surface. From a position of the actual physics of the specimens, whether thin (0.7 mm) or relatively thick (3.2 mm) compared to the laser spot (0.25 mm),

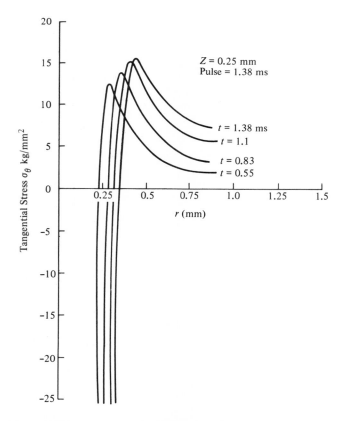

Figure 4-65   *Tangential stress distribution in r direction at $Z = 0.25$ mm.*

the ceramic substrates are very much like thin plates. Because of this, the curves are developed for the case of a plane stress where the tangential stress component at the wall of the laser drilled hole is found by the expression

$$\sigma_\theta = \frac{\alpha E}{r^2} \left(\int_a^r Tr \, dr - Tr^2 \right) \tag{4-6}$$

where α is the coefficient of linear thermal expansion, E is Young's modulus, and a is the radius of the laser spot.

The above thermal and stress analysis provides one with a greater insight into the significance of the hole drilling parameters of power and pulse duration in laser drilling processes. The theory indicates that shorter pulse lengths generally give lower stresses. Longer pulses will generate higher stresses simply because the heat will penetrate or diffuse further into the material. Since the magnitude of the stress is governed essentially by the temperature profile, the desirable condition for hole drilling is to maintain a sufficiently high beam intensity for a minimum time to remove (theoretically by sublimation) a given mass of material. Furthermore, the theory can be used to predict the hole profile.[67]

4.3 micromachining

In the area of micromachining, the laser has perhaps been used to its fullest advantage in thin-film and semiconductor circuit processing. The laser is a promising tool for both the formation of, and trimming of, passive components such as resistors and capacitors. Fabrication of gap capacitors has been demonstrated. The thin-film-on-silicon technology coupled with laser adjustment of resistors can accommodate requirements that fall within the 0.1 percent to 1 percent accuracy range. Line scribing for the purposes of subsequent substrate separation, both in the thin-film and semiconductor areas, has proven practical from a production standpoint. Selective removal of fine lines of conducting material for conductor path or circuit generation also looks promising.

The primary advantages to be gained through use of the laser in micromachining can be listed as follows:

1. Localized or confined heat affected zones
2. Short time reactions (specifically for pulsed and Q-switched lasers)
3. Noncontact
4. Capability for "post-fabrication" component adjustment

To minimize damage to the substrate in laser machining of thin films, the substrate should absorb less readily at the laser wavelength than does the film. As in other application areas, many laser types are readily available and have been successfully employed. Among the more important are the Nd:YAG, pulsed argon ion, and CO_2. The high repetition rates and short pulse durations obtainable from the continuously pumped, repetitively Q-switched YAG make it particularly well suited for high-speed machining.

4·3·1   resistor trimming

The first application considered is the adjustment of Ta_2N thin-film resistors. Figure 4-66 illustrates one possible configuration for such a resistor. The resistance between conductors, being a function of both the film properties and its cross-sectional area (i.e., the area normal to the current flow), can be adjusted by either an alteration of the material's properties or by a reduction in the effective cross-sectional area. Laser trimming of resistors is a noncontact process that can be used to adjust small resistors and can be used at almost any step in the sequence of circuit fabrication.[68]

Three methods are possible when using the laser. These are:

1. Trimming by producing holes
2. Adjusting the resistance by shaping or altering the area
3. Trimming by thermal oxidation

1. Vaporizing small spots of material to produce a hole array in the interior of the resistor in a regular fashion offers distinct advantages over other techniques in that it minimizes changes in inductance and capacitance and maintains the same resistor substrate area, hence minimizing hot spots. A Q-switched YAG laser can be used to produce uniform

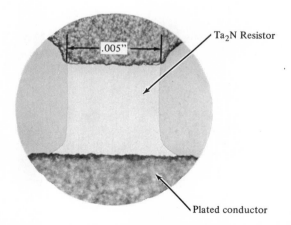

.005"
Ta₂N Resistor
Plated conductor

Figure 4-66   Typical configuration for tantalum nitride thin-film resistors.[68]

holes in Ta$_2$N film from less than 8 μm in diameter to a maximum exceeding 40 μm in diameter (see Figure 4-67). For a nominal 10 Ω resistor, changes of less than 0.01 percent per hole can be achieved for holes less than 20 μm in diameter on 50–75 μm spacings when a small number of holes are vaporized. When hundreds or thousands of holes are produced, a room temperature drift or aging condition is often seen which increases the resistance more than the increase resulting from a single hole. A typical drift characteristic is shown in Figure 4-68a. The drift is most likely a result of the heat-affected zone adjacent to the areas actually evaporated. Small diameter holes produce greater drifts than larger holes for the same overall resistance change since the heat-affected area is greater for a given resistance change produced with small holes than with the same change produced with larger holes. Thus, to reduce post-trimming drift, a hole diameter as large as possible should be used. Figure 4-68b shows a typical aging characteristic as a function of hole diameter.

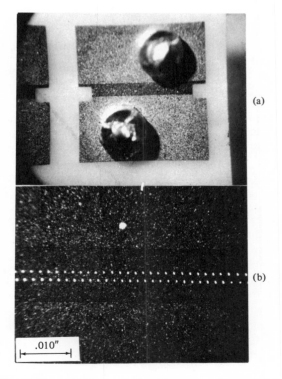

(a)

(b)

Figure 4-67   Uniform holes vaporized in a tantalum nitride resistor. (a) Overall view of resistor.   (b) Magnified view of the tantalum nitride showing individual laser evaporated areas.

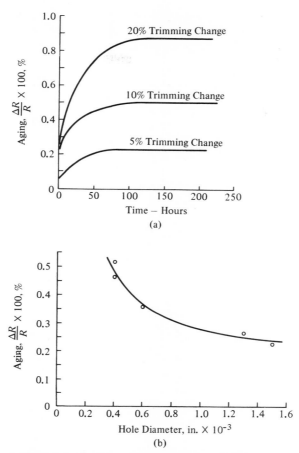

Figure 4-68 **(a) Drift characteristic of laser-trimmed tantalum nitride resistors.** **(b) Effect of hole size on the drift of tantalum nitride resistors.**[68]

2. The second method of laser trimming of resistors is patterning or reshaping the resistor.   Examples of very large changes made in 125 μm square resistors are shown in Figure 4-69.   In Figure 4-69a, the machined serpentine geometry increased the resistance by a factor of ten; a factor of three increase in resistance was achieved for the resistor shown in Figure 4-69b.

The post-trimming drift observed with machined resistors is generally less than that experienced by resistors trimmed by vaporizing an array of holes.   For instance, a 300 Ω serpentine resistor showed a 0.2 percent drift after a 10 percent trimming change by vaporizing an array of 25 μm diameter holes on 125 μm centers.   The same resistor showed less than 0.03 percent drift in several experiments in which the laser machined lines across the current path, normal to the resistor edge, to produce a similar

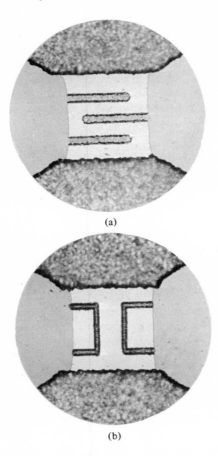

(a)

(b)

Figure 4-69   Reshaping resistor geometry by laser machining.[68]

increase in resistance. It is believed that the reason for this difference is that the peripheries of the lines were less than the total periphery associated with the array of holes.

3. A third method of trimming resistors is by using the laser as a heat source to oxidize the tantalum film. Very stable power-aging results with relative insensitivity to various processing parameters have been reported and should apply to laser thermally trimmed resistors as well. The use of a laser as a heat source has two advantages over other heat sources. First, the laser beam can be focused to very fine areas for the trimming of small resistors, and it can be used in a raster fashion to cover large components.

In the compatible thin-film-on-silicon technology, a vacuum deposited "Cermet" of chromium and silicon monoxide (Cr-SiO) has been used as the resistive material.   The Cermet film is about 30 nm thick and has a specific resistivity of 3×10^{-3} Ω-cm which provides a sheet resistance of 1000 $\Omega/\square$.   The composition of the film is 58 percent Cr, 42 percent SiO by weight, and is generally used where higher power dissipation is required.[69]   The resistors are adjusted by using localized laser heating with the package completely sealed with a transparent glass cover before the adjustments are made.   A pulsed argon-ion laser providing an energy density of 100 J/cm² and pulse widths between 15 and 150 μs was used with a resulting resistor film surface temperature of $\sim 1000°C$.   In this case, a decreasing resistivity was found to occur and was attributed to an annealing effect resulting in a more ordered structure and, hence, consistent with a lower resistivity.

The processes utilized in the adjustment or trimming of thick-film components are much the same as those with thin-film circuits, except that different lasers might be utilized.   For instance, a small Q-switched Nd:YAG laser (maximum of 1.5 kW peak power in 300 ns pulses) appears ideally suited to trimming thin-film circuits.   It is relatively inexpensive to operate, it is reliable, and it can controllably remove areas as small as a few square micrometers.   With thick films, more material must normally be vaporized; thus more energy must be absorbed.   This requires a larger laser or a laser having an output more readily absorbed by the workpiece.

Laser systems are commercially available for the purpose of trimming thick-film resistors.   One system has an automatic work table for locating the resistor under the focused laser beam and a Q-switched CO_2 laser for removing the thick-film resistor material.   With such a system, it should be possible to trim in the same manner as with thin-film circuits, using the YAG laser, except for two considerations.

First, the CO_2 laser wavelength is 10.6×10^3 nm, whereas the Nd:YAG laser wavelength is 1.06×10^3 nm.   The shorter Nd:YAG wavelength allows its output to be focused to a spot diameter approximately one tenth that of the CO_2 laser.   Second, most substrate materials, such as aluminum oxide or glass, do not absorb a large percentage of 1.06×10^3 nm radiation, whereas they do absorb 10.6×10^3 nm radiation quite well. Thus it appears that greater substrate damage can be expected when using the CO_2 laser.

A procedure was developed for adjusting glass encapsulated deposited carbon resistors to a tolerance of ± 1 percent automatically (Figure 4-70). Because encapsulation caused a random change in value, trimming could not be obtained by other techniques.   The system used contains a Q-switched ruby laser which delivers 1/2 J, 30 ns pulses at a rate of 1 pps. The optical system consists of a mask to shape the laser beam, a telescope to control the focused beam size, and a lens to project the beam onto the resistor surface.   The projection lens also serves as the objective lens of a CCTV system used for observing the resistor when it is in the work

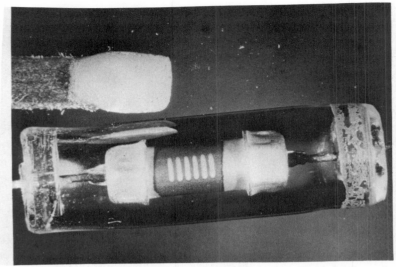

Figure 4-70   Deposited carbon resistor adjusted to value by a laser after glass encapsulation.

station. This technique utilizes the laser's ability to perform useful operations without physical contact, its ability to vaporize high boiling point materials, and its ability to selectively vaporize materials (i.e., to evaporate the carbon while having no detrimental effect on the ceramic core and glass envelope).

4·3·2   capacitor adjustment and fabrication

Trimming of thin-film capacitors with the laser has been attempted but success has been somewhat limited. The ideal capacitor trimming technique should not degrade the capacitor dielectric in any way; however, currently this is impossible. It is expected in the future that mode-locked lasers will be available which will deliver extremely short, high peak power pulses; it is possible that these can be used to remove only the top electrode material with little if any degradation of the dielectric material.

   Although the process of trimming thin-film capacitors is not developed at the moment, an alternate technique of making thin-film capacitors with the laser has been successful.[70] A Q-switched Nd:YAG laser has been used to vaporize extremely narrow lines in a gold conducting film to form gap capacitors and capacitance values of 4000 pF/cm^2 with line (gap) widths as narrow as 6 μm (Figure 4-71). These capacitors could easily be trimmed to value by using the laser to cut one of the meanders at the proper point.

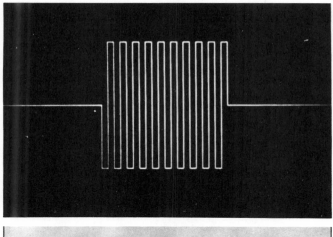

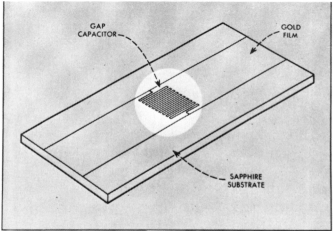

Figure 4-71   Gap capacitor formed by laser machining of gold film on sapphire. [70]

4·3·3   scribing

Scribing is an effective way in which materials may be separated or shaped, especially brittle materials such as silicon, glass, and ceramic.   In scribing, it is desired to remove material along a path on the surface.   Conventional methods generally accomplish this by mechanically traversing a diamond point along the surface of the material.   When the material is stressed sufficiently, a fracture will occur along the scribed path.

It was proposed that the laser be used for the purpose of scribing materials, [71] and recent developments have shown that the ideal method is by the use of a repetitively Q-switched or repetitively pulsed laser which vaporizes the material with little excess heating and melting. The specific example of using a Q-switched YAG laser in scribing semiconductor devices is treated in detail in Section 4.3.4.

One application for high-power CO_2 lasers is in the scribing and cutting of ceramic substrates. Diamond scribing tools used in the "scribe and break" process are expensive and suffer a high wear rate on ceramics. The focused high-power CO_2 laser beam, on the other hand, provides an effective zero wear rate tool for scribing or cutting ceramics.

Laser radiation at 10.6×10^3 nm is absorbed well by all ceramics. However, ceramics do present a problem for thermal cutting processes. They have moderate thermal conductivities and low tensile strengths coupled with high elastic moduli. As a result, continuous beam laser cutting tends to result in melting damage due to overheating near the cut, and fracturing due to high thermal stresses. Hence, as mentioned above, substrate scribing is best accomplished with a pulsed beam. The scribe is produced by drilling a series of small holes. Figure 4-72a shows a 0.64 mm thick alumina substrate which has been scribed at a speed of

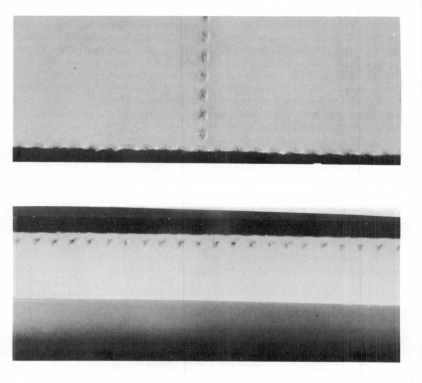

Figure 4-72   Alumina substrate after separation along a laser-scribed line.   Mag. 25X.   (a) Surface view.   (b) Edge view.

6 cm/s.   The system was pulsed at a frequency of 333 pps with a pulse period of 3 ms at a power level of 20 W.   The width of the damage area is approximately 100 μm.   Figure 4-72b shows an edge view of the same substrate.   Hole depth is approximately 125 μm with a hole-to-hole spacing of 190 μm. CO_2 systems capable of delivering 50 W of continuous TEM_{00} power make possible a scribing speed of 10 cm/s with a minimum focused spot size of 50 μm.[61]

4.3.4   detailed analysis and solution for a micromachining application—silicon scribing

Many unique and challenging manufacturing problems arise as a result of miniaturized circuit components.   One of these is the separation into individual components of many hundreds of discrete electronic devices, such as diodes or transistors, which have been fabricated on a single wafer or substrate.   Figure 4-73 shows a portion of such a wafer on which silicon transistors have been made.   The devices themselves are approximately 0.4 mm by 0.4 mm square and are separated from each other by a series of grid lines each 50 μm wide.   Conventional separation techniques consist of traversing a pre-oriented diamond point, under mechanical pressure, along these inactive grid lines to cause material removal, thus generating a scribe line.   After the complete wafer, typically from 2.5 to 7.5 cm in diameter, is scribed in this manner, chip separation is accomplished by the application of sufficient force to cause fracture along these lines.

So long as process variables, such as the amount of wear of the diamond point, its orientation with respect to the material surface, applied pressure, etc., are known and controlled, this process can result

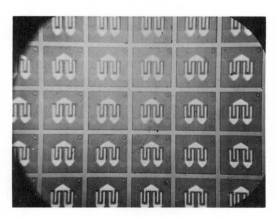

Figure 4-73   Portion of a silicon wafer showing discrete transistors.

in high device yield, i.e., the recovery after breaking of essentially all devices on the original wafer. In practice, however, it has proven difficult, if not impossible, to control and monitor these variables, and hence an acceptable yield is not always achieved.

It has been found that good wafer-scribing results can be achieved using the laser to cause evaporation within the grid lines. There are a number of advantages to be gained through use of the laser, the most important of which is the ability to generate a consistent and uniform scribe line as a result of the precise control one has over a laser process. Being continuously able to monitor the laser output is the single most important factor leading to this control. No such monitoring is possible when diamond scribing.

Specific Requirements—Laser Selection   The possible use of the laser for this application requires careful examination of several factors. From a manufacturing standpoint, the process must prove to be economical. The component cost of the laser and associated equipment required for this application exceeds by a factor of 4-5 the cost of conventional diamond-scribing equipment. Hence, from economic considerations, the laser process should result in higher yield, be faster, etc., in order to be practical. In addition, a stable and reliable laser should be available to accomplish the evaporation process with no resulting thermal or other damage to the electronic devices themselves.

In selecting the laser with its specific output requirements and mode of operation, the single most important item to be considered is one of thermal damage to active devices located adjacent to the area of material evaporation (in some cases, less than 25 μm from the affected area). From this fact alone, CW lasers and pulsed lasers with relatively long temporal pulse widths would be ruled out due to the short thermal time constants of the material involved. The flow of heat in matter is governed by solutions to the basic heat flow equation (see Chapter 3 and (3-25)). From solutions presented and discussed in Chapter 3, it can be seen that to minimize any possible damage due to excessive amounts of heat flow, the time duration of the laser pulse should be minimized. At present, Q-switched lasers are the most practical sources of such radiation, specifically the ruby (694.3 nm), Nd:glass (1.06×10^3 nm), and Nd:YAG (1.06×10^3 nm) lasers. For intrinsic silicon (ignoring for the moment effects due to doping, oxide layers, etc.), optical absorption due to valence-conduction band transitions at room temperature occurs below 1130 nm.[72] Also, there is no significant difference in surface reflectivity in the 700 nm to 1100 nm range (at room temperature). Thus, from wavelength considerations, it would appear that any of the three lasers could conceivably be used. Each possesses sufficient power to vaporize silicon. However, the ruby and Nd:glass are limited in repetition rate and hence would limit the scribing speed. With recent advances in acousto-optic modulators, the Nd:YAG has the capability of being Q-switched at rates exceeding 10 kHz. It is primarily for these reasons that the continuously pumped, repetitively Q-switched Nd:YAG is used in this application.

Theoretical Analysis The basic question to be answered is: What effect will focused Q-switched radiation at 1060 nm have on silicon? Both the depth to which material can be removed and the temperature gradients developed in the material are required information.

Material removal was discussed in Section 3.3.4. Applying the simplified steady-state analysis presented there to this problem (assuming an incident laser pulse as shown in Figure 3-22), a penetration depth of at least 37 μm is predicted. The experimentally measured depth is 25 μm. Thus, with outputs easily attainable from Q-switched YAG lasers, penetration depths of at least 25 μm are predicted and verified by experiment. For a nominal 0.15 mm thick silicon wafer, this single-pulse depth results in an adequate scribe line when repetitive pulses are overlapped. This topic is treated in more detail in the following section.

Knowing that material removal to sufficient depths is possible, consider the thermal damage problem from an analytical viewpoint. If possible, estimates should be made of radial or transverse temperature distributions present during and after the laser pulse. This is done by applying the thermal model discussed in Section 3.3.4 (Figure 3-23) and specifically by obtaining solutions to (3-68). The following conditions are imposed to obtain the solution:

1. A semi-infinite body is assumed. Thus

$$T \to 0 \quad \text{as} \quad Z \to \infty$$

2. The intensity distribution across the focused spot is Gaussian, with the distance between $1/e^2$ points being approximately 12 μm.
3. Unfocused peak power is 1 kW and the pulse duration is 150 ns.

As was the case in the example previously discussed for laser drilling of Al_2O_3, the calculation of the temperature distribution is dependent on the velocity of sublimation. In this case, an average value is chosen consistent with the experimentally observed depths and laser pulse lengths. Figure 4-74 shows the solution to (3-71) under the above conditions. The temperature as a function of radial distance from spot center is shown with time as a third parameter. The temperature is seen to remain at its room temperature value beyond 30 μm from spot center, thus leading to the conclusion that for a nominal grid line width from 50 μm to 75 μm damage due to excessive temperature rises would not be expected.

In summary, from the theoretical calculation just reviewed, it appears that the output available from a Q-switched YAG laser is well suited for silicon machining.

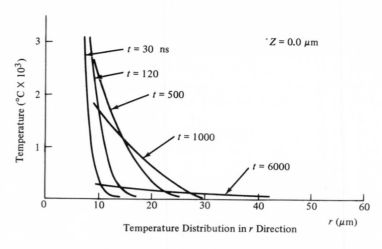

Temperature Distribution in r Direction

Figure 4-74   Surface temperature versus radial position with time as a parameter.

Equipment Characterization, Preliminary Investigations, and System Implementation   In this section procedures for determining operating parameters for a laser-scribing system are described. In general, these parameters are subdivided into those which are considered static, i.e., relating specifically to the laser and its output, and those which are considered dynamic and relate to the actual formation of a continuous scribe line.

A typical Q-switched YAG laser considered for this application consists of a 3 mm by 50 mm Nd:YAG rod optically pumped by two 1500 W tungsten-bromine lamps in a double ellipse configuration. CW output is 10 W. Q-switching is accomplished acousto-optically. The cavity is internally apertured for transverse mode selection. The laser head (consisting of YAG rod, pump lamps, etc.) is water cooled to maintain an operating temperature of 70°F to 80°F.

The output of such a laser, when operated in the Q-switched mode, is characterized by its average and peak power, pulse width, and beam divergence. Average power measurements of pulsed outputs are made by an integrating or averaging type detector. (As indicated in Chapter 9, a number of devices are available for such measurements at 1.06×10^3 nm, a typical example being the EG&G Radiometer.) The pulse width, or more specifically the temporal pulse shape, is monitored with a device whose response time is adequate to follow the pulse. Rise times of 5 ns to 30 ns are typical and any number of solid-state detectors or vacuum phototubes can provide adequate response. From a measure of average power and pulse width, the peak power can be calculated, as illustrated by the following example.

A typical laser pulse shape, as monitored by a photodiode, is shown in Figure 4-75a.   Although calibrated photodiodes can be used to make peak power measurements, the most common method is to approximate the pulse by a square wave of height equal to the peak and width equal to the half-amplitude width, as measured on the monitoring oscilloscope. Referring to Figure 4-75b, the peak power is then calculated as:

$$P_{\text{peak}} \times \text{pulse width} = P_{\text{avg}} \frac{1}{\text{rep rate}}$$

Typical values are:

$$P_{\text{avg}} = 600 \text{ mW, rep rate} = 1 \text{ kHz, pulse width} = 240 \text{ ns}$$

$$\therefore P_{\text{peak}} = 2.5 \text{ kW}$$

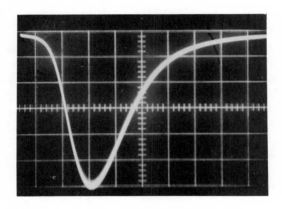

(a) Photodiode output depicting pulse shape of Q-switched laser

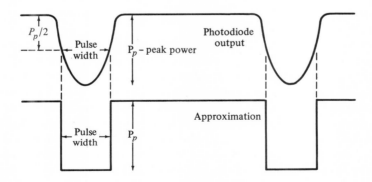

(b) Approximation used to calculate peak power

Figure 4-75

The energy per pulse can likewise be estimated from the square-wave approximation to be

$$\text{Energy/pulse} = \int_0^{240 \text{ ns}} P_{\text{peak}} \, dt = 0.6 \text{ mJ}$$

Typical characterization results are shown in Figure 4-76, where peak power is plotted versus repetition rate for different internal cavity aperture sizes, and hence transverse modes.

Beam divergence is defined as a measure of the angular spread of the beam after it emerges from the cavity (see Section 3.1*).   It can be found from a straightforward geometrical measurement with the aid of viewing devices, such as infrared phosphors, since 1.06×10^3 nm radiation is not visible to the eye.   Such viewing devices are also required for physically locating the beam for alignment of optical components and the like.

In practice, the lens parameters which can be controlled should be optimized, and followed by experimental determination of actual working parameters, such as spot size and depth of focus.   In the following discussion, an $f/1.4$ focusing lens with a focal length of 50 mm is used.   For a minimum spot size, the beam is expanded to fill the aperture of the lens. This also results in a minimum depth of focus.   If, however, a larger depth of focus is required, the effective f/number of the lens could be

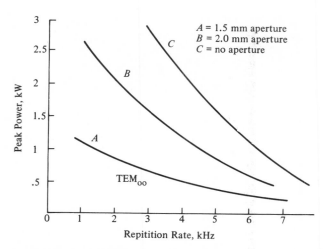

Figure 4-76   Peak power versus repetition rate for Q-switched Nd:YAG.

* Section 3.1 is devoted to a consideration of focusing optics required for material working applications.   The important relations among lens and beam parameters are considered and specific examples illustrated.   It is assumed that all lens elements are diffraction limited and the laser is operated in the fundamental TEM_{00} mode with a resultant transverse intensity distribution that is Gaussian.

increased by reducing the beam diameter and hence not completely filling the lens aperture (resulting in a corresponding increase in spot diameter).

For silicon scribing, a spot size no larger than 25 μm is required; and due to possible wafer thickness variations, a depth of focus of at least ± 25 μm is also necessary. In this context, depth of focus is defined as that distance over which the same maximum penetration depth is obtained, in contrast to (3-8). It was found that at $f/2$ (i.e., the beam diameter expanded to approximately 2.5 cm), a satisfactory effective spot size of 20 μm and depth of focus of ± 25 μm resulted. Figure 4-77 illustrates the setup used to establish these parameters.

A significant advantage of the acousto-optic Q-switch is the ability to externally control the modulator and generate, for example, a single Q-switched pulse from the laser. Both penetration depth and depth of focus can be determined in one experiment. By either moving the lens with respect to the sample or vice versa, a curve such as that shown in Figure 4-78 can be obtained where each data point represents a measure of the penetration depth obtained from a single pulse at the particular lens to sample spacing. The maximum pentration depth occurs at the lens position resulting in a minimum spot diameter (greatest focused power density) and is seen to occur over a range of approximately 50 μm, therefore resulting in a depth of focus of ± 25 μm for this lens system.

Having reviewed the more important static characteristics associated with the application, the actual formation of a continuous scribe line will now be considered. Because Q-switching results in a series of discrete pulses, each focused to approximately a 20 μm diameter, it is necessary to overlap pulses in order to create a continuous scribe line. As a result, one of the more important dynamic parameters is the amount of pulse overlap. This directly determines the resultant penetration depth and amount of force required to cause fracture along the line as well as the operating economics.

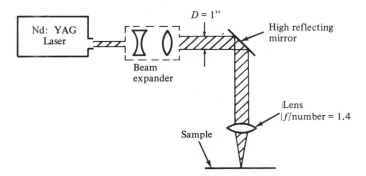

Figure 4-77 Typical schematic representation of an experimental micromachining setup.

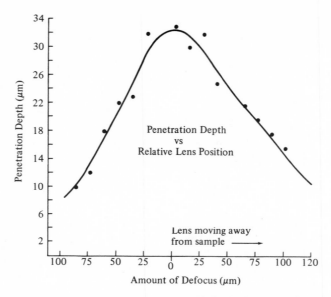

Figure 4-78 *Variation of single-pulse penetration depth with changes in lens to sample spacing for silicon using a Q-switched Nd:YAG laser.*

Percent overlap is defined geometrically as shown in Figure 4-79. There are two methods to investigate and characterize this parameter. One consists of a visual examination of the resultant line (cross sections, e.g.) to determine width, penetration depth, contour, and the like, i.e., its geometrical shape. The second is by measuring the force required to cause fracture along the line for various amounts of overlap or equivalently, various penetration depths. Percent overlap is investigated at constant power with laser pulse rate and/or the mechanical speed with which the sample is moved as the parameters to be varied. Experimental results are shown in Figures 4-80a and 4-80b. The data were obtained with a power density of approximately 10^9 W/cm^2.

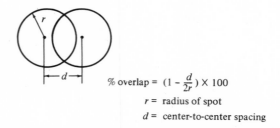

$$\% \text{ overlap} = \left(1 - \frac{d}{2r}\right) \times 100$$

$r =$ radius of spot

$d =$ center-to-center spacing

Figure 4-79 *Percent overlap defined geometrically.*

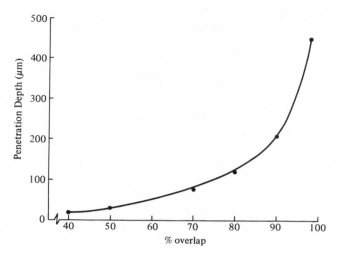

Figure 4-80a.   Penetration depth versus percentage overlap for laser-scribed lines on silicon using a Q-switched YAG laser.   Peak power density was approximately 10^9 W/cm², pulse width 100 ns.

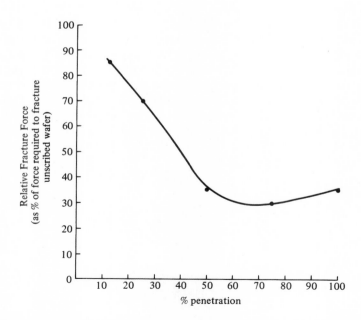

Figure 4-80b   Relative fracture force versus percent penetration. Same conditions as Figure 4-80a.

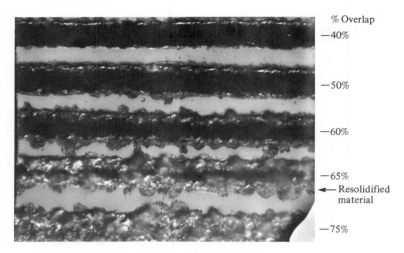

% Overlap

—40%

—50%

—60%

—65%
←— Resolidified
   material

—75%

Figure 4-81   Surface view of laser-scribed lines on silicon for the
percent overlaps indicated.

The dependence of penetration depth on pulse overlap is shown in Figure 4-80a and the variation of fracture force versus percent penetration for a wafer thickness of 0.25 mm is shown in Figure 4-80b. Arguments would predict a general trend toward decreasing fracture force as the amount of pulse overlap (or equivalently penetration) increases. However, the distinct minima in the curve at approximately 70 percent penetration can only be predicted by a study of the laser material interaction itself.[73] The basic reason for its existence is a buildup of resolidified material which subsequently effects the resultant scribe line. Figure 4-81

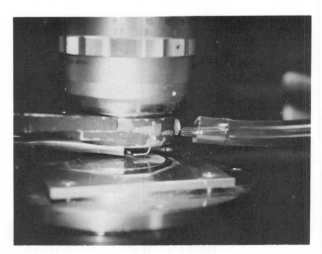

Figure 4-82   Photo showing components used in particle pickup
technique.

shows a surface view of lines scribed at the percent overlaps indicated. The buildup of resolidified matter is clearly shown.

As yet no mention has been made regarding specific selection of operating parameters such as laser repetition rate and table speeds. From the previous discussions, however, the nature of their interdependence should be clear.   In most cases the particular method used to fracture and separate the devices will dictate the required fracture force; then the corresponding amount of pulse overlap can be estimated from Figure 4-80b.   Knowing the single-pulse spot size, the laser repetition rate and linear table speed are adjusted to achieve this operating condition.   Practical limitations in such parameter selection are the maximum achievable table speed and the laser peak power (which is a decreasing function of repetition rate above a few kilohertz).

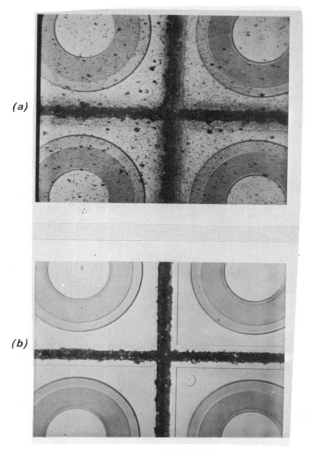

(a)

(b)

Figure 4-83 Laser-scribed silicon wafer. (a) Results without particle pickup scheme.   (b) Corresponding results using particle pickup.

These discussions and results have assumed undoped silicon. All practical devices, and especially the grid lines separating the active devices, are generally coated with oxide or nitride layers (e.g., SiO_2, Si_3N_4). In addition, the substrate itself is not intrinsic but impurity doped. However, it has been found that with the power densities being used neither the amount or type of impurity donor nor the various surface layers have any significant effect.

Another consideration in using laser scribing in device processing is the possibility of circuit damage due to the generation of and depositing of particulate matter on the surface of the wafers. Any number of vacuum pickup schemes can be used to prevent such deposits from occurring. One such technique, which has been successfully used, employs an air jet and vacuum suction as shown in Figure 4-82. The conventional laminar flow vacuum pickup is enhanced through turbulence caused by the air jet blowing into the immediate area. Figure 4-83 shows the results using this particular "pickup" technique followed by an ultra-sonic cleaning of the wafer.

Figure 4-84 is a photograph of a prototype laser-scribing system developed for use in production. Because of operator safety require-ments, the entire system is enclosed and interlocked. Viewing of the devices for alignment purposes prior to scribing is done using a CCTV system similar to that illustrated in Figure 4-22.

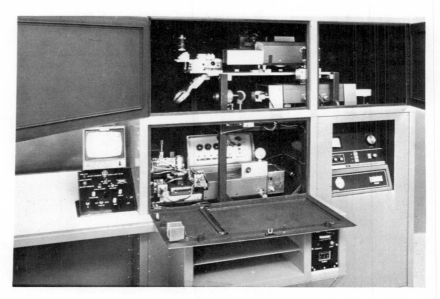

Figure 4-84   Laser-scribing system.

4·4   miscellaneous applications

4·4·1   controlled fracturing

Controlled fracturing is a technique for separating materials such as electronic circuits or components which are batch processed, or for the generation of special shapes in brittle materials.[74]   This technique, which uses the laser to controllably fracture or break, has one inherent advantage over other separation techniques; i.e., controlled fracture allows a sample to be separated into two or more parts with no evaporation or loss of material.   Figure 4-85 shows miscellaneous ceramic pieces generated by controlled fracture with a laser.

   In the controlled fracture process, the laser's energy is applied to a small area of the surface of the material (Figure 4-86).   The absorption of the beam creates thermal gradients which, in turn, create mechanical stresses sufficient to fracture the material.   If the material is moved with respect to the laser beam, the fracture follows.   This technique works because the laser creates stresses sufficient to cause fracture but over a region so small that the fracture does not propagate uncontrollably.   In Figure 4-87 data are plotted for the minimum power as a function of parting rate to reliably fracture a high alumina material using a CO_2 laser.

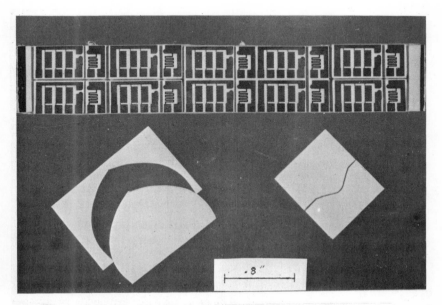

Figure 4-85   Various shaped pieces of high alumina ceramic formed by controlled fracture technique.

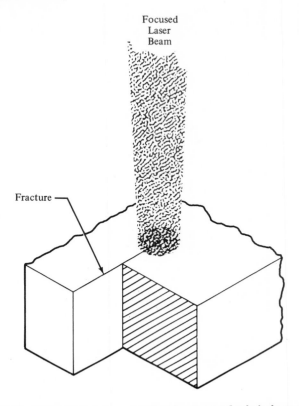

Focused
Laser
Beam

Fracture

Figure 4-86 Schematic of controlled fracture of a brittle material by a laser beam.

Many brittle materials such as high alumina ceramic, ferrite sheet, single-crystal quartz, sapphire, soda-lime glass, and Corning 7059 glass have been controllably fractured. Fused quartz was the only material that could not be fractured.

When using the laser to controllably fracture single crystals, the effects of cleavage planes are usually notable because of the preference of the crystals to fracture along these planes. Possibly the greatest advantage of cleaving crystals is that the crystal itself is the primary control of the direction of separation and, therefore, the tool or device to initiate the cleavage need not have fine control. For instance, single-crystal quartz (0.6 mm thick, 8 mm wide) can be cleaved by focusing the energy of a CO_2 laser (40 W) into a line along the desired cleavage direction. Alternately, applying the laser's energy to a circular spot on the crystal surface achieves the same result. The location of the spot determines the location of the plane along which the cleavage will occur, and the crystal itself determines the path along which the fracture will occur.

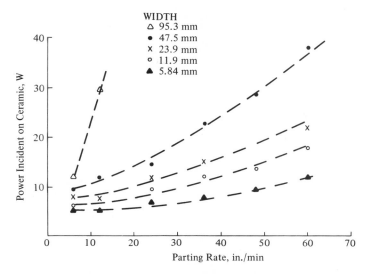

Figure 4-87   Laser power versus parting rate for high alumina ceramic. Ceramic thickness 0.7 mm, length 11.4 cm, and width as indicated. [74]

Some evidence indicates that focusing the laser energy into a line may not be desirable, for if the line is not perfectly aligned with the cleavage plane, it may force the fracture to deviate from the desired path.

4·4·2   evaporation

Conventional evaporation processes for the deposition of thin films involve:

1. A vacuum enclosure which provides a suitable environment for the evaporation process.
2. A vapor source, where the material to be evaporated can be held and heated.
3. The substrates, which are to be coated with evaporant.
4. A substrate holder and heater.

Heat sources consist of resistance heated wire, strips, and boats containing or supporting the evaporants. Electron beam bombardment has also been used because of the high-energy flux available resulting in a very high evaporation rate. In certain applications, however, the use of a laser offers several unique advantages over these more common sources.

1. The vapor can be generated in any atmosphere transparent to the laser radiation. It should be noted that vacuum is still generally used for film deposition.

2. No contaminants are introduced by the laser radiation.
3. Essentially all of the laser energy may be used for evaporation with little of it being absorbed by the substrate.
4. Small selected areas of the source material may be evaporated.
5. The evaporant source may be located very close to the substrate.
6. Compounds may be evaporated with little change in composition.
7. The laser can be located outside the vacuum chamber.

A CW YAG laser has been used as a replacement for an electron beam energy source in the vapor deposition of platinum onto silicon.[75] Specifically, MOS device fabrication requires platinum deposition for the formation of the silicide layer for making low-resistance contacts to the silicon, and the barrier layer for isolating layers of titanium and gold. Use of the electron beam resulted in a space charge buildup at the metal oxide interface. A laser heat source did not produce electrically charged particles or other ionizing radiation in the vacuum chamber and was shown to eliminate the associated problems in the MOS devices themselves.

Figure 4-88 schematically shows the experimental setup. A 20 W CW YAG laser was chosen over pulsed systems, since use of the latter generally results in splattering and/or an ionized plume of the target material. Either or both of these effects are undesirable in a process intended to deposit a very thin, uniform, and defect-free film. Since platinum does not develop an appreciable vapor pressure unless heated above its melting point (1775°C), it was necessary physically to support a melt in the vacuum chamber. As shown in Figure 4-89, the molten

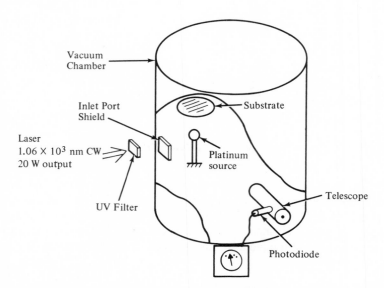

Figure 4-88   Experimental apparatus for evaporation using a laser.[75]

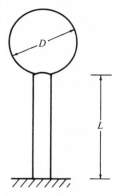

Figure 4-89   Molten sphere supported by platinum wire.[75]

platinum wire was supported by surface tension on the tip of an upright platinum wire.   Through proper parameter adjustment, the bulk remains static and molten.   Evaporation rates achieved with a 20 W YAG were 12 Å/h at a 6 cm source-to-substrate distance.   Although quite slow, this is only a consequence of the limited output power of the laser used. No theoretical limitation to the utilization of a laser was encountered in this example.

Another example of thin-film deposition has been reported.[76]   A transparent substrate coated completely with a thin film of some material is placed adjacent to a blank substrate on which it is desired to obtain a pattern.   A laser is then focused through the first substrate onto the thin film.   As the two substrates are moved with respect to the laser beam, the material is vaporized from the one substrate and redeposited on the second substrate in a pattern which duplicates the movement of the substrates with respect to the laser beam.

An investigation of the applicability of lasers in evaporation processes resulted in the following conclusions:[77]

1. Pulse radiation of bulk materials can produce congruent evaporation of alloys and compounds.
2. Films produced by laser evaporation have a degree of crystallinity which is normally only achieved by external heating of the substrate.
3. Films of refractory materials can be produced without the normal problems of contamination by simply evaporating from the surface of a bulk specimen.

4.4.3   cutting

Except in the case of controlled fracturing (Section 4.4.1), when substances are cut, material is removed through either the vaporization or sublimation process.   Although this process can be used effectively for many materials, the majority of industrial applications of laser cutting have employed a gas stream coaxial with the laser (Figure 4-90). Two basic types of gas-jet cutting have been used, one employing a reactive gas for metal cutting and the other an inert gas used generally for flammable materials. By far the most common laser used to date for continuous cutting is the CO_2 due to the relatively high CW powers that can be achieved. At present, commercial systems capable of delivering 500 W are available, with the prospect good for >1000 W in the near future.

In the reactive gas-jet assisted laser-cutting process, the incoming gas jet chemically reacts with the material being cut. Consider the specific case of an oxygen jet employed in cutting a highly reactive metal such as titanium. Normally, kilowatts of continuous power would be required for cutting significant thicknesses. However, through application of the oxygen jet, the highly exothermic reaction

$$Ti + O_2 \rightarrow TiO_2 + heat$$

occurs from which most of the energy required for the cutting process is obtained. The laser serves to raise the metal to an elevated temperature, thus enhancing the speed of the reaction. The gas jet also serves to expel the molten material produced from the cut.

Materials that have been successfully cut using this method are titanium, low-carbon steel, stainless steel, and zircaloy. Table 4-10 summarizes typical "oxy-laser" cutting results for various metals using a CW CO_2 laser with the power levels indicated. Figure 4-91 shows a 302 stainless steel cut at a speed of 2.3 m/min using this method.

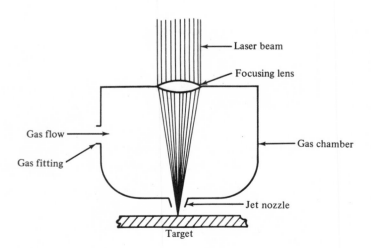

Figure 4-90 Schematic diagram of gas-jet laser material cutting system.

TABLE 4-10 Oxygen Jet Assisted CO_2 Laser Cutting [a]

Material	Thickness (cm)	Cutting Rate (m/min)	Max. Kerf Width (cm)	Laser Power on Material (W)	Gas-Jet Assistance	Remarks
Titanium 6A14Va	1.0	2.5	0.16	260	O_2	0.005 in. thick heat-affected zone
Titanium 6A14Va	0.64	2.8	0.10	250	O_2	0.005 in. thick heat-affected zone
Titanium 6A14Va	0.22	3.8	0.08	210	O_2	
Titanium 6A14Va	0.13	7.6	0.08	210	O_2	
Titanium Com. Pure	0.05	15.2	0.04	135	O_2	
Steel C1010	0.32	0.6	0.10	190	O_2	
Stainless Steel 321	0.13	0.8	0.05	165	O_2	
Zircaloy	0.05	15.2	0.05	230	O_2	

[a] With permission of Coherent Radiation Laboratories.

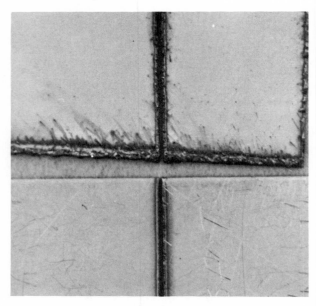

Figure 4-91   Oxygen-laser cut 302 type stainless steel.   (With per-mission of Coherent Radiation Laboratories.)

The second type of gas-jet assisted laser cutting makes use of an inert gas jet, concentric with the focused laser beam.   In this case, no chemical reactions occur.   The gas is used only to purge the melted or evaporated material from the laser cut, to cool the edges of the material, and to minimize oxidative reactions.   In this technique, all energy to melt and/or evaporate the material being cut must be supplied by the laser.   For the CO_2 laser at 10.6×10^3 nm, the technique works best with materials which are highly absorbant at this wavelength, such as ceramics, glass, plastic, cloth, paper, wood, etc.   Unassisted laser cutting of these materials would generally result in fracture, melting, or burning damage. Table 4-11 lists results for the CO_2 laser on various materials using this method.

Acrylic plastic cut at a speed of 41 cm/min with a N_2 gas assist is shown in Figure 4-92.   Kerf width is 0.08 cm.   Burning was eliminated by the use of nitrogen.

The above examples show the ability of the laser to shape by "cutting."   Although the discussion concerned itself primarily with flat planes of materials, the processes or techniques can be extended to almost any shaping process.   For instance, the cutting of wire is easily accomplished with the laser.   Figure 4-93 shows a 0.64 mm diameter tantalum wire which was cut by a 20 J, 1 ms pulse from a ruby laser.   In this case, the cut was circular, duplicating the shape of the beam.

TABLE 4-11   Inert Gas Jet Assisted CO₂ Laser Cutting[a]

	Thickness (cm)	Cutting Rate (m/min)	Kerf Width (cm)	Incident Power	Type Gas
Boron fiber composite	0.13	0.8	0.08	260	N_2
Alumina 99.5 percent	0.06	1.3	0.03	250	N_2
Carpet, polyester	0.95	3.0	0.05	200	Ar
Carpet, polyester	0.64	3.0	0.05	200	Ar
ABS plastic	0.25	3.8	0.08	240	N_2

[a] With permission of Coherent Radiation Laboratories.

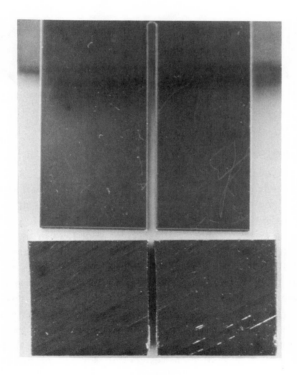

Figure 4-92   Acrylic plastic cut using a CO_2 laser with N_2 gas assist. (With permission of Coherent Radiation Laboratories.)

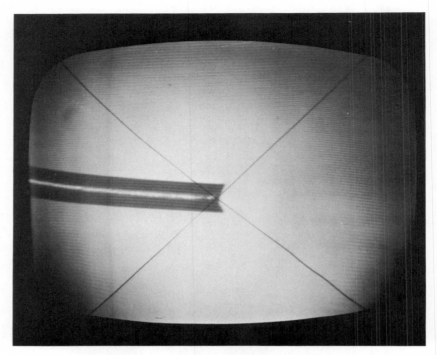

Figure 4-93   Tantalum wire cut by a single pulse of energy from a ruby laser.

4.4.4   pattern generation

Defining or generating intricate and highly complex patterns has been successfully demonstrated using the laser. Two applications of laser pattern generation are discussed in this section. The first, a device generally referred to as the Primary Pattern Generator (PPG), uses the focused beam from an argon laser to expose a photographic plate for IC and thin-film mask production.[78] The second application uses a Q-switched Nd:YAG for selective removal of a conductive layer of material (e.g., gold) in order to generate or repair a conductor circuit pattern.

In the Primary Pattern Generator (Figure 4-94), the main coordinates of the pattern to be formed are processed by an automated design program on a large computer and transmitted through an interface for storage on magnetic tapes. This enables a designer to arrange circuit components on various levels and provides all associated interconnecting points that are required.

Using the stored information as input to a smaller computer to control an argon laser, IC masks are produced automatically by exposing

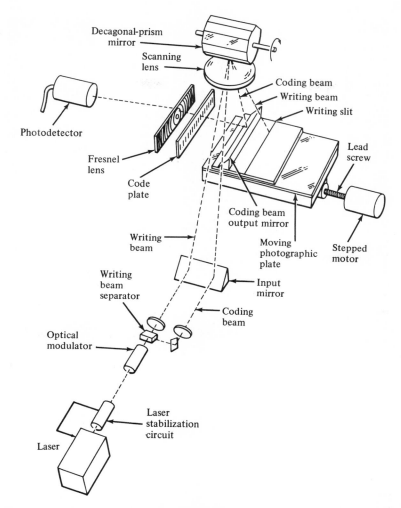

Figure 4-94 Schematic representation of PPG system.[78] *(With permission of Bell System Tech. J.)*

select portions of a mask blank. The laser beam is focused to a spot diameter of 7 μm.

The mask blank consists of a photographic plate with an orthochromatic emulsion. The plate is exposed by the focused beam from the laser which is reflected from a 10-sided, rotating mirror that scans the beam over the plate. The blank is mounted on an 8 in. by 10 in. table that moves in discrete steps under computer control. The computer also controls the optical modulator which switches the laser "on" or "off" as required.

To maintain accuracy, the PPG system is operated in a specially controlled environment chamber. The temperature inside the chamber is held within 0.25 °F, and each cubic foot of air contains fewer than 100 dust particles larger than 1 μm.

At present, a highly sophisticated circuit mask, an example of which is shown in Figure 4-95, requires only about 12 min to complete. Formerly, it required more than 12 h.

The PPG laser mask-making system eliminates many of the errors found in conventional methods. For example, identical devices can be drawn differently on composite masks, coordinates can be improperly transferred from drawings to cut-and-peel materials, essential cuts can be omitted, or properly cut sections might not be peeled. The PPG automatic laser mask-making system eliminates these usual errors.

As mentioned, conductor or circuit patterns have also been generated and/or repaired by selective removal of a conductor material deposited on a nonconducting substrate. The first example to be cited involves the use of a Q-switched Nd:YAG laser for repair of shorts which may occur between conductor paths. Figure 4-96a shows a portion of an IGFET

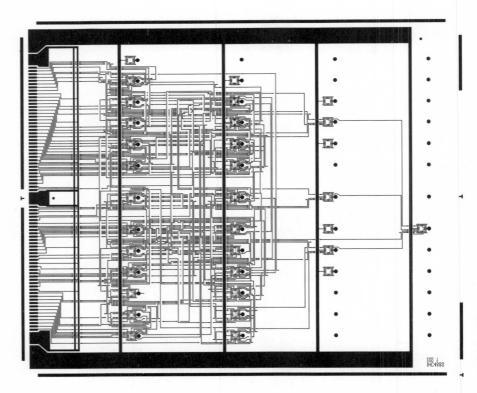

Figure 4-95   Circuit mask typical of the type generated by the PPG.

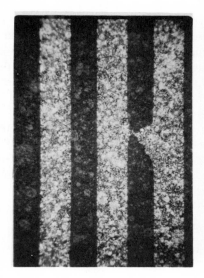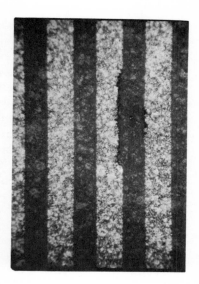

Figure 4-96   Repair of shorted gold conductor paths via material removal using the laser.   The short is seen in (a).

memory circuit where a short exists between conductor paths.   The same unit is shown after repair in Figure 4-96b, i.e., after the unwanted material has been removed by exposure to the focused laser beam.   Typical dimensions in the photographs are 50 μm lines and spaces.   Contact or conductor material is approximately 500 Å of titanium and 10,000 Å to 14,000 Å of gold on ceramic.

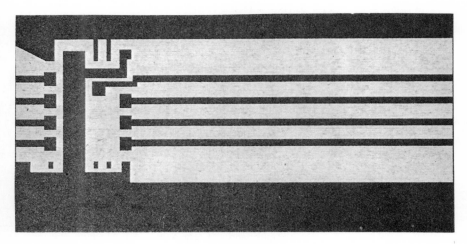

Figure 4-97   A pattern laser machined in a thin film of gold.

When machining gold in this fashion, two extreme conditions can be observed. The first is found when the power is marginal and results in the gold not being completely vaporized, but being melted and resolidified in small nodules. The second extreme is observed when too much power is used. In this case some gold is evaporated and some is driven into the substrate. One technique to optimize the power is to locate the workpiece far enough below the focused beam to minimize driving gold into the substrate, but not so far below the focus point as to create gold nodules.

Figure 4-97 is an illustration of a pattern machined from a conductor "blank" consisting of a uniform deposit of 500 Å of titanium and 10,000 Å of gold on ceramic. As before, a Q-switched YAG laser system was used. Patterns of this complexity require precise control of both the laser's output and its positioning with respect to the part being machined.[79]

References

1. F. P. Gagliano, "Laser Welding Techniques as Applied to Electronic Industry," presented at the Design Engineering Conference, Design Engineering Division, American Society of Mechanical Engineers, Chicago, May 11–14, 1970.

2. E. K. Pfitzer and R. Turner, "Quartz Working with a CO_2 Laser," *J. Sci. Instr. (J. Phys. E)*, Series 2, **1**, 360 (1968).

3. H. S. McCracken, "Parameters Effecting Laser Welding," presented at the 1967 Materials Engineering Exposition and Congr., Cleveland, Ohio, *ASM Tech. Report C7-19.1.*

4. R. H. Fairbanks and C. M. Adams, "Laser Beam Fusion Welding," *Welding J.* **43**, 97s–102s (March 1964).

5. W. N. Platte and J. F. Smith, "Laser Techniques for Metals Joining," *Welding J.* **42**, 481s–489s (November 1963).

6. C. O. Brown and C. M. Banas, "Deep Penetration Laser Welding," presented at the American Welding Society 52nd Annual Meeting, San Francisco, Calif., April 26–29, 1971.

7. E. V. Locke, E. D. Hoag, and R. A. Hella, "Deep Penetration Welding with a High Power CO_2 Laser," *IEEE J. Quantum Electronics* **QE-8**, 132–135 (1972).

8. K. K. Kelly, Contributions to the Data on Theoretical Metallurgy, U.S. Dept. of the Interior, *Bureau of Mines Bulletin 584.*

9. M. S. Baranov, L. A. Metashop, and I. N. Geinrikhs, "Laser Welding of Some Dissimilar Metals," *Svar. Proiz.*, No. 3, 13–15 (1968).

10. W. G. Alwang, L. A. Cavanaugh, and E. Sammartino, "Continuous Butt Welding Using a Carbon Dioxide Laser," *Welding J.* **48**, No. 3, 110s–115s (1969).

11. F. Horrigan, C. Klein, R. Rudko, and D. Wilson, "Windows for High-Power Lasers," *Microwave Mag.* (January 1969).

12. K. J. Miller and J. D. Ninnikhoven, "Laser Welding," *Machine Design*, pp. 120–125 (August 1965).

13. C. M. Banas, "The Role of the Laser in Material Processing," presented at The Canadian Materials and Processing Technology Conference, Toronto, Canada, Sept. 29 to Oct. 2, 1969.

14. C. G. Young, "Glass Lasers," *Proc. IEEE* **57**, No. 7, 1267–1289 (July 1969).

15. Laser Report, *Laser Focus* **6**, No. 5 (May 1970); also see H. C. Eckbreth and J. W. Davis, "Cross Beam Electric-Discharge Convection Laser," *IEEE J. Quantum Electronics* **QE-8**, 139–144 (1972).

16. A. J. Beaulieu, "Transverse Excitation Atmospheric Pressure Lasers," presented at the IEEE Conference on Laser Engineering and Applications, Washington, D.C., June 2–4, 1971. Digest of paper in *IEEE J. of Quantum Electronics* **QE-7**, 281 (1971).

17. Laser Report, *Laser Focus* **6**, No. 5 (May 1970).

18. A. R. Fluger and P. M. Mass, "Laser Beam Welding Electronic-Component Leads," *Welding J.* **44** (6), 264s–269s (1965).

19. M. I. Cohen, F. J. Mainwaring, and T. G. Melone, "Laser Interconnection of Wires," *Welding J.* **48**, No. 3, 191–197 (1969).

20. C. Chiou *et al.*, "Laser Welding," U.S. Patent 3,485,966, December 23, 1969.

21. A. D. Battista and M. A. Ponti, "Laser Welding of Microcircuit Interconnections—Simultaneous Multiple Bonds of Aluminum to Kovar," 1968 Microelectronics Packaging Conference Proceedings, p. 27, Society of Automotive Engineers, Inc., New York.

22. F. P. Gagliano, R. M. Lumley, and L. S. Watkins, "Lasers in Industry," *Proc. IEEE* **57**, No. 2, 114–147 (February 1969).

23. F. P. Gagliano and J. F. Carr, "Laser Line Welding of Beam-Lead Integrated Devices to Thin Films," presented at the IEEE Conference on Laser Engineering and Applications, Washington, D.C., May 26–28, 1969. Digest of paper in *IEEE J. of Quantum Electronics* **QE-5**, 336 (1969).

24. F. J. Jannett, "Method for Holding Workpieces for Radiant Energy Bonding," U.S. Patent 3,520,055, July 14, 1970.

25. J. F. Carr and S. S. Charschan, "Obtaining Near Gaussian Intensity Distribution from Multimode Pulsed Ruby Lasers," *Appl. Optics* **10**, 684 (1971).

26. F. P. Gagliano and D. H. Lockhart, "Pulsed Laser Welding of Transistor and Other Electronic Component Parts," presented at the IEEE International Convention, New York, 1969, *IEEE Digest*, 69C-14-IEEE, pp. 150–151 (1969).

27. J. E. Anderson and J. E. Jackson, "An Evaluation of Pulsed Laser Welding," *Engineering Proc. P-44*, published by the Pennsylvania State University, College of Engineering, University Park, Pa. (May 1966).

28. F. J. Lavoie, "Laser Welding—A State-of-the-Art Report," *Machine Design*, pp. 136–140 (February 20, 1969).

29. F. E. Harper and M. I. Cohen, "Properties of Si Diodes Prepared by Alloying Al into n-Type Si with Heat Pulses from a Nd : YAG Laser," presented at the IEEE Conference on Laser Engineering and Applications, Washington, D.C., May 26–28, 1969. Digest of paper printed in *IEEE J. of Quantum Electronics* **QE-5**, 335 (1969).

30. *EDN Magazine* (January 1969).

31. F. P. Gagliano, "Laser Microwelding of Uncommon Metal Combinations," presented at the 1969 International Electronic Circuit Packaging Symposium,

Western Electronic Show and Convention, August 20–21, 1969, San Francisco, California, *IECP Symposium Record*, Vol. 10.

32. J. M. Ney Company, Bloomfield, Connecticut, *Data Sheet*, Ney-Scope, Vol. 7, No. 3 (May–June 1965), Paliney 7 (registered trademark for a commercial precious metal alloy).

33. American Society for Metals, *Metals Handbook*, Vol. 1, 8th Ed., Metals Park, Ohio (1969).

34. F. N. Rhines, *Phase Diagrams in Metallurgy*, pp. 38–39, McGraw-Hill Book Co., New York (1956).

35. C. J. Smithells, *Metals Reference Book*, Vol. 1, 3rd Ed., Butterworth and Co., Ltd., London, England (1962).

36. American Society for Metals, *Metals Handbook*, 1948 Ed., p. 1241, Metals Park, Ohio.

37. C. M. Adams, Jr., and G. A. Hardway, "Fundamentals of Laser Beam Machining and Drilling," *IEEE Trans. on Industry and General Applications*, IGA-1, 90 (1965).

38. D. L. Williams, "The Laser as a Drilling Tool," *Engineering Proc. P-44*, published by the Pennsylvania State University, College of Engineering, University Park, Pa. (May 1966).

39. D. S. Young, "The Laser as an Industrial Machining and Welding Tool," *Engineering Proc. P-44*, published by the Pennsylvania State University, College of Engineering, University Park, Pa. (May 1966).

40. J. P. Epperson, R. W. Dyer, and J. C. Grzywa, "The Laser Now a Production Tool," *Western Electric Engineer* 10, 2–9 (April 1966).

41. J. C. Grzywa and A. Chesko, "Laser Piercing and Reworking of Diamond Dies," *Wire and Wire Products* 41 (September 1966).

42. G. Rauscher, "Recent Production Techniques Using Laser Beams" (in German), *Werkstattstechnik* 59, No. 1 (June 1969).

43. D. R. Whitehouse and W. Prifti, "State-of-the-Art of Laser Applications in Manufacture," presented at the 1970 IEEE International Convention, March 23–26, 1970, New York, *IEEE Digest* 70C15, pp. 270–271.

44. N. N. Bicky, "Simultaneous Recording of Near-Field and Far-Field Patterns of Lasers," *Appl. Optics* 8, No. 11, 2249–2253 (November 1969).

45. J. F. Ready, "Effects Due to Absorption of Laser Radiation," *J. Appl. Phys.* 36, 1522 (1965).

46. R. D. Haun, Jr., "Laser Applications," *IEEE Spectrum* 5, 82–92 (May 1968).

47. K. G. Nichols, "Review of Laser Microwelding and Micromachining," *Proc. IEE* 116, No. 12, 2093–2100 (December 1969).

48. M. K. Chun and K. Rose, "Interaction of High Intensity Laser Beams with Metals," *J. Appl. Phys.* 41, No. 2, 614–620 (February 1970).

49. F. W. Dabby and U. C. Paek, "High Intensity Laser Induced Vaporization and Explosion of Solid Material," *IEEE J. Quantum Electronics* QE-8, 106 (1972).

50. J. F. Ready, "Interaction of High Power Laser Radiation with Absorbing Surfaces," *1964 Proceedings of the National Electronics Conference*.

51. F. P. Gagliano and U. C. Paek, "High Speed Photographic Investigation of Explosive Material Removal Induced by a Laser" (to be published).

52. J. G. Sickman and R. E. Morijn, "The Mechanism of Welding with a Sealed-Off Continuous CO_2 Gas Laser," *Philips Research Projects* **23**, R673, 367–374 (1968).

53. S. I. Anisimov, "Evaporation of a Light-Absorbing Metal," translated from *Teplofizika Vysokikh Temperatur* **6**, No. 1, 116–120 (January/February 1968).

54. M. I. Cohen, "Laser Beams and Integrated Circuits," *Bell Labs. Record*, **45**, 247–251 (September 1967).

55. M. I. Cohen and J. P. Epperson, "Applications of Lasers to Microelectronic Fabrication," in *Advances in Electronics and Electron Physics*, A. B. El-Kareh, Ed., Academic Press Inc., New York (1968).

56. G. Bellows, "Import of Nonconventional Material Removal Processes on the Surface Integrity of Materials," *Technical paper MR68-518*, presented at the 1968 Conference on Material Removal, American Society of Tool and Manufacturing Engineers, Dearborn, Mich.

57. R. S. Otstat *et al.*, "Method for Machining with Laser Beam," U.S. Patent 3,440,388, April 1969.

58. J. C. Boyle and C. M. Pleass, private communication.

59. "Laser Metal Removal Aids Dynamic Balancing," *Steel* **159**, 28–29 (July 1966).

60. "On-Line Balancing Systems," *Laser Focus* **4**, 3 (June 1968).

61. "The Laser as a Production Tool," *Electro-Optical Systems Design* (April 1970).

62. J. Longfellow, "Production of an Extensible Matrix by Laser Drilling," *Rev. Sci. Instr.* **41**, No. 10, 1485–1486 (October 1970).

63. R. M. Lumley, "Controlled Separation of Brittle Materials Using a Laser," presented at the 70th Annual Meeting of American Ceramics Society, Chicago, Ill., Paper 13-E-68 (April 1968).

64. R. Bakish, "Industrial Material Processing with CO_2 Lasers," *Engineering Proc.*, published by the Pennsylvania State University, College of Engineering, University Park, Pa., p. 46 (August 1970).

65. A. Goldsmith *et al.*, *Handbook of Thermophysical Properties of Solid Materials*, Vol. III, *Ceramics*, Armour Research Foundation, The Macmillan Company, New York (1961).

66. M. I. Cohen and T. G. Melone, private communication.

67. U. C. Paek and F. P. Gagliano, "Thermal Analysis of Laser Drilling Processes," *IEEE J. Quantum Electronics* **QE-8**, 112–119 (1972).

68. B. A. Unger and M. I. Cohen, "Laser Trimming of Thin Film Resistors," *Proc. Elect. Components Conf.* (May 1968).

69. L. Braun and D. Breuer, "Laser Adjustable Resistors for Precision Monolithic Circuits," *Solid State Technology* (May 1969).

70. B. A. Unger, M. I. Cohen, and J. F. Milkosky, "Laser Machining of Thin Film and Integrated Circuits," *Bell System Tech. J.* **47**, 385 (1968).

71. D. J. Garibotti, "Dicing of Micro-Semiconductors," U.S. Patent 3,112,850, December 3, 1963.

72. W. R. Runyan, *Silicon Semiconductor Technology*, Texas Instruments Electronics Series, McGraw-Hill Book Co., New York (1965).

73. V. J. Zaleckas, "Laser System for Scribing Semiconductor Devices," NEREM 70 Record, 176–177, Boston, Mass. (November 1970).

74. R. M. Lumley, "Controlled Separation of Brittle Materials Using a Laser," *Ceramic Bulletin* **48**, 850 (1969).
75. M. Hess and J. F. Milkosky, private communication.
76. T. M. Jackson, A. D. Brisbane, and C. P. Sandbank, "Automated Interconnections Processes for Semiconductor Integrated Circuit Slices," *Proc. Conference Integrated Circuits*, Eastbourne, England (May 1967).
77. P. D. Zavitsanos, L. E. Brewer, and W. E. Sauer, "Evaporation Processes by Laser Beams," *Proc. National Electronics Conf.* **24**, 864–869 (1968).
78. M. J. Cowan *et al.*, "The Primary Pattern Generator, Part 1—Optical Design," *Bell System Tech. J.* **49**, 2033 (1970).
79. W. W. Weick, "Laser Generation of Conductor Patterns," *IEEE J. Quantum Electronics* **QE-8**, 126–131 (1972).

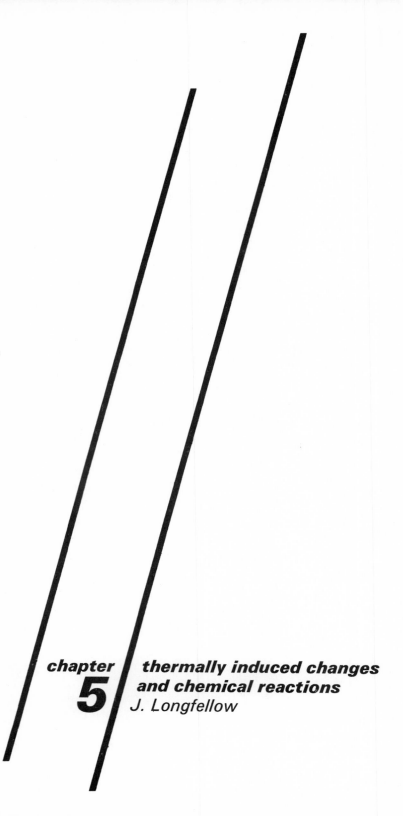

chapter 5

thermally induced changes and chemical reactions
J. Longfellow

5.0 introduction

The advent of laser radiation has provided practicing engineers and scientists with a readily controlled source of energy. Within the area encompassed by focused laser light incident on a target, one may achieve energy densities which may exceed millions of watts per square centimeter with resulting temperatures comparable to those to be found within the interior segments of stars. In addition, pressure changes attributable to laser beam-induced phenomena may be expected to reach several million kilograms per square centimeter.

Before considering ways to exploit laser phenomena in thermal reactions, it behooves an engineer to consider primary boundary conditions which are imposed automatically by physical limitations of available lasers. Namely, one may induce extreme pressure, temperatures, and/or energy densities via a laser beam only at the expense of accepting small working areas (~ 1 mm^2), small working volumes (~ 1 mm^3), and low average power inputs (~ 1 kW maximum). Normally, energy densities are nonuniform across the diameter of a beam. Consequently, one must always consider nonuniformity in energy densities which are distributed on the target area.

The use of lasers for heat treating and for inducing permanent changes in materials has lagged far behind the use of lasers for machining, welding, and related work. This is due largely to practical considerations, i.e., most of the attainable processes for effecting thermally induced changes are simply not profitable to industry. Consequently, there are available to the engineer few experimental data upon which practical thermal processing can be predicted. Thus, the physical attributes of available lasers must be used to predict future applications for lasers in the matters of thermally inducing changes in materials.

In order to describe the boundary conditions which govern the applications of lasers to thermally inducing changes in materials, it is necessary first to consider a laser beam in three-dimensional space. Figure 5-1 is a photograph of a section of Lucite® which has been exposed to a beam of CW energy from a commercial CO$_2$ laser. The wavelength of the radiated wave was 10.6×10^3 nm and the power level was 180 W. The cross-sectional distribution of energy density in the beam is Gaussian, i.e., the energy density at the center of the beam is high and the energy density at the rim of the beam is low. The diameter of a laser beam is commonly given as the distance at which the maximum energy falls to the $1/e^2$ value, e being the base of natural logarithms. The diameter of the illustrated beam is about 17 mm.

The nonuniform, nonsymmetrical distribution of energy density which may be found in a laser beam is illustrated in Figure 5-2. The heavily burned areas of the paper are described in the vernacular as "hot spots," and they represent areas of higher energy density than the interspersed areas within the diameter of the beam.

When the beams illustrated in Figures 5-1 and 5-2 are compressed

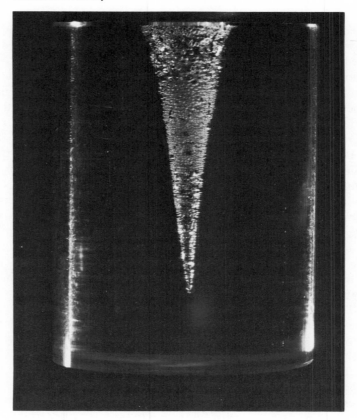

Figure 5-1   Radiation pattern of a laser beam.   The plastic block was irradiated by the beam from a 250 W CO_2 laser.

through focusing optics, the resulting patterns on a target will be unchanged from the unfocused patterns, assuming that the optics introduce no distortions.   However, with the same optics used for each beam, the beam illustrated in Figure 5-1 can be focused to a much smaller area than can the beam illustrated in Figure 5-2.   This is true because the divergence of a beam with a low-order modal structure (Figure 5-1) is less than the divergence of a beam with a higher-order modal structure (Figure 5-2). In any case, the ultimate diameter of a focused laser beam can be no less than approximately λ, λ being equal to the wavelength of the laser radiation.   This limitation was detailed in Chapter 3.   Practically speaking, the diameter will be several times larger than λ.   About 1 mm or less may be taken as the working diameter of a focused beam, whereas an unfocused beam may range up to 25 mm.   Thus, it may be seen that the laser beam is hardly a practical competitor for commercial heat treating furnaces.   However, it may be used to good effect on parts or sections with dimensions less than the diameter of an unfocused laser beam.

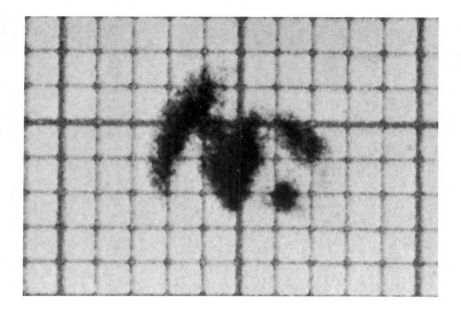

Figure 5-2 Cross section of a laser beam. The heat-sensitive paper was irradiated with a single pulse from a CO_2 laser.

Consideration must also be given to the total energy outputs which are available from commercial lasers when one wishes to compare the effects of laser beams upon materials with the effects of conventional thermal processing equipment. The maximum power radiated by a commercial laser (CW) is about 1 kW. Focused upon a target, the beam from such a laser might indeed yield a power density of approximately 200 MW/cm^2, yet the total power input would remain at 1 kW. A pulsed ruby laser might yield a peak power output of 1000 MW (focused approximately 10^{18} W/cm^2); yet this high power level would endure for a few nanoseconds (10^{-9} s) only over a target area of some 2×10^{-8} cm^2. In conclusion, the reader may note the power density (or energy density) from conventional devices can hardly be compared with the power density (or energy density) attained via a laser.

5·1 heat treating

The laser is a useful instrument for heat treating metals for two reasons. First, the beam can be focused on an extremely small area within a surrounding matrix. In the same vein, very small discrete particles can be singled out for heat treating. Second, heating rates of 10^{6}°C/s may be realized, and the times for heat treating may be varied from a few nanoseconds to hundreds of hours at the same power level.

When a metal is worked, it becomes harder and progressively non-workable. Therefore, it must be softened before it can be worked further. Softening by heat treating is termed annealing. Annealing occurs via any one or combination of three phenomena; namely, (1) recovery, (2) recrystallization, and (3) grain growth.

5·1·1   recovery

Recovery is defined as the softening by heating of a previously worked metal by the process of polygonization and/or annihilation of dislocations.[1] Recovery takes place before and at lower temperatures than does recrystallization.

There are in the literature no direct references which describe recovery *per se* in metals via laser heating, although a conventional diffusion furnace has been used[2] for low-temperature annealing of 70:30 brass prior to laser heating specimens to higher temperatures, i.e., recrystallization temperatures. Also, several micrographs have been published which show recovery concurrent with recrystallization.[3,4] The paucity of information is probably due to the supposition that laser-heating phenomena in the recovery range of temperatures for common metals would not prove to be different from phenomena effected by conventional heating devices.

In the matter of annealing metals, however, laser heaters may offer significant advantages as they are compared with conventional devices. As examples, the annealing of small, discrete particles and/or moving wire certainly seems feasible. The advantages to be realized include the application of energy upon the workpiece alone, whereas the surrounding atmosphere plus supports remain at a fixed temperature, i.e., low temperature. It is expected that such applications may require low-powered lasers operating in the CW fashion. YAG, CO_2, and ion lasers appear to be suitable instruments for such work since the wavelengths cover the electromagnetic spectrum from the ultraviolet through the intermediate infrared.

5·1·2   recrystallization

Recrystallization is defined as the replacement of a deformed lattice (by heating) with a new, unstrained one by means of a nucleation and growth process.[1] As far as recrystallization by laser heating is concerned, fairly extensive studies have been conducted on 70:30 brass[2] and on iron, iron-carbon, gold, and $3\frac{1}{4}$ percent silicon steel.[3,4]

Zone refined iron (90 percent cold worked) was completely recrystallized (100 percent) by laser heating for 0.050 s at 755°C.[3] For $3\frac{1}{4}$ percent silicon steel, a linear growth rate for recrystallizing grains, G, is given by the following equation:[4]

$$G = K_G/t$$

$$K_G = \text{constant} = 0.85 \times 10^{-3} \text{ cm}$$

$$t = \text{time of heating in seconds}$$

The constant, $K_G = 2.29 \times 10^{-2}$ cm was calculated[2] for 40 percent cold-worked 70:30 brass which was 50 percent recrystallized.

Specimen reflectivity has been reported[2,4] as being a significant problem in laser annealing. Consequently, one researcher[2] treated specimens by means of an oxidation process, whereas others[4] coated the laser target with a layer of iron which was subsequently oxidized. The oxidized regions served as highly absorbing regions for laser light. The reflectivity of the oxide layer on 70:30 brass with incident ruby laser light ($\lambda = 694.3$ nm) was $\simeq 0.25$.

Insofar as the future of recrystallizing metals by laser is concerned, it appears that the techniques originally developed[3] can be effectively utilized in solving many problems related to metallographic studies wherein very high heating rates on small, thin specimens are required. In production applications it would seem that metal powders and moving wires might be suitable targets on which to apply laser radiation for recrystallization. However, for massive pieces, laser treatment would establish localized thermal gradients, thus precluding the use of the laser for treating the entire piece uniformly.

5·1·3   grain growth

When a strained lattice has been replaced by an unstrained lattice, a metal may lower its energy further by reducing the total area of grain surface, i.e., by the process of inducing the growth of some of the grains at the expense of smaller grains. This phenomenon is defined as grain growth.[1]

Unfortunately, none of the works involving lasers which have been published to date have listed any experimental data for grain growth other than the primary grain growth which occurs during recrystallization. The reason for this situation lies in the fact that ruby lasers have been used to furnish the energy for thermally inducing changes, and a ruby laser can be operated normally only in the pulsed or Q-switched fashion, not with a CW output. Consequently, grain growth was rather impractical since the growing of grains requires a low, steady input of thermal energy. It may very well be that YAG lasers, CO_2 lasers, and ion lasers (all of which can be operated readily in the CW fashion) will prove to be adequate instruments for controlled grain-growth studies in the future.

But there exist at the present time no definitive data upon which to base such a conclusion. If such work were to be done, it seems logical to assume that the technique could become quite valuable. For instance, very small samples of metal could be processed in controlled atmospheres to produce single crystals from small bits of polycrystalline materials.

5·1·4   quenching

It has been stated previously that very high heating rates ($10^6°C/s$) can be attained in laser-heated specimens. By the same token, cooling rates on laser-heated specimens were $10^3°C/s$, $10^4°C/s$, and $10^5°C/s$, respectively, when the specimens were quenched with static air, flowing helium, and flowing helium plus water vapor.[3] These rates are decades higher than the rates obtained with conventional quenching methods.

The fact that very high heating and quenching rates may be achieved via a laser can be a considerable merit for treating many alloys. When a metal B is alloyed to a metal A, the metal B can sometimes be absorbed (in a limited range of temperature) to such a high degree of solubility that a new phase which differs in some significant way (say crystal structure) from that of both parent metals is formed. The new phase is generally termed an intermediate phase, or a secondary solid solution, or an intermetallic compound. Since many of these intermediate phases exist only in a limited range of temperature, it is important that this range be passed quickly, i.e., by rapid heating, if one wishes to suppress the formation of an intermediate phase. Conversely, if one wishes to "freeze" an intermediate phase and prevent its dissociation, it is important that one have the capability of rapid quenching from the limited range of temperature in question to room temperature.

Although it is not at all clear now where the uniquely fast heating and quenching rates attainable via laser might best be employed, it seems likely that the formation of small particles of intermetallic compounds could be the most useful application for lasers. Indeed, it is entirely possible that some intermediate compounds can be formed in no other fashion.

5·1·5   microstructures

Most of the micrographs published to date[2,3,4] lead one to believe that the microstructures developed during recrystallization by laser heating are not radically different from microstructures developed by conventional heating methods. However, it must be noted that most of the work was done by using defocused beams. The distribution of energy

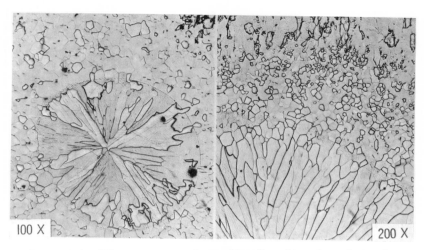

Figure 5-3   Microstructure of metal irradiated by a laser beam drawn to a fine point focus.[4]   *(With permission of United States Steel Corporation.)*

in the beam pattern was "smeared" so that a fairly uniform temperature was achieved across comparatively large areas of interest.

By way of contrast to the defocused beam, others[4] have demonstrated graphically that the microstructure is not uniform within an area encompassed by a laser beam drawn to a fine point focus.   Their micrographs of areas heated with a laser spot 100 μm in diameter show columnar (elongated) grains growing out from the center of the laser spot where the energy density is presumably at the highest level.   The columnar grains are surrounded with a ring of more equiaxed (symmetrical) recrystallized grains.   The microstructure is illustrated in Figure 5-3.   These phenomena serve to demonstrate that nonuniform energy densities must always be considered when a laser light is employed as a source of energy.

5·2   diffusion

The motion of atoms as they wander from one lattice site to another in a solid is called diffusion.[5]   Common examples of diffusion processing in industry include diffusion welding, diffusion hardening of alloys, and semiconductor junction formation.   Normally, diffusion as a means of processing materials in industry is effected at an elevated temperature, i.e., above ambient room temperature.   Since a primary effect which occurs when a laser beam interacts with a material is an elevated temperature at the point of intersection, it follows naturally that the laser be considered as an energy source for diffusion processes.

5·2·1   metals and insulators

At the present time there is little or no definitive information in the literature regarding diffusion processing in metals or insulators by means of a laser beam. As was the situation in heat treating, diffusion by laser is restricted to the extremely small areas encompassed by the laser spot. Consequently, the laser offers no competition, economically speaking, with conventional sources of energy, e.g., resistance heating diffusion furnaces. However, the laser may very well prove competitive when the material to be processed exists in the form of small discrete volumes. Examples of materials wherein laser diffusion processing might prove effective include dots on recording tape, thermistor blanks, magnetic memory elements, and microminiature relay contacts.

5·2·2   semiconductors

The limitations imposed by the nature of a focused laser beam work to advantage when the laser is used to initiate diffusion processes in semiconductor materials. That is to say, the active regions in semiconductor devices occupy volumes that approach in cross-sectional dimensions the area of a laser spot, e.g., 0.025 mm to 0.05 mm. Further, the diffused layers in some semiconductor devices approach in thickness the normal penetration depths of laser-induced energy.

Nielsen[6] suggested, after a series of experiments with strip heaters, that recrystallization of silicon and germanium thin films (i.e., forming single crystals in the films) was possible if very steep temperature gradients could be created. His conclusions suggest the use of a laser beam to generate the steep temperature gradients. Nielsen[6] speculated that recrystallization occurred by the removal of oxide from grain boundaries via diffusion, thus allowing silicon or germanium to react with alloy zones by means of thin alloy zone crystallization.

Resistivity changes in silicon which occur after irradiation with a ruby laser have been described.[7] In general, the resistivity of n-type material decreases after irradiation, whereas the resistivity of p-type material increases. These changes in resistivity were attributed to the clustering of oxygen impurities, and this clustering suggests that diffusion occurred at about 400°C.

A process for forming junctions or circuit elements in silicon or gallium arsenide immersed in a doping atmosphere of arsenic or antimony has been described.[8] It is claimed that the doping material is diffused at the spot locally heated by the application of a laser beam.

Silicon diodes made by irradiation using a ruby laser with a 5 ms pulse width have been described.[9] The illuminated surface area was

2×10^{-3} cm^2, whereas the total energy density per pulse was about 2×10^{-2} J/cm^2. The base material was silicon doped with boron on which was painted a thin layer of phosphorus. The authors claimed that *p-n* junctions were formed to depths of up to 1 μm where localized melting occurred. However, it is difficult to escape the conclusion that some diffusion occurred, since the authors stated that single crystallinity was maintained. This point leads one to visualize the diffusion of phosphorus to a very limited depth within a matrix of silicon.

By way of summary, it appears that laser-produced diodes may figure profitably in future semiconductor processing by industry. Such a diode can be made on an integrated circuit chip without causing damage by heat in the remainder of the chip. Thus a manufacturer of chips could establish a much higher degree of circuit versatility than is available through present techniques.

5·3 *zone melting*

The technique of zone melting finds primary industrial applications in refining materials and in the fabrication of single crystals from polycrystalline forms. When it is desired to melt a zone in a refractory* material, the technique is difficult to apply simply because the achievement of a high temperature in a source of radiant energy is difficult in itself to accomplish. Then, the temperature of the target can be no higher than the temperature of the source. For this reason alone, the laser can be considered as an excellent source of radiant energy. A laser beam can be considered as emanating from a point source of energy, and the blackbody equivalent temperature of a laser can be extremely high, e.g., 10^{23}°K.[10] The ultimate temperature which can be generated by the point focus of a laser beam is limited only by the laws of diffraction.

5·3·1 *conventional methods*

Excellent reviews of energy sources which have been used to zone refine and zone melt refractory materials have been written.[11] In order of both historical and practical importance, these energy sources are the following ones:
1. The sun. In a solar furnace one may approach the apparent surface temperature of the sun (6000°K). The intensity of the radiation from a solar furnace has been recorded as stable within 5 percent for 6 h. The one great disadvantage of a solar furnace lies in the fact that energy is not always available when it is needed.

---

* The term *refractory* is arbitrarily applied to those elements and compounds that have fusion temperatures (T_f) higher than the fusion temperature of iron (1539°C).

2. The carbon arc.   In the familiar carbon arc one may achieve a temperature at atmospheric pressure which is close to the sublimation temperature of carbon ($\sim 4600°K$).   Pressurized arcs can, of course, be operated at higher temperatures.   Major disadvantages of the carbon arcs include instability, wander, and short lives.

3. The electric resistor.   Temperatures of 2840°K have been achieved with electrically heated carbon resistors.   As with the carbon arc, the temperatures that can be achieved are limited by the fusion/sublimation temperatures of the heated materials.

4. The high-pressure compact arc.   This device consists of a glass or metal bulb which houses two electrodes.   A gas under pressure (e.g., xenon, mercury, or mercury-xenon) fills the bulb and serves to constrict the arc.   This type of source is relatively stable in the output intensity, but the arc tends to wander and the overall efficiency is low.

5. The plasma generator.   Plasma temperatures of 7000°K under pressures of 17 atm have been reported for plasma generators.   The chief disadvantage of the plasma generator appears to be its inherent complexity.

6. The electron beam.   Generally speaking, the use of this device is confined to the melting of materials which are electrically conductive.   In addition, the electron beam chamber must be evacuated.

Researchers who have employed the image furnace technique in zone refining and zone melting are numerous, but they can be grouped as taking a few basic approaches.

A carbon-arc image furnace has been used for building up single crystals from fused powders which were fed into the focal area, i.e., the Verneuil technique.[12]   Rutile, sapphire, and magnesium ferrite crystals were grown.

More recent work[13] has extended the arc image–fused powder technique to growing crystals of stabilized zirconia and hafnia, and others[14] have extended the arc image furnace–floating zone technique to growing iron-nickel oxide spinel single crystals.   A xenon lamp, floating-zone technique has been used to produce single crystals of neodymium-doped garnets.[15]

An RF induction heated, floating-zone process has been used to make single crystals of hafnium diboride and zirconium diboride.[16]   A carbon-arc fusion apparatus was used for growing crystals of hafnium carbide and tantalum carbide.[17]   The authors claimed temperatures in excess of 3500°C and pressures to 1 atm.

Melting techniques which employed energy sources other than imaged arc furnaces and electrically heated zone furnaces for processing refractory materials are few in number.   They are limited to one variation or another of the Czochralski pulling technique, wherein a solidifying crystal is withdrawn from a pool of liquid refractory which may or may not contain a low melting point flux. Examples of refractory processing by the Czochralski technique include making sapphire monocrystals[18] and making tungsten carbide monocrystals.[19]

5.3.2   laser zone melters

Although it has not yet become a viable production instrument, it seems appropriate at this time to discuss the laser zone melter. The reason for discussing it is to list the apparent advantages and disadvantages of the laser as compared with energy sources presently used for zone refining and zone melting refractory materials. The laser zone melter offers significant advantages from the following points of view:

1. Unlimited temperature capability. Since laser light is coherent, directional, and very intense, energy densities in the point focus may exceed millions of watts per square centimeter. Suffice it to say that metals and nonmetals placed in a laser beam may easily be heated to any temperature within the range of 300°K to 10,000°K. This range is sufficiently wide to allow fusion-evaporation-sublimation of any material known to man.
2. Absorption of energy. High-powered CW lasers (e.g., CO_2, CO, and YAG) radiate in the infrared portion of the electromagnetic spectrum. With few exceptions, dielectric materials absorb this type of radiated energy very strongly. Most metals reflect this type of radiated energy. As metals are heated, however, they become more absorbing.
3. Wavelength selection. It has been pointed out that a pyrometer which views a heated zone in a material sees a combination of light scattered by the zone and light emitted from the zone.[20] Most optical pyrometers measure the intensity of radiation within the visible portion of the electromagnetic spectrum, i.e., emitted light. If a CO_2 laser is used as an energy source, the scattered radiation would have a wavelength of 10.6×10^3 nm. This latter wavelength is sufficiently far removed from the visible portion of the spectrum to preclude false indications of temperature.
4. Conversion efficiency. The conversion efficiency of the CO_2 laser may exceed 30 percent. Although it is difficult to generalize the comparable efficiencies of conventional devices, it may be noted that listed figures[11] indicate an average efficiency of less than 1 percent in carbon-arc devices.
5. Concentration of energy. Since a laser beam is highly directional and the light in the beam is coherent, the focusing optics may have cross-sectional dimensions which are approximately equal to the beam diameters, i.e., about 25 mm. By way of contrast, searchlight reflectors used with imaged arcs commonly have diameters of 1–2 m. In addition,

all of the energy in the beam can be played directly on the surface of the target rather than being dissipated into the surrounding spaces.

6. Ambient atmosphere. Few, if any, common gases attenuate laser radiation to any appreciable degree. Consequently, processing in hydrogen or oxygen is feasible. The electron beam furnace, in contrast, commonly requires a chamber pressure of 10^{-3} to 10^{-6} torr (mm of Hg) for efficient operations.

7. Energy control. The CW power output of a laser can be controlled within 1 percent of the set point or even less. Also, beam wander from a center set point within a distance of several meters can be controlled to less than a few hundredths of 1 mm.

The disadvantages of the lasers as sources of energy for zone melting/refining must also be listed in turn. The optical materials suitable for use in the CO_2 wavelength, 10.6×10^3 nm, are few in number, expensive, and fragile. Finally, alignment of the laser beam is difficult and quite critical.

A typical schematic drawing for a proposed laser zone melter is shown in Figure 5-4. The reader may note that the optical system is quite simple, being only one generation removed from an elementary point focusing system or an unfocused beam. It is quite possible, of course, to split the laser beam as many times as may be considered desirable in order to ring the entire perimeter of the target with radiated energy.

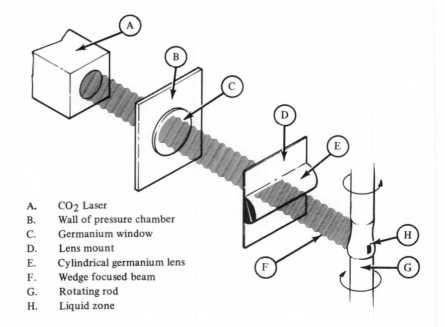

A. CO_2 Laser
B. Wall of pressure chamber
C. Germanium window
D. Lens mount
E. Cylindrical germanium lens
F. Wedge focused beam
G. Rotating rod
H. Liquid zone

Figure 5-4   Schematic illustration of a laser zone melter.

5·3·3   rod crystals

The laser zone melter and rod crystals grown therein have been described briefly in the literature.[21]   Geometrical considerations favor the formation of single crystals from solid cylinders of polycrystalline materials, i.e., rods, with the laser zone melter.   In Figure 5-5, a sapphire rod crystal which was grown by zone melting a polycrystalline rod with a CO_2 laser is shown.   Three zone passes were made to purify the material and form a seed crystal.   A final pass at the rate of 38 mm/h with 40 W of applied power served to form the single crystal, which has a diameter approximating 1.5 mm.

Emission spectrographic analyses of starting and final materials indicated that such impurities as titanium and calcium had been reduced by

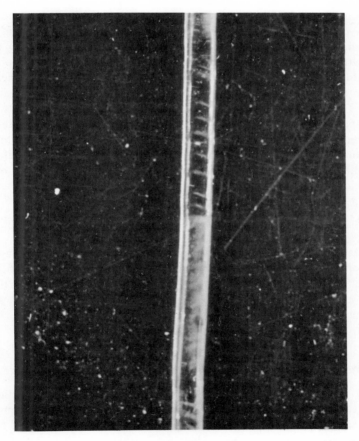

Figure 5-5   Sapphire rod crystal grown from polycrystalline alumina by a laser zone melter.

TABLE 5-1

Material	Temperature of Fusion, $^\circ K$
Alumina (Al_2O_3)	2303
Zirconia (ZrO_2)	2973
Magnesia (MgO)	3073
Hafnia (HfO_2)	3063
Hafnium carbide (HfC)	4223
Tantalum carbide (TaC)	~ 4273
Silicon carbide (SiC)	~ 2973

two orders or more of magnitude during the three zone refining passes on the rod shown in Figure 5-5. This fact serves to suggest applying the technique to zone refining and zone leveling other types of materials in rod forms. Although the rod illustrated in the photograph was processed in an atmosphere of air, there appear to be no technical reasons for not using other atmospheres. For instance, it appears that magnetic metal rods might be zone refined and purified simultaneously in an atmosphere of hydrogen. Second, an atmosphere of oxygen might be employed to minimize reduction of refractories (e.g., barium titanate) during crystal growth. Third, crystals of compounds which include elements of different volatilities, e.g., carbon in hafnium carbide, could be grown under inert gases at high pressures to minimize diffusion of the more volatile element.

The materials listed in Table 5-1 include some of the crystals which can probably be zone refined/melted quite adequately by the laser zone melter. The list is neither exhaustive nor exclusive. It is merely confined to some materials that have high temperatures of fusion. Therefore, in forming these materials, the high intensity of light in a laser beam offers a distinct advantage over present sources of energy.

5·4   chemical reactions

It has been stated that in focused laser beams, electric field strengths in the optical wave may equal 10^9 V/cm, which is in the range of fields by which valence electrons are held in atoms.[10]   For this reason, plus the fact that materials can be heated to extremely high temperatures with a laser beam, the laser is considered an excellent tool for forcing chemical and photochemical reactions.

5·4·1   thermally induced reactions

Perhaps the simplest examples of thermally induced chemical reactions by lasers are oxidation of metals and decomposition of inorganic metallic compounds. Burning a metal by applying heat plus a stream of oxygen is a universally accepted procedure for cutting. The adaptation of the laser to cutting metals has been accomplished by the British Welding

Research Association.[22] The device is called a gas-jet laser cutter. It consists of a 300 W CO_2 laser, the beam of which is combined with a jet of pure oxygen gas. Cutting rates of 100 cm/min in high-carbon steel 0.25 cm thick have been reported.

An example of thermal oxidation by laser to change resistance of a thin-film resistor *in situ* has been reported briefly.[23] A laser spot about 25 μm diameter was used, and the tantalum thin-film resistor surface (125 μm square) was swept past the beam. The resistance changed from 16.96 Ω to 17.98 Ω via oxidation of tantalum.

Laser beam decomposition of inorganic metallic compounds has been studied extensively.[24] The researchers have concluded that oxides of silver and copper can be decomposed and the metals deposited simultaneously in line forms on nonconducting substrates. The object of the study was to adapt the technique to "writing" conductive patterns on ceramics for use in microminiature electronic circuits. The technique of laser "writing" appears to be a promising one.

The degradation of aromatic compounds which were irradiated with a focused beam from a ruby laser has been studied.[25] The results indicate that the reaction products (methane and acetylene) were probably formed by pyrolysis (thermal degradation), but the results are by no means unequivocal.

5.4.2 photochemically induced reactions

One of the ways in which an excited molecule can rid itself of energy is to undergo a chemical transformation. This type of reaction is a photochemical reaction and only the simplest of them are understood in detail.[26] To date, laser-induced photochemical reactions have been confined largely to the irradiation of photochromic paper for imaging laser pulses.[27,28] It has been suggested that laser beams could be used as energy sources for exposing photoresist materials in thin-film processing. This technique, however, has not yet been implemented, probably because lasers with high-power outputs at the wavelengths desired have not been developed.

The most fascinating application proposed for laser-induced photosynthesis is the rapid growth of plants irradiated with laser light.[29] Here again, development of suitable lasers has precluded adopting the technique on a large scale.

5.4.3 photolysis

Another way in which an excited molecule can dissipate its energy is to be torn apart, i.e., photolysis.[26] Photolysis by laser has been reported,[30,31] but the process to date has been confined to the study of short-lived intermediate states.

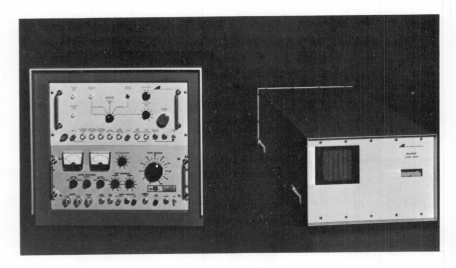

Figure 5-6   An ultraviolet laser.   (With permission of Avco Everett Research Laboratories.)

It would be very desirable if laser-induced photolysis could be accomplished on a large scale.   One of the many applications for a process of this type would be in reducing air pollution from industrial stacks.   Unfortunately, photolysis of the common gases (H_2, O_2, NO) requires quanta of such high-energy content that the lasers emitting them radiate in the ultraviolet range of the spectrum.   High-energy lasers of this type have not yet been developed to the degree required.

A start toward development of a high-energy laser which radiates in the ultraviolet range has been made.[32]   The pulsed nitrogen laser which was developed is pictured in Figure 5-6.   The wavelength is 337.1 nm, which is in the near ultraviolet, a slightly longer wavelength than is needed for dissociating common diatomic gases.

References

1. R. E. Smallman, " Modern Physical Metallurgy," pp. 230ff, Butterworths, London (1963).
2. D. A. Mehta, "A Study of Recrystallization of 70 : 30 Brass by Laser Irradiation," unpublished master's thesis, Lehigh University, Bethlehem, Pa. (June 1968).
3. G. R. Speich, A. Szirmae, and R. M. Fisher, "A Laser Heating Device for Metallographic Studies," *Advances in Electron Metallography* 6, ASTM STP 396, Am. Soc. Testing Mats., pp. 97–114 (1966).

4. G. R. Speich and R. M. Fisher, "Recrystallization of a Rapidly Heated $3\frac{1}{4}\%$ Silicon Steel," *Recrystallization, Grain Growth, and Textures*, Ed. by H. Margolin, American Society for Metals (Metals Park, Ohio), pp. 563–598 (1966).

5. C. A. Wert and R. M. Thomson, *Physics of Solids*, p. 54, McGraw-Hill Book Co., New York (1964).

6. S. Nielsen, "Recrystallization of Thin Films of Germanium and Silicon," *J. Electrochem. Soc.* **112**, No. 5, 534–535 (May 1965).

7. D. V. G. L. Narasimha Rao, "Laser-Induced Resistivity Changes in Silicon," *J. Appl. Phys.* **39**, No. 10, 4853 (September 1968).

8. R. Solomon and L. F. Mueller, "Method of Using Laser to Coat or Etch Substrate," U.S. Patent 3,364,087 (January 16, 1968).

9. J. M. Fairfield and G. H. Schwuttke, "Silicon Diodes Made by Laser Irradiation," *Solid-State Electronics* **11**, 1175–1176 (December 1968).

10. C. H. Townes, "Production of Coherent Radiation by Atoms and Molecules," *IEEE Spectrum* **2**, No. 8, 30–43 (August 1965).

11. T. S. Laszlo, "Image Furnace Techniques," Interscience, Inc., New York (1965).

12. R. E. DeLaRue and F. A. Halden, "Arc-Image Furnace for Growth of Single Crystals," *Rev. Sci. Instr.* **31**, No. 1, 35–38 (January 1960).

13. G. J. Goldsmith, M. Hopkins, and M. Kestigian, "A High Intensity Carbon-Arc-Image Furnace and Its Application to Single Crystal Growth of Refractory Oxides," *J. Electrochem. Soc.* **111**, No. 2, 260–262 (February 1964).

14. E. A. Weaver, H. D. Merchant, and R. P. Poplawsky, "Growth of Fe-Ni Oxide Spinel Single Crystals by Arc Image Techniques," *J. Am. Ceram. Soc.* **52**, No. 4, 214–215 (April 1969).

15. H. M. O'Bryan, Jr., and P. B. O'Connor, "Growth of Rare Earth Aluminum Garnets by Floating Zone Technique," *Am. Ceram. Soc. Bull.* **45**, No. 6, 578–581 (June 1966).

16. J. S. Haggerty, J. F. Wenckus, and D. W. Lee, "Orientated Growth and Defect Structures of Single Crystal Transition Metal Diborides," a paper presented at the Third International Symposium, High Temperature Technology, Asilomar, Calif. (September 1967).

17. R. W. Bartlett, F. A. Halden, and J. W. Fowler, "High Temperature Verneuil Crystal Growth by Arc Melting," *Rev. Sci. Instr.* **38**, No. 9, 1313–1315 (September 1967).

18. B. Cockayne, M. Chesswas, and D. B. Gasson, "Single Crystal Growth of Sapphire," *J. Mater. Sci.* **2**, No. 1, 7 (January 1967).

19. A. P. Gerk and J. J. Gilman, "Growth of Tungsten Carbide Monocrystals," *J. Appl. Phys.* **39**, No. 10, 4497–4500 (September 1968).

20. S. Stecura, "Evaluation of an Imaging Furnace as a Heat Source for X-ray Diffractometry," *Rev. Sci. Instr.* **39**, No. 5, 760–765 (May 1968).

21. F. P. Gagliano, R. M. Lumley, and L. S. Watkins, "Lasers in Industry," *Proc. IEEE* **57**, No. 2, 114–147 (February 1969).

22. "Laser Combines With Oxygen Jet to Make a New Cutting Tool," *Product Eng.* **39**, No. 8, 101 (April 8, 1968).

23. M. I. Cohen, B. A. Unger, and J. F. Milkosky, "Laser Machining of Thin Films and Integrated Circuits," *Bell System Tech. J. (USA)* **47**, No. 3, 385–405 (March 1968).

24. A. J. Martin *et al.*, "The Production of Electrically Conductive Tracks by the Electron or Laser Beam Decomposition of Inorganic Metallic Compounds I. Oxide Systems," *Thin Solid Films* **2**, 253–269 (1968).

25. R. H. Wiley and P. Veeravagu, "Focused, Coherent Radiation (Laser) Induced Degradation of Aromatic Compounds," *J. Phys. Chem.* **72**, No. 7, 2417–2421 (July 1968).

26. G. Oster, "The Chemical Effects of Light," *Sci. American* **219**, No. 3, 158–170 (September 1968).

27. J. A. Sousa and R. A. Kashnow, "Photochromic Paper for Imaging Ultraviolet Laser Pulses," *Rev. Sci. Instr.* **40**, No. 7, 966–967 (July 1969).

28. R. B. Jablonski, "High-Speed Data Recording Device," *IBM Tech. Disclosure Bull.* **10**, No. 10, 1601–1602 (March 1968).

29. A. P. Pedrick, "Laser Ray Beam Gun, or Concentrator, for use in Polar Regions, Accelerating Crop Growth, and Promoting Nuclear Fusion Reactions," British Patent 1,119, 948 (July 17, 1968).

30. J. A. Sousa and R. A. Kashnow, "Laser Photolysis: A Versatile New Technique," *Optical Spectra* **3**, No. 4, 48–51 (July/August 1969).

31. I. Tanaka *et al.*, "Photolysis of Methylene Blue by a Giant-Pulse Ruby Laser," *J. Phys. Chem.* **72**, No. 7, 2684–2686 (July 1968).

32. D. A. Leonard, "Design and Use of an Ultraviolet Laser," *Laser Focus* **3**, No. 3, 26–32 (February 1967).

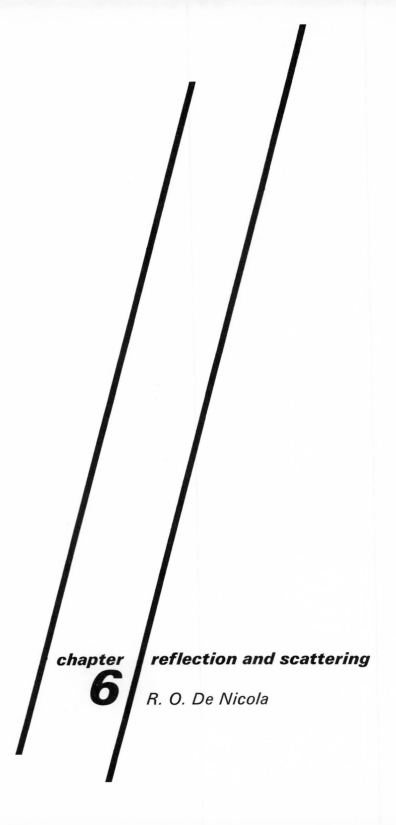

chapter 6   reflection and scattering

R. O. De Nicola

6·0 introduction

The physical phenomena of reflection and scattering of light have long been known and used to varying degrees in measurement. Some techniques that use these phenomena are ellipsometry, Raman spectroscopy, Doppler velocity measurements, and small particle measurement by Rayleigh light scattering. Only recently has the application of these phenomena been greatly increased and expanded in scope. The underlying factors are the laser and the properties of laser light, i.e., spatial and temporal coherence, intensity, small angular divergence, some or all of which can be exploited to give an excellent measurement tool.

This chapter will examine some of the optical measurement processes that use reflection and scattering of laser light for measurement and control.

6·1 reflection of light and its applications

6·1·1 general equations

Whenever an electromagnetic wave is incident upon a boundary separating two media of different optical properties, there results both a reflected and a transmitted (refracted) wave. According to classical optics, well-defined relationships exist between the directions, intensities, polarization, and phases of the incident, reflected, and refracted waves. Figure 6-1 defines the angles of incidence, reflection, and refraction as they will be referred to in this chapter. In addition, it serves to illustrate some of the following classical relationships between all three waves.[1]

1. *The law of reflection* states that the angle of incidence is equal to the angle of reflection; furthermore, the normal to the reflecting surface and the directions of propagation of the incident, reflected, and refracted waves all lie in the same plane.
2. *Snell's law* relates the angle of incidence to the angle of refraction. Mathematically expressed,

$$n_1 \sin \theta_i = n_2 \sin \theta_t \qquad (6\text{-}1)$$

   where n_1, n_2 are the indices of refraction of medium 1 and medium 2, θ_i is the angle of incidence, and θ_t the angle of refraction. In the general case, n_1, n_2, θ_i, and θ_t may all be complex quantities.
3. *Fresnel formulas* give the relationships between the amplitudes of the components of the incident, reflected, and transmitted waves that are polarized* parallel and perpendicular to the plane of incidence (the

---

* See Chapter 2 for a treatment of polarization. Polarization components are treated in Section 6.1.2.

317

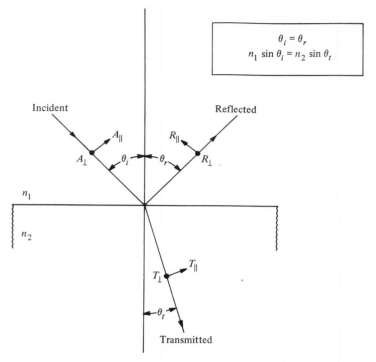

Figure 6-1   Reflection and refraction of a plane wave incident on an optical boundary.

plane formed by the reflecting-surface normal and the propagation direction of the incident beam).

$$T_{\parallel} = \frac{2n_1 \cos \theta_i}{n_2 \cos \theta_i + n_1 \cos \theta_t} A_{\parallel} \tag{6-2}$$

$$T_{\perp} = \frac{2n_1 \cos \theta_i}{n_1 \cos \theta_i + n_2 \cos \theta_t} A_{\perp} \tag{6-3}$$

$$R_{\parallel} = \frac{n_2 \cos \theta_i - n_1 \cos \theta_t}{n_2 \cos \theta_i + n_1 \cos \theta_t} A_{\parallel} \tag{6-4}$$

$$R_{\perp} = \frac{n_1 \cos \theta_i - n_2 \cos \theta_t}{n_1 \cos \theta_i + n_2 \cos \theta_t} A_{\perp} \tag{6-5}$$

where $A_{\parallel}$, $T_{\parallel}$, $R_{\parallel}$ are the incident, transmitted, and reflected amplitudes, respectively, of the component of the wave polarized parallel to the plane of incidence, and $A_{\perp}$, $T_{\perp}$, $R_{\perp}$ are the amplitudes of the components polarized perpendicular to the plane of incidence.

4. *Total internal reflection* can occur since, for light incident on a boundary from an optically dense medium to an optically less dense medium,* there exists a certain angle beyond which the wave is totally reflected. This follows from Snell's law (Equation 6-1), with $\sin \theta_i = (n_2/n_1) \sin \theta_t$. If n_2/n_1 is greater than 1, then for some angle θ_t, $\sin \theta_i$ will be greater than 1. This can be interpreted physically to mean that light is totally reflected at the boundary, with no light transmitted across the boundary.

By knowing certain characteristics of the incident wave—i.e., wavelength, polarization, degree of collimation, intensity, phase, and direction— and by measuring changes in these quantities after reflection from a surface, one may obtain valuable information about the reflecting material, such as thin-film presence and thickness, doping levels in semiconductors, and optical constants. In addition, distance, surface flatness, contamination, and surface stress can all be measured by reflection techniques.

The properties of the incident light that one might want to control, detect, and measure depend upon the classification of the reflecting object (dielectric, metal, semiconductor, amorphous film, etc.) as well as the particular information desired and the physics of the interaction between the surface and the incident light. Table 6-1 provides a brief summary of the parameters of light that undergo changes on reflection and some of the typical applications using these changes for measurement purposes. The characteristics of light reflected from the different classifications of materials will be reviewed below.

The importance of the laser as a light source for these types of measurements cannot be overstated, especially where properties such as monochromaticity, collimation, and intensity are required. Certain types of reflection studies in the near and far infrared have been made possible by the laser since, in many cases, it has eliminated the energy limitations imposed by noncoherent sources.

TABLE 6-1   Some Optical Measurement Techniques and Applications Using Various Characteristics of Light

Light Characteristic	*Typical Reflection Applications*
Polarization	Ellipsometry
Intensity	Imaging, ranging, spatial filtering, velocity measurement, absorption studies
Spatial coherence	Spatial filtering, ellipsometry, polarimetry, imaging, ranging
Temporal coherence	Doppler effect (velocity measurement), interferometry

* Region 2 is said to be optically more dense than region 1 if $n_2 > n_1$, where n is the index of refraction of the region.

Among the applications of reflection of light that will be described are:

1. Ellipsometry as a measurement tool in semiconductor processing
2. Doppler effect and some applications
3. Static distance measurements

6·1·2 polarization components

The general concepts of polarization were treated in Section 2.1.3.   It is convenient, particularly when dealing with the reflection of plane-polarized light, to speak of components of light polarized parallel and perpendicular to a particular reference plane, the plane of incidence.   Figure 6-2 represents a plane-polarized wave propagating out of the paper.   The E-vector, representing the direction of oscillation of the electric field, is oriented at an angle θ with respect to the plane $y = 0$, i.e., the plane of incidence.   We can treat this plane-polarized wave as the sum of two plane-polarized waves, one polarized in the x direction (parallel to the plane of incidence) and one polarized in the y direction (perpendicular to the plane of incidence).   The parallel component is called the p *component* and is given by

$$E_\| = E \cos \theta$$

The perpendicular component is called the s *component* (from " senkrecht," the German word for " perpendicular") and is given by

$$E_\perp = E \sin \theta$$

When convenient to do so, the individual components of circularly or elliptically polarized light may also be resolved into p and s components in the same manner.

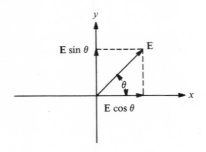

Figure 6-2   *Decomposition of a single plane-polarized beam into two orthogonal plane-polarized components.*

6·1·3   reflection from dielectrics

The properties of light reflected from an ideal dielectric can readily be described by the classical equations presented earlier.   An ideal dielectric is characterized as having a real refractive index n.   If a beam of plane-polarized light is incident from air onto a dielectric surface, at an angle θ_i, then the angle θ_r that the reflected beam makes with the normal to the surface is equal to θ_i.   The angle θ_t that the refracted wave makes with the surface normal is given by Snell's law as:

$$\sin \theta_t = \frac{n_1}{n_2} \sin \theta_i \qquad (6\text{-}6)$$

where n_1 and n_2 are the indices of refraction of air and dielectric, respectively, and θ_i is the angle of incidence.

Further aspects of reflection become clear from Fresnel's equations. Again considering the case of a beam of plane-polarized monochromatic light incident from air onto a dielectric, Fresnel's equations for the reflected components of light polarized parallel and perpendicular to the plane of incidence are:

$$R_{\parallel} = \frac{n_2 \cos \theta_i - n_1 \cos \theta_t}{n_2 \cos \theta_i + n_1 \cos \theta_t} A_{\parallel} \qquad (6\text{-}7)$$

and

$$R_{\perp} = \frac{n_1 \cos \theta_i - n_2 \cos \theta_t}{n_1 \cos \theta_i + n_2 \cos \theta_t} A_{\perp} \qquad (6\text{-}8)$$

The numerator in (6-7) becomes zero when $\cos \theta_i = (n_1/n_2) \cos \theta_t$, whereas the numerator in (6-8) can never become zero under the case being considered (i.e., $n_1 < n_2$).   Thus we see that for any true dielectric, there exists a certain angle θ_p, called the *polarizing angle,* for which light, incident at θ_p onto the dielectric, is reflected in a plane-polarized state, vibrating perpendicular to the plane of incidence.   The dielectric can be used as a polarizer.   Furthermore, the numerator in (6-8) is negative for any angle of incidence, indicating an abrupt 180° phase shift on reflection for the perpendicular (s) component. The numerator in (6-7) changes from positive to negative at the polarizing angle, indicating a zero phase shift in the reflected parallel (p) component up to the polarizing angle and a 180° phase shift as θ is increased beyond θ_p.   Figures 6-3, 6-4, and 6-5 show the reflectances and phase changes of the p and s components of light reflected in air ($n = 1$) from a dielectric of index $n \simeq 1.5$.   The reflectances are defined as

$$R_p = \left| \frac{R_{\parallel}}{A_{\parallel}} \right|^2 \qquad (6\text{-}9)$$

and

$$R_s = \left| \frac{R_{\perp}}{A_{\perp}} \right|^2 \qquad (6\text{-}10)$$

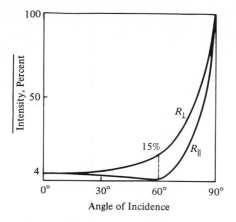

Figure 6-3   Reflectances for p and s waves from a dielectric of index $n = 1.5$.[2]   (**With permission of McGraw-Hill Book Co.**)

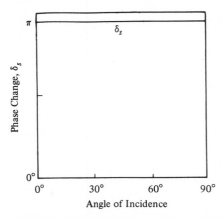

Figure 6-4   Phase shift for s wave upon reflection from a dielectric surface.[2]   (**With permission of McGraw-Hill Book Co.**)

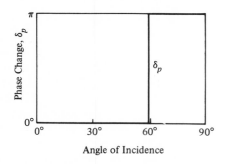

Figure 6-5   Phase shift for p wave upon reflection from a dielectric of $n = 1.5$.[5] (**With permission of McGraw-Hill Book Co.**)

For the special case of normal incidence, i.e., $\theta_i = 0$, there is no distinction between parallel and perpendicular components of the beam, and the expression for the reflected amplitude is given as

$$R = \frac{n-1}{n+1} A \tag{6-11}$$

6·1·4   reflection from metals

The characteristics of light reflected from metals can also be derived from Snell's law and Fresnel's equations. The important difference between this case and reflection from dielectrics is that because of absorption the index of refraction is now complex and is given by

$$\mathbf{n} = n - i\kappa \tag{6-12}$$

where n characterizes the velocity of the wave in the material and κ is the attenuation of the wave in the material per vacuum wavelength.* To describe reflection from an air-metal boundary, we rewrite Snell's law as

$$n_1 \sin \theta_i = (n - i\kappa) \sin \theta_t \tag{6-13}$$

Notice that θ_t is complex and cannot be interpreted simply as an angle of refraction. Actually, for a wave within a metal, the surfaces of constant amplitude and the surfaces of constant phase do not coincide. The "complex angle" θ_t is used in deriving the angular relationship between these constant-phase and constant-amplitude surfaces.[1] By substituting the "complex angle" θ_t into Fresnel's equations, they become complex expressions and are not easily treated. We will briefly describe metallic reflection from a qualitative viewpoint to show the basic differences between light reflected from metals and light reflected from dielectrics.

We have seen that, for plane-polarized light reflected from a dielectric, the s component undergoes a 180° phase shift upon reflection, while the p component undergoes no phase shift up to the polarizing angle θ_p, and an abrupt 180° phase shift thereafter. In this case the reflected light is always plane polarized. For a metal the situation is different. Assume plane-polarized light is incident at an angle θ_i and polarized at a 45° angle to the plane of incidence. Upon reflection, both p and s components will undergo relative phase and amplitude changes so that, in general, the reflected beam will be elliptically polarized. For a given angle of incidence, the degree of elliptical polarization will depend upon the cleanliness of the surface, the reflecting material, and its optical constants. For each metal there is a certain angle of incidence ϕ, called the *principal angle*. Plane-polarized light incident on the metallic surface at

---

* Chapter 2 describes how absorption gives rise to a complex index.

TABLE 6-2[a] **Principal Angle and Angle of Restored Polarization Measured at $\lambda = 5893$ nm for Some Metals**[3]

	ϕ	ψ
Bi	77° 3′	31° 58′
Hg	79° 34′	35° 43′
Au	72° 18′	41° 39′
Ag	75° 42′	43° 35′
Cu	71° 35′	38° 57′
Ni	76° 1′	31° 41′
Al	79° 55′	37° 34′
Mg	77° 57′	42° 42′
Pt	78° 30′	32° 35′

[a] With permission of Longmans Group, Essex, England.

this angle is such that the p and s components undergo exactly a 90° relative phase shift, and the reflected light is, in general, elliptically polarized but with the ellipse axes parallel and perpendicular to the plane of incidence.   By use of a quarter-wave plate* to restore the original phase relation, the reflected beam becomes plane polarized at an angle ψ, called the *angle of restored polarization*.   Once the principal angle ϕ, and the angle of restored polarization ψ have been determined, one can calculate the optical constants of the reflecting surface by using (6-30) and (6-31), with Δ set equal to $\pi/2$.   Table 6-2 lists the principal angle and the angle of restored polarization for some metals.   In general, both ϕ and ψ depend on wavelength, ϕ increasing and ψ decreasing as λ increases.

6·1·5   reflection from semiconductors

The basic characteristics of radiation reflected from semiconductor materials depend upon the wavelength of the radiation and the free carrier concentration of the material.   A number of different absorption mechanisms,[4] the most important of which are intrinsic absorption and free carrier absorption, act over different portions of the spectrum with the result that a semiconductor can show reflection characteristics ranging from those of metals to those of weakly absorbing dielectrics.   Optical test techniques that take advantage of these characteristics are currently becoming of interest in the semiconductor industry because they are non-destructive and potentially very accurate.

* See Glossary.

   The most familiar mode of absorption in semiconductors is *intrinsic absorption*. An electron in the valence band will be excited into the conduction band upon absorption of an amount of energy E equal to or greater than the band gap E_g. Thus the optical photons of energy $h\nu \geq E_g$ will be absorbed and will create two charge carriers in the semiconductor—a conduction electron and a hole. There are certain rules which the absorption process must fulfill, principally conservation of energy and momentum.[5,6] The point we wish to make here is that for any semiconductor there exists a frequency of radiation above which there is large absorption and the creation of hole-electron pairs.

   A second type of absorption, *free carrier absorption*, is becoming important in measurements. This type of absorption can also be termed metallic absorption since absorption by free electrons also characterizes absorption in metals. As developed in Section 2.6.4, the index of refraction of a semiconductor of free carrier concentration N_c is obtained from the expressions

$$n^2 - \kappa^2 - \varepsilon_\infty = \frac{-N_c e^2}{\varepsilon_0 m_c^*} \times \frac{1}{\omega_i^2 + \Gamma^2} \qquad (6\text{-}14)$$

and

$$2n\omega_i \kappa = \frac{N_c e^2}{\varepsilon_0 m_c^*} \times \frac{\Gamma}{\omega_i^2 + \Gamma^2} \qquad (6\text{-}15)$$

where ε_0 = permittivity of free space,
   m_c^* = effective mass of free carriers,
   ω_i = angular frequency of incident radiation,
   Γ = a damping coefficient, defined as $\Gamma \equiv e/m_c^* \mu_c$, where μ_c is carrier mobility,
   ε_∞ = lattice contribution to the dielectric constant,
   n = real part of index of refraction,
   κ = absorption index or imaginary part of refractive index.

By using the standard definition of absorption coefficient

$$\alpha = \frac{4\pi\kappa}{\lambda} \qquad (6\text{-}16)$$

and the fact that $\Gamma = e/m_c^* \mu_c$, we can write

$$\alpha = \frac{e^3 \lambda^2}{4\pi^2 c^3 n \varepsilon_0} \times \frac{N_c}{m_c^* \mu_c} \qquad (6\text{-}17)$$

where c = velocity of light, and μ_c = mobility of charge carriers. For a given sample whose free carrier concentration is N_c, carrier mobility is μ_c and effective carrier mass is m_c^*, the absorption coefficient due to free carriers increases as the wavelength of the incident light increases.

The fact that below the intrinsic absorption edge the optical constants are functions of free carrier concentration can be used to develop optical test techniques that use these differences in optical constants to measure resistivity and thickness of epitaxial layers.

In summary, semiconductors exhibit reflection properties characteristic of both metals and insulators, depending upon the wavelength of radiation used and the particular absorption mechanism that is dominant.

6·1·6 applications of reflection

<u>Ellipsometry</u>   Ellipsometry is the study of the changes in the polarization states of light after reflection from a surface.   By measuring the ellipsometric parameters Δ and ψ, explained below, one can do such things as:

1. Measure the optical constants of semiconductors and metals;
2. Measure the optical constants and thicknesses of thin films on semiconductor or metallic substrates, or of metallic films on dielectric substrates;
3. Inspect films and surfaces for the presence of undesired material phases or contamination.

These are just a few examples of areas where ellipsometry can be applied and are not intended as a total survey of possible ellipsometric applications.   The laser is an ideal light source for ellipsometry because of the collimation and monochromaticity of its output and promises applications using the infrared portion of the spectrum.   An example of such an application to epitaxial layer thickness measurement in integrated circuit manufacture will be described later in this section.

A schematic of a typical ellipsometry setup is shown in Figure 6-6. The laser provides the required source of collimated monochromatic light.

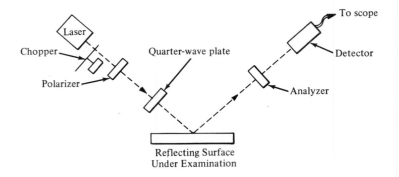

Figure 6-6   Schematic diagram of a typical ellipsometric arrangement.

The polarizer and analyzer are mounted in graduated circles capable of providing angular rotational measurements to at least 0.1°. An optical compensator (usually a quarter-wave plate) is mounted either before or after the reflecting surface and provides a means for adjusting polarization of the incident light or analyzing polarization of the reflected light. For purposes of this discussion, assume the quarter-wave plate has been placed before the reflecting surface. The detector used will depend upon the wavelength of measurement.

Operation of the instrument is described for reflection from a clean metallic surface. As stated in the section treating metallic reflection, the p and s components of the plane-polarized incident light undergo different phase and amplitude changes upon reflection so that, in general, the reflected beam is elliptically polarized. By properly adjusting the elliptical polarization of the incident beam, the reflected beam will be plane polarized at some azimuth and can be prevented from reaching the detector by rotating the analyzer. The combination of the polarizer and quarter-wave plate enables adjustment of the polarization of the incident beam to any desired degree of ellipticity, and specifically to that value which yields a plane-polarized reflected beam. This is accomplished by setting the quarter-wave plate with fast or slow axis at 45° to the plane of incidence and rotating the polarizer to an appropriate angle.

The polarizer and analyzer, then, are adjusted for minimum signal at the detector. The adjustment of the polarizer effectively selects the polarization of the incident light to yield a plane-polarized reflected beam. The adjustment of the analyzer effectively prevents this plane-polarized reflected beam from reaching the detector. Once the minimum signal is obtained, the azimuth of both polarizer and analyzer (i.e., the angles the planes of transmission make with the plane of incidence) are recorded. These readings are generally referred to as P and A readings, respectively.

There are a number of different P and A settings that yield a minimum detector signal, corresponding to settings in four different zones. The explanation of these zones and the procedures to be followed in taking measurements are presented in Ref. 7. For convenience, the procedure is outlined here.

Zone 1—The fast axis of the quarter-wave plate is set at $-\pi/4$. The polarizer plane of transmission makes an angle of $+P$ with the plane of incidence. The analyzer plane of transmission makes an angle of $+A$ with the plane of incidence.

Zone 2—The fast axis of the quarter-wave plate is set at $+\pi/4$. The polarizer plane of transmission makes an angle of $\pi/2 - P$ with the plane of incidence. The analyzer plane of transmission makes an angle of $+A$ with the plane of incidence.

Zone 3—The fast axis of the quarter-wave plate is set at $-\pi/4$. The polarizer plane of transmission makes an angle of $\pi/2 + P$ with the plane of incidence. The analyzer plane of transmission makes an angle of $-A$ with the plane of incidence.

Zone 4—The fast axis of the quarter-wave plate is set at $+\pi/4$. The polarizer plane of transmission makes an angle of $-P$ with the plane of incidence. The analyzer plane of transmission makes an angle of $-A$ with the plane of incidence.

If all optical components of the ellipsometer were ideal, then all four P and A readings obtained by the above procedure would be identical, and one could calculate Δ and ψ from the relations[7]

$$\Delta = 2P + 90°$$

and

$$\psi = A$$

In practice, however, polarizers are not ideal and quarter-wave plates can exhibit retardations different from 90°. Furthermore, multiple reflections in the quarter-wave plate and improper alignment of the components will cause these readings to differ. Generally, by using the average of the four P and A readings, the equations given above for Δ and ψ can be used. For extremely accurate work, detailed correction and averaging procedures are necessary.[7-10] Having obtained the values of Δ and ψ, one can now use these in various expressions relating Δ and ψ to the thickness and index of refraction of thin films or to the optical constants of a film-free substrate. These applications are described below.

Optical Constants   In this section, the ellipsometric parameters Δ and ψ are used to obtain optical constants of a film-free absorbing surface. The derivations start from the simple form of Snell's law, presented earlier, i.e.,

$$n_1 \sin \theta_i = n_2 \sin \theta_t \tag{6-18}$$

Here, the ambient medium is assumed to be air of index $n_1 = 1.0$. The complex index of the metal or semiconductor surfaces is $n_2 = n - i\kappa$. The angle of incidence is θ_i, and θ_t is the "complex angle" of refraction,

$$\sin \theta_t = \frac{\sin \theta_i}{n - i\kappa} \tag{6-19}$$

Fresnel's equations, presented earlier, give the ratios of reflected amplitude to incident amplitude for both p and s waves. The equations can be put in the form

$$\frac{R_\parallel}{A_\parallel} = \frac{\tan (\theta_i - \theta_t)}{\tan (\theta_i + \theta_t)} \tag{6-20}$$

and

$$\frac{R_\perp}{A_\perp} = \frac{\sin(\theta_t - \theta_i)}{\sin(\theta_i + \theta_t)} \tag{6-21}$$

where θ_i and θ_t are angles of incidence and complex angle of refraction, respectively, and $R_\parallel$, $A_\parallel$, $R_\perp$, $A_\perp$ are as defined previously.

Since θ_t is complex, both of the quantities $R_\parallel/A_\parallel$ and $R_\perp/A_\perp$ are complex and can be expressed as

$$\frac{R_\parallel}{A_\parallel} = r_\parallel = p_\parallel e^{i\Delta_\parallel} \tag{6-22}$$

and

$$\frac{R_\perp}{A_\perp} = r_\perp = p_\perp e^{i\Delta_\perp} \tag{6-23}$$

If the incident light is polarized at $45°$ to the plane of incidence, then $A_\parallel = A_\perp$. Define α to be the azimuth of the reflected light,

$$e^{i\Delta}\tan\alpha = \frac{R_\parallel}{R_\perp} = \frac{p_\parallel e^{i(\Delta_\parallel - \Delta_\perp)}}{p_\perp} = pe^{i\Delta} \tag{6-24}$$

where α is in general complex, and $\Delta = (\Delta_\parallel - \Delta_\perp)$. To evaluate (6-24) for p,

$$\tan\alpha = p = \frac{p_\parallel}{p_\perp} \equiv \tan\psi \tag{6-25}$$

Note that Δ is the relative phase difference between parallel and perpendicular components of the reflected beam. If Δ is made zero by compensation (i.e., a suitably oriented quarter-wave plate), both components will be in phase, will combine to form linearly polarized light, and can be extinguished by the analyzer. The azimuth of the analyzer is read as A. The amount of compensation required, Δ, is determined from the polarizer setting. To determine the optical constants n and k in terms of Δ and ψ, it is convenient to form the quotient

$$\frac{1 - pe^{i\Delta}}{1 + pe^{i\Delta}} = \frac{\cos\theta_i \cos\theta_t}{\sin\theta_i \sin\theta_t} \tag{6-26}$$

But

$$\sin\theta_t = \frac{\sin\theta_i}{n - i\kappa} \tag{6-27}$$

Thus

$$\cos\theta_t = \sqrt{1 - \frac{\sin^2\theta_i}{(n - i\kappa)^2}} \tag{6-28}$$

Then

$$\frac{1 - pe^{+i\Delta}}{1 + pe^{+i\Delta}} = \frac{\sqrt{(n - i\kappa)^2 - \sin^2 \theta_i}}{\sin \theta_i \tan \theta_i} \tag{6-29}$$

Let $p = \tan \psi$.   Then

$$\frac{1 - \tan \psi \, e^{+i\Delta}}{1 + \tan \psi \, e^{+i\Delta}} = \frac{\cos 2\psi - i \sin 2\psi \sin \Delta}{1 + \sin 2\psi \cos \Delta} \tag{6-30}$$

and

$$\frac{\sqrt{(n - i\kappa)^2 - \sin^2 \theta_i}}{\sin \theta_i \tan \theta_i} = \frac{\cos 2\psi - i \sin 2\psi \sin \Delta}{1 + \sin 2\psi \cos \Delta} \tag{6-31}$$

If $\mathrm{Re}[(n - i\kappa)^2] \gg 1$, as is usually the case, then $\sin^2 \theta_i$ can be neglected in the numerator and this gives approximate expressions for n and κ as

$$n \simeq \frac{\sin \theta_i \tan \theta_i \cos 2\psi}{1 + \sin 2\psi \cos \Delta} \tag{6-32}$$

and

$$\kappa \simeq \frac{\sin 2\psi \sin \Delta \sin \theta_i \tan \theta_i}{1 + \sin 2\psi \cos \Delta} \tag{6-33}$$

If this assumption, $(n - i\kappa)^2 \gg 1$, is not made, the exact expressions are

$$n^2 = \kappa^2 + \sin^2 \theta_i + \frac{\sin^2 \theta_i \tan^2 \theta_i (\cos^2 2\psi - \sin^2 2\psi \sin^2 \Delta)}{(1 + \sin 2\psi \cos \Delta)^2} \tag{6-34}$$

and

$$\kappa = \frac{\sin^2 \theta_i \tan^2 \theta_i \sin 4\psi \sin \Delta}{2n(1 + \sin 2\psi \cos \Delta)^2} \tag{6-35}$$

It must be emphasized that in making measurements of optical constants of bare surfaces, the ellipsometer must be accurately aligned and the surface must be essentially film free, a condition that is not easily obtained. Fortunately, for thin-film measurements, these requirements can be somewhat relaxed.

Thin-Film Thickness Measurement

If the optical constants of a substrate are known, one can use ellipsometry to obtain the thickness and index of refraction of a thin film present on the substrate surface. The only requirement is that the thickness of the film being measured be much less than the wavelength of light being used.   The technique relies on the fact that the ellipsometric parameters Δ and ψ are very sensitive to the presence of thin films and will change from the film-free surface values by an amount determined by the thickness and index of refraction of the film. The equations relating the changes in the Δ and ψ readings to the thickness and index of refraction of the film are given as[11]

$$\tan \psi \, e^{i\Delta} = \frac{r_{1p} + r_{2p} e^{-2i\delta}}{1 + r_{1p} r_{2p} e^{-2i\delta}} \times \frac{1 + r_{1s} r_{2s} e^{-2i\delta}}{r_{1s} + r_{2s} e^{-2i\delta}} \qquad (6\text{-}36)$$

where

$$\delta = \frac{360}{\lambda} d(n_1^2 - \sin^2 \theta_i)^{1/2} \text{ deg} \qquad (6\text{-}37)$$

and r_{1p}, r_{1s} = Fresnel reflection coefficients for light reflected at air-film boundary,

r_{2p}, r_{2s} = Fresnel reflection coefficients for light reflected at film-substrate boundary,

n_1 = index of film,

θ_i = angle of incidence,

d = thickness of film,

λ = wavelength of light.

One general procedure in solving for the index of the film and its thickness is to assume a value of n_1 and then calculate Δ and ψ for a range of film thicknesses, d. If there are no values of Δ and ψ on this theoretical curve that match the experimental values, then another theoretical curve is generated by assuming a different value of n_1. The experimental values are then compared against this curve. This procedure continues until the experimental point falls on the theoretical curve. When this happens, n_1 is taken as the index of the film.

The technique is well suited for use with a computer, and there are a number of programs available to the experimenter. Of particular value are the NBS programs.[12] These provide a computational capability for quickly obtaining optical constants and even multiple film thicknesses.

An example that ties together much of what has been covered on reflection is the ellipsometric measurement of semiconductor epitaxial layer thickness (typically 5 μm to 15 μm).[13] Silicon epitaxial layers deposited on silicon substrates generally have doping levels of about 10^{15} impurities/cm^3, while the substrate is doped typically from 10^{18} to 10^{19} impurities/cm^3. Thus, the free carrier concentrations in the layer and the substrate differ by a factor of 10^3 to 10^4. Use of (6-14), (6-15), (6-16), and (6-17) show that their corresponding optical constants will be different and depend both on impurity concentrations N_c and wavelength of measurement. By measuring Δ and ψ at a long wavelength, one can:

1. Accentuate the difference between the optical constants of substrate and epitaxial layer by taking advantage of the λ^2 dependence shown in (6.17).

2. Satisfy the ellipsometric requirement that the wavelength used be much longer than the film thickness being measured.

TABLE 6-3   Measured Values of
Δ and ψ for a Series
of Epitaxial Wafers

Sample	Δ Average	ψ Average
1	82.0	35.6
2	69.2	37.7
3	230.6	35.5
4	173.8	37.5
5	270.6	35.5
6	180.6	37.4
7	193.3	37.2

The laser provides a truly satisfactory source for ellipsometric measurements at far-infrared wavelengths. Two particularly useful types are the water-vapor laser and the HCN laser. The water-vapor laser provides radiation at various lines out to 220×10^3 nm, whereas the HCN emits at lines out to over 300×10^3 nm in the far infrared.

Table 6-3 lists some typical ellipsometry data obtained from measurement of silicon epitaxial layer thickness at the 118.6×10^3 nm line of a water-vapor laser. The data were taken in the four zones previously mentioned, and averaged.

These values of Δ and ψ are compared with a graph that shows how Δ and ψ vary with epitaxial layer thickness. Figure 6-7 shows the theoretical curve that applies to an epi-substrate system in which the epitaxial layer resistivity is 5 Ω-cm and the substrate resistivity is 0.01 Ω-cm. The data of Table 6-3 are also plotted. The fit between theory and experiment is excellent. Table 6-4 compares the results of thickness measurement by both ellipsometry and the standard near-infrared scan technique.[14] Notice that the thickness measured by far-infrared ellipsometry is consistently less than the thickness measured by the near-infrared scan. This is due to the fact that the epilayer-substrate junction is graded as shown in Figure 6-8. Because of the N_c and λ^2 dependence of the optical constants, as the wavelength of measurement increases, the effective optical boundary

TABLE 6-4   Comparison of Thickness Measured by Ellipsometry and Conventional Near-Infrared Techniques

Sample	Far-Infrared Ellipsometry	Near-Infrared Scan
1	4.7	6.0
2	5.3	6.6
3	11.1	12.0
4	16.0	17.2
5	8.6	9.3
6	15.5	16.5
7	14.1	15.0

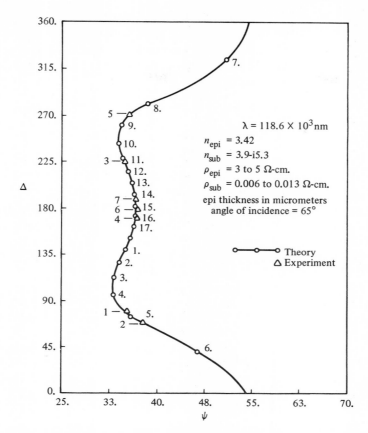

Figure 6-7   A typical Δ versus ψ curve characteristic of silicon epitaxial wafers.

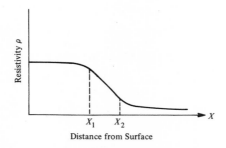

Figure 6-8   Resistivity profile at the interface between a substrate and an epitaxial layer.

between epitaxial layer and the substrate occurs at points close to the "knee." For example, near-infrared scan might measure epitaxial thickness to X_2 as labeled on Figure 6-8, whereas at the longer wavelength of far-infrared ellipsometry, the thickness measured would be X_1. One can immediately draw two conclusions:

1. As the junction becomes more abrupt, both methods will yield the same thickness.
2. The difference in thickness measured by each of the techniques gives an indication of junction grading.

Ellipsometry at such long wavelengths poses its problems. Specialized optical components such as wire grid polarizers,[15] and polyethylene lenses to collimate the beam, are required. Detectors must be operated at liquid helium temperatures, although work is being done on room temperature far-infrared detectors. Overall sensitivity is not as good as it is for visible light detectors. As new and better optical components are developed, such far-infrared techniques will become more common.

Optical Constants at Normal Incidence   In the previous sections it was shown how optical constants are obtained by reflecting light at nonnormal incidence. There are other common techniques that one can use to determine n and κ at a desired wavelength.[16] For example, if the sample is somewhat transparent, transmission can be measured by comparing the intensity of light before and after it propagates through the sample at normal incidence. Assuming the surrounding medium to be air, the transmittance T is given by (2-61) as

$$T = \frac{4n_2}{(1 + n_2)^2 + \kappa_2^2} \tag{6-38}$$

Normal reflectance is then measured, and is given by (2-60) as

$$R = \frac{(1 - n_2)^2 + \kappa_2^2}{(1 + n_2)^2 + \kappa_2^2} \tag{6-39}$$

With these two equations in two unknowns, one can solve for both n and κ of the sample.

Although transmittance measurements generally do not present too much of a problem, measurements are most conveniently made if the sample thickness t is such that

$$\alpha t \simeq 1$$

where $\alpha \equiv 4\pi\kappa/\lambda$ and κ is the extinction coefficient. Otherwise, the measurement becomes less precise.

Normal reflectance is usually measured by reflecting off the surface at a slight angle of incidence, say 7°. This is done to avoid the use of beam splitters which can adversely affect measured reflectance.

Total Internal Reflection and Measurement of Carrier Concentration

A use of the laser for nondestructive measurements of carrier concentrations in silicon epitaxial layers has been described.[17] The technique is based on (6-4) and the principle of total internal reflection. Using a HeNe laser operating at 3390 nm wavelength, radiation polarized parallel to the plane of incidence is focused just outside of a germanium hemisphere. Germanium is chosen because its index of refraction is greater than that of the silicon epilayer. Radiation enters the germanium and propagates through it in a collimated beam. A silicon epitaxial wafer is placed in near contact with the back side of the germanium hemisphere (within one wavelength of the radiation used). The result is a collimated beam of light traveling from an optically dense medium (germanium) to an optically less dense medium (silicon). The angle of incidence is then varied and the reflected light intensity is monitored with a detector. Since the light is traveling from an optically dense to a less dense medium, reflectivity changes from almost 0 percent to 100 percent between the Brewster (polarizing) angle and the critical angle. As carrier concentration changes, both the Brewster angle and the critical angle change. An accurate measurement of epi-resistivity is obtained by measuring the critical angle. The minimum detectable change in carrier concentration is quoted as 1×10^{17} atom/cm^3 for a wavelength of 3390 nm. At 10.6×10^3 nm, the change in critical angle is about one minute for a carrier concentration change from 1×10^{16} to 2×10^{16} atoms/cm^3.

Surface Diagnostics The use of a small 3 mW HeNe laser in a flying light-spot system for rapidly detecting defects on ceramics and semiconductor surfaces and pinholes in thin metal films has been described.[18] A pictorial schematic of the general instrument is shown in Figure 6-9. The laser beam is first expanded and is incident upon a beam deflector. Different types of beam deflectors, such as acousto-optic and rotating mirror deflectors were considered, but based upon cost, size, and convenience, a torsionally oscillating mirror was selected and shown to be quite satisfactory. The deflector directs the beam onto a lens which focuses the beam to a small spot. The lens must be sufficiently large to intercept the beam over its entire deflected range. As the mirror oscillates, causing the expanded beam to scan back and forth across the lens, the focused spot effectively becomes a fine focused line. The surface to be inspected is moved perpendicular to this scan line. Depending upon the nature of the inspected surface, there will be a specular reflection, a diffuse reflection, or both, or a transmission of light. Detection is obtained by placing detectors in the appropriate positions.

In the selection of focusing optics, it is well to consider that a maximum signal-to-noise ratio at the detector will be achieved when the beam spot size on the surface is a minimum. This means that the lens, in addition to being large enough to intercept the beam over its entire scan width,

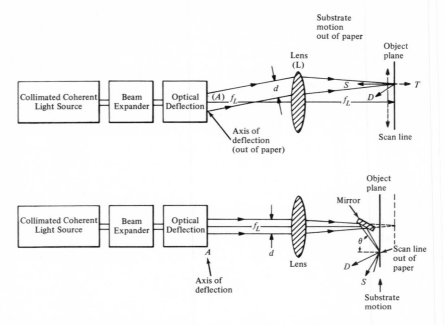

Figure 6-9 Schematic diagrams of the flying light-spot surface inspection system.[18]

must also have a low f/number. Any mirrors (such as the scanning mirror) should be flat to a fraction of a wavelength to achieve the best results. Depth of focus is generally not critical and in most cases need not be of concern.

Some practical applications, as discussed in Ref. 18, are repeated below.

1. Pinhole Detection A scheme for detecting pinholes in film deposited on translucent substrates is shown in Figure 6-10. It is presently being evaluated in studies of pinholes in sputtered Ta_2N and chromium. In the first of these applications a 3 mW HeNe laser is employed with a beam expanded to 1.5 cm, incident on a lens 5 in. in diameter, 12 in. focal length, producing a spot size of 15 μm over a scan of 4 in.   Pinholes with diameters greater than 2 μm can be readily detected.

For those applications where it is desired to inspect films for the presence of pinholes above a certain critical size, it is necessary to use a sufficiently tight raster to ensure that the intensity of light reaching all parts of the substrate result in a signal from the detector above threshold for pinholes greater than the critical size.   The location of these pinholes is then indicated on the storage oscilloscope.

In order to reduce rejection to a minimum in a given application, selective inspection may be necessary and can be accomplished by covering

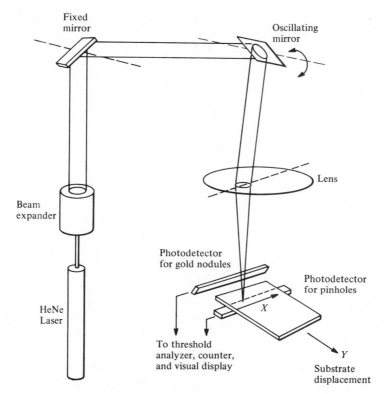

Figure 6-10   Inspection scheme for pinholes and gold nodules in thin films.[18]

the metallized substrate directly with a mask transparent in the region to be inspected.

2. Gold Nodule Detection   The simple scheme shown in Figure 6-10 has been demonstrated to be very effective in detecting gold nodules on smooth surfaces, such as glass or silicon wafers, or on rough ceramic surfaces covered with gold film.   Detection is based on the theoretical and experimental facts that evaporated gold nodules, generally spherical in shape, scatter light isotropically, whereas the substrate, rough or smooth, scatters relatively little light at large angles.   This, therefore, accounts for the location of the detector in Figure 6-10.   Some indication of the capabilities are provided by comparison, in Figure 6-11, of a microscope picture of an area of ceramic covered with gold nodules and the picture presented on a CRT, intensity modulated using the focused laser beam scanner.   Under these conditions, a $3\frac{3}{4}$ in. $\times$ $4\frac{1}{2}$ in. substrate can be scanned in 20 s to give the location and number of nodules ~ 1 mil in diameter.

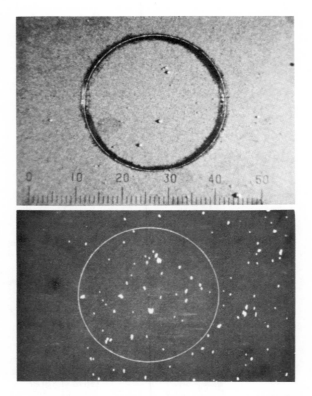

Figure 6-11   Storage oscilloscope pictures showing surface defects.[18]

3. Detection of Pits, Burrs, and Scratches   Efforts to detect the presence of pits, burrs, and scratches on ceramic have centered on the use of glazed ceramics, because in the method described below, the surface must have a significant specular reflectivity in the normal direction.   The glaze normally applied to ceramics is only a few micrometers thick and therefore contours those defects damaging to the fabrication of circuits. The major factor complicating the detection of these defects is the long-ranged waviness always associated with ceramics.   The scheme devised to accommodate tolerable waviness and still be sensitive to defects is shown in Figure 6-12.

In this scheme the line scan of the focused laser is achieved by the same arrangement as shown in Figure 6-10.   To collect the specular light basically only four more components are required, as shown in Figure 6-12.   For parallel light, the variable aperture becomes a virtual aperture by reflection in the beamsplitter and oscillating mirror.   It can be considered as located in the plane of the large lens and to scan along directly above the focused laser spot.

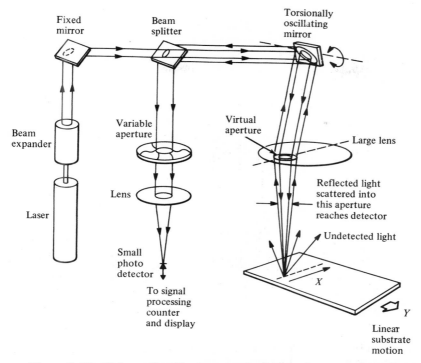

Figure 6-12   Schematic of instrument for inspecting ceramic surfaces for burrs, scratches, and pits.[18]

Provided there are no burrs, and the waviness is sufficiently small for the reflected light to pass through the variable scanning aperture, a constant signal will be registered by the photodetector. When a localized surface defect is encountered by the beam, some of the light is scattered outside the aperture, causing a reduction in the intensity of light received by the detector. The sensitivity may be increased by stopping down the aperture consistent with the demands on aperture size made by the limit of acceptable waviness. With suitable electronic signal processing the scheme has been demonstrated to be capable of detecting burrs 5 μm high and 10 μm in diameter.

4. Conductor Pattern Inspection   A comparative scheme for conductor pattern inspection is shown in Figure 6-13. The great merit of the comparative method is that it circumvents the need for a dynamic memory. In the present arrangement, the two circuits, one known to be acceptable, the other under study, are located in optically equivalent positions relative to the two tracking focused light spots. They are mounted on a common carriage, which moves linearly perpendicular to

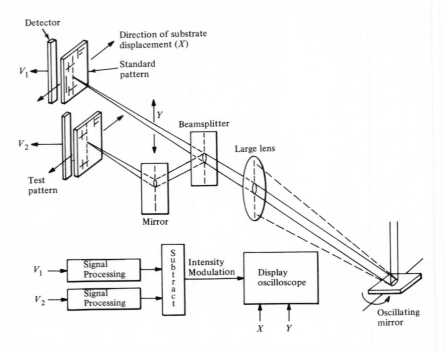

Figure 6-13   Scheme for comparing a conductor pattern on a test piece with that on a standard.

the two synchronized line scans.   For translucent substrates, the photo-detectors are placed directly behind the two line scans and pick up the transmitted light.   Unwanted opens and shorts are indicated as differences in the photodetector outputs and used to intensity modulate the storage CRT.   The X and Y displacements of CRT beam are proportional to the laser spot and carriage locations, respectively.

All of the above examples refer to the detection of defects in thin-film rather than in silicon technology, where all dimensions, including the size of tolerable defects, are much smaller.   These techniques, however, can readily be adapted to detection of defects on silicon wafers.

Doppler Effect   The Doppler effect can be used to measure veloc-ity by detecting the frequency shift of laser light after reflection (or scatter-ing) from a moving surface.   The Doppler frequency shift is detected by impinging the reflected light together with a reference beam taken from the same laser onto a square-law detector.   From a knowledge of this frequency shift, one can compute the velocity of the moving object.   The resolution of this technique is excellent, allowing one to detect frequency changes of a few cycles in 10^{14} Hz.   Velocities as low as 10^{-3} cm/s can be measured.   We now derive the relationships between object velocity and wavelength shift.

Figure 6-14 shows a stationary point source of spherical waves.[19]   At a certain distance, d_2, from the source, the wavefront is one wavelength ahead of the wavefront at d_1, so that $d_2 - d_1 = \lambda$, the wavelength of the light.   If the source now moves with velocity, v, toward an observer, then the wavefront at d_2, observed at time t_2, is actually at a distance $d_2' = d_2 - vt_2$ from the source, whereas the wavefront observed at t_1 will be at a distance $d_1' = d_1 - vt_1$.   The observer will record the wavelength as $\lambda' = d_2' - d_1' = d_2 - vt_2 - d_1 + vt_1$.   But $t_2 - t_1 = 1/v = \lambda/c = T$,   the period of the wave emitted by the source.   During the time interval, T, the source has moved a distance $vT = v(\lambda/c)$, so that now the distance from the wavefront at d_2 to the wavefront at d_1 is decreased by the distance $\lambda(v/c)$, i.e.,

$$\lambda' = \left(1 - \frac{v}{c}\right)\lambda \qquad (6\text{-}40)$$

The corresponding frequency is given as

$$v' = \frac{c}{\lambda'} = \frac{c/\lambda}{1 - v/c} = \frac{v}{1 - v/c} \qquad (6\text{-}41)$$

Thus, by knowing v, the frequency of the reference or incident radiation, and by determining v', the Doppler-shifted frequency of the detected beam, one can calculate the velocity of the source or reflecting object.   The general expressions for the Doppler-shifted frequency observed at an angle θ to the source motion is obtained from consideration of Figure 6-15.

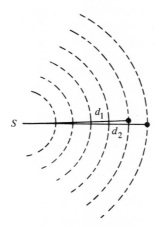

Figure 6-14   Spherical waves emanating from source S.

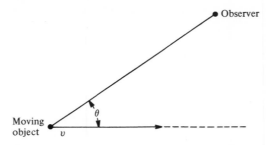

Figure 6-15   Figure showing general velocity relationships between observer and a moving source.

Because the change in frequency is due to the relative velocity between observer and source, the velocity component in the direction of the observer should be used in (6.41).   Hence,

$$v' = \frac{v}{1 - \frac{v}{c} \cos \theta} \tag{6-42}$$

Optical Heterodyning—Detection of the Doppler Shift   In order to apply the theory developed in the previous section, one must accurately measure the shift in the frequency of light emitted by the moving source.   To do this, optical heterodyning is used.   A laser beam is split and part (the reference beam) is sent directly to an intensity-sensitive detector.*   The other part of the beam (the signal) is reflected or scattered off the object whose velocity one is trying to measure.   The light returned by the moving source is then collected and sent to the same detector as the reference beam.   The signal beam has undergone a frequency shift as described above.   Whenever two signals of different frequencies are mixed on a square-law detector, there results, in addition to the signal frequencies, both sum and difference frequencies.   If, for example, the signals

$$E_1 = A \cos \omega_1 t \tag{6-43}$$

and

$$E_2 = B \cos \omega_2 t \tag{6-44}$$

are incident on the cathode, then the response is

$$I \propto (E_1 + E_2)^2 = E_1^2 + E_2^2 + 2E_1E_2 \tag{6-45}$$

or

$$I \propto A^2 \cos^2 \omega_1 t + B^2 \cos^2 \omega_2 t + 2AB \cos \omega_1 t \cos \omega_2 t \tag{6-46}$$

* Detectors, such as a photomultiplier tube, that respond to incident light intensity (square of amplitude) are called *square-law detectors*.

The factor $\cos \omega_1 t \cos \omega_2 t$ can be written as

$$\cos \omega_1 t \cos \omega_2 t = \tfrac{1}{2}[\cos(\omega_1 - \omega_2)t + \cos(\omega_1 + \omega_2)t] \qquad (6\text{-}47)$$

The total response is then written as

$$I \propto A^2 \cos^2 \omega_1 t + B^2 \cos^2 \omega_2 t + AB[\cos(\omega_1 - \omega_2)t + \cos(\omega_1 + \omega_2)t]$$

$$(6\text{-}48)$$

The frequencies ω_1, ω_2, and $(\omega_2 + \omega_1)$ are much too rapid for the detector to follow and a dc signal proportional to their time average will result. However, the frequency $(\omega_1 - \omega_2)$ typically will be in the tens of megahertz range and the detector signal will have a component at this frequency.

There are a number of factors to consider before efficient heterodyning can be achieved. For example, when reference beam and signal are superimposed on the photocathode, an area of the cathode of diameter many times greater than the wavelength emits photoelectrons, and each element of this area contributes to the total current. For maximum response, the signal and the reference beams must maintain the same relative phase relationship across this entire area.

Other factors to consider are that for efficient detection: (1) the laser supplying both signal and reference should be operated in the TEM_{00} mode, (2) both beams should be coincident and of the same size, (3) the wavefronts should be identical, and (4) polarization should be the same. For a discussion of these and other fine points associated with optical heterodyning, a very readable and thorough treatment is presented in Ref. 20.

The Laser as a Light Source for Doppler Measurements

The equations used to describe the optical heterodyne process assume that the interfering beams are strictly monochromatic, i.e., single frequency. If each beam contains considerable bandwidth, then the velocities that can be measured are limited to high velocities, since resolution on the low-velocity scale becomes extremely poor and ultimately impossible. For example, using the Doppler equations and the fact that, for conventional light sources, the bandwidth is of the order of 10^9 Hz, the minimum velocity that can be resolved is, from (6-41),

$$v = \frac{v' - v}{v'} c \qquad (6\text{-}49)$$

For $v \simeq 5 \times 10^{14}$, the velocity must be of the order of 600 m/s. This limitation arises from the continuous bandwidth of the conventional source.

For a laser, the situation is considerably different. Gas lasers are available that have a bandwidth of 10^6 Hz or less. Velocities of the order of 10 cm/s can be measured with these lasers, and use of specially

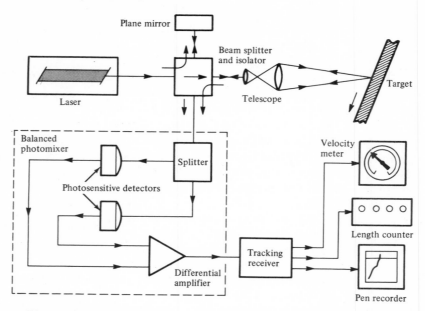

Figure 6-16   Diagram of a laser Doppler velocity measurement system.[21]   (*With permission of* **The Engineer.**)

stabilized single-frequency lasers enables one to measure velocities down to 10^{-3} cm/s.   The laser is thus indispensable for low-velocity measurements using the Doppler technique.

   Applications   Laser Doppler velocimeters incorporating the principles of the previous sections are being used to measure the speed of aluminum extrusions, sheet metals, and hot steel rod.[21]   One such system* uses a 1 mW HeNe laser (632.8 nm) and has been in operation for 8000 h with the original plasma tube and with no maintenance other than to correct a minor power supply fault.   A schematic of this system is shown in Figure 6-16.   Speeds between 0.75 and 150 m/min are measured by this equipment.   The Doppler effect also forms the basis for a device called a Portable Electronic Traffic Analyzer† which measures speeds between 16 and 130 km/h (10 to 80 mph).   In one mode of operation, the speed of a particular vehicle is held on the meter for $1\frac{1}{2}$ s, so that signals received from other cars are not measured.   Another system,‡ completely portable and weighing 13.3 kg (29 lb), has a speed measurement range of 8 to 160 km/h (5 to 100 mph).

   Other applications of speed measurements using the Doppler effect include the measurement of fluid flow rates, particle flow rates, and the

* Decca Radar, Ltd.
† Marconi Company, Ltd.
‡ Ekco Avionics.

speed of large objects, such as trains and jet-propelled sleds. It is only necessary to receive a reflected or scattered signal from the target of interest.

Ranging and Distance Measurements   Lasers are being used for distance measurements and tracking in such diverse applications as military ranging to testing of the general theory of relativity. Applications such as maintaining distances during airborne refueling operations, critical altitude information (accurate to within centimeters in distances of 100 m or more) during lunar landings and maintaining distances between cars and trucks or trains moving in a common line are being suggested.[22]   The accuracy of geodetic surveys will be greatly improved by use of laser surveying instruments.

In order to use light to measure distances, at least two requirements must be met.   First, the light must be sufficiently intense so that the returned signal is sufficiently strong to be detected.   In this way, signal degradation due to atmospheric propagation loss and multi-angular scattering by the target can be offset.   Second, a means of comparison between the light emitted at the laser and that returned by the target must be selected.

There are several techniques that can be used for laser distance measurements.   One involves measuring the time elapsed between emission of a pulse and the reception of a portion of its diffuse reflection.   Ruby lasers, operating in the Q-switched mode, have been used to generate the pulses, which are typically 30 ns long.   The factor which limits the accuracy of such a system is the value assumed for the velocity of light and the accuracy of elapsed-time measurement.   For example, electronic instrumentation can measure elapsed-time to an accuracy of about 1 ns. With an assumed velocity of 3×10^8 m/s, light travels a distance of about 30 cm, so a range measurement error of about 15 cm can result.   In addition, the speed of light is accurate to about 1 part in 10^5.   Considering these factors, range measurement accuracies of 1 part in 10^3 for distances of several hundred meters to 1 part in 10^5 for distances longer than 160 km (100 miles) are possible.[23]

A second highly accurate method of ranging involves the amplitude modulation of a light beam at a modulation frequency ω_m in the range of 30 MHz.   The phase of the modulation envelope of the returned light is then compared with the phase at the transmitter.   The detection circuit is arranged so that when the optical path from the modulator to the reflector and back is $(\frac{1}{2}M + \frac{1}{4})$ wavelengths of the modulation frequency, a null is obtained.   The distance is obtained by varying ω_m and measuring the values for which the detection circuit gives a null.   By measuring a number of nulls, the ambiguity in the value of the integer M is resolved. Under good atmospheric conditions, it has been estimated that sensitivities of one part in 10^7 over distances of 30 km or more are possible.[24]

6·2 scattering

A number of different scattering effects result from different types of interaction between incident radiation and a scattering system. These effects allow one to use the special properties of laser radiation to obtain specific information about a scattering system. The three particular types of scattering treated in this section are Rayleigh, Brillouin, and Raman.

For our purposes, scattering is defined as a process whereby a physical system extracts energy from a beam of light and re-emits this energy at the same or at a different wavelength, in the same or different directions from the incident beam. There are two general types of scattering: elastic and inelastic. Scattering in which a definite phase relation exists between incoming and scattered waves is called *elastic* or *coherent scattering*. Interference then occurs between waves scattered by two or more scattering centers. Scattering in which the scattering elements act independently so that there are no definite phase relationships between different parts of the scattered beam is termed *inelastic* or *incoherent scattering*. The intensity of the scattered radiation at any point is determined by adding the intensities of the scattered radiation reaching the point from the independent scattering elements.

6·2·1 general concepts of scattering

We have seen in Chapter 2 that the interaction between an applied electric field $\bar{E}$ and a material body results in an induced polarization $\bar{P}$ and is described by a physical parameter called the *polarizability*. In an isotropic material, the expression for the polarizability is given as

$$\alpha_0 = \frac{P}{E} = \sum_k \frac{N_k e^2}{m_k(\omega_{0k}^2 - \omega^2 - i\Gamma_k \omega)} \tag{6-50}$$

where α_0 = scalar polarizability,

N_k = number of particles of type k,
m_k = mass of each particle of type k,
ω_{0k} = resonance frequency for particle type k,
Γ_k = damping term associated with particle of type k,
ω = frequency of the incident radiation.

This expression is derived classically by assuming that the incident electric field causes a displacement of the electron charge cloud with respect to the nuclei, with the nuclei remaining stationary. However, the actual situation is more complex. Any molecule, whether in a liquid, solid, or gas, is constantly undergoing vibration (and/or rotation) due to thermal energy. In crystalline solids, thermal energy causes atoms to vibrate about their mean lattice positions.   These thermally induced vibrations alter the polarizability and cause the polarization to exhibit frequencies other than that of the incident radiation.

Consider, for example, a material medium at a temperature T.   Within the medium, assume atoms are undergoing simple harmonic motion with respect to their center of charge and with respect to their equilibrium lattice positions.   Atomic motion with respect to the center of charge gives rise to a modulation of the polarizability of the individual atoms and hence of the polarizability of the material.   Atomic motion with respect to equilibrium lattice position gives rise to modulation of the dielectric constant of the material due to slight local modulation in density, and also results in a polarizability modulation.

Consider first the periodic modulation of polarizability due to vibration of the atoms or molecules about their charge centers.   The polarizability α can be expressed as

$$\alpha = \alpha_0(1 + b \cos \omega_T t) \tag{6-51}$$

where ω_T is the vibration frequency of the atom and b is a first-order term involving the nuclear position and the rate of change of the polarizability with respect to nuclear position evaluated at the equilibrium nuclear position.   The complete expansion contains higher-order terms, and the reader is referred to Section 2.6.1 for a further discussion of the origin of these terms.   Considering only the first-order terms, the polarization of the medium under the influence of an applied electric field $E = E_0 \cos \omega_E t$ is given as:

$$P = N\alpha E = N\alpha_0 E_0(1 + b \cos \omega_T t) \cos \omega_E t \tag{6-52}$$

or

$$P = N\alpha_0 E_0 \cos \omega_E t + \frac{N\alpha_0 bE_0}{2} [\cos(\omega_E - \omega_T)t + \cos(\omega_E + \omega_T)t] \tag{6-53}$$

The polarization will radiate energy at the frequency of the incident radiation ω_E.   This component is called the *Rayleigh scattered component*. The other two components of scattered light at frequencies $(\omega_E - \omega_T)$ and $(\omega_E + \omega_T)$ are the sum and difference-frequency scattered components. The light at the difference frequency $(\omega_E - \omega_T)$ is called the *Stokes component* of the scattered light and light at the sum frequency $(\omega_E + \omega_T)$ is called the *anti-Stokes component*.

Consider next the lattice vibrations of the medium (acoustic and optical modes).   The vibrations result in a slight modulation of polarizability.   Consequently, scattering occurs with the scattered light shifted in frequency by an amount equal to the frequency of the lattice vibration. Monatomic lattices have only acoustic vibrational modes, whereas diatomic lattices have both an acoustic and an optical vibrational mode.   If scattering is from an acoustic mode, it is called *Brillouin scattering*. If scattering is from an optical mode, it is called *Raman scattering*.

The existence of first-order or higher-order terms for a particular scattering system depends on the values of the coefficients such as *b*. These values in turn depend upon such factors as molecular symmetry and crystallographic point-group symmetry. Again, a brief discussion of these points is given in Chapter 2.

6·2·2   Rayleigh scattering

The previous section described how the scattering of light incident on a material medium could result in scattered beams of frequencies equal to, less than, or greater than, the incident beam frequency. By far the largest amount of scattering occurs at the frequency of the incident beam. In this section the term Rayleigh scattering will be used to denote scattering in which no change in wavelength results, and the object will be to show how information about the presence, size, and density of scattering particles can be obtained.

The salient features of Rayleigh scattering can be derived from (6-50) and (6-52). Since Rayleigh scattered light has the same frequency as the incident light, the effects of polarizability modulation can be disregarded. For simplicity, absorption is also neglected (i.e., set the imaginary term in Equation 6-50 to zero). The polarization for a single atom is then

$$P = \frac{e^2 E}{m(\omega_0^2 - \omega^2)} \tag{6-54}$$

The power per square meter radiated in the direction θ by an accelerating charge is given by[25]

$$S = \frac{e^2 a^2 \sin^2 \theta}{16\pi^2 \varepsilon_0 \, r^2 c^3} \tag{6-55}$$

where a is the acceleration given the oscillating charge by the incident E field and r is the distance from the charge. The expression for a is obtained from (2-81) by taking the second derivative. This yields

$$a = \frac{-e\omega^2 E}{m(\omega_0^2 - \omega^2)} \tag{6-56}$$

Substituting (6-56) into (6-55), we get

$$S = \frac{e^4 \omega^4 E^2 \sin^2 \theta}{16\pi^2 \varepsilon_0 \, r^2 c^3 m^2 (\omega_0^2 - \omega^2)^2} \tag{6-57}$$

Thus, the power per square meter scattered in a particular direction θ, where θ is measured as in Figure 6-17, is inversely proportional to the square

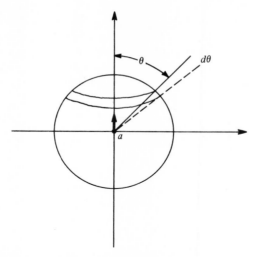

Figure 6-17   Figure showing how θ is measured.   θ is used in expressions to calculate power per square meter radiated in direction θ by an oscillating dipole.[25]   (With permission of Addison-Wesley Publishing Company.)

of the distance from the scattering particle, directly proportional to the intensity (E^2) of the incident radiation, and inversely proportional to the fourth power of the incident radiation wavelength (directly proportional to ω^4).*   In addition, for a fixed point of observation, the power scattered by isotropic scattering systems will depend on the polarization direction of the incident beam, since this determines the direction of oscillation of the dipoles.

The above relationships apply strictly only when the scatterer is much smaller in diameter than the wavelength of light.   For particles whose size is greater than a wavelength, scattering is generally independent of wavelength.   For particles whose size is approximately equal to a wavelength, there is no simple expression for light scattered.   Reference 1 contains a thorough treatment of the Mie theory of scattering of light from spheres of arbitrary size.

Rayleigh Scattering with a Laser Light Source   The high intensity and directionality of laser light can be used to good advantage in Rayleigh light scattering from particles suspended in liquids, gases, or transparent solids.   The CW HeNe and argon-ion lasers are convenient sources.

---

* Scattered power is directly proportional to ω^4 provided $\omega_0^2 \gg \omega^2$.   For bound electrons, this is generally the case, as shown in Section 2.5.4.

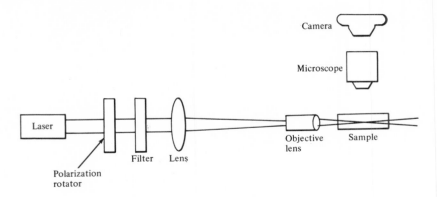

Figure 6-18   Laser ultramicroscope arrangement.

Laser Ultramicroscope   A device called the laser ultramicroscope has been developed to study 90° scattering from imperfections in transparent samples.   The instrument uses a 1 mW HeNe laser, equipped with a polarization rotator which enables adjustment of the polarization to any angle.   The light is focused onto the sample by a lens, and scattered light is observed in a microscope.   A pictorial schematic is shown in Figure 6-18.

Care is taken to obtain maximum contrast by viewing the scattered light against a darkened background and by providing an optically polished exit face on the crystal.   In addition, optically polished faces are required for admitting the beam into the crystal and for viewing the scattered light. An alternative would be to submerge the sample in an index-matching liquid.

Studies have been performed to determine what the theoretical limits of detectability for this instrument are by suspending spherical latex particles in a liquid and photographically recording the scattered light intensity.[26]   For a 1 h exposure with a 1 mW HeNe laser as a source, the theoretical limit of detectability is quoted at 300 Å.   With the use of more powerful lasers (1 W, CW) this theoretical limit can be extended to 100 Å. It should be noted that these figures give only an estimate of the size of the smallest detectable latex particle.   In an actual crystal, the shape and index of refraction of the scattering particle will affect scattered intensities, and hence exposure time will be different.   Nevertheless, such particles can be sized by comparing their scattered light intensity, for a given exposure time, with that of the latex particles.   The size is then given in "equivalent latex diameters" or e.l.d.'s.   Figure 6-19 shows defects in a synthetic ruby crystal that were observed using 90° light scattering in a laser ultramicroscope.   Figure 6-20 shows a commercially available instrument.*

* Tem-Press Research, Inc., State College, Pa.

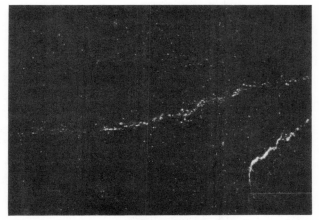

Figure 6-19   Defects in synthetic ruby, recorded on a laser ultra-microscope.   (With permission of Tem-Pres Research, Inc.)

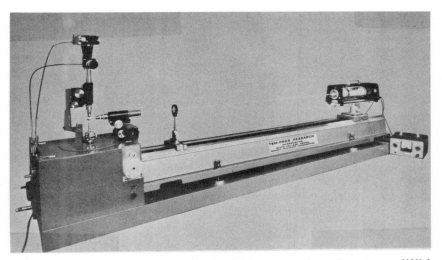

Figure 6-20   Commercially available laser ultramicroscope. (With permission of Tem-Pres Research, Inc.)

Particle Counters   Integrated circuit manufacture requires stringent environmental contamination control with particular attention paid to the number and size of airborne particles in clean rooms.   Commercially available instruments for detecting and sizing such airborne particles by light scattering techniques have been available and in general have proved satisfactory.   However, the air sampling rates are small, in the range of one half of 1 cu ft/min.   A high-volume particle counter that demonstrates high sensitivity at sampling rates 50 to 100 times that of standard monitors has been described.[27]   This instrument, shown schematically

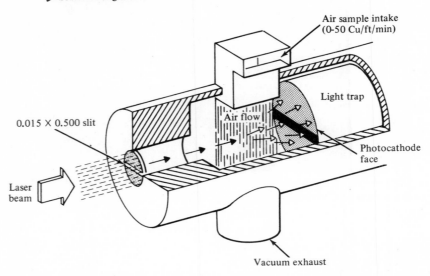

—▶ Primary Laser Beam
—▷ Scattered Light Path

Air sample intake
(0-50 Cu/ft/min)

Light trap

0.015 × 0.500 slit

Air flow

Photocathode
face

Laser
beam

Vacuum exhaust

Figure 6-21   Schematic diagram of Sandia Corporation's high-volume particle counter.[27]

in Figure 6-21, uses a 1 mW HeNe laser as a light source.   It is the laser that permits a large light-sensing zone, which in turn allows the greater sampling flow rates.

The laser emits a 2 mm diameter beam which passes through a spatial filter, beam expanding lens, straightening lens, slit lens, and a series of three slits.   The result is a beam that is 0.015 in. thick and 0.5 in. wide. The beam then passes through a light-sensing zone in which the column of intake air forms the length dimension.   The width of the air column is such that all of the sample air passes through the light beam, thus assuring that particles in the sample air stream will be counted and sized.   Detection of particles as small as 0.3 μm appears to be feasible, and the large sampling rates provide a means for real-time monitoring, i.e., elimination of the long lag in pickup detection and recording, characteristic of low-volume monitors.

6·2·3   Raman scattering

Raman scattering is an inelastic scattering of light which results in a change of frequency of the scattered light.   The energy change per photon is $\Delta E = h(v_s - v_0)$, where v_s is the frequency of the scattered photons and v_0 the frequency of the incident photons.   If the incident photons give net energy to the scattering system, then the scattered photons have lower energy and constitute what are called the *Stokes lines*.   If the scattering system is initially in a high-energy state, it can yield energy to the photon. The scattered photons then have a higher frequency and constitute the *anti-Stokes lines*.   The frequencies of the Stokes and anti-Stokes lines are symmetrically located around the incident photon frequency.   Since in thermal equilibrium the proportion of scattering systems in high-energy states to those in low-energy states follows the Boltzmann distribution, the Stokes lines are generally stronger than the anti-Stokes lines.

Raman scattering studies yield information about the structure of molecules and the effects of molecular rearrangement.   Such information is generally obtained from energy changes corresponding to transitions in the infrared portion of the spectrum.   Although this somewhat duplicates ordinary infrared spectroscopy, both techniques are complimentary in that certain modes of molecular vibration interact only with infrared radiation, whereas other modes are only Raman active.

Before the laser, Raman scattering was generally avoided as a common analytical tool because of the extreme care and long exposure time needed to obtain a photographic record of the Raman shifted lines.   The laser has since changed this.   Using such lasers as CW HeNe, typically operating at 50 mW, or argon-ion, operating at 1 W or more power output, the researcher can work in the visible portion of the spectrum where sensitive detectors and relatively large S/N ratios are readily obtainable.   The great increase in intensity of incident radiation afforded by the laser over such conventional sources as the mercury arc results in a corresponding increase in the intensity of Raman scattered lines.   The inherent collimation of the laser beam, the narrow spectral output, and the availability of a multitude of different lines all make the laser a very suitable source for Raman studies.

Models for Raman Scattering   Consider first a quantum system which can have only discrete energy states, such as a molecule or an atom. Any molecule, whether in a solid, a liquid, or gas, is constantly undergoing vibration and rotation due to thermal energy.   According to quantum mechanics, the vibrational and rotational energies of these molecules are quantized and can take on only discrete values.   The energy differences between the quantized states of vibration or rotation generally correspond to photon energies in the infrared portion of the spectrum.   A molecule can be induced to undergo a transition from a lower to a higher vibrational or rotational energy state by extracting energy from an incident photon. Regardless of the frequency of the incident light, the frequency shifts caused by a particular quantum system are always the same.   Since the incident photon loses energy, this process gives rise to the Stokes line.   With any quantum system, there will always be a certain number of members in an excited energy state.   The populations are generally exceedingly small compared to the ground-state population. Nevertheless, these higher energy molecules can be induced to undergo a transition to a lower energy state by a passing photon. The photon gains this energy and this process gives rise to the anti-Stokes lines. Each type of molecule has a characteristic Raman spectrum which serves as a fingerprint for identification.

Chapter 2 describes from a more theoretical viewpoint the origins of Raman scattering from the optical vibrational modes of diatomic crystals. Scattering arises because an optical vibrational mode propagating in a crystal will alter the polarizability of the material as described in Section 6.2.1. When a light beam interacts with these vibrational modes, the resulting polarization will radiate at ω_E and at $(\omega_E - \omega_p)$ and $(\omega_E + \omega_p)$, where ω_E is the incident light frequency and ω_p the optical phonon frequency.

Stimulated Raman Scattering   In Raman scattering processes, light is scattered randomly in all directions by each scattering molecule or unit cell. Scattering efficiencies are very low, a typical number being 10^{-6} scattered photons for each incident photon. Under certain conditions, however, a stimulated Raman effect occurs. The stimulated effect differs from the normal Raman effect in that (1) it is threshold dependent; (2) the Stokes line is coherent and highly directional; (3) conversion efficiencies in the range of 30 percent are obtainable. In stimulated Raman scattering, the presence of a particular Stokes mode influences neighboring molecules to break into oscillation in the same mode so that there exists in effect a gain mechanism at the Raman frequency. Depending upon the input radiation, the stimulated effect provides a means for obtaining coherent signals over a number of wavelengths from infrared to visible.

Raman Systems   In order to perform Raman scattering studies, a system of specialized components is needed. First, the light source should be considered. The most common nonlaser source for Raman spectroscopy is the so-called Toronto light source—a low-pressure mercury arc source. It has been estimated that under normal operating conditions as many as 50 W is radiated in the 435.8 nm line which is frequently used for Raman studies.[28]   However, not more than about 1 W of this power can be collected in the collimated beam and made available for Raman excitation. Further, since the intensities of the emitted radiation are subject to variation, it is difficult to measure intensities and intensity ratios. In contrast to this, a laser source has its energy contained in a highly directional narrow beam that can easily be manipulated. Intensity can be well controlled so that absolute intensity measurements can be made with confidence.

The intensity of Raman scattered light was stated previously as being very low. However, some optimization can be achieved by proper wavelength selection. This is due to the fact that the scattering efficiency increases as the fourth power of the frequency of the incident light. Thus, purely from incident beam wavelength considerations, an argon-ion laser would provide better scattering efficiency than a HeNe laser.

The sample is generally mounted in a special cell specifically designed for gas, liquid, or solid samples. Provisions for sample cooling can be incorporated into these cells if desired. Light from the source is focused onto the sample with a lens. Light scattered by the sample at 90°, both Raman and Rayleigh components, are then collected by a lens and focused onto the slit of a monochromator.

The monochromator is the single most important part of the system, since it enables the separation and detection of the Raman scattered components from the more intense Rayleigh scattered components. Precision Raman equipment uses a double monochromator, Figure 6-22, in which light undergoes diffraction from two separate gratings to provide a somewhat optimized wavelength discrimination capability. Once this wavelength selection has taken place, the problem of detecting the weak Raman scattered lines must be considered.

Detection is usually accomplished by using a photon-counting system, which essentially is a high gain photomultiplier tube, or by a lock-in detection system (synchronous detection) in which the exciting laser line is modulated at a frequency at which the noise level of the photomultiplier tube has small amplitude. For very low light levels, photon counting is superior.

Applications   To date, Raman scattering has been used primarily as a laboratory instrument for studies of molecular vibrations and chemical identifications. However, prospects for introducing it as a tool for industrial applications are gradually appearing. Of particular interest is

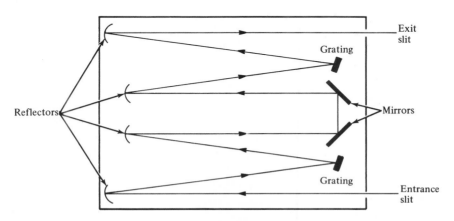

Figure 6-22   Schematic diagram of a double monochromator typical of those used in Raman systems.

the application of Raman scattering to air-pollution monitoring.[29]   In this technique, a laser beam is directed to a sample volume of air, which can be as far away as 1 mile.   Some light scattered from the molecular constituents within the laser-irradiated sample undergoes a Raman frequency shift that is characteristic of the Raman-active molecules in the sample.   The Raman-scattered light is collected by a telescope whose field of view is collinear with the laser beam and then enters a double monochromator, where the spectral content of the radiation is analyzed. A number of lines will be recorded, each shifted in frequency from the frequency of the incident laser beam by an amount characteristic of the scattering substance.   Figure 6-23 shows the Raman spectrum of a sample volume containing sulfur dioxide.   Incident upon this volume was a 337.1 nm beam from an N_2 laser giving a 1 W average power output.   A peak in the scattered spectrum occurs at about 350.8 nm. The wavelength shift from 337.1 nm to 350.8 nm is due solely to the presence of SO_2.   Shifts of this nature occur for other types of pollutants present in the sample volume, the magnitude of each shift characteristic of each individual pollutant.   Among some of the pollutants detected in various sample volumes are carbon tetrachloride, benzene, ammonia, carbon dioxide, methane, hydrogen sulfide, and methanol.

Figure 6-24 shows a schematic of the system.   Accuracy of a few parts-per-million concentration at distances up to 1 mile can be quoted with this technique.

A number of factors must be kept in mind if an optimum system is to be constructed for Raman scattering applications.   For example, the λ^{-4} dependence of the Raman scattered intensity was discussed above.   However, wavelength selection should also take into account the wavelength region in which the detector has the greatest quantum efficiency.   Atmospheric absorption bands will also influence the choice of a particular laser.

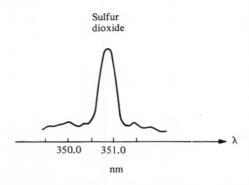

Sulfur
dioxide

350.0   351.0

nm

Figure 6-23   Raman spectrum of a sample volume containing SO_2.[29] (**With permission of** Proceedings of the 1969 Electro-Optical Systems Design Conference, p. 425.   Copyright © 1969 by Industrial & Scientific Conference Management, Inc.)

LASER REMOTE RAMAN SPECTROGRAPH

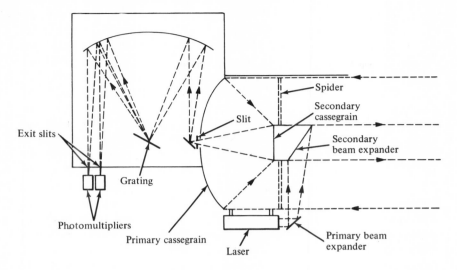

Figure 6-24   Schematic diagram of a remote Raman system for monitoring air pollutants.[29]   *With permission of* **Proceedings of the 1969 Electro-Optical Systems Design Conference.** *Copyright © 1969 by Industrial & Scientific Conference Management, Inc.*)

Some current research is being performed on the use of Raman scattering to obtain carrier concentrations in semiconductor material.[30] Using argon- and krypton-ion lasers, with emission frequencies near the band gap of CdS, a relationship was obtained between carrier concentration and observed frequency shifts of the incident light.   The frequency shifts were due to Raman scattering from coupling excitations between phonons and the plasma of free carriers (these coupling excitations are usually termed plasmons).

6·2·4   Brillouin scattering

Brillouin scattering is the scattering of light resulting from the interaction between acoustic waves and light waves.   The acoustic waves usually range from 10^6 to as high as 10^{12} Hz and can be externally introduced into a material medium, can be already present in the material in the form of thermally activated phonons, or can be stimulated in the medium by the light beam itself (stimulated Brillouin scattering).   Although the term Brillouin scattering has been applied to denote the interaction of sound waves and electromagnetic waves, in general, we will reserve the term Brillouin scattering to denote scattering from acoustic phonon modes.

Scattering from an externally introduced acoustic column will be described as Debye-Sears and Bragg scattering.

Applications that take advantage of acousto-optic interactions of the Brillouin, Debye-Sears, or Bragg type are appearing. For instance, using the acousto-optic interaction, it is possible to phase and amplitude modulate a light beam, change its frequency and direction, Q-switch a laser, and obtain information about thermal vibration (phonon) modes in solids.

The laser is the best available light source for acoustic scattering studies because of its coherence properties. Use of conventional sources is unsatisfactory because their spectral width makes it difficult to resolve Brillouin scattered components and to determine the spectral line widths of these Brillouin components.

<u>Models for Acoustic Scattering</u> In order to describe how the interaction between an electromagnetic wave and an acoustic wave in a solid arises, we will take the example of Bragg scattering from a column of coherent acoustic waves. The traveling acoustic column, with wave vector $\mathbf{k}_s$, is introduced externally by coupling a high-frequency acoustic source to the solid by means of a piezoelectric transducer. Once in the material, the acoustic wave sets up alternating regions of compression and dilatation. These regions of compression and dilatation present small alternating changes in the refractive index to a light beam and act basically as a moving diffraction gration. In Figure 6-25, a beam of light of wavelength λ_1 is incident from the left at an angle θ. Since regions of lattice compression and dilatation have different optical constants, light is reflected from each compression peak and interferes constructively only if the optical path difference for each reflection is an integral number of wavelengths. This condition is identical to the familiar Bragg condition for reflection of X-rays from the planes of a crystal lattice. However, since the acoustic wave is moving, the scattered wave will also undergo a Doppler shift.

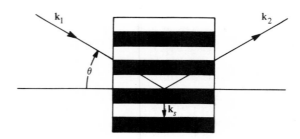

Figure 6-25   Bragg scattering of light.

The Bragg condition

$$2\lambda_s \sin \theta = n\lambda_1 \qquad (6\text{-}58)$$

indicates that if λ_1 and λ_s are fixed, considerable reflection will occur only for values of θ close to the Bragg angle. Alternatively, if θ and λ_1 are fixed, only certain acoustic wavelengths will reflect to any great extent. The Doppler shift can be shown to be

$$\Delta\omega = \omega_1 - \omega_s = 2\omega_1 v_s \frac{n}{c} \sin \theta \qquad (6\text{-}59)$$

where v_s is the velocity of the acoustic wave in the material, and c/n is the velocity of light in the medium. Using (6-58) and (6-59) we can show that if θ is the Bragg angle, the frequency of the scattered wave is just equal to the frequency difference between the incident optical wave and the receding acoustic wave.

The Debye-Sears effect, Figure 6-26, results when a plane wave is incident upon an acoustic column moving across the beam. As the beam enters the column, it sees an index of refraction that varies sinusoidally as the acoustic signal. This varying index varies the time taken by the beam to traverse the column and hence the beam emerging from the column is phase modulated. One can write the mathematical expression for the emerging beam as[31]

$$E = E_0 \sin(\omega_1 t + B \sin \omega_s t) \qquad (6\text{-}60)$$

where $B \sin \omega_s t$ is the sinusoidal phase variation due to the acoustic wave. This signal can be expanded to the form

$$E = E_0 J_0(B)\sin \omega_1 t$$

$$+ J_1(B)[\sin(\omega_1 + \omega_s)t + \sin(\omega_1 - \omega_s)t]$$

$$+ J_2(B)[\sin(\omega_1 + 2\omega_s)t + \sin(\omega_1 - 2\omega_s)t] + \cdots \qquad (6\text{-}61)$$

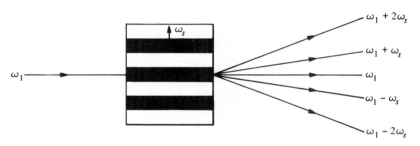

Figure 6-26   Debye-Sears effect.

where the J_n are Bessel functions. There result sidebands, spaced in frequency from the carrier frequency by integral multiples of the acoustic frequency ω_s. The directions into which the sidebands radiate are given by[32]

$$\theta = \frac{N\lambda_1}{\lambda_s} \tag{6-62}$$

where θ is the angle between the direction of propagation of the Nth sideband and the carrier, and λ_1 and λ_s the light and acoustic wavelength, respectively.

Stimulated Brillouin Scattering   Use of the laser as a light source has resulted in a stimulated effect. If the incident beam is an intense beam of frequency ω_1, a coherent acoustic wave of frequency ω_s is produced within the material while simultaneously a scattered optical beam of frequency $\omega_1 - \omega_s$ is generated.[33] For stimulated Brillouin scattering to occur, the input energy of the beam must be above a well-defined threshold. It must be sufficiently intense so that an induced electrostrictive pressure wave is built up within the solid. Thus, low-power lasers such as the HeNe would not produce this effect, but a giant pulse ruby laser would. In the original experiment, a giant pulse ruby laser giving about 50 MW during a 30 ns interval was used.

Applications   Applications of light-sound interactions generally make use of Bragg or Debye-Sears effects for laser beam deflection and modulation. For example, a laser can be acoustically Q-switched by introducing a Bragg-scattering cell within the cavity (Figure 6-27). Sufficient power is applied to scatter the beam acoustically and prevent laser oscillations. During that period, the laser medium is pumped until a desired level of population inversion is achieved. Once this level is achieved, the acoustic signal is removed and gain is restored in the time

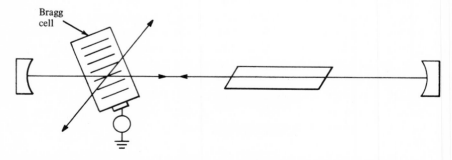

Figure 6-27 Acoustical Q-switching by insertion of a Bragg cell within the laser cavity.

it takes the acoustic wave to travel from the transducer to the far side of the laser beam. Within a few hundred nanoseconds the gain is restored and the energy is "dumped" in a short high-energy pulse.

In order to achieve efficient acousto-optic Q-switching, there are a number of factors that must be considered. For example, a practical situation might require the Q-switching of a Nd : YAG laser. To do this, an acousto-optic modulator that provides sufficient diffraction efficiency and a high transmittance at the laser wavelength must be selected. For Bragg scattering, the diffraction efficiency is defined as the ratio of scattered light to incident light and is given by

$$\frac{I_s}{I_1} \simeq \sin^2 \sqrt{\eta} \qquad (6\text{-}63)$$

The parameter η is given by

$$\eta = \frac{\pi^2}{2} \frac{n^6 p^2}{\rho v_s^3} \frac{1}{\lambda_1^2} \frac{W}{H} P_a \qquad (6\text{-}64)$$

where ρ is the modulator density, p is the appropriate elasto-optic coefficient, v_s is the acoustic velocity, n the index of refraction, λ_1 the laser wavelength, W the width of the acoustic wave, H the height of the acoustic wave, and P_a the acoustic power. H is selected to be at least twice the diameter of the light beam, and W is chosen so that the diffraction angles of both light and sound are approximately equal, or

$$\frac{\lambda_s}{W} \simeq \frac{\lambda_1}{D} \qquad (6\text{-}65)$$

where D is the light beam diameter at the acoustic column.

Next, one must consider how much of the cavity radiation it is desired to deflect. Sufficient acoustic power, P_a, must be applied so that the single-pass gain of the cavity is overcome and the medium does not lase. For $\eta \simeq 1$, about 70 percent diffraction efficiency is obtained. This is more than sufficient to keep the optical energy within the cavity essentially at zero. (A 10 percent diffraction efficiency is considered large enough to block laser action in a Nd : YAG.) Once laser action is prevented, a large population inversion is built up in a time approximating the relaxation time of the upper level, which for Nd : YAG is about 230 μs. The acoustic drive signal is removed either by a train of pulses with the desired repetition rate, or, for a single-laser pulse, by a manually keyed pulse. Removal of the acoustic drive signal restores the high Q of the cavity and a short (about 300 ns) high-energy pulse is emitted from the laser.

Because of the large amount of power in the Nd : YAG cavity, fused quartz is generally selected as the acousto-optic material. Quartz has a relatively high acoustic loss, so that fairly large amounts of RF power are needed to drive the modulator. Such units are commercially available, with typical specifications as below.

Wavelength	1060 nm
Cell transmission	99.5 percent
Beam diameter	Up to 5 mm
Q-spoiled light loss	>45 percent round trip
Acoustic drive frequency	50 MHz
Electrical power	50 W
Size (including mechanical enclosure)	2½ in. by 2¾ in. by 2¾ in.

A second, quite different application of Bragg scattering is the generation of two-dimensional arrays, for example, in TV display systems.[35] Such a system makes use of two Bragg cells, one for horizontal and one for vertical deflection. The direction of the Bragg-scattered beam will vary as the frequencies of the applied acoustic waves vary. This can be seen by writing the Bragg equation for small deflection angles so that $\sin \theta \simeq \theta$. Then

$$2\theta = \frac{\lambda_1}{\lambda_s} = \frac{\lambda_1 v_s}{v_s} \tag{6-66}$$

where v_s is the velocity of the sound wave in the medium and v_s is the acoustic frequency. By varying v_s, one can vary θ:

$$2\Delta\theta = \frac{\lambda_1}{v_s} \Delta v_s \tag{6-67}$$

The capacity of the system, defined as the total number of positions in the array, can be obtained by dividing the total swing of deflection angle, $2\Delta\theta$, by the spot size of the laser beam at the plane of the array. The spot size is determined by diffraction effects. The minimum diffraction spread of a light beam of diameter D is $\alpha \simeq \lambda_1/D$. Hence capacity C is given as

$$C \simeq \frac{\Delta v_s}{v_s} \alpha \tag{6-68}$$

It should be evident that if the frequency changes of the acoustic signal are large, then the Bragg condition will not be satisfied. There are a number of techniques available such as changing the acoustic beam direction as a function of frequency, so that the Bragg condition is maintained. The efficiency of such a system is dependent upon the material supporting the acoustic wave. Materials with high indices of refraction are best. Readers interested in pursuing this entire topic further should consult Refs. 32 and 35.

The Debye-Sears effect can be used for intensity modulation of a light beam. As shown in Figure 6-28, an acoustic column traveling through a liquid will diffract some of the incident light past the stop. The intensity of the optical output signal is thus a function of the acoustic

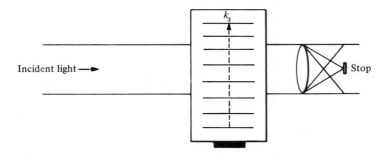

Figure 6-28   Intensity modulation of a light beam by an acoustic signal.

power.   Equation (6-62) shows that the angle at which the diffracted side-bands diverge is a function of the acoustic frequency.   If several acoustic frequencies are simultaneously present, each frequency will produce its own effect.   This principle has been used to describe an instantaneous spectrum analyzer.[36]

References

1. M. Born and E. Wolf, *Principles of Optics*, Rev. Ed. 4th Ed., Pergamon Press, Inc., New York, Chapter 1 (1970).
2. F. A. Jenkins and H. E. White, *Fundamentals of Optics*, 3rd Ed., McGraw-Hill Book Co., New York (1957).
3. J. R. Partington, *An Advanced Treatise on Physical Chemistry*, Vol. 4, p. 507, John Wiley and Sons, Inc. (1954).
4. T. S. Moss, *Optical Properties of Semiconductors*, Academic Press Inc. (1959).
5. J. L. Moll, *Physics of Semiconductors*, McGraw-Hill Book Co., New York (1964).
6. W. R. Beam, *Electronics of Solids*, McGraw-Hill Book Co., New York (1965).
7. F. L. McCrackin *et al.*, "Measurement of the Thickness and Refractive Index of Very Thin Films and the Optical Properties of Surfaces by Ellipsometry," *J. Res., NBS* **67A**, No. 4 (July–August 1963).
8. W. G. Oldham, "Ellipsometry Using a Retardation Plate as Compensator," *J. Opt. Soc. Amer.* **57**, No. 5, 617–624 (May 1967).
9. D. A. Holmes and D. L. Feucht, "Formulas for Using Wave Plates in Ellipsometry," *J. Opt. Soc. Amer.* **57**, No. 4, 466–472 (April 1967).
10. T. Yolken *et al.*, "Ellipsometric Errors Due to Multiple Reflections in Mica Quarter-Wave Plates," *J. Opt. Soc. Amer.* **57**, No. 2, 283–284 (February 1967).
11. R. J. Archer, *Ellipsometry*, Gaertner Scientific Corporation, Chicago, Ill. (1968).
12. F. L. McCrackin, "A FORTRAN Program for the Analysis of Ellipsometer Measurements," *NBS Technical Note 479* (April 1969).

13. A. R. Hilton and C. E. Jones, "Measurement of Epitaxial Film Thickness Using an Infrared Ellipsometer," *J. Electrochem. Soc.* **113**, No. 5, 472–478 (May 1966).

14. W. G. Spitzer and M. J. Tannenbaum, "Interference Method for Measuring the Thickness of Epitaxially Grown Films," *J. Appl. Phys.* **32**, 744 (1961).

15. G. R. Bird and M. Parrish, "The Wire Grid as a Near-Infrared Polarizer," *J. Opt. Soc. Amer.* **50**, No. 9, 886–891 (September 1960).

16. J. Tauc, Ed., *The Optical Properties of Solids*, Academic Press Inc., New York (1966).

17. D. Gupta, "Non-Destructive Determination of Carrier Concentration in Epitaxial Silicon Using a Total Internal Reflection Technique," *Solid-State Electronics* **13**, 543–552 (1970).

18. D. F. Munro and J. D. Cuthbert, "Surface Topography Diagnostics Using Scanned Focused Laser Beams in the Manufacture of Hybrid Integrated Circuits," *Proc. Electro-Optical Systems Design Conference*, 71/WEST, May 18–20, Anaheim, Calif. (1971).

19. B. Rossi, *Optics*, Addison-Wesley Publishing Co. (1965).

20. O. E. DeLange, "Optical Heterodyne Detection," *IEEE Spectrum* **5**, No. 10, 77–85 (October 1968).

21. B. Cooper, "Speed Sensing can be Fast and Accurate," "Principles of the Decca Laser Doppler System," *The Engineer*, pp. 22–25 (April 23, 1970).

22. J. Vollmer, "Applied Lasers," *IEEE Spectrum*, **4**, No. 6, 66–70 (June 1967).

23. H. A. Elion, *Laser Systems and Applications*, Pergamon Press, Inc., New York (1967).

24. P. L. Bender, "Laser Measurements of Long Distances," *Proc. IEEE* **55**, 1039 (1967).

25. R. P. Feynman *et al.*, *Lectures on Physics*, Vol. 1, Chapter 32, Addison-Wesley Publishing Co., Reading, Mass. (1965).

26. V. Vand *et al.*, "The Laser as a Light Source of Ultramicroscopy and Light Scattering by Imperfections in Crystals. Investigation of Imperfections in LiF, MgO and Ruby," *J. Appl. Phys.* **37**, 2551 (1966).

27. W. E. Nietzel, "A High-Volume, Real Time Aerosol Monitor," SC-DR-69-56 (June 1969).

28. H. A. Syzmansky, *Raman Spectroscopy*, Plenum Press, New York (1967).

29. T. Hirschfeld *et al.*, *Proc. Tech. Prog.*, *Electro-Optical Systems Design Conference*, New York (1969).

30. J. F. Scott *et al.*, "Light Scattering from Plasmas and Simple-Particle Excitations in Cadmium Sulfide Near Resonance," *Phys. Rev. B.* **1**, 4330 (1970).

31. A. Hund, *Frequency Modulation*, p. 350, McGraw-Hill Book Co., New York (1942).

32. R. Adler, "Interaction Between Light and Sound," *IEEE Spectrum* **4**, No. 5, 42–54 (May 1967).

33. R. Y. Chiao *et al.*, "Stimulated Brillouin Scattering and Coherent Generation of Intense Hypersonic Waves," *Phys. Rev. Lett.* **12**, 592 (1964).

34. A. Korpel *et al.*, "A Television Display Using Acoustic Deflection and Modulation of Coherent Light," *Proc. IEEE* **54**, 1429–1439 (October 1966).

35. E. I. Gordon, "A Review of Acousto-Optical Deflection and Modulation Devices," *Proc. IEEE* **54**, 1391–1401 (October 1966).

36. L. B. Lambert, "Wide Band Instantaneous Spectrum Analyzers Employing Delay-Line Light Modulators," *1962 IRE International Convention Record*, Pt. 6, pp. 69–98.

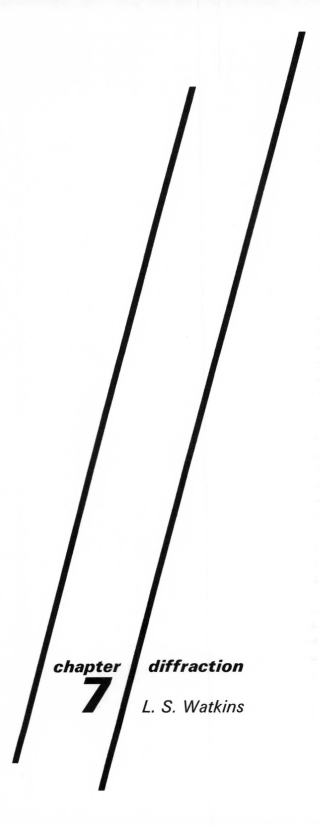

chapter
7

diffraction

L. S. Watkins

7·0 introduction

The term diffraction may conveniently be defined[1] as "any deviation of light rays from rectilinear paths which cannot be interpreted as either reflection or refraction." Thus, the lack of very well-defined borders between shadow and light regions when the pattern of light is observed on a screen through an aperture, as illustrated in Figure 7-1, is such a phenomenon, and it is attributable to the wave nature of light. The field of geometric optics is incapable of explaining these diffraction phenomena, and a satisfactory explanation requires the use of techniques from the realm of physical optics, where the wave nature of light is taken into account.

Although diffraction effects have been observed and studied for many years, their applications in optics for measurement purposes have until recently been limited in scope. The limitation was imposed primarily as a result of the absence of an adequate source of spatially coherent light. Before the advent of the laser, the only available source of spatially coherent light consisted of a high-intensity lamp whose radiation was passed through a very small pinhole. Under such an operation, the spatial coherence is improved by reducing the pinhole size, ideally to the size of a wavelength of the radiation. Such an increase in spatial coherence is achieved only at the expense of intensity, and, since the emission from a blackbody source is limited by its temperature, good spatial coherence could only be achieved at very low intensities. Thus, only patterns of low intensity and small complexity could be obtained, and good diffraction patterns were restricted to small objects.

The laser with its inherent spatial coherence and high intensity permits the observation of much more complex diffraction phenomena with greater accuracy, and diffraction patterns from objects as large as the laser beam are readily obtained. The higher intensity of the spatially coherent laser facilitates the detection procedure, and the temporal coherence allows more complicated operations and measurement to be performed on the phase of the observed pattern, as well as its amplitude.

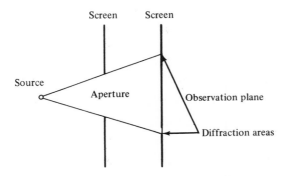

Figure 7-1   Observing diffraction of light.

367

The laser, with its spatial coherence and small divergence, has thus brought about rapid development of new techniques and applications in areas ranging from alignment, to pattern recognition and optical signal processing. Although diffraction phenomena and applications constitute the major part of this chapter, other applications which rely on the spatial coherence of the laser are also discussed.

7·1   alignment, surveying, and geodetic systems

Before proceeding to explore in detail diffraction phenomena and measurement techniques utilizing these effects and the spatially coherent laser as the source, we wish to examine briefly the simplest application of a spatially coherent collimated* laser beam, namely, that as an alignment and surveying tool.

7·1·1   alignment telescopes

General alignment instruments have been developed,[2] are commercially available, and find use, especially in the aerospace industry.   They are simpler and easier to use than an autocollimator, and require only one person to operate since they feature a passive reference (laser) and an active target (detector) rather than the active reference and passive target of conventional autocollimator and alignment telescope.

Alignment tools usually employ a low-power HeNe laser operating in the lowest order transverse mode (TEM_{00}) at 632.8 nm.   The beam is expanded and collimated to a relatively large diameter (e.g., 10 mm or even more) with the use of diffraction limited lenses.†   The laser and expander are mounted in a rugged housing with alignment screws for beam alignment.   Since the beam direction is critical, the stability of the laser resonator is important, and the cavity and housing must be designed in such a way that the beam does not wander.   Achieving such stability may require a long warm-up period lasting up to an hour.   However, the presence of the beam expander is helpful, since it reduces the wander angle in direct proportion to the magnification.   Thus, a requirement of 10^{-6} rad directional stability translates into a 10^{-5} rad stability for the laser using a 10:1 beam expander.

The beam may be displayed on a diffusing surface and visually examined where low resolution alignment is sufficient.   However, a more

---

* See Section 1.5.2 and 3.1.1 and Glossary for discussions on spatial coherence, beam expanders, and collimator.
† See the Glossary for a definition of diffraction limited lens.

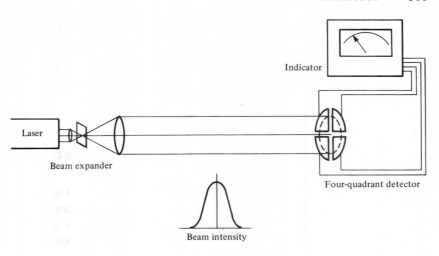

Figure 7-2   Alignment system employing four-quadrant detector.

accurate and reliable operation uses a quadrant detector arrangement, as shown in Figure 7-2.   Any misalignment would vary the amount of light falling on each quadrant, thereby giving an indication of misalignment. The indicator shows when the spot is misaligned in both the vertical and horizontal directions, and the meters are scaled to indicate the amount of lateral displacement of the detector.   Since the beam intensity profile is Gaussian, the detector will still indicate the center of the beam even though the beam has diverged to a diameter larger than the detector.

Accuracies claimed for these instruments range up to 10^{-6} rad (0.8 μm/m) at large distances.   At large distances the accuracy is limited by the laser beam wander and atmospheric turbulence, whereas at short distances, the accuracy is limited by the lateral resolution of the detector which is approximately 25 μm.   An illustration of an actual shop setup of an alignment laser is given in Figure 7-3.

Table 7-1 lists the typical specifications for an alignment laser.

TABLE 7-1   Typical Specifications for an Alignment Laser

Power output TEM_{00} Mode	1 mW at 632.8 nm
Output beam diameter	10 mm
Beam divergence	0.2 mrad
Beam concentricity	0.025 mm
Beam alignment	10 arc s
Beam stability	0.0002 in. $+$ 0.2 arc s/°C/h

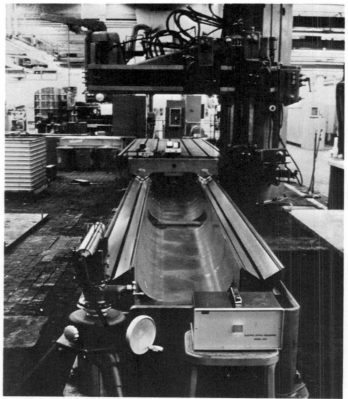

Figure 7-3   Measurement setup for the determination of straightness of travel of a Rockford planing machine. (Courtesy Grumman Aircraft Engineering Corporation with permission of Electro Optics Associates.)

7·1·2   accelerator alignment system

A much more sophisticated alignment system[3] than the one described above is used in the Stanford Linear Accelerator to measure a misalignment of 10^{-7} rad or greater.   To achieve such accuracies, the laser beam is diverged by a lens, creating a virtual point source as shown in Figure 7-4, and is imaged onto a detector using a Fresnel lens.*   The alignment line is that between the laser and the detector, and the various parts of the accelerator (to which the Fresnel lenses are attached) are aligned to image the point source onto the detector.   The Fresnel lenses are retractable, and the alignment is made with one lens at a time.   To achieve the accuracy of 10^{-7} rad, it is necessary to enclose the laser beam path and partially evacuate it, thus reducing air turbulence.

* See Glossary for a description of a Fresnel lens.

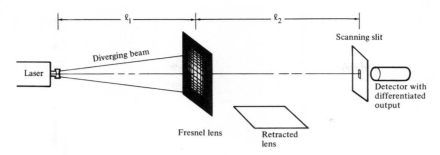

Figure 7-4 Stanford accelerator alignment system.

As can be seen from the diagram, the present alignment system differs considerably from the previous one. In the first system, elements (detectors) are aligned to an optical line generated by one point. In the second system elements (Fresnel lenses) are aligned to an optical line defined by two points. The accuracy depends on the resolution of the lenses and the detector. If the detector (and lens) can resolve the position of the image on the scanning slit to an accuracy of Δs, then by using geometric optics the positional accuracy of the lens ΔP is given by

$$\Delta P = \frac{\ell_1}{\ell_2} \Delta s \tag{7-1}$$

where Δs is the width of the scanning slit, and ℓ_1 and ℓ_2 are the distances between the lens and the laser and detector, respectively.

7·1·3 surveying and geodetic systems

The small divergence of the laser beam suggests several additional applications similar in origin to alignment, and indeed uses of lasers in surveying and geodetic applications in such tools as plummets and levels have been reported.[4]

Schematic diagrams of two different laser plummets designs are shown in Figure 7-5. In the one in part (a) dubbed a laser optical plummet, the laser light reflected from the mercury pool is made to coincide with the light reflected from the mirror with the use of an autocollimator. Accuracy obtained by this device is of the order of 0.5 arc s. In the plummet depicted in part (b), a plate possessing a circular slit is photoelectrically positioned in the center of the laser beam. The laser light projected on this plate is diffracted, and the pattern (which is schematically illustrated by the rings in the figure) is reflected from the mercury bath back toward another photodetector system at the bottom of the plate. The laser is

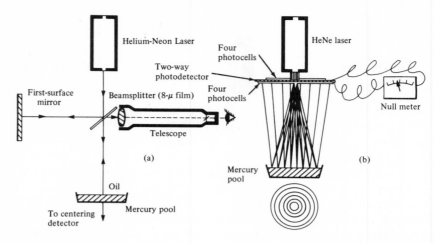

adjusted so that both incident and reflected lights are centered on the plate. The accuracy obtained by this plummet is somewhat higher (0.2 arc s).

Laser levels measuring differences in elevation between two points separated by 1 to 100 m and possessing accuracies of 0.1 mm have also been developed.   Reflection from a mirror floating in a mercury pool may be used as a reference horizontal beam, and the laser is usually placed about halfway between the points whose difference in elevation is desired.

7·2 far-field diffraction effects

When an obstacle or aperture is placed within the cross section of a beam of light and the transmitted light is observed on a screen, the resulting distribution of light is called a *diffraction pattern*.   If both source and observation screen are at a finite distance from the diffracting obstacle, the pattern is termed *Fresnel diffraction pattern*.   If, on the other hand, the observation screen is placed very far from the obstacle, the pattern is called *Fraunhofer diffraction pattern*.   The Fraunhofer diffraction pattern may also be observed by placing a lens immediately behind the diffracting object and observing the pattern on a screen at the focal plane of the lens, and this approach is the one most commonly followed in practice.   Both diffractions are manifestations of the same basic principle, originally formulated by Huygen and now carrying his name, which states that the propagation of light from a given wavefront may be obtained by viewing each element of the wavefront as a source of the secondary spherical disturbance, and the wavefront at any later instant of time may be found by constructing the envelope of the secondary wavelets. Such a construction is illustrated in Figure 7-6. The construction depicted in Figure 7-6 suffers from one major drawback in that it yields an equally strong backward traveling wave in the reverse direction to the actual direction of propagation. This backward wave which physically does not exist resulted from the tacit assumption that the secondary wavelets had uniform amplitudes in all directions. This assumption has to be modified, and in order to take account of the variation in the amplitudes of the secondary wavelets with direction, an obliquity factor in the form of $1 + \cos \theta$ (where θ is given in Figure 7-6) is introduced into the amplitude of the wavelets. This factor ensures a maximum amplitude in the forward direction, and a vanishing of the backward traveling wave.

A mathematical formulation of Huygen's principle will be the backbone of our analysis throughout the chapter. However, it should be noted that such an analysis suffers from one major simplification, namely, the light is treated as a scalar phenomenon and only the scalar amplitude of one transverse component of either the electric or the magnetic field is considered. This treatment tacitly assumes that other components of the field can be similarly treated in independent fashion. This approach thus neglects the obvious fact that the various electromagnetic field vectors are coupled through Maxwell's equations (see Chapter 2) and cannot be regarded as independent quantities. However, under circumstances where the diffracting object (aperture or obstacle) is large compared to a wavelength, and where the observed field is not too close to the diffracting object, the scalar formulation does result in a very good approximation.

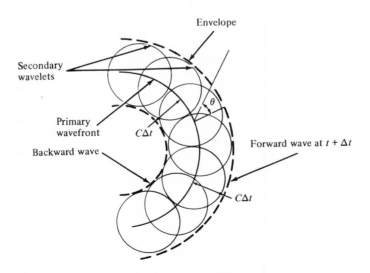

Figure 7-6   Huygen's envelope construction.

7·2·1 *Fresnel zones*

To gain further insight into the wave nature of light, Huygen's principle will be employed to examine qualitatively the behavior of light when obstructed by various opaque objects.   A more quantitative analysis must await the rigorous mathematical presentation of the principles, which is given in Section 7.2.3.

Perhaps the simplest case where Huygen's principle may be used to compute the light amplitude at a particular point in space consists of a monochromatic spherical wave diverging from a point source O (see Figure 7-7) and whose effect at the observation point P is to be ascertained. The source of secondary waves in this case is a spherical wave of radius r', which is smaller than the separation between the source and observation points, and the elemental areas dS on this spherical surface give rise to the secondary wavelets.   The sum total of the contributions from the entire closed surface constitute the light amplitude at the observation point.   If r is the distance between the secondary source dS and the observation point P, the time it takes light to transverse that distance is given by r/c (c is the velocity of light), so that the relative phases of the secondary waves is given by $2\pi r/\lambda$, where λ is the wavelength of the wave.

The relative amplitudes of the secondary waves are harder to compute since they depend on three factors: (1) they are proportional to the infinitesimal area dS, (2) they are inversely proportional to r, and (3) they depend on the angle θ through the obliquity factor $1 + \cos\theta$.   In this particular case, the secondary waves from all elements of areas dS except those in a small region around P' mutually destroy each other by interference at P so that the net effect is identical to that of light traveling in a straight line from the source to the observation point.

If an obstacle such as an opaque screen is now inserted between the source and the observation point as illustrated in Figure 7-8, the possibility of mutual cancellation of secondary waves amplitudes at P is removed, and

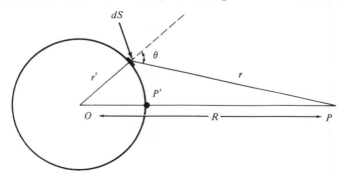

Figure 7-7 Use of Huygen's principle to compute light amplitude from a spherical wave.

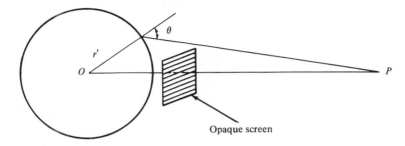

Figure 7-8 *Diffraction of spherical wave caused by an opaque screen.*

diffraction occurs. These diffraction effects' may manifest themselves by either a higher or lower light intensity at P than in the absence of the obstacle, depending on the relative positions of the screen and observation point.

The task of computing the total amplitude in the presence of a diffracting object, such as an opaque screen, involves an integration over the entire surface, giving rise to the secondary wavelets. In general, this is a rather complicated process; however, a procedure first proposed by Fresnel may be used to approximate the resultant amplitude without resorting to complicated mathematical integration. This procedure will be outlined here for the computation of the amplitude at a point P ahead of a plane wave, which will be the source of secondary wavelets, as is shown in Figure 7-9.

The procedure entails the construction of a series of circles about point O as a center of radii $r_1, r_2, r_3, \ldots$, so that the distance between the observation point P and the circles increases by half a wavelength in going from one circle to its neighbor. This procedure thus divides the secondary source surface into a series of zones called Fresnel zones consisting of a

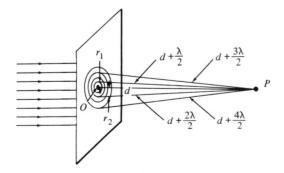

Figure 7-9 *Construction of Fresnel zones.*

circle surrounded by a series of annular rings, whose location depends on the point of observation. Since the difference in distances to point P between consecutive circles is $\lambda/2$, the difference in phase between waves arriving from the edge of one zone and the next will be 180°. The phases of wavelets from a given zone will not differ by more than 180°, and since each zone is on the average $\lambda/2$ further away from the observation point, successive zones will produce amplitudes at P which differ in phase by 180°. A change of 180° in phase is tantamount to a reversal in the sign of the amplitude, and the resultant amplitude from the entire secondary wave is given by

$$A = A_1 - A_2 + A_3 - A_4 + \cdots + A_N \qquad (7\text{-}2)$$

where A_1, A_2 are the contributions from the respective Fresnel zones. The magnitude of a contribution from a zone will vary in general due to three factors: (1) the zone areas change slightly from one zone to the next; however, to a good approximation the area of a zone is independent of the zone number when the wavelength is much smaller than the distance between the observation point and the surface of secondary sources; (2) the distance between zones and the observation point increases with increasing zone number; (3) the angle θ of the obliquity factor increases with zone number. The total effect of all these factors is to slowly decrease the magnitude of the contribution from a particular zone with increasing zone number.

The sum of the alternating series of (7-2) may be approximated by

$$A = \frac{A_1 + A_N}{2} \qquad (7\text{-}3)$$

where N is the index number of the last contributing zone, and where it has been assumed that N was odd. For N even, A_N in (7-3) must be replaced by $-A_N$. Equation (7-3) may be arrived at by noting that the magnitude of the amplitude from each zone is very nearly equal to the average of the amplitude of the preceding and following zones, but of opposite sign; therefore, only an average of the first and last terms is left unpaired and contributes to the resultant at the observation point. The geometrical construction illustrated in Figure 7-10 may be used to help clarify the above

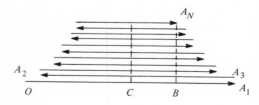

Figure 7-10   Vectors representing contributions from various Fresnel zones.

result. The vectors representing contributions from successive zones have been placed side by side and end to tip, so that the resultant is represented by the length OB which is the sum of OC and CB which is just the sum given by (7-3).

When a screen containing an aperture is placed in front of the observation point, it is assumed that the amplitude of light within the aperture is the same as if the diffracting aperture were absent, and the contributions due to secondary waves emitted from within the aperture are computed. An approximate method based on the Fresnel zone procedure may be employed where the Fresnel zones are constructed in the plane of the diffracting screen, and only those zones that fall within the aperture contribute to the total field amplitude at the observation point. To obtain the total diffraction pattern, the point of observation has to be varied, and consequently the corresponding system of Fresnel zones varies with it. The actual diffraction pattern will depend on which zones are uncovered and which become obscured as the observation point moves around.

With the help of the above we may explain some interesting observable phenomena for which geometric optics are inadequate. For example, consider the case of an opaque circular obstacle the size of the first Fresnel zone placed in front of a plane wave, as shown in Figure 7-11. If the extent of the light at the plane of the object is large, the contribution from the last Fresnel zone may be neglected, and since in our case $A_1 = 0$ the total amplitude at the observation point P is approximately $-A_2/2$, and we obtain the surprising result of a bright spot in the center of the geometrical shadow. This result, which has been observed experimentally, can thus be explained only by the wave nature of the light.

Another interesting consequence of Fresnel zones becomes evident if the diffracting screen is designed to obscure the light from every other

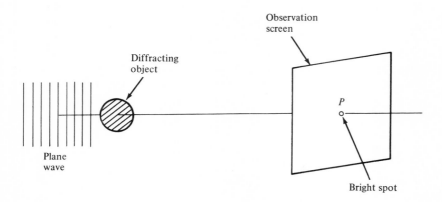

Figure 7-11 Diffraction by an opaque object the size of the first Fresnel zone.

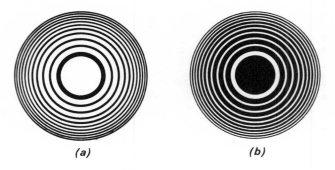

(a)   *(b)*

Figure 7-12   Zone plates.

zone, as is illustrated in Figure 7-12.   The diffracting object in this case is termed a *zone plate*.   The effect of the zone plate is to eliminate all the positive or all the negative terms in (7-2), and, since destructive interference no longer occurs, the amplitude at the observation point increases to a value many times that observed without the plate.   The bright spot produced that way is so intense that the effect is very much like that of a lens.   This is again a direct result of the wave nature of light.

7·2·2   diffraction by a rectangular aperture

Further insight into the wave nature of light may be obtained by examining the Fraunhofer diffraction pattern of a single rectangular aperture.   This result will be used later in applications involving diffraction from various different objects.   For the sake of simplicity let the diffracting screen containing the aperture be perpendicular to the incident plane wave of monochromatic light.   The pattern is observed on a screen very far from the aperture, or by placing a lens in back of the diffracting aperture and observing the pattern on a screen placed in the focal plane of the lens as in Figure 7-13.   Thus the intensity at any point P of the pattern is due to the superposition of all the diffracted rays leaving the various points of the aperture in a given direction.   All the rays leaving the aperture at an angle θ with the normal to the plane of the slit are brought to a focus at the point P on the observation screen as shown in Figure 7-13.

Calculation of the diffraction pattern makes use of a coordinate system, as shown in Figure 7-14, with the origin at the center of the rectangular aperture of width a and length b.   The observation screen is placed at a finite but very long distance z_0 from the aperture, and the wave arriving at P (coordinates x_0, y_0, z_0) is considered as the superposition of elementary secondary waves coming from the various infinitesimal elements of area dS of the aperture.

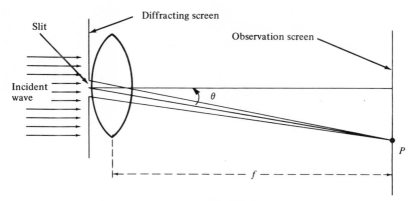

Figure 7-13 Use of a lens to focus diffraction pattern.

A spherical wave emanating from the origin has the form

$$U(r_0) = \frac{1}{r_0} \exp[i(kr_0 - \omega t)] \tag{7-4}$$

where $k = 2\pi/\lambda$ and ω is the angular frequency of the light. Thus the contribution at (x_0, y_0, z_0), due to one elementary secondary wave emanating from dS at $(x, y, 0)$ in the plane of the aperture, is given by

$$dU(x_0, y_0, z_0) = C\, dS \exp[i(k\sqrt{(x_0 - x)^2 + (y_0 - y)^2 + z_0^2} - \omega t)]$$

$$\Big/ \sqrt{(x_0 - x)^2 + (y_0 - y)^2 + z_0^2} \tag{7-5}$$

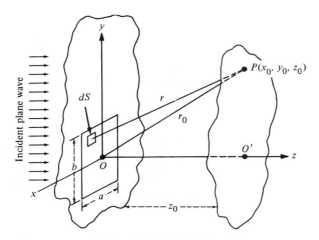

Figure 7-14 Diffraction from rectangular aperture.

In (7-5), C is a proportionality constant, and it has been assumed that the effect of angle variation (obliquity factor) is negligible. This assumption will hold true for observation points at large distances away from the diffracting screen and close to the center of the diffraction pattern at O', which are the points in which we are interested. The total light amplitude at the observation point is therefore given as an integral of (7-5) over the entire aperture area in the form

$$U(x_0, y_0, z_0) = \iint_A \frac{C \exp[i(k\sqrt{(x_0 - x)^2 + (y_0 - y)^2 + z_0^2} - \omega t)] \, dS}{\sqrt{(x_0 - x)^2 + (y_0 - y)^2 + z_0^2}}$$

(7-6)

where A denotes integration over the aperture. Evaluation of (7-6) is considerably aided by defining r_0 to be the distance between the origin and the point of observation, so that $r_0^2 = x_0^2 + y_0^2 + z_0^2$, and if r is the distance between the elemental area dS and the point of observation, we readily find that

$$r^2 = r_0^2 - 2xx_0 - 2yy_0 + x^2 + y^2$$

(7-7)

Noticing that x_0/r_0 and y_0/r_0 are direction cosines which may be denoted by ℓ and m, respectively, (7-7) may be written as

$$r^2 = r_0^2\left(1 - \frac{2\ell x + 2my}{r_0} + \frac{x^2 + y^2}{r_0^2}\right)$$

(7-8)

For the points of observation in which we are interested, the last term in the above parentheses is much smaller than unity and may be neglected (Fraunhofer case); thus expansion of the square root according to the binomial theorem as required by (7-6) yields $r \simeq r_0 - (\ell x + my)$. The denominator in (7-6) does not vary much with the actual source position in the aperture and may be approximated by r_0, so that the variations in amplitude in the diffraction pattern will only be due to relative phase differences among the various waves given by the exponential term in (7-6). That equation may therefore be approximated to a good degree by

$$U(x_0, y_0, z_0) = \frac{C \exp[i(kr_0 - \omega t)]}{r_0} \int_{-a/2}^{a/2} \int_{-b/2}^{b/2} \exp[-ik(\ell x + my)] \, dx \, dy,$$

(7-9)

and the integration may readily be carried out now to yield

$$U(x_0, y_0, z_0) = \frac{abC}{r_0} e^{i(kr_0 - \omega t)} \frac{\sin(k\ell a/2)}{k\ell a/2} \frac{\sin(kmb/2)}{kmb/2}$$

(7-10)

Since the quantity usually observed is the intensity of light which is proportional to the square of the amplitude, we obtain

$$I = I_0 \frac{\sin^2(k\ell a/2)}{(k\ell a/2)^2} \frac{\sin^2(kmb/2)}{(kmb/2)^2} \tag{7-11}$$

where I_0 is the intensity at the center of the diffraction pattern (ℓ, $m = 0$ or $x_0 = y_0 = 0$).

Since the variation in the xz plane (transverse to the length of the aperture) is identical with that in the yz plane (along the length of the aperture), it will suffice to examine the intensity variation in the xz plane. For all points in this plane, $m = 0$, since the angle between r_0 (Figure 7-14) and the y axis is 90°.   Thus

$$\frac{\sin(kmb/2)}{kmb/2} = 1$$

and for this case (7-11) becomes

$$I = I_0 \frac{\sin^2(k\ell a/2)}{(k\ell a/2)^2} \equiv I_0 \frac{\sin^2 \alpha}{\alpha^2} \tag{7-12}$$

which is plotted in Figure 7-15.

The maximum intensity occurs at the center, falls off to zero at $\alpha = \pm\pi$, $\pm 2\pi$, $\pm 3\pi$, etc., with secondary maxima approximately halfway between.   The positions of the maxima are assumed to be the points

$$\alpha = \frac{k\ell a}{2} = \frac{\pi \ell a}{\lambda} = \pm \frac{3\pi}{2}, \pm \frac{5\pi}{2}, \cdots$$

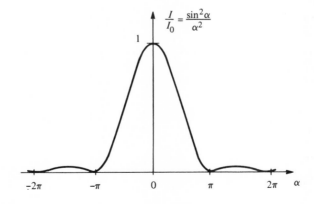

Figure 7-15   One-dimensional diffraction pattern from rectangular aperture.

the relative intensities at these points are

$$\left(\frac{2}{3\pi}\right)^2, \left(\frac{2}{5\pi}\right)^2, \ldots, \quad \text{or} \quad 0.045, 0.016, \ldots$$

Thus we see that the intensities of the secondary maxima fall off very rapidly as one proceeds away from the central maximum, so that practically all the light is concentrated in the central diffraction band. The half angle θ subtended at the aperture by this band is given by

$$\sin \theta = \ell = \frac{\lambda}{a}$$

or, for small angles,

$$\theta = \frac{\lambda}{a}$$

This is shown in Figure 7-16, in which the reader may imagine the aperture dimension b to be so large compared to a that essentially a one-dimensional pattern exists. Note that the diffraction pattern becomes more extended with narrower aperture dimensions, or longer wavelengths.

The general expression for the location of the minima is given by

$$\frac{\pi \ell a}{\lambda} = \pm k\pi \qquad (k = 1, 2, 3, \ldots)$$

or for the angles

$$\sin \theta = \ell = \pm k\frac{\lambda}{a} \qquad (k = 1, 2, 3, \ldots)$$

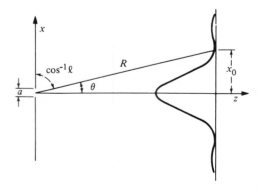

Figure 7-16   Illustration of the diffraction angle θ.

7·2·3 *Fresnel-Kirchhoff diffraction formula*

The previous sections dealt with the diffraction of plane waves only. A more general mathematical formulation of diffraction, treating arbitrarily shaped apertures illuminated by nonuniform fields, places the Huygens principle on a much firmer mathematical foundation. This formulation is due to Kirchhoff and results in what is usually referred to as the Fresnel-Kirchhoff diffraction formula. A reader who is primarily interested in the physical *rather than* mathematical understanding of the problem may wish to proceed directly to Section 7.2.6 with little loss in continuity.

Consider the diffraction geometry presented in Figure 7-17, where it is assumed that monochromatic light is incident upon an aperture in an infinite opaque planar screen.

A rectangular coordinate system (x, y) is attached to the plane of the aperture, and a similar coordinate system (x_0, y_0) to a parallel plane where the observation is taking place. The coordinate axes (x, y) are parallel to (x_0, y_0) and both are normal to the z direction along which the separation between the two planes is measured. The scalar field in the plane defined by (x_0, y_0) is then obtained by summing up the contributions of all the individual points P, within the aperture in the form

$$U(x_0, y_0) = \frac{1}{2i\lambda} \iint U_0(x, y) \frac{\exp(ikr)}{r} (1 + \cos \theta) \, dx \, dy \qquad (7\text{-}13)$$

In (7-13) $U_0(x, y)$ denotes the scalar field at a point P, within the aperture with

$$r^2 = z_0^2 + (x_0 - x)^2 + (y_0 - y)^2 \qquad (7\text{-}14)$$

and θ is defined as the angle between the line connecting the observation point P_0 to the contributing point P and the normal in the z direction. The

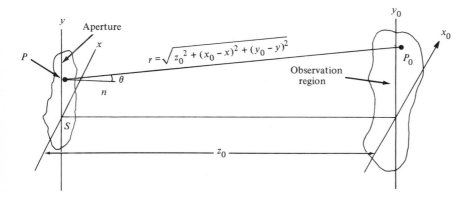

Figure 7-17 Diffraction geometry.

integration in (7-13) is carried out over the entire aperture area, and the formula is valid only when the dimensions of the aperture are much greater than a wavelength and much smaller than the separation between the planes. A close scrutiny of (7-13), which is the Fresnel-Kirchhoff integral, reveals that it carries a sample interpretation of the Huygens principle. It may again be interpreted to imply that the total field at an observation point P_0 arises from an infinite number of fictitious secondary point sources located within the aperture, as expected. However, the secondary field source differs from the original field $U_0(x, y)$ at the point by a factor of $1/2i\lambda (1 + \cos \theta)$, which includes the obliquity factor $(1 + \cos \theta)$, an amplitude constant of $1/2\lambda$, and a phase factor of $90°$. This interpretation is readily arrived at if one recalls once more that a monochromatic scalar field emitted by a point source is given by a spherical wave of the form

$$U(r, t) = \frac{A}{r} \exp[i(kr - \omega t)] \qquad (7\text{-}15)$$

where the complex constant A is a measure of the amplitude and phase of the wave, and r is the distance from the observation point to the point source.

In the following analysis, the diffraction of relatively narrow and highly collimated laser beams propagating in the z direction, thus involving only small angles of θ, will be examined. In this case, the obliquity factor $(1 + \cos \theta)$ can be approximated by 2, and distance r, appearing in the denominator, can be replaced by z_0. Equation (7-13) thus reduces to

$$U(x_0, y_0) = \frac{1}{i\lambda z_0} \iint U_0(x, y)\exp(ikr)\, dx\, dy \qquad (7\text{-}16)$$

Note that r appearing in the exponent *cannot* be simply replaced by z, since any resulting error will be multiplied by $k = 2\pi/\lambda$ which is a very large number ($\sim 10^5$ cm^{-1}) and may give rise to substantial phase errors (greater than 2π).

However, further simplification is possible if (as has been assumed) both the aperture and the observation regions are much smaller in size than the separation between the planes. When this condition is taken into account,

$$r = z_0\sqrt{1 + \left(\frac{x_0 - x}{z_0}\right)^2 + \left(\frac{y_0 - y}{z_0}\right)^2}$$

$$\simeq z_0\left[1 + \frac{1}{2}\left(\frac{x_0 - x}{z_0}\right)^2 + \frac{1}{2}\left(\frac{y_0 - y}{z_0}\right)^2\right]. \qquad (7\text{-}17)$$

This approximation, called the Fresnel approximation, is valid for the Fresnel diffraction region and leads to a diffraction integral of the form

$$U(x_0, y_0) = \frac{e^{ikz_0}}{i\lambda z_0} \iint U(x, y)\exp\left\{i\,\frac{k}{2z_0}\,[(x_0 - x)^2 + (y_0 - y)^2]\right\} dx\,dy$$

(7-18)

Even further simplification results from an additional assumption which greatly facilitates the computation of diffraction patterns. When the condition

$$z_0 \gg \frac{k(x^2 + y^2)_{max}}{2}$$

(7-19)

is satisfied (this is the so-called Fraunhofer or far-field approximation) the quadratic exponent in the Fresnel approximation of (7-18) may be expanded to yield the Fraunhofer diffraction pattern given by

$$U(x_0, y_0) = \frac{\exp(ikz_0)}{i\lambda z_0}\,\exp\left\{i\,\frac{k}{2z_0}\,(x_0^2 + y_0^2)\right\}$$

$$\times \iint U_0(x, y)\exp\left[-\frac{i2\pi}{\lambda z_0}\,(x_0 x + y_0 y)\right] dx\,dy \quad (7\text{-}20)$$

which by making use of the definitions

$$\omega_x = \frac{2\pi x_0}{\lambda z_0} \quad \text{and} \quad \omega_y = \frac{2\pi y_0}{\lambda z_0}$$

may be reduced to

$$U(x_0, y_0) = \frac{\exp(ikz_0)}{i\lambda z_0}\,\exp\left[i\,\frac{k}{2z_0}\,(x_0^2 + y_0^2)\right]$$

$$\times \iint U_0(x, y)\exp(-i\omega_x x - i\omega_y y)\,dx\,dy \quad (7\text{-}21)$$

Implicit in the derivation of the Fresnel-Kirchhoff formula was the assumption that the scalar function describing the field in the (x, y) plane was identically zero outside the aperture. Because of this the limits of integration in (7-21) may be extended to infinity yielding

$$U(x_0, y_0) = \frac{\exp[ikz_0]}{i\lambda z_0}\,\exp\left[i\,\frac{k}{2z_0}\,(x_0^2 + y_0^2)\right]$$

$$\times \int_{-\infty}^{\infty}\int_{-\infty}^{\infty} U_0(x, y)\exp[-i\omega_x x - i\omega_y y]\,dx\,dy \quad (7\text{-}22)$$

where the dependence of the integral on x_0 and y_0 is contained in ω_x and ω_y, respectively. A one-dimensional Fourier transformation is defined as[5]

$$\mathcal{F}\{f(t)\} = F(\omega) = \int_\infty^\infty f(t)\exp(-i\omega t)\,dt \tag{7-23}$$

where $F(\omega)$ is called the frequency domain Fourier transform of the time function $f(t)$. This Fourier transform function $F(\omega)$ may be expressed as

$$F(\omega) = A(\omega)\exp[i\phi(\omega)] \tag{7-24}$$

where $A(\omega)$ is known as the amplitude of the Fourier transform and $\phi(\omega)$ its phase.

Similarly, a two-dimensional Fourier transform of a function of space $g(x, y)$ may be defined in the form

$$\mathcal{F}\{g\} = G(\omega_x, \omega_y) = \int_{-\infty}^\infty \int_{-\infty}^\infty g(x, y)\exp[-i\omega_x x - i\omega_y y]\,dx\,dy \tag{7-25}$$

where ω_x and ω_y are referred to as spatial frequencies. Then the Fraunhofer diffraction pattern is simply given by

$$U(x_0, y_0) = \frac{\exp(ikz_0)\exp\left[i\dfrac{k}{2z_0}(x_0^2 + y_0^2)\right]}{i\lambda z_0}\,\mathcal{F}\{U_0(x, y)\}\,\Biggr|_{\substack{\omega_x = \frac{2\pi x_0}{\lambda z_0} \\ \omega_y = \frac{2\pi y_0}{\lambda z_0}}} \tag{7-26}$$

The notation used in the last equation denotes that the Fourier transform has to be evaluated at the spatial frequencies $\omega_x = 2\pi x_0/\lambda z_0$ and $\omega_y = 2\pi y_0/\lambda z_0$.

One important property of this integral may now be pointed out. Any variation in the position of the aperture will only add a phase term to $U(x_0, y_0)$, so that the position of the aperture (within the approximations) will not change the amplitude of the diffraction pattern. This is an important property which is very useful.

When a plane wave impinges on a rectangular aperture as given in Figure 7-14 with $U_0(x, y)$ constant, then the Fraunhofer diffraction pattern reduces to

$$U(x_0, y_0) = \frac{\exp(ikz_0)\exp\left[i\dfrac{k}{2z_0}(x_0^2 + y_0^2)\right]}{i\lambda z_0}\,C\int_{-a/2}^{a/2}\int_{-b/2}^{b/2}\exp(-iw_x x)$$

$$\times \exp(-iw_y y)\,dx\,dy \tag{7-27}$$

and

$$I(x_0, y_0) = I_0 \frac{\sin^2 \dfrac{\pi x_0 a}{\lambda z_0}}{(\pi x_0 a / \lambda z_0)^2} \frac{\sin^2 \dfrac{\pi y_0 b}{\lambda z_0}}{(\pi y_0 b / \lambda z_0)^2} \tag{7-28}$$

which is identical to (7-12) within the approximations employed.

7·2·4 *Fraunhofer diffraction pattern by a lens*

When light passes through an optical material whose index of refraction is greater than that of air, its propagation velocity in the medium is reduced below its value in air. If such a material (e.g., lens) is thin, light rays passing through it will undergo no translation motion within the medium and emerge with the same coordinates as they entered the opposite face of the lens. The effect of the thin lens will merely be to delay the wavefront of the light by an amount proportional to the thickness of the optical element at each point. If such a lens is positioned in the path of a laser beam and attention is restricted to the region around the axis of the lens, the effect of the lens may be viewed as the addition of a quadratic phase factor to the light field immediately in front of the lens. Mathematically, the effect of the lens may be accounted for by a factor $L(x, y)$ multiplying the light distribution impinging upon it. This factor may be expressed in the form

$$L(x, y) = \exp\left(-ik \frac{x^2 + y^2}{2f} \right) \tag{7-29}$$

where f is the focal length of the lens. When such a lens is placed immediately in back of a diffracting object, the field in the Fresnel region may be obtained from (7-18) in the form of

$$U(x_0, y_0) = \frac{\exp(ikz_0)}{i\lambda z_0} \int_{-\infty}^{\infty} \int_{-\infty}^{\infty} U_0(x, y) \exp\left(-ik \frac{x^2 + y^2}{2f} \right)$$
$$\times \exp\left\{ \frac{ik}{2z_0} [(x_0 - x)^2 + (y_0 - y)^2] \right\} dx\, dy \tag{7-30}$$

where the limits of integration were again extended to infinity in accordance with the assumptions contained in the derivation of the Fresnel-Kirchhoff integral. When the second quadratic phase factor is expanded and the integral evaluated in the focal plane of the lens ($z_0 = f$), the resulting field disturbance $U(x_f, y_f)$ is given by

$$U(x_f, y_f) = \frac{\exp(ikf)}{i\lambda f} \exp\left[i\frac{k}{2f}(x_f^2 + y_f^2) \right]$$
$$\times \int_{-\infty}^{\infty} \int_{-\infty}^{\infty} U_0(x, y) \exp\left[-i\frac{2\pi}{\lambda f}(x_f x + y_f y) \right] dx\, dy \tag{7-31}$$

where it is assumed that the aperture of the lens is at least as large as that of the diffracting object.   An inspection of (7-31) reveals that it is identical to (7-22) with $z_0 = f$.   Thus the Fraunhofer diffraction pattern is obtained at a finite distance from the diffracting aperture.   The diffraction pattern in the focal plane of the lens differs from the exact Fourier transform of the field disturbance by the quadratic phase factor preceding the integral in (7-31).   (The term $\exp(ikf)/i\lambda f$ is a constant for all points in the focal plane and thus has essentially no real effect on the Fourier transform.)   However, it can be shown[6] that, when the diffracting object is placed in the front focal plane of the lens (a distance f in front of the thin lens), the quadratic phase factor disappears, yielding exact Fourier transforms between the field $U_0(x, y)$ and the diffraction pattern in the focal plane $U(x_f, y_f)$.   In most cases, interest centers around the intensity of the disturbance in the focal plane, which yields information about the power spectrum of the incident disturbance $U_0(x, y)$.   In these cases, the phase factor is of no consequence, and it is therefore unnecessary to keep the diffracting object in the front focal plane to obtain the information on intensity in the back focal plane.

The use of a lens to form the diffraction pattern might be essential for large objects because the distance demanded by the far-field approximation used in (7-18) may become prohibitively large.   For example, for an aperture with maximum dimension of 1 in. and HeNe laser light at 632.8 nm, the far-field observation point without a lens has to satisfy the condition $z \gg 1600$ m or 1 mile.

7·2·5 Fraunhofer diffraction pattern of a circular aperture

When a circular aperture of radius a is illuminated by a normally incident plane wave of amplitude A, the far-field diffraction pattern in polar coordinates (r_0, θ_0) in the observation plane is given by

$$U(r_0) = A \frac{\exp(ikz_0)}{i\lambda z_0} \exp\left(\frac{ikr_0^2}{2z_0}\right)\left(\frac{a^2 J_1(kar_0/z_0)}{ar_0/\lambda z_0}\right) \tag{7-32}$$

where J_1 is a Bessel function of first kind order one, and its intensity $|U(r_0)|^2$ is given by

$$I(r_0) = \left(\frac{ka^2}{2z_0}\right)^2\left(\frac{2J_1(kar_0/z_0)}{kar_0/z_0}\right)^2 \tag{7-33}$$

and is usually referred to as the Airy pattern.   A one-dimensional cross section of the Airy pattern is illustrated in Figure 7-18, and it is seen that the first minimum occurs at $r_0 = 1.22\ (\lambda z_0/2a)$.

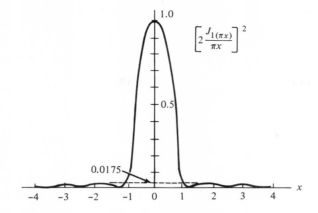

$$\left[2\frac{J_{1(\pi x)}}{\pi x}\right]^2$$

Figure 7-18   One-dimensional cross section of the Airy pattern.

7·2·6   Fraunhofer diffraction pattern of a narrow slit

Consider a rectangular slit of width a and length b upon which a collimated expanded laser beam is normally incident.   It is assumed that the laser is operating in the fundamental transverse mode (TEM_{00}) and consequently possesses a Gaussian electric field distribution in the plane of the slit. Figure 7-19 depicts such an arrangement where it is further assumed that

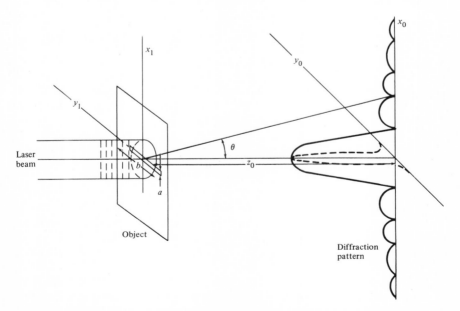

Figure 7-19   Diffraction of a laser beam by a long narrow aperture.

the width of the laser beam, $2w$ (w is the spot size of the Gaussian beam as defined in Equation 3-1), is much greater than the width of the slit, a, and much smaller than the length of the slit, b.

In the plane of the slit, the field disturbance $U_0(x, y)$ is given by

$$U_0(x, y) = A \exp\left[\left(-\frac{x^2 + y^2}{w^2}\right)\right] \tag{7-34}$$

where the complex parameter A is independent of x and y.   Since $a \ll 2w$, the field is assumed independent of x and is approximated by its value along the y axis for use in (7-22) to obtain the expression for the far-field diffraction pattern,

$$U(x_0, y_0) = \frac{Aa}{i\lambda z_0} \frac{\sin(\pi x_0 a/\lambda z_0)}{\pi x_0 a/\lambda z_0} \exp(ikz_0)\exp\left[i\frac{k}{2z_0}(x_0^2 + y_0^2)\right]$$

$$\times \int_{-\infty}^{\infty} \exp\left[-\frac{y^2}{w^2}\right]\exp\left[-\frac{i2\pi y_0 y}{\lambda z_0}\right] dy \tag{7-35}$$

where the finite limits of integration have been extended to infinity without introducing an appreciable error.   The integral in the above expression is immediately recognized as the Fourier transform of a Gaussian, which is again a Gaussian,[5] and finally

$$U(x_0, y_0) = \frac{Awa\sqrt{\pi}}{i\lambda z_0} \frac{\sin(\pi x_0 a/\lambda z_0)}{(\pi x_0 a/\lambda z_0)} \exp(ikz_0)$$

$$\times \exp\left[i\frac{k}{2z_0}(x_0^2 + y_0^2)\right]\exp\left[-\left(\frac{\pi w y_0^2}{\lambda z_0}\right)\right] \tag{7-36}$$

The intensity of the diffraction pattern is also illustrated in Figure 7-19, where it is seen to consist of a series of maxima and minima in the x_0 direction and is Gaussian in the y_0 direction.   Since the minima position are defined by the zeros of the sine function, they are seen to satisfy

$$\frac{\pi x_0 a}{\lambda z_0} = n\pi \tag{7-37}$$

or

$$x_{0_{min}} = \frac{n\lambda z_0}{a} \tag{7-38}$$

Since the angle θ given in Figure 7-19 is defined by $\tan \theta = x_0/z_0$, in the limit of small angles $\theta \simeq x_0/z_0$ and the minima are defined by a series of angles satisfying the relation

$$\theta_{min} = \frac{n\lambda}{a} \text{ rad} \tag{7-39}$$

By measuring the separation of the intensity minima, a determination of slit width may be obtained.

7·2·7   Babinet's principle

If U_1 is the diffracted field for the case when the slit (Figure 7-19) is in place, and U_2 is the diffracted field using the opposite, i.e., a screen which is transparent except for an opaque area of width a and length b, then the sum of these two is equal to the field without any screen at all.

$$U = U_1 + U_2 \qquad (7\text{-}40)$$

This is Babinet's principle, which will be used here to calculate the diffraction pattern of an opaque rectangular object in a laser beam.

The procedure is demonstrated in Figure 7-20.   Figure 7-20a shows the laser beam and its diffraction pattern.   Figure 7-20b shows the

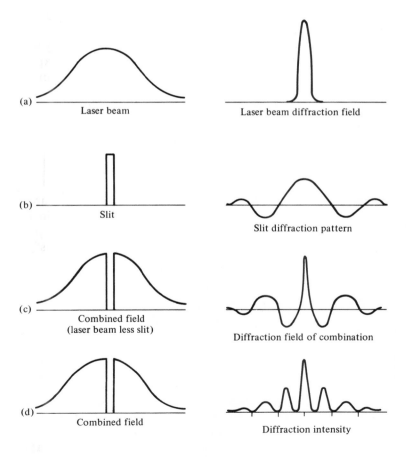

(a)   Laser beam   Laser beam diffraction field

(b)   Slit   Slit diffraction pattern

(c)   Combined field (laser beam less slit)   Diffraction field of combination

(d)   Combined field   Diffraction intensity

Figure 7-20   Use of Babinet's principle to obtain diffraction patterns.

diffraction pattern of a slit.   Figure 7-20c is the combined effect, where the slit field is subtracted to obtain the field of a laser beam with the central part blocked.   The diffraction pattern is thus the laser beam pattern plus the negative of the slit diffraction pattern.   Figure 7-20d shows the intensity pattern and is the one normally detected.   This diffraction pattern is identical to the slit diffraction intensity except for the bright spot in the center.   For the central peak not to affect the minima of the slit pattern, at $(\pi x_0 a)/\lambda z_0$ the peak must be small in width.   This corresponds to a large laser beam spot size and implies that the spot size should be many times larger than the slit width.

Using (7-38), the width of the opaque object may be obtained by measuring the separation of the minima, except those adjacent to the central peak.

7·2·8 diffraction and measurement of objects other than slits

Diffraction can be applied to measuring sizes of wires and other objects within certain limitations.   The advantages of using diffraction are that the measurement is noncontact and does not require any critical transverse positioning of the object.   (It only requires rotary alignment.)   Opaque objects, such as wires with a diameter greater than 2.5 μm, produce diffraction patterns that can be measured; however, as the diameter becomes smaller, detection becomes increasingly more difficult.   The reason for the above is shown in Figure 7-21a where it is seen that light is reflected from the sides of the wire and interferes with the diffraction pattern produced by the wire profile.

The objects must be opaque to produce diffraction patterns; if they are not opaque, the field at the object is not zero, and a different pattern is produced (see Figure 7-21b).   Experiments have demonstrated that to measure glass-fiber diameters accurately using diffraction, the fibers must be coated with metal.[7]   It is possible to calculate diameters of transparent objects by measuring the diffraction (forward scattered) radiation; however, the pattern is no longer simple and the full scattering theory must be used.[8]

Diode Array for Monitoring Diffraction Patterns   Dynamic wire diameter monitoring instruments have been constructed using diffraction of collimated light from a HeNe laser at 632.8 nm wavelength.[9]   As illustrated in Figure 7-22, an array of photodiodes was used to detect the various parts of the pattern.   Outputs of the diodes were then analyzed to determine the position of one of the minima.   Gain of each diode was

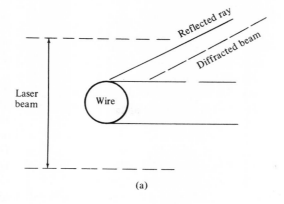

(a)

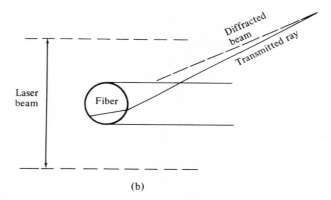

(b)

Figure 7-21 Interference of reflected and transmitted beams with diffracted beam in transparent objects.

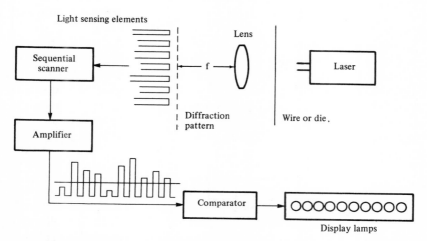

Figure 7-22 Diode array detection system showing formation of diffraction pattern, its detection by the diodes, and the display indicating wire size.

compensated to offset the decreasing intensity of the pattern with increasing angle θ.   Accuracy of the method depends on the precision with which the minimum position can be determined.   To increase accuracy, the separation between a number of minima rather than adjacent minima were measured, and the intensity zeros at as large an angle as possible were observed.

TV Detector for Monitoring Diffraction Patterns

An alternate method for detecting the diffraction minima is shown in Figure 7-23.   In this setup, the diffraction pattern is imaged onto a vidicon camera, and the signal is analyzed electronically to measure the distance between the minima.   With the help of (7-38), the wire diameter is obtained.   Once again by measuring the distance between a number of minima rather than adjacent minima, better accuracy is obtained.   Accuracies achieved with this system are 0.3 percent, and wires up to 2.5 mm can be measured.   The smallest measurable diameter is of the order of a few wavelengths and, with the use of a HeNe laser at 632.8 nm, is about 2.5 μm.

In summary, diffraction can be used to measure sizes of one or two dimensional opaque objects with good accuracy; the measurement is noncontact and is not critically dependent on the transverse position of the object (it is, however, dependent on the angular orientation).   Thus, moving or vibrating objects can be monitored.   In addition, it should be noted that the size of the diffraction pattern is inversely proportional to the size of the object.   Therefore, small objects can be measured with greater accuracy than large objects.

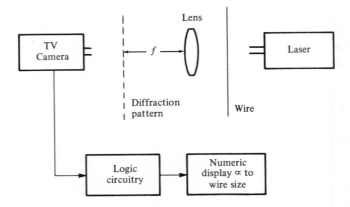

Figure 7-23   TV detection system showing the formation of the diffraction pattern, its detection, and analysis by the TV camera and logic circuits, and a numeric display proportional to wire size.

7·2·9   laser requirements

In calculating the diffraction pattern the incident wave used was a plane-parallel wave.   Producing this in practice requires a single-mode laser of relatively low power, such as a HeNe laser.   In addition, a beam expander may be required for illuminating large objects.

The main stability requirement, apart from reasonable amplitude stability, is that of beam direction.   A variation of beam direction, $\delta\alpha$, gives a positional variation of the diffraction pattern of $\delta\alpha \times f$.   (f is the lens focal length which is thus the distance from the lens to the diffraction pattern.)   Thus, if the detector is sensitive to positional variations, errors in wire diameter measurements will result.   However, this stability requirement is not as critical as that for the alignment lasers discussed earlier.

7·2·10   reconstruction of slit profiles

In the previous measurement techniques, the separation of the diffraction minima was used to give the size of binary (i.e., opaque or transparent) objects with sharp edges.   It is possible to extend this process one step further, by making a more critical study of the diffraction pattern.

Ideally, if the amplitude and phase of the diffraction pattern could be measured and its inverse Fourier transform calculated, the result would be the field produced by the object.   The Fourier transform may be calculated using a digital computer and a fast Fourier transform routine.[10]

Measuring the amplitude and phase usually entails a very involved experiment, using either an interferometer or a holographic recording technique.   However, if the illumination across the object is real and symmetric, some simple predictions can be made about the phase by comparing it with the ideal diffraction pattern, since the Fourier transform is also real,[5] and the phase will be either 0 or π.   For example, a slit or line diffraction pattern has the well-known $\sin x/x$ amplitude characteristic and there is a phase change of π radians between adjacent lobes. Once the phase change and amplitude are known, the original object can be reconstructed by calculations.

Figure 7-24 shows a result obtained using this technique on a Fourier transform diffraction pattern of a slit recorded on low-resolution photographic emulsion.   Figure 7-24a depicts the diffraction pattern amplitude, and 7-24b displays the calculated inverse transform which is plotted on a logarithmic intensity scale in the center of the graph.

It can be seen that the reconstructed slit possesses a large edge gradient; however, as shown by the noisy result, the diffraction pattern measurements were not very accurate and the dotted line is, therefore,

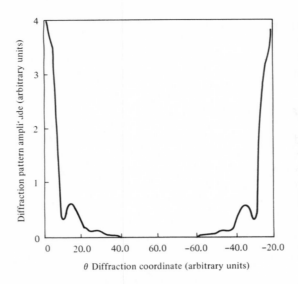

Figure 7-24a   Diffraction pattern amplitude of a slit as recorded on a low-resolution photographic emulsion.

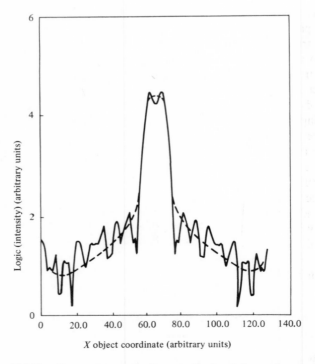

Figure 7-24b   Reconstructed slit as obtained from inverse Fourier transform.

chosen to show an average profile of the object. This technique is obviously also applicable to the measurement of very small photographic line images, and experiments conducted at the Western Electric Engineering Research Center suggest that it may be possible to obtain line profiles with a resolution of better than 0.5 μm using a HeNe laser at 632.8 nm.

7·3   spatial filtering

The preceding section on simple diffraction effects describes the Fraunhofer diffraction pattern for single slits and apertures. This section enlarges on the action of a converging lens in forming a Fourier transform of the light amplitude distribution across the object and describes more complex diffraction pattern forms. It then demonstrates uses of this operation and shows how pattern analysis and inspection can be accomplished by operating on (filtering) the diffraction pattern and subsequently reforming the modified pattern image.

7·3·1   Fourier transform property of a lens and its electronic analogue

In (7-31) it was shown that a converging lens forms the far-field diffraction pattern at its focal plane and that within a phase factor, this is a Fourier transform of light amplitude distribution across the object. It was also stated that the complex image at the back focal plane is the Fourier transform in both amplitude and phase of the illumination across an object at the other focal plane. Since a lens can be employed to form the two-dimensional Fourier transform of an object transparency, lenses are finding increasing use in applications involving real time signal processing, some of which will be discussed later.

The analogue between the lens and an electronic spectrum analyzer helps in understanding the nomenclature used. An electronic spectrum analyzer uses a Fourier transform in determining the frequency components of an electronic signal. In forming the diffraction pattern, the "signal" is now the amplitude of the light at the object, which is normally a function of transverse distances x and y. The lens, in forming the diffraction pattern, determines the spatial frequency spectrum of this signal. There are two frequency dimensions, ω_x and ω_y, since there are two signal dimensions, x and y.

7·3·2   illumination

In the discussion of simple diffraction effects, the illumination was considered to be a plane-parallel beam. This made the solution straightforward and yielded a diffraction pattern independent of the transverse position of the object.   For precisely the same reason, in spatial filtering applications the illumination is also normally plane-parallel wave.   However, a variation, which will be briefly discussed below, can be used for adjusting the size of the diffraction pattern.

If the beam is slightly diverging or converging, the diffraction pattern is still formed after going through the lens; however, it is no longer at the focal plane but at a distance slightly greater or smaller, respectively. The resultant size of the pattern is, therefore, increased or reduced in the same proportion.   The distance at which the pattern is formed is governed by R, the wavefront radius of the assumed Gaussian beam (of the illuminating beam with no object) after passing through the lens,* and the pattern is still independent of the position of the object provided the divergence is relatively small.

Although some experiments have been reported on incoherent spatial filtering systems,[11] most research and development work has been confined to using spatially coherent illumination employing collimated light or a laser source.   The remainder of the discussion will, therefore, be limited to coherent spatial filtering only.

7.3.3   spatial filtering arrangement

The spatial filtering system is completed by adding a second lens behind the diffraction pattern, as shown in Figure 7-25.   This has the effect of taking the light from the diffraction pattern and reforming an image of the object.   However, the image will be inverted since two successive Fourier transformations are involved rather than a Fourier transform and its

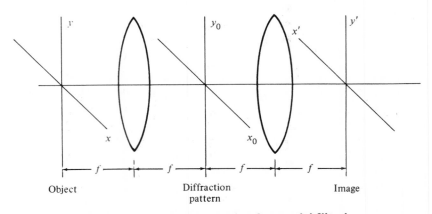

Figure 7-25   Lens configuration for spatial filtering.

* See Section 3.1.1 for discussion of Gaussian beam optics.

inverse. As stated before, to obtain a diffraction pattern which is a Fourier transform both in amplitude and phase, the arrangement shown would be used with the distance f, the focal length, separating object, lenses, and images. For an amplitude diffraction pattern, separation distances are not critical, except for the distance between the first lens and the diffraction pattern. The image is then reformed by proper positioning of the second lens as dictated by the standard geometrical optics formula for a two-lens imaging arrangement.

7·3·4 optical processing

There are now numerous applications of the Fourier transform property of lenses to both image processing and other signal processing problems,[12,13] and some of these will be described to demonstrate the kinds of problems that may be treated by means of optical signal processing.

Optical processing was first demonstrated in 1950[14] when the process was called double diffraction, although, in fact, an analysis of the microscope for periodic objects using this principle was carried out in 1873.[15] Later work[16] has shown how both amplitude and a combination of amplitude and phase filtering can improve an image from a badly aberrated lens. The filter is used to compensate the modulation transfer function[6] of the aberrations. The compensation is not perfect and one or more spatial frequencies are missing. Also, just as in communications, the filter cannot retrieve frequencies that are beyond the cutoff of the lens.

Comprehensive discussions on spatial filtering are available in the literature,[17] and some give examples of recovering otherwise indiscernible images from very noisy backgrounds.[18] Recently, a review of optical data processing techniques was presented, which includes matched filter types[19] of optical signal processing.[11]

7·3·5 examples of other spatial filtering arrangements and operations

Figure 7-26 shows some alternate configurations for spatial filtering which can be used. In all cases the diffraction pattern is an exact Fourier transform in terms of amplitude only. The phase term is modified by a factor which is a function of the distance between the object and the diffraction lens.[20] However, this does not mean that phase filtering cannot be performed.

Figure 7-26a depicts an arrangement in which only one lens is required. The distance between the object and the lens is increased to ℓ_1, so that a magnified image is produced. The diffraction pattern is still

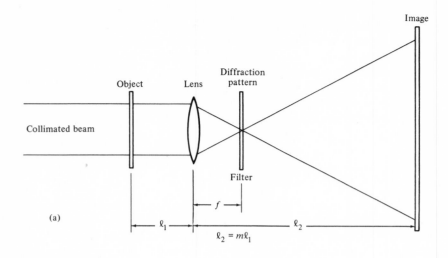

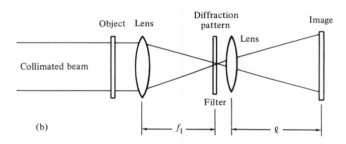

Figure 7-26   Spatial filtering configurations.

formed at the back focal plane.   This arrangement can be used in inspection applications where a magnified image is required.

Figure 7-26b illustrates a double-lens arrangement which makes the system more compact.   In addition, the second lens does not vignette the image, and this may be important when observing large images.   The first lens, however, has to be sufficiently large to cover the subject, as in the other configurations.   The setup of an actual system using this arrangement in the inspection of integrated circuits photomasks, which is discussed in Section 7.3.14, is shown in Figure 7-27.

Figure 7-28 is a modification of Figure 7-26b which can be used when a high-quality image is required with low-resolution filtering.   In this case the diffraction pattern is distorted at the higher frequencies; the second lens only performs the imaging, and thus this arrangement does not require two high-quality lenses of special design.   This is treated in greater detail in a later section.

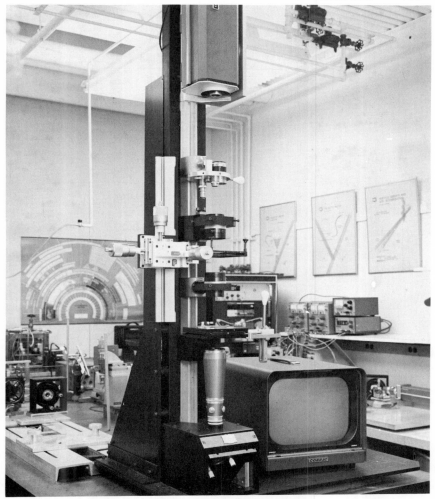

Figure 7-27   Actual spatial filtering setup (laser is behind tower).

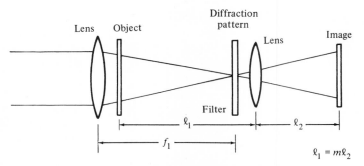

Figure 7-28   Alternate spatial filtering configuration.

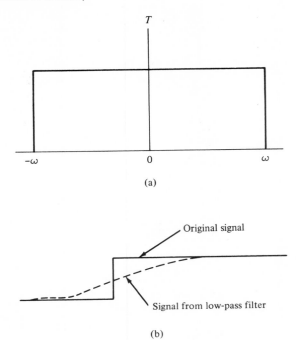

(a)

(b)

Figure 7-29   Low-pass filter and its response.

Simple Filtering Operations: Low-Pass Filter   Figure 7-29a shows, one dimensionally, a low-pass filter with cutoff frequency ω. This type of filter is easy to construct because it is binary, being transparent or opaque. The effect on an image is to stop the high-frequency information resulting in the blurring out of small images and sharp edges, as seen in Figure 7-29b. Therefore, this low-pass filter is useful in the detection of large objects in a noisy background.

High-Pass and Band-Pass Filters   The opposite of the low-pass filter is the high-pass filter which transmits spatial frequencies above ω and is illustrated in Figure 7-30a. There are two operations this filter can effect; the first is differentiation for signals of period L larger than $1/\omega$, and the second operation is the dc (zero frequency) bias removal. Because the image is seen as intensity, for the sinusoidal signal depicted, the frequency of the latter would be double the original frequency, as seen in Figures 7-30c and 7-30d. Applications of this type of filter to detect the small images by removing the background (dc) light will be detailed later.

A band-pass filter is a combination of these filters resulting in a transparent section between the spatial frequencies ω_1 and ω_2. Such a filter is shown in Figure 7-31.

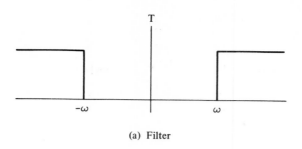

(a) Filter

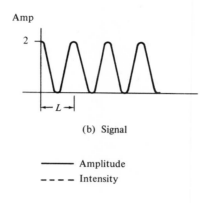

(b) Signal

——— Amplitude
- - - - Intensity

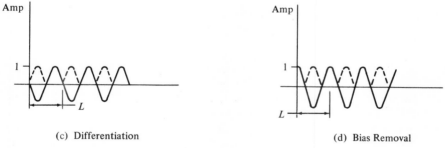

(c) Differentiation

(d) Bias Removal

Figure 7-30   High-pass filter and its functions.

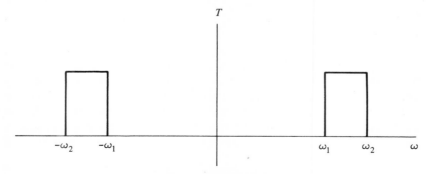

Figure 7-31   Band-pass filter.

403

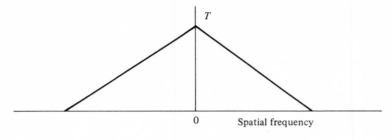

(a) Camera frequency response

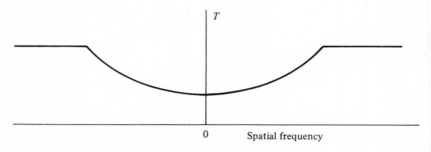

(b) Compensating filter transmission

Figure 7-32   Amplitude filters.

Amplitude Filter   An amplitude filter which is neither transparent nor opaque but possesses transmission that varies with position is more difficult to make and can be used to enhance or reduce certain spatial frequencies in an image.   For example, if a picture is taken by a camera with a spatial frequency response shown in Figure 7-32a, then the use of a filtering process of amplitude response shown in Figure 7-32b would result in a more faithful reproduction of the original image.   However, the amount of light reaching the detector will be reduced.   In addition, for accurate control of the filtering, the correct filter transmission needs to be constructed for the particular γ* of the photographic recording process of the original image.

Phase Filter   A filter that operates on the amplitude and phase can make compensations for images formed where the response goes negative for certain spatial frequencies.   The construction of a combined amplitude and phase filter is rather involved, but once it is obtained it may be used effectively to compensate for images from aberrated or defocused lenses.[16]

* γ is the relation between optical density of a developed photographic plate and the exposure to light.[21]

Directional Filter   The above filters were described in one dimension only; the spatial frequency plane, however, is two dimensional, and therefore directional filtering can be obtained.

For example, in an earlier section the diffraction pattern from a slit was described, and the result is reproduced in Figure 7-33a.   The pattern in the x_0 direction is given by $(\sin x_0/x_0)^2$ and in the y_0 direction by the Gaussian form for laser beams in a TEM_{00} mode, since the beam diameter is much smaller than the slit length.   If the slit were rotated, the diffraction pattern would rotate with it.   Figure 7-33b shows a line filter which could be used to filter out (stop) the diffraction pattern.   The diffraction pattern from either a slit or opaque strip will always lie along the x_0 axis and so will be blocked.   Figure 7-33c shows the diffraction pattern from a much shorter slit, and it can be seen that the pattern is much wider and the intensity variation in the y_0 direction is now given

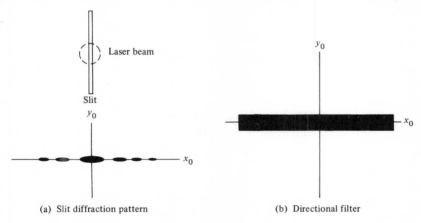

(a) Slit diffraction pattern   (b) Directional filter

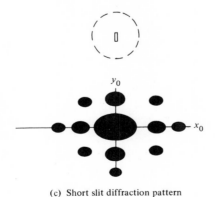

(c) Short slit diffraction pattern

Figure 7-33   Slit diffraction patterns and directional filter.

by $(\sin y_0/y_0)^2$.   To block this slit, the filter would need to be made much wider in the y_0 direction.   Obviously, the end result of trying to block narrower and narrower slits will be to block all spatial frequencies.   In this case, a compromise has to be reached to block edges down to a certain length while still allowing some light to the images which are to be detected.

7·3·6 defect detection

An application for a high-pass filter can be found in the system shown in Figure 7-34 to inspect semiconductor wafer surfaces.

The system uses a 5 mW HeNe laser operating in a TEM_{00} mode, whose beam is expanded to some convenient diameter.   This highly collimated beam is then reflected off the surface under inspection at an angle of incidence of about 12.5°.

A lens is used to collect the reflected light from the wafer surface. This lens will form a two-dimensional Fourier transform of the light amplitude reflected from the surface of the object (wafer) that is incident upon the lens, which may be represented by an illumination function $U_0(x, y)$.   It is assumed that the collimated beam incident upon the semiconductor wafer is of uniform intensity and possesses a plane wavefront.

If no imperfections (i.e., pits, projections, haze) are present on the surface, the light amplitude across the surface will be a constant, i.e.,

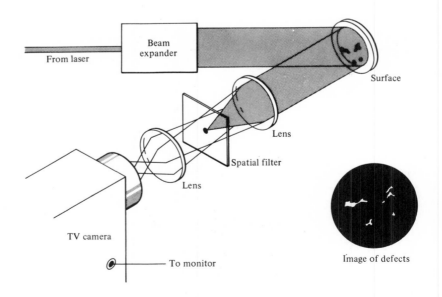

Figure 7-34   Spatial filtering system for surface inspection.

$U_0(x, y) = A$, and the lens will form the Fourier transform of this constant amplitude distribution in its focal point. The transform in this case is a two-dimensional impulse function[20] centered at the origin of the spatial frequency coordinate system and representing in the spatial frequency domain the bias mentioned previously. By placing a high-pass spatial filter consisting of an opaque central dot on a glass plate at the focal point of the lens, the constant information is blocked. Using a second lens to obtain a second Fourier transform, the final image, which in this case is a blackened field, or no image at all, is obtained. Thus, for a surface free of defects, no visible image will be obtained as a result of the spatial filtering process. However, $U_0(x, y)$ is not in general a constant, but varies with position along the surface. For example, assume that at various points on the surface there are small rectangularly shaped regions over which the light intensity is lower than on the rest of the surface. This condition, although idealized, is an approximation for a pit, projection, or some surface defect which scatters light away from the primary beam. In one dimension, this would be analogous to Figure 7-35, where the same light intensity for all imperfections is assumed.

In this case $U_0(x, y)$ can be expressed as

$$U(x, y) = A - \sum_i B_i [\mu(x - x_i + \Delta_i)\mu(y - y_i + \Delta_i) + \mu(x - x_i - \Delta_i)$$

$$\times \mu(y - y_i - \Delta_i) - \mu(x - x_i + \Delta_i)\mu(y - y_i - \Delta_i)$$

$$- \mu(x - x_i - \Delta_i)\mu(y - y_i + \Delta_i)] \tag{7-41}$$

where $\mu(x)$ and $\mu(y)$ are unit step functions (functions that are unity for positive argument and zero for negative arguments), and the other parameters are defined in Figure 7-35.

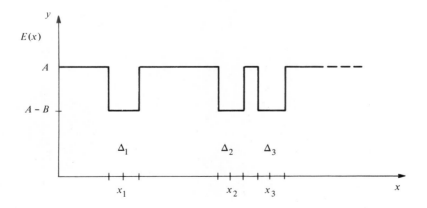

Figure 7-35 **One-dimensional model of light amplitude from an imperfect surface.**

The Fourier transform in this case consists not only of a two-dimensional impulse function centered at the origin of spatial frequency coordinates, but also a series of terms, in form similar to the one-dimensional function sin x/x, containing also the high spatial frequencies in the signal $U_0(x, y)$. By using the same type spatial filter (central opaque dot), the low-frequency information (bias) will be blocked, while the high-frequency information is passed. Again, using a second lens to take a second transform, an image of just the defects on the wafer is obtained. Removal of the null spatial frequency (bias) while transmitting the high spatial frequencies results in the defects being imaged as bright spots on a blackened background. Figure 7-36 shows a typical semiconductor substrate surface whose filtered image was detected by a vidicon and displayed on a TV monitor.

Once the filtered image is detected by the TV system, an electronics package similar to the one described subsequently in Section 7.3.15 can be used to count the number of defects or to give a percentage of area covered

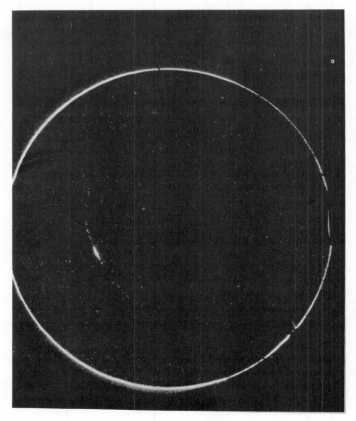

Figure 7-36   Defects observed on a semiconductor substrate with use of spatial filtering.

by defects.   By magnifying and viewing small portions of the wafer, micron-size defects can be detected and counted.

7·3·7   use of a directional filter

Directional filters can be used for simple pattern recognition or inspection. One such application, the inspection of integrated circuit photomasks[22] (used in the photolithographic process for making integrated circuits), will be discussed below.   It relies on the generally applicable condition that the pattern features are of the "Manhattan" type, i.e., they have edges only in two orthogonal directions.

The application uses a standard spatial filtering arrangement with the photomask in the object plane illuminated by a spatially coherent HeNe laser.   The filter is shown in Figure 7-37 and is an opaque cross that blocks the light from the features with lines along the orthogonal axes.   As explained earlier, the cross arms have to be wide enough to block the small correct features but narrow enough to pass the errors, i.e., details that are to be detected.

The errors in this case constitute features that do not have edges in only two orthogonal directions and are pinholes, scratches, dust, and other contamination of the pattern.   One of the consequences of the filter is that it also acts as a high-frequency pass filter, and therefore the errors are manifested by their edges only.   In addition, if a large part of the low-frequency spectrum is removed, the images become very blurred.

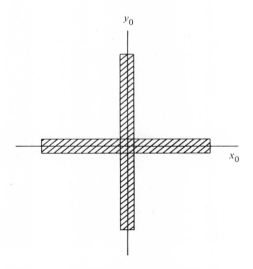

Figure 7-37   Cross-directional filter.

7·3·8 phase contrast and Schlieren effects

Although phase contrast and Schlieren effects are well known and documented techniques,[23] it is pertinent to describe them here briefly, since they are spatial filtering operations.

The phase contrast method is used to enable small phase objects (i.e., transparent objects) to become visible by transforming phase variations in the object into amplitude variations in the image. If, using the standard spatial filtering arrangement, a small phase object is illuminated with collimated light, the spatial light distribution leaving the object can be written (in one dimension only, for simplicity) as

$$U(x) = A \exp(i\phi(x)) \simeq A(1 + i\phi(x)) \tag{7-42}$$

where A is the amplitude of incident wave and ϕ is the phase acquired by the wave passing through the transparent phase object and is real and small.

The light amplitude distribution at the spatial frequency plane will then be the Fourier transform of (7-42) given by[5]

$$V(\omega) = A[2\pi\delta(\omega) + i\Phi(\omega)] \tag{7-43}$$

In (7-43), $\delta(\omega)$ is the delta function resulting from the constant incident light, and $\Phi(\omega)$ is the Fourier transform of $\phi(x)$. Since ϕ is small, the function $\Phi(\omega)$ will be spread over a large range of frequencies ω.

The filter used has a transmission characteristic given below

$$\begin{aligned} T(\omega) = i = e^{i\pi/2} &\qquad |\omega| < \varepsilon \\ = 1 &\qquad |\omega| > \varepsilon \end{aligned} \tag{7-44}$$

where ε is made relatively small so that only a negligible part of $\Phi(\omega)$ is affected.

Such a filter usually consists of a very thin transparent plate of lateral dimension corresponding to a frequency ε, which retards the light passing through it by a quarter wavelength. After passing through the filter, the light amplitude will have the Fourier transform given by

$$V'(\omega) = A(2\pi i\delta(\omega) + i\Phi(\omega)) \tag{7-45}$$

since only the impulse function will be affected by the $\pi/2$ phase introduced by the filter. The intensity of the image will be the square of the amplitude of the inverse Fourier transformation of $V'(\omega)$ in (7-45) which is given by

$$I(x) \simeq A^2(1 + 2\phi(x)) \tag{7-46}$$

and the effect of the filtering is to suppress the factor i in (7-42) leading to an intensity which is linearly related to the phase of the object. Amplitude filtering of the constant term by reducing its transmission through the filter further improves the contrast between the image and the background.

Similar but less effective results could be achieved by simply blocking the impulse term (central dark ground method) or by blocking the $-\omega$ spectrum and passing the ω frequencies. The latter is denoted as the Schlieren method.

7.3.9 spatial frequency spectrum of periodic patterns

One type of pattern which effectively lends itself to analysis by spatial filtering is an array-type structure consisting of identical features repeated on a constant separation. Consequently, spatial filtering has recently been applied to photomask inspection,[24-26] grid inspection,[27] and to an array pattern smoothing.[28]

Consider the simple example of a periodic pattern consisting of an array of slits shown in Figure 7-38. Since Fourier transformation is a linear process,[5] the diffraction pattern of this array will be the superposition of the respective diffraction patterns from each slit. This is shown

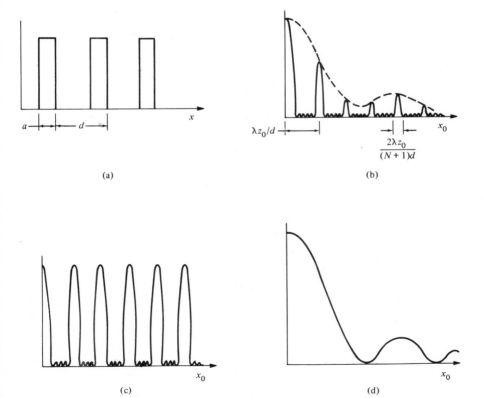

(a)

(b)

(c)

(d)

Figure 7-38 Periodic slits and their diffraction pattern.

in the equation below which is the sum of the slit diffraction patterns described in (7-27).

$$U(x_0, y_0) = \frac{\exp(ikz_0)\exp[i(k/2z_0)(x_0^2 + y_0^2)]}{i\lambda z_0}$$

$$\times C \sum_n \iint_{A_n} \exp\{-i(k/z_0)[x_0(x_n + x) + y_0(y_n + y)]\}\, dx\, dy \quad (7\text{-}47)$$

In this equation the array of slits is assumed to be illuminated by a constant light amplitude C, (x_n, y_n) are the coordinate points of each aperture, and x, y are coordinate frames set at each aperture. The integration extends over each aperture area A_n.

Equation (7-47) can be rewritten in the form

$$U(x_0, y_0) = C \sum_n \exp[-i(k/z_0)(x_0 x_n + y_0 y_n)]$$

$$\times \frac{\exp(ikz_0)\exp[i(k/2z_0)(x_0^2 + y_0^2)]}{i\lambda z_0} \iint_A \exp[-i(k/z_0)(x_0 x + y_0 y)]\, dx\, dy$$

$$(7\text{-}48)$$

where A is now the integral over any aperture. Equation (7-48) is seen to be simply a product of the diffraction pattern of one slit and the exponential sum.

When the integral is evaluated and the result simplified to the one-dimensional case, the intensity of the diffraction pattern assumes the form

$$I(x_0) = \frac{I_0}{(N + 1)^2} \left\{ \frac{\sin[(N + 1)(k/2z_0)x_0\, d]}{\sin(kx_0\, d/2z_0)} \right\}^2 \left\{ \frac{\sin(kx_0\, a/2z_0)}{kx_0\, a/2z_0} \right\}^2 \quad (7\text{-}49)$$

where $N + 1$ is the total number of slits in the x direction, d is the periodic separation between slits in that direction, and I_0 is the intensity at $x_0 = 0$. This intensity pattern is shown in Figure 7-38b. The diffraction pattern is the product of two terms. The first term $\{\sin^2[(N + 1)(k/2z_0)x_0\, d]/\sin^2[(kx_0\, d/2z_0)]\}$ is depicted in Figure 7-38c and represents the interference term for $N + 1$ slits, whereas the second term is the single-slit diffraction pattern (Figure 7-38d). The diffraction pattern of an array of slits is thus an array of spots whose separation is determined by the separation of slits. The intensity of the spots is modulated by the form of the single slit diffraction pattern. For a more complicated array, the result will be very similar, the separation of the spots (i.e., the interference function) will depend on the feature spacing in the array, and the modulation of the intensity will follow the diffraction pattern of one feature.

The size of the spot is governed primarily by the interference function. The first minimum for this function occurs for x_0 satisfying the relation

$$(N + 1)\frac{kx_0 d}{2z_0} = \pi \tag{7-50}$$

or

$$x_{0\,min} = \frac{\lambda z_0}{(N + 1)d}$$

By defining the spot diameter as $2x_{0min}$,

$$S = 2x_{0min} = \frac{2\lambda z_0}{(N + 1)d} \tag{7-51}$$

The separation of the spots is also governed by the interference function and is given by the inverse of the spatial frequency of repetition $2\pi d/\lambda z_0$.

Thus the separation h is given by

$$h = 2\pi \left/ \frac{2\pi d}{\lambda z_0} = \frac{\lambda z_0}{d} \right. \tag{7-52}$$

The analogy between spatial frequency spectrum and an electronic frequency spectrum helps in the clarification. The array of slits is a periodic square wave whose spectrum contains a fundamental frequency plus harmonics. The periodicity gives rise to an interference function whose various spots represent the fundamental frequency and its harmonics. The spot at zero is the constant term, i.e., a bias level. The modulation function, on the other hand, contains the frequency components of an individual pulse. The diameter of the spots represents the resolution of the spectrum analyzer and compares to the resolution of a diffraction limited lens which might be used to form the diffraction pattern. This will limit the total number of slits $N + 1$.

As a final result, the information pertaining to array structures is contained in very restricted and discrete areas of the spatial frequency spectrum. This implies that spatial filtering can be used effectively to discriminate between periodic structures and nonperiodic (i.e., random) structures, since the latter normally contain a frequency spectrum distributed over the whole or a large area of the spatial frequency plane.

7·3·10   types of filtering: periodic stop filters

There are two basic spatial filtering operations which may be performed on a periodic array. The first involves filtering out the periodic structure frequencies while transmitting the rest, and the second entails the opposite, transmitting only the periodic frequency spectrum.

The principal application of a stop filter is in the inspection of array patterns where the array pattern is suppressed by the filter leaving images of all the errors. Applications have been reported for photomask inspection and electron tube grid inspection.[27]

The operation is shown schematically in Figure 7-39 where the spatial filtering arrangement is depicted at the top (in one dimension) and the various states of the signal in going through the elements of the spatial filter are presented below. The array pattern is depicted as an array of slits and an error is added, in this case, as an extra slit. The diffraction pattern is shown as two separate parts: the diffraction pattern of the array, with the array of spots (the secondary minima have been neglected in this drawing) and the diffraction from the error slit. The combined effect would be their superposition, taking account of the phase relationships between the patterns. The filter is constructed to attenuate the array diffraction pattern, and, as can be seen, this will also stop a small part of the error diffraction pattern. On reforming the image with the second lens, the filtered diffraction pattern, which is due to the error, gives rise to an image of the error. In addition, the filter also generates secondary errors; these, however, are of significantly lower intensity than the primary error intensity.

It is important to note here that a light image is always produced, whether the error is a transmission defect or an opaque defect. This is due to the fact that the central bright spot, i.e., the zero frequency, is stopped and any bias is removed. This is in accordance with the result

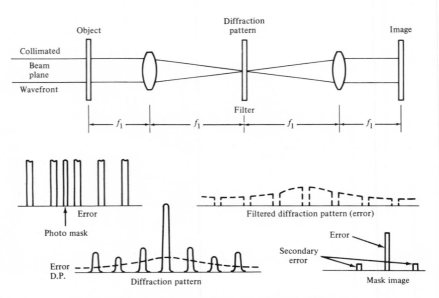

Figure 7-39   Schematic diagram of spatial filtering.

obtained in the section on simple diffraction patterns, where it is shown that the patterns for a narrow slit and its inverse, the wire, were the same except for the central bright spot which is due to the diffraction of the laser beam itself.

A picture of an actual spatial filter employed in the detection of grid errors is shown in Figure 7-40.   The grid to be inspected consisted of a 12.5 cm square mesh having 40 lines per mm.   Using spatial filtering all 25 million squares may be inspected simultaneously since the pattern array is periodic.   Figure 7-41a depicts the grid to be inspected, Figure 7-41b shows the corresponding diffraction pattern, whereas Figure 7-41c presents the reconstructed image containing errors which are obtained after the filtering operation.

Another very similar application of the spatial filter has been demonstrated in the inspection of the collimating grid used in the diode array vidicon for the Picturephone® set.   This grid also has a line spacing of 25 μm, and the width of the lines is less than 7.5 μm.   The grid can be either totally viewed for a general look, with the result shown in Figure 7-42, or scanned under reduced field conditions.   A resolution of 2.5 μm was obtained for a small field and 5 μm for a larger one.   A TV scanning system was constructed to automatically count the number of errors within a specified field, and it was shown that the technique could readily be adapted to conform with the inspection criteria of separation of at least 1 mm between defects affecting two or more holes.

The simplest method of constructing a filter is by direct photography. In this case, a relatively perfect array is placed at the object and a negative photographic plate is exposed to the diffraction pattern.   After developing, this plate can be used as the filter.   If a linear filter is desired, then the developments should be done with a γ of 1.   However, in most cases,

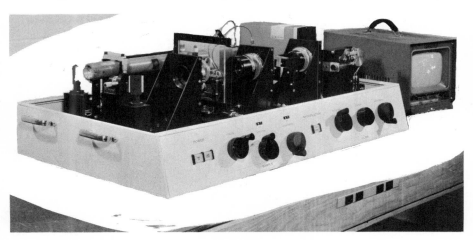

Figure 7-40   Spatial filter for the detection of errors in a 12.5 cm × 12.5 cm grid.[27]   *(With permission of Machine Design.)*

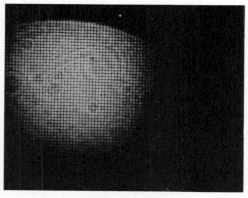

(a) Grid to be inspected

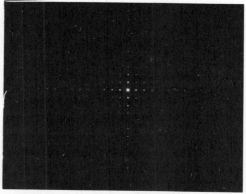

(b) Diffraction pattern of grid

(c) Errors displayed as a result of
the filtering

*Figure 7-41   States of signal (illuminated grid) in going through
spatial filter.*[27]   *(With permission of Machine Design.)*

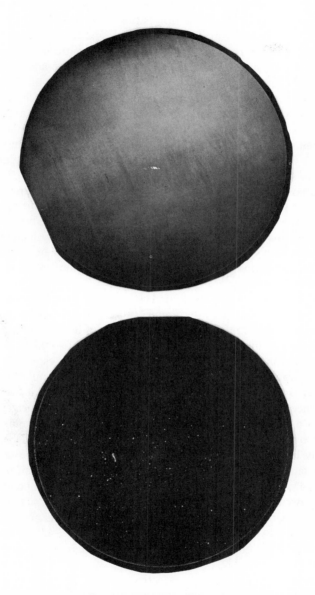

Figure 7-42   Picturephone grid and an image displaying its errors.

only strong attenuation of the array diffraction is required, and so the γ is not critical. Early experiments on mask inspection[24] and grid inspection[27] used this type of filter. However, as has been pointed out,[24] the intensity range of the diffraction pattern is so great that it is difficult to obtain a correct exposure over the entire pattern, and therefore the method is efficient only for simple diffraction patterns. Assuming the achievement of a linear filter, this method does have an advantage which is contained in the fact that all the intensity information on the diffraction pattern is recorded on the filter. This fact means that the filter should detect arrays of the same period but of different features and points out that the features are not correct even though they have similar frequency components. However, the kinds of differences detectable tend to be gross. It would be similar to the kinds of amplitude filtering described in the earlier sections.

A second type of periodic filter is the interference function filter,[26] which has also been employed for mask inspection. In this case, a binary filter is made in the form of the interference function and comprises an array of opaque spots. The size of the dots is normally made larger than the diffraction pattern spot size for reasons that will be explained later. (The secondary side maxima are not considered since most of the light is in the primary maxima.)

Figure 7-43 shows an integrated circuit mask imaged through a spatial filtering system using the interference function filter. This type of filter has the advantage of not containing the effects of the exposure problems of the first type of filter; however, it needs relatively sophisticated drafting and photographic reduction techniques to construct, especially for image arrays of large periods where the number of dots in the filter is very large. This filter operates in a slightly different manner; since it attenuates the interference function it blocks all spatial frequencies corresponding to a certain array period. Thus, any feature repeated on the array will be stopped by the filter. This makes the filter more versatile in the sense that only one filter is required to inspect any array of the same period. It is not sensitive to details of repetitious features. This can be seen from Figure 7-43; the apparent error in the second row, second column feature, is in fact not an error at all. That element in the array actually contains the correct features; however, it is the element which is not repeated, and is thus shown as an error. Notice also in Figure 7-43 the fact that the errors show up light whether they are transmission errors or opaque errors.

This kind of filtering is an effective method for inspecting array patterns such as IC masks and electron tube grids by allowing the observation of nonperiodic errors. The procedure of inspection only requires rotary alignment of the array, and means that it can be scanned through the laser beam. Finally, using the interference function filter, only a single filter is required for each set of arrays of the same period.

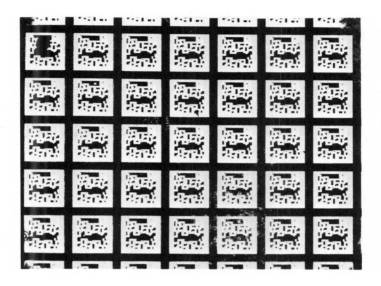

Figure 7-43 Integrated circuit photomask and its errors displayed through spatial filtering.

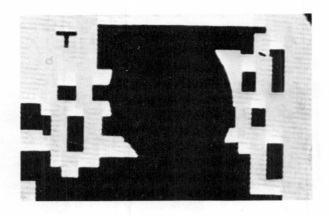

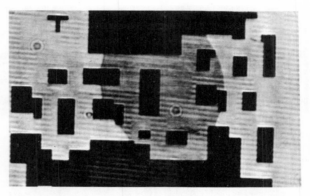

Figure 7-44   Defective feature and its reconstructed image.

7·3·11   periodic transmission filters

The effect of a filter which transmits the interference function or the periodic diffraction pattern is to block most of the light from nonperiodic features.   This can be used to " clean up " a periodic array by removing defects, producing an array of identical features.   Figure 7-44 shows one feature of an array where a transmission filter filled in, to a large extent, the defect shown.   A filter of this form has also been used for smoothing or averaging noisy periodic images,[28] and Figure 7-45 shows an electron micrograph image which was smoothed using a periodic filter.

7·3·12   auxiliary filters

Other simple filters can be used with the periodic filter to improve the detection of errors; e.g., a high-pass filter can be used if it is known that the defects are all small.

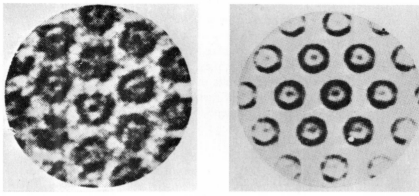

MICROGRAPH

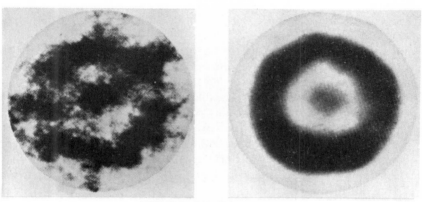

EFFECT OF SMOOTHING FILTER

Figure 7-45 Electron micrograph image smoothing with periodic filter.[28] *(With permission of* **Scientific American.**)

7·3·13 limitations

Up to now, no mention has been made of limitations due to lens aberrations and how they and other effects limit resolution of the spatial filter. The remainder of the section on periodic filters will be devoted to a discussion of some of these problems.

<u>Coherence Requirements</u> The degree of spatial coherence limits the spectral resolution of the spatial filter. Normally, using a single transverse mode laser, the spatial coherence is nearly perfect. However, for some filtering applications, a well-collimated, nonlaser source may be sufficient; but its limited spatial coherence will significantly affect the spatial filter performance.

In Section 3.1.1 the collimation property of an unknown mode structured beam was expressed in terms of the divergence of the beam. When this beam passes through the lens, it forms a spot of radius $w = \theta \times f$ in the diffraction pattern plane, where f is the lens focal length, and θ is the divergence half angle. This spot may be viewed as a spread in the zero frequency and the spot thus results in a frequency width of $4\pi w/\lambda f$. In terms of angle (assuming small diffraction angles) the resolution is thus 2θ and means that any spatial frequency will be displayed at the diffraction pattern plane with an angular spread of 2θ. Thus filtering to bandwidths smaller than $4\pi\theta/\lambda$ is not possible.

Limitations of a Lens Due to Aperture and Aberrations   Since the lenses are the primary elements of the spatial filter, their performance governs the efficiency of the system. In a normal imaging system the lens is required to transfer an image from one plane to another. These planes are called the *conjugate planes*, and the lens will be optimized for operation at these planes. For spatial filtering a lens is required to operate at four planes: the two conjugate image planes and the two conjugate diffraction planes. For example, in the standard spatial filtering setup, the object is at the left focal plane and, therefore, its image will be at infinity to the right. The diffraction pattern is at the focal plane on the right and is thus the imaging pattern from an imaginary object at infinity to the left. These are the two pairs of conjugates for which the lens should be designed, and they call for a symmetrical lens designed for infinite conjugates. Since most off-the-shelf lenses are optimized for only one pair of conjugates, the best operation of a spatial filter requires a custom designed lens.

In Figure 7-26a the lens would need to be designed for the imaging conjugates of magnification m and the diffraction conjugate, which is the infinite conjugate. This is why the system in Figure 7-28 should offer the highest quality image, provided only low-resolution filtering is required, since the second lens only has to operate at the one pair of imaging conjugates.

Resolution of Imaging   The definition of a diffraction limited f/number lens, at specified conjugate planes, is given in the Glossary; and, when light passes through such a lens, it may be focused to a minimum spot radius of w_0. The minimum spacing between point images that are just resolved by the lens is w_0 and even though features giving rise to frequencies greater than that corresponding to w_0 may exist in the object, they will not be resolved in the image. Normally they will add a background noise in the image plane, so that a low-pass filter is sometimes helpful in reducing this problem.

Applying a common criterion to the definition of resolution,* for uniform illumination the separation between two just resolved central diffraction discs formed by an aperture of radius w, of a diffraction limited

---

* See Glossary for a definition of diffraction limit of a lens.

lens of focal length f is given by*

$$w_0 = \frac{1.22\,\lambda f}{2w} \tag{7-53}$$

It is important to know this resolution not only in the center but over the entire field of the image, since resolution usually deteriorates at the edge of the field.

Resolution of Diffraction Pattern   The same kind of criterion that was applied to imaging above may be used in stating the lens performance for diffraction; however, it is instructive to discuss these effects on the filtering and the filtered image.

The resolution w_0 in terms of the diffraction pattern now defines the spectral resolution, so that discrimination between spatial frequencies smaller than that corresponding to w_0 represents images with a period larger than the diffraction limited lens aperture.   Figure 7-46 shows the

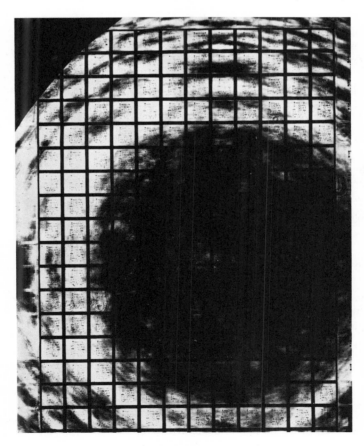

Figure 7-46   Result of filtering with a lens of insufficient aperture.

* See also Section 3.1.1.

result of using a periodic filter on an IC photomask where the lens had a diffraction limited aperture of $f/8$, and thus only the center portion is filtered. If an increase in the field is desired and lower resolution of filtering can be tolerated, the actual lens aperture can be increased. This will improve detectability, but since the imaging properties of a lens deteriorate with increased aperture, the size of the opaque spots of the filter will have to be increased. This increases the field over which filtering is achieved but decreases the resolution.

The field of view of the lens determines the highest spatial frequency that can be resolved. The resolution deterioration toward the edge of the diffraction pattern means that the higher frequencies will be displayed with lower resolution. This will not necessarily imply any limitation on image resolution at these frequencies; however, it will affect how well these frequencies can be detected or filtered.

7.3.14 practical inspection system

As was mentioned earlier, periodic filters have been suggested for use in applications involving IC mask inspection and grid inspection, with both being readied for full use as production-line techniques.

A practical problem with the former or any other pattern which is supported on a substrate is the quality of the transmitting substrate material. The diffraction pattern is a function of both amplitude and phase of the light illuminating the object; therefore, any phase changes caused by glass unevenness modifies the diffraction pattern. For example, consider a simple slit diffraction pattern. If a piece of glass of small wedge angle α is introduced in front of the slit, as depicted in Figure 7-47, the wedge produces a change in the angle of the incident plane wavefront of $\theta = (n - 1)\alpha$, where n is the index of refraction of the substrate. The diffraction pattern of the slit (in one dimension) then becomes

$$U(x_0) = \frac{\exp(ikz_0)\exp\left(i\dfrac{k}{2z}x_0^2\right)}{i\lambda z_0} C \int_{-a/2}^{a/2} \exp(ik\theta x)\exp[ik(x_0/z_0)x]\, dx \quad (7\text{-}54)$$

where use has been made of the one-dimensional analog of (7-37). Performing the integration gives the following expression for the intensity of the diffraction pattern:

$$I(x_0) = I_0 \frac{\sin^2\left[\dfrac{ka}{2}\left(\dfrac{x_0}{x_0} + \theta\right)\right]}{\left[\dfrac{ka}{2}\left(\dfrac{x_0}{z_0} + \theta\right)\right]^2} \quad (7\text{-}55)$$

In (7-55) expression I_0 is once more the peak intensity, and the equation has a form identical to the one-dimensional analog of a simple slit diffraction given in (7-28) except for the shift by an angle of $ka\theta/2$.

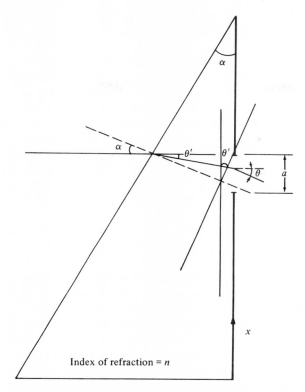

Figure 7-47   Diffraction geometry of a slit preceded by wedged glass.

The effect of varying substrate thickness can be seen in Figure 7-43 where some of the correct features appear as errors.   One standard method of eliminating this difficulty consists of the use of a liquid gate where the object is immersed in a tank containing transparent liquid whose refractive index matches that of the substrate,[6] as is illustrated schematically in Figure 7-48.

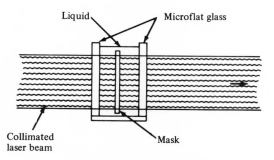

Figure 7-48   Liquid gate.

7·3·15   TV detection system

For the inspection applications described, the only light images produced were those which constituted the errors.   In this form they can be analyzed with a simple TV detection system which will count the number of errors present and also make size estimates, etc.   A short description is given below of the features built into such a system for both mask inspection and surface inspection.

Figure 7-49 is a block diagram of the circuits.   The camera is placed so that an image on the spatial filter output falls onto the vidicon.   The video signal from the camera consists of a sequence of the sweeps of the electron beam across the vidicon face, and the signal voltage is proportional to the light intensity on the vidicon at the position of the electron beam.   Normally there are 525 separate sweeps across the vidicon to cover the entire area, each lasting 63 μs and thus giving a total frame period of 32 ms.   The analyzing circuit following the camera selects a frame of video signal and records when the electron beam sweeps through an error, as indicated by a change in signal voltage.   With a large error (greater than one scan width), the electron beam may scan across it more than once and so may give more than one record or count.   The rest of the analyzing circuit can process these records in a number of ways.

A. Total Count—Counter is made to increment for each detected error giving a total count of the number of errors scanned by the electron beam.   This will be larger than the number of errors because, with a large error, the electron beam will scan through it more than once.

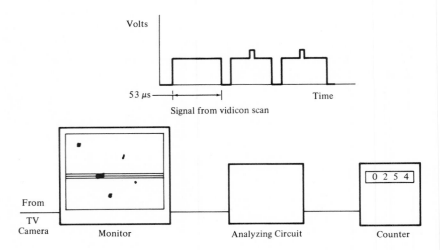

Figure 7-49   TV detection system for counting errors.

B. Error Magnitude—Counter is made to increment an amount corresponding to the size (in the scan direction) of the error, each time
an error is recorded. This is achieved by starting and stopping a
clock during the time the error is being scanned. This gives a count
proportional to the light area on the vidicon.

In addition, the above modes can be used where a variable number of
scan lines are monitored, such as one scan line or a block of scan lines
in a critical part of the image. This kind of detection provides a quick
quantitative estimate of the image; however, it is severely limited because
of the poor resolution of the TV camera. Resolution of much better than
1000×1000 counts is difficult to achieve, whereas the image from the
spatial filtering system has a much better resolution than this.

7·4   complex spatial filter

In the previous discussion the filters have all been relatively simple, being
primarily amplitude filters. The major reason has been the lack of a
simple effective technique for making a filter of a complex signal spectrum
$S(x_0, y_0)$ containing both amplitude and phase information. This
problem has been overcome[29] using the holographic principle, and its use
is demonstrated here in a character recognition problem.

7·4·1   matched filter

The concept of a matched filter is familiar to communication engineers
where it has long been recognized as an optimum detection scheme for a
known signal buried in uniform (white) noise. If a particular electronic
signal to be detected has a frequency spectrum given by $S(\omega)$, the matched
filter which provides the linear operation that maximizes the ratio of
instantaneous signal power to average noise power will have a frequency
response given by[30] $H(\omega) = S^*(\omega)$ (the complex conjugate of the signal
spectrum $S(\omega)$). In our treatment the optical signal will be considered
noiseless, and the matched filter is used as an element in a character
recognition problem.

When a matched filter is used in a two-dimensional character recognition system, such as the one depicted schematically in Figure 7-50, we
note that incident upon the filter will be a light distribution which is
proportional to $S(x_0, y_0)$, the Fourier transform of the light distribution
at the input plane. If the filter is matched to that signal, the field distribution transmitted by it is proportional to $S(x_0, y_0) S^*(x_0, y_0)$. Since
$|S(x_0, y_0)|^2$ is a real quantity, it implies that the filter exactly cancels the
wavefront curvature introduced by the optical input signal, and the

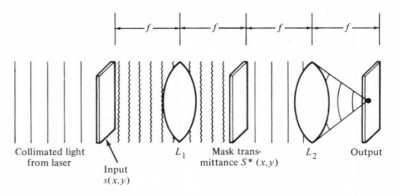

Figure 7-50   Optical interpretation of the matched-filtering operation.

transmitted wavefront is planar.   This planar wave will be focused to a bright spot by the second lens in the system at the output plane.   When another signal is present at the input plane, the product of its Fourier transform and $S^*(x_0, y_0)$ will not in general be real, which means that its wavefront curvature will not be exactly canceled by the matched filters. The light transmitted by the filter will thus not be brought to a bright focus at the output plane, and the presence or absence of a known signal at the input may be deduced by measuring the intensity of light at the focal point of the second lens.

7·4·2   constructing matched filters

Figure 7-51a shows one of the methods of constructing a complex filter. The lower arm of this modified Mach-Zehnder interferometer corresponds to the first half of the spatial filter with the collimated beam going through the object, and lens, and then forming the diffraction pattern at its focal plane.   The top arm of the interferometer introduces a collimated beam onto the diffraction pattern to interfere with it.   The beam is introduced at an angle θ to the spatial filter axis.   The recording photographic plate thus records the interference (or product) of these two beams.   The plate records the intensity of the light to give $I(x_0, y_0)$ the filter plate transmission.

$$I(x_0, y_0) = R^2 + |S(x_0, y_0)|^2 + RS(x_0, y_0) \exp(-ik \sin \theta\, y_0)$$

$$+ RS^*(x_0, y_0) \exp(+ik \sin \theta\, y_0) \quad (7\text{-}56)$$

where $S(x_0, y_0)$ is the signal spectrum and $R \exp(+ik \sin \theta\, y_0)$ is the interfering beam at angle θ to the x_0 axis with an amplitude R.   The last

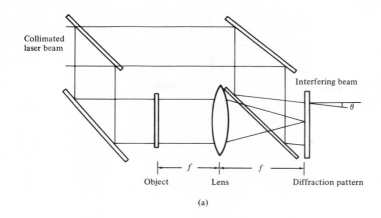

(a)

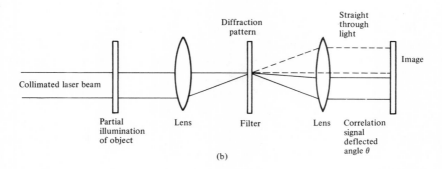

(b)

Figure 7-51   Methods for constructing and using a complex spatial filter.

term of the equation is proportional to the required matched filter frequency response.

The effect of the phase term $\exp(ik \sin \theta \, y_0)$ is to deflect the output away from the axis when a matched filter constructed in this fashion is used. This is essential since it isolates it from the effects of the other terms in the equation. For a fuller account of the holographic technique of wavefront recording and reconstruction, see Chapter 8.

The method of filtering is shown in Figure 7-51b using a standard spatial filtering arrangement. The output, as shown, is deflected by angle θ, where the small angle assumption has once more been made. The illumination as shown is somewhat restricted to prevent the signal detection output from overlapping the images from other terms in (7-56) which are not deflected. By increasing the angle θ, a larger part of the object can be illuminated.

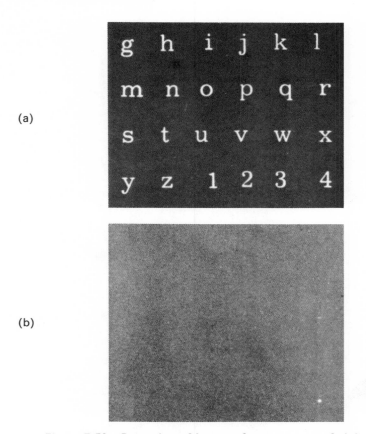

(a)

(b)

**Figure 7-52   Detection of letter g from an array of alphanumerics.[29]
(With permission of IEEE, Inc.)**

Figure 7-52 shows an example of the detection of a letter g from an array of alphanumerics. Just as in the previous spatial filtering applications, the image (in this case the light spot) is in the same relative position as the object. Here, too, there is no need to critically align the object transversely; however, it does have to be aligned in rotation. This technique is very important in enabling any passive type of filter to be constructed and should add numerous applications to spatial filtering.

7.5 Fresnel correlation

In the previous spatial filtering examples, the illumination of the object was always a normally incident plane whose spatial frequency was zero. In this last section, spatial filtering will be explored a step further; in this case, the illumination beam is no longer normally incident and its Fourier transform will contain some spatial frequency or a number of frequencies.

A complete account of the theory and range of possible applications is beyond the scope of this section and so an example will be given to illustrate the technique.

7·5·1   step and repeat measurement

By comparing two amplitude signals, one of which is a standard, accurate high-resolution tests on the other signal can be made.   This method has been applied to the checking of photomask array feature registration against a reference fringe pattern.[31]   The product of the two signals was passed through a low-pass filter to display a correlation signal.

Figure 7-53 shows a schematic of the spatial filtering arrangement. A collimated beam is split into two equal intensity beams and brought onto the mask at angle θ.   If λ is the light wavelength, this arrangement creates an interference fringe pattern on the mask with period $\lambda_F = \lambda/(\sin \theta/2)$, and the corresponding frequency is at a multiple of the repetition frequency of the periodic pattern.   Since both incident waves are plane waves, the fringe pattern is sinusoidal, and the fringe pattern intensity has a wavelength $\lambda_F/2$.   A mask of simple features, an array of slits, is used to discuss the result of combining the fringe pattern and a periodic pattern.

The mask transmits portions of the fringe pattern whose spatial frequency spectrum is displayed at the focal plane of the lens.   This frequency spectrum shows the carrier (the fringe pattern) modulated by the mask spectrum.   This is manifested by two diffraction patterns of the mask centered about the fringe pattern frequencies ω_F and $-\omega_F$, as shown in Figure 7-53.

To observe the relation between the fringe pattern and the mask, a low-pass filter is placed to block frequencies greater than or equal to ω_F (the pass bandwidth is optimized for the effects which are to be discussed).

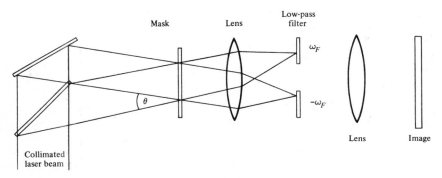

Figure 7-53 Spatial filtering configuration for step and repeat measurements.

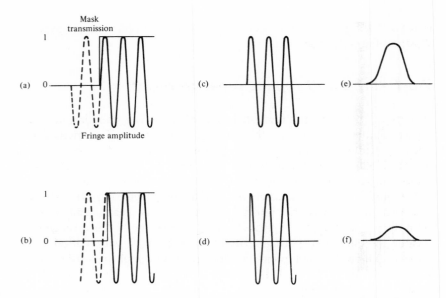

Figure 7-54   Relations between fringe and mask and their effect on the output image.

The result can be explained with the help of Figure 7-54.   The aim is to detect where a mask feature edge is located with respect to the fringe pattern.   The two extreme cases shown are: (a) when the edge coincides with the fringe maximum (positive or negative), and (b) when the edge is at a fringe zero.   The signals are shown in (c) and (d).   The effect of taking these through a low-pass filter is shown in (e) and (f) and is seen to produce a low-frequency pulse whose intensity depends on the cutoff position of the edge.   A maximum value exists when the edge is at a fringe zero and vice versa.   This follows from the fact that the high-frequency components at the plane of the low-pass filter depend on the relative positions of the pattern edge and the fringe maximum.   Thus, the position of the edge can be determined within one period of the fringe pattern by observing the pulse intensity.

Figure 7-55 shows the result for an array, the lines being the pulses from the feature border edges.   In case (a), the array is correct and all the edges coincide with a fringe zero.   In case (b), the array has errors showing variations in the pulse intensity.   In these pictures HeNe laser wavelength was 632.8 nm and the interference fringe period λ_F was 10 μm, giving a distance of 2.5 μm between the pulse maximum and minimum. One point to note is that only the position of the edge within one half-fringe period can be detected; i.e., the pulse does not indicate which fringe the edge is aligned with.   For a complete check of edge position a

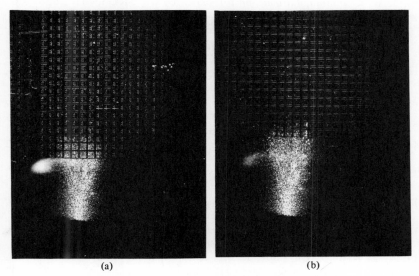

(a) (b)

Figure 7-55 Results of step and repeat measurement.

number of fringes have to be used, starting with low frequencies and working up.

An obvious advantage of this technique lies in the fact that it quickly displays the difference in one look over a large array area. In addition, lenses need not be of high quality since they only have to deal with a low-frequency signal. It is the beam collimation and the beamsplitting optics which establish the standards that have to be very accurate. A disadvantage of the method results from the fact that a well-formed distinct edge, such as a border, is required to easily observe the pulse. In a complex feature there will be many pulses, all of different intensities, for all of the feature edges.

References

1. A. Sommerfeld, *Optics Lectures on Theoretical Physics*, Vol. IV, Academic Press Inc., New York (1954).
2. P. A. Hickman, "Optical Tooling Viewed in a New Light," *Laser Focus* **4**, No. 5, 22 (1968).
3. W. B. Herrmannsfeldt *et al.*, Precision Alignment Using a System of Large Rectangular Fresnel Lenses," *Appl. Opt.* **7**, 995 (1968).
4. A. Chrzanowski *et al.*, "New Laser Applications in Geodetic and Engineering Surveys," *IEEE J. of Quantum Electronics* **QE-7**, 304 (1971).
5. A. Papoulis, *The Fourier Integral and Its Applications*, McGraw-Hill Book Co., New York (1962).

6. J. W. Goodman, *Introduction to Fourier Optics*, McGraw-Hill Book Co., New York (1968).

7. L. A. Jeffers, *IEEE Conference on Laser Engineering and Applications*, paper THAM 11.5, "Determination of the Diameter of Small Fibers by Diffraction of a Laser Beam," Washington, D.C. (May 1967).

8. W. A. Farone and M. Kerker, "Light Scattering from Long Submicron Glass Cylinders at Normal Incidence," *J. Opt. Soc. Amer.* **56**, 481 (1966).

9. L. S. Watkins and V. J. Zaleckas, *IEEE Conference on Laser Engineering and Applications*, paper 9.9, "Dynamic Wire Measurements by Automatically Monitoring the Laser Diffraction Pattern," Washington, D.C. (May 1969).

10. W. T. Cochran *et al.*, "What Is the Fast Fourier Transform?" *Proc. IEEE* **55**, 1664 (1967).

11. A. Van der Lugt, "A Review of Optical Data-Processing Techniques," *Optica Act* **15**, 1 (1968).

12. D. K. Pollack, C. J. Koester, and J. T. Tippett, Eds., *Optical Processing Information*, Spartan Books, New York (1963).

13. J. T. Tippett *et al.*, *Optical and Electro-Optical Information Processing*, Massachusetts Institute of Technology Press, Cambridge, Mass. (1965).

14. A. Marechal, "Un Filtre de Frequences Spatiales pour L'Amelioration du Contrast des Images Optiques," *Comptes Rendus Acad. Sci.* **237**, 607 (1953).

15. E. Abbe, *Archiv. f. Mikroskopesche Anot.* **9**, 413 (1837).

16. J. Tsujiuchi, "Correction of Optical Images by Compensation of Aberrations and by Spatial Frequency Filtering," *Progress in Optics* (E. Wolf, Ed.), Vol. 2, p. 133 (1963).

17. L. J. Cutrona *et al.*, "Optical Data Processing and Filtering Systems," *IRE Trans. Infor. Theory* **6**, 386 (1960).

18. E. L. O'Neill, "Spatial Filtering in Optics," *IRE Trans. Infor. Theory* **2**, 56 (1956).

19. J. H. Van Vleck and D. Middleton, *J. Appl. Phys.* **17**, 940 (1946).

20. A. Papoulis, *Systems and Transforms with Applications in Optics*, McGraw-Hill Book Co., New York (1968).

21. J. B. DeVelis and G. O. Reynolds, *Theory and Application of Holography*, Addison Wesley Publishing Co., Inc., Reading, Mass. (1967).

22. N. Axelrod, "Improved Defect Detection for Photolithographic Masks," *IEEE International Electron Devices Meeting*, Washington, D.C. (October 1969).

23. M. Born and E. Wolf, *Principles of Optics*, Rev. Ed. 4th Ed., Pergamon Press, Inc., New York (1970).

24. L. S. Watkins, "Inspection of Periodic Patterns with Intensity Spatial Filters," *Solid State Technology* **12**, No. 2, 35 (1969).

25. L. S. Watkins, "Integrated Circuit Photomask Inspection by Spatial Filtering," *Solid State Technology* **12**, No. 9, 29 (1969).

26. L. S. Watkins, "Inspection of Integrated Circuit Photomasks with Intensity Spatial Filters," *Proc. IEEE* **57**, 1634 (1969).

27. R. Kohl, "Optical Computers," *Machine Design* **41**, No. 19, 116 (1969).

28. R. D. B. Fraser, "Keratins," *Sci. American* **221**, No. 2, 86 (1969).

29. A. Van Der Lugt, "Signal Detection by Complex Spatial Filtering," *IEEE Trans. Infor. Theory* **10**, 139 (1964).

30. M. W. Brown, *Analysis of Linear Time Invariant Systems*, McGraw-Hill Book Co., New York (1963).
31. L. S. Watkins, " Integrated Circuit Step and Repeat Inspection Using Spatial Filtering," *IEEE International Electron Devices Meeting*, Washington, D.C. (October 1969).

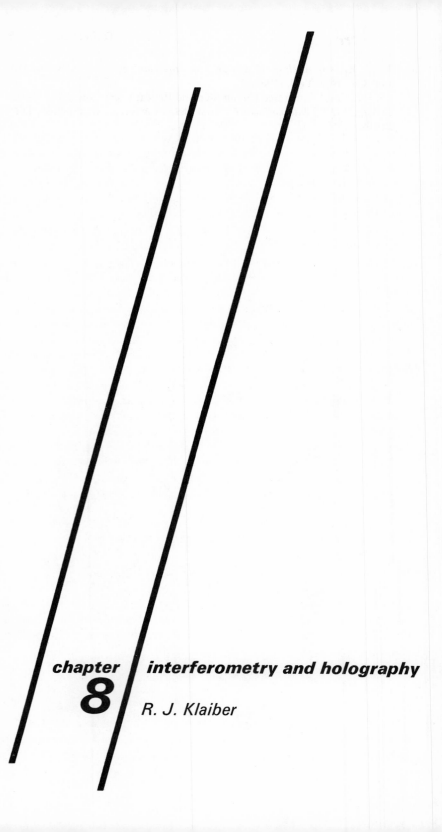

chapter 8   *interferometry and holography*

R. J. Klaiber

8·0 introduction

Interferometry, the study of the interference of coherent radiation, stems from the first experiments of Thomas Young in 1801. Early experiments were simple; the sun was the primary source and two small, closely spaced pinholes in a foil were the secondary or interfering sources. Young observed a dark and light pattern on a screen at some distance from the pinholes. This work was the first experimental indication of the wave nature of light. During the next hundred years the wave nature of light was conclusively proved by a series of experiments, the most notable of which was the confirmation by Arago of predictions based on Fresnel's wave theory explaining diffraction. A significant theoretical advance came when Maxwell presented his equations governing electromagnetic fields and his deduction that light is composed of electromagnetic waves.

Another milestone was passed early in the twentieth century when Michelson invented his two-beam interferometer. This device made possible very accurate measurement of optical path lengths. From this point on, the science of interferometry became very well developed as an indispensable measuring tool. However, the limited coherence of conventional sources restricted interferometry to those tasks where high coherence was not required, i.e., those areas where the optical path lengths of the interfering radiations were essentially equal. The coherence properties of the laser now allow appreciably unequal path two-beam and multiple-beam interferometry. In addition, the laser prompted the rebirth of holography, since the long coherence length allows the examination and recording of volume objects and subsequent reconstruction of an identical image of the object. Since the phase of the recorded object wave is related to the contour of the object it is obvious that this phase must be recorded by the hologram. Phase is recorded by the conversion to intensity information; the mechanism is interference, the subject of this chapter.

8·1 temporal and spatial coherence

We will briefly extend the basic concepts of coherence outlined in Section 1.5. There the interference effects were observed with radiation from quasi-monochromatic sources provided that the paths traversed by the radiation do not differ in time by an amount greater than the coherence time, $\Delta\tau(1 - 40)$. The maximum optical path difference corresponding to this coherence time is the coherence length,

$$l \simeq c\Delta\tau \simeq \frac{c}{\Delta\nu} = \frac{\bar{\lambda}^2}{\Delta\lambda} \tag{8-1}$$

where $\bar{\lambda}$ is the mean wavelength of the wave train of dispersion $\Delta\lambda$. The best conventional sources have a bandwidth $\Delta\nu = 10^8$ Hz corresponding to line widths of about $\Delta\lambda = 10^{-4}$ nm. However, the laser provides much greater flexibility since the bandwidth is considerably smaller, i.e., as low as 10^2 Hz, and therefore interference can be observed when the paths traversed by two beams from the same source are appreciably unequal. This is especially important in holography where the three-dimensional character of objects precludes matching of the signal and reference path lengths.

If we are interested in the spatial coherence of radiation from a highly monochromatic source of finite size, the complex degree of coherence (1-46) can be used to find the correlation between two points in the field, except now there is no interest in the coherence time $\Delta\tau$. For almost perfect coherence, the separation between two points located a distance D from a source of radius ρ is[2]

$$S \le \frac{0.16D\lambda}{\rho} \qquad (8\text{-}2)$$

As an example of the restrictions imposed by conventional sources, let us suppose that we are focusing the light from a mercury discharge lamp at $\lambda = 546$ nm through a 5 μm pinhole and observing interference at a distance of 0.5 m. The diameter of an area over which interference can be demonstrated is given by (8-2) and is calculated to be

$$S = \frac{0.16(0.5)(546 \times 10^{-6})}{2.5 \times 10^{-6}} \simeq 77 \text{ mm}$$

a fairly small dimension. In order to extend the coherence region it is necessary to remove the observation point very far from the source or, alternatively, to decrease the source size. Both situations significantly reduce the energy available for experiments. In any event, a conventional source cannot approach the temporal or spatial coherence of the laser.

8·2   interference

8·2·1   interference of two coherent plane waves

We have been briefly exposed to the conditions of the source that are necessary to observe interference. Now assume complete temporal and spatial coherence, an assumption not unwarranted in most cases in which a laser is the source. To start, consider the superposition of two plane waves traveling in the same direction:

$$E_1 = A_1 e^{i[\omega t - \phi_1(r)]}$$

$$E_2 = A_2 e^{i[\omega t - \phi_2(r)]} \qquad (8\text{-}3)$$

The quantities $A_1 e^{-i\phi_1(r)}$ and $A_2 e^{-i\phi_2(r)}$ are called the complex amplitudes where the phase, ϕ, and the amplitude, A, are functions of spatial co-ordinates. The term $e^{i\omega t}$ denotes the time variation of the electric field oscillating with angular frequency, ω. Two important facts about (8-3) will be stated here (proof can be found in Chapter 2):

1. They are solutions of the wave equation derived through Maxwell's equations.
2. They represent the amplitude and phase variations of the electric field; the square of the amplitude is the intensity, the only directly measurable field quantity of interest in interferometry.

Since only monochromatic signals observed over long times are of concern, the time variation in (8-3) will be dropped. The total electric intensity is the square of the sum of the electric field amplitudes,

$$I(r) = (E_1 + E_2)^2 = (A_1 e^{-i\phi_1(r)} + A_2 e^{-i\phi_2(r)})$$

$$+ (A_1 e^{-i\phi_1(r)} + A_2 e^{-i\phi_2(r)})*$$

$$= |A_1|^2 + |A_2|^2 + 2A_1 A_2 \cos(\phi_1 - \phi_2)$$

$$= I_1 + I_2 + 2\sqrt{I_1 I_2} \cos(\phi_1 - \phi_2) \tag{8-4}$$

where I_1 and I_2 are the intensities of the two waves and * indicates complex conjugate.

The physical significance of (8-4) may be demonstrated as follows. Suppose a laser beam is expanded by means of an inverted telescope so that a large diameter beam of intensity I_0 results. The wave can be sub-divided with a beamsplitter to obtain two beams of intensities I_1 and I_2 such that

$$I_1 + I_2 = I_0$$

If the beams are recombined in a Michelson interferometer, as shown subsequently in Figure 8-4, and the combination strikes a ground glass screen, $I(r)$ will be displayed. Equation (8-4) shows that the intensity $I(r)$ may vary between wide limits depending on the phase difference $(\phi_1 - \phi_2)$ and the relative intensities of I_1 and I_2. The phase difference is related to the optical path difference traversed by each beam expressed in radians:

$$(\phi_1 - \phi_2) = \frac{2\pi}{\lambda} n\ell \tag{8-5}$$

where n is the index of refraction of the medium, ℓ is the measured distance, and λ the wavelength. If the two beams have the same intensity, then the screen display will consist of a disc whose intensity lies between zero and $2I_0$, depending on the value of $(\phi_1 - \phi_2)$.

8·2·2 interference of two angularly separate plane waves

The situation of interference of two angularly separate plane waves is illustrated in Figure 8-1, where the amplitudes of the waves are represented with the same form as (8-3) except now the treatment of the phases, ϕ_1 and ϕ_2, must be a little more explicit.   The XY plane is chosen as the observation plane (perpendicular to paper).   Examination shows that the positive X axis is in the direction of advancing phase of beam one, i.e., a new position on the wavefront is attained which is advanced from $x = 0$ by an amount

$$\phi_1 = \frac{2\pi}{\lambda} x \sin \theta_1 \text{ rad} \tag{8-6}$$

In an analogous fashion, beam two is retarded from $x = 0$ by an amount

$$\phi_2 = \frac{-2\pi}{\lambda} x \sin \theta_2 \text{ rad} \tag{8-7}$$

There is no alteration of the phases in the Y direction.   The two coherent beams are then written,

$$E_1 = A_1 e^{-i(2\pi x \sin \theta_1)/\lambda}$$
$$E_2 = A_2 e^{+i(2\pi x \sin \theta_2)/\lambda} \tag{8-8}$$

The resultant superposition in the XY plane yields an intensity,

$$I(x) = I_1 + I_2 + 2\sqrt{I_1 I_2} \cos \frac{2\pi}{\lambda} x(\sin \theta_1 - \sin \theta_2) \tag{8-9}$$

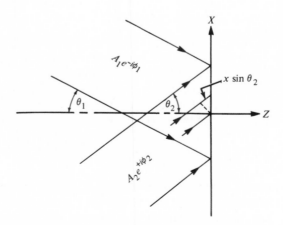

Figure 8-1   Interference of two plane waves.

There will be destructive interference (dark areas) whenever

$$\frac{2\pi}{\lambda} x(\sin\theta_1 - \sin\theta_2) = 2\pi(m + \tfrac{1}{2})$$

or

$$x(\sin\theta_1 - \sin\theta_2) = (m + \tfrac{1}{2})\lambda \qquad (8\text{-}10)$$

where m is an integer.   Similarly, bright areas are observed whenever

$$x(\sin\theta_1 - \sin\theta_2) = m\lambda \qquad (8\text{-}11)$$

Examination shows that these bright and dark areas are alternating bands, lying parallel to the Y axis.   They are called interference *fringes*.   The fringes vary sinusoidally in intensity as indicated by (8-9).   Equation (8-11) is identical to the grating formula of diffraction theory.

8·2·3   interference of spherical waves—Young's experiment

Description of the interference of spherical waves is carried out in an analogous fashion to the preceding examples, except now the fields are represented by functions of the form,

$$E_1(x) = \frac{A_1}{S_1} e^{-i(2\pi x \sin\theta_1)/\lambda}$$

$$(8\text{-}12)$$

$$E_2(x) = \frac{A_2}{S_2} e^{-i(2\pi x \sin\theta_2)/\lambda}$$

where S_1 and S_2 are the distances of the point sources (Figure 8-2), and A_1 and A_2 are amplitudes at a unit distance from the source.   A one-dimensional form is used which does not result in any loss of generality.

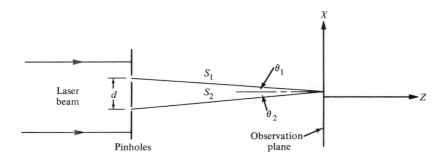

Figure 8-2   Young's experiment using a laser.

It can be seen that the intensity, I_2, falls as the inverse square of the distance.   This can be easily derived from the fact that the intensity is the energy flow per unit area perpendicular to the wave propagation and that this flow is inversely proportional to the surface area of a sphere with its center at the source point.

Young's experiment was briefly described in Section 1.5.2.   Figure 8-2 shows a modern equivalent of Young's arrangement.

Since the phases of the interfering light waves determine the intensity distribution in the fringes, our task is to write the phase of each wave in terms of the geometry.   If we wish to make an unaided visual observation of the interference fringes, the distance, d, between the pinholes will be small and so will the angle $(\theta_1 + \theta_2)$ between two rays at the observation plane.   Therefore, the mathematics is simplified by writing

$$\sin \theta_1 = \theta_1$$

$$\sin \theta_2 = \theta_2$$

The angles θ_1 and θ_2 are related by the geometry:

$$\theta_2 = \frac{d - S_1\theta_1}{S_2} \tag{8-13}$$

Using (8-9), (8-13), and the sine approximation, the intensity at the observation plane is

$$I(x) = I_1 + I_2 + 2\sqrt{I_1 I_2} \cos \frac{2\pi}{\lambda} x\left(\theta_1 + \frac{d}{S_2} - \frac{S_1\theta_1}{S_2}\right) \tag{8-14}$$

The fringes lie on the locus of points for which the phase difference is 2π,

$$\frac{2\pi}{\lambda} \Delta x\left(\theta_1 + \frac{d}{S_2} - \frac{S_1\theta_1}{S_2}\right) = 2\pi \tag{8-15}$$

so that in the vicinity of $x = 0$, where $S_1 \simeq S_2$, the fringe spacing is

$$\Delta x = \frac{\lambda S_2}{d} \tag{8-16}$$

It should be noted that the locus of points described by (8-16) are *approximately* straight lines near $x = 0$, but are actually hyperboloids with the pinholes as foci as shown in Figure 8-3.   As an example of the practical requirements involved for the visual observation of fringes, let us calculate from (8-16) the pinhole separation necessary for a fringe spacing of 1 mm at a distance of 0.5 m, using a HeNe laser.   The pinhole separation is

$$d = \frac{0.633 \times 10^{-3} \times 500}{1} = 0.32 \text{ mm}$$

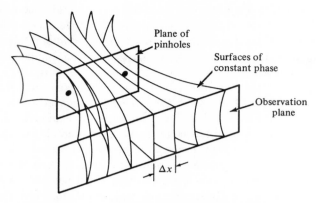

Figure 8-3 Loci of fringes in Young's experiment.

a fairly close spacing. In interference experiments using conventional sources it is necessary to use two closely spaced slits in order to have sufficient fringe illumination. The slits are easily produced in a dense photographic film by making two cuts with a razor blade.

8·3 two-beam interference

In two-beam interference, the wavefront is first divided (as shown in Figure 8-4) and the resulting beams recombined at some other location. This is called *amplitude division*, since each beam is reduced in amplitude. The chief advantage of this arrangement is that it allows a disturbing medium (some test object) to be conveniently placed in one of the beams. The Michelson interferometer[3] (Figure 8-4) is the best known instrument for producing two-beam interference.

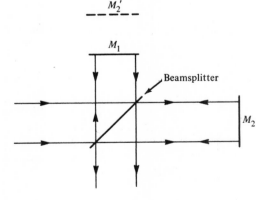

Figure 8-4 The Michelson interferometer.

In the original Michelson interferometer, an extended monochromatic source was used. In this case, the observed interference fringes are circular,[1] provided that the image of mirror M_2 is parallel to mirror M_1. Michelson first used this interferometer to compare the standard meter to the wavelength of the red cadmium spectral line. The method was to use shorter substandards as the mirrors in the interferometer and to measure their lengths in terms of fringes. The Michelson interferometer is now chiefly used in classroom instruction. However, if a laser source with collimated beams in the interferometer is used, a broad class of modified interferometers that have great practical utility will result.

First, let us consider the use of collimated beams as shown in Figure 8-4. If the optical elements of the interferometer are perfect, interference at the beamsplitter will be observed due to the superposition of the two reflected plane waves from mirrors M_1 and M_2. In this case the interference is described by (8-4). If the intensities are adjusted to be equal, the observed intensity will pass through maxima and minima as one mirror of the interferometer is displaced. The mirror displacement, d, between successive maxima, is given by

$$2d = m\lambda \qquad (m = 0, 1, 2, \ldots) \qquad (8\text{-}17)$$

If the optical elements in the interferometer are not perfect, but have phase distortions arising from spherical aberrations, glass nonuniformity, mirror curvature, etc., then these will be displayed as intensity variations at the output and the total error can be measured. This is the basic principle behind the measurement of nonhomogeneous objects and the measurement of the optical transfer function of lenses.[3]

8·3·1   an application to linear length measurement

A practical situation in which this interferometer can be used to measure very small mechanical displacements is shown in Figure 8-5. Here one

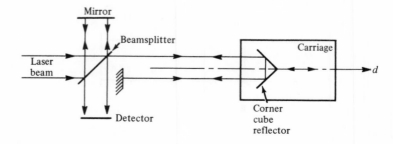

Figure 8-5   Length measuring interferometer.

mirror is mounted on the movable carriage of an XY table that is part of a step and repeat camera used to produce photomasks for microminiature circuits. The spacing between each microcircuit is extremely important, since there may be 1000 circuit arrays on each mask that must accurately align to the same number on each of, perhaps, a dozen masks. In the system of Figure 8-5, the amount of linear traverse of the table is measured by a count of fringes. If the interfering beams are coincident (see Section 8.2.1), a simple detection scheme can be provided to measure the bright and dark fringes of the interfering beams. Figure 8-5 shows a corner cube reflector mounted on the moving platform. This reflector serves two functions: the first is to increase the optical path by a factor of two owing to the dual passage of light back through the reflector; and the second function is to negate the disastrous effects of small angular displacements of the moving carriage that would preclude the use of a conventional flat mirror Michelson interferometer. (The Glossary has a description of the operation of a corner cube reflector.) It can be seen that a displacement, d, of the corner cube reflector changes the phase by

$$\phi = \frac{8\pi d}{\lambda} \text{ rad}$$

owing to the dual passage of the reflected beam through the corner cube. Hence, it is obvious that the displacement between successive bright and dark fringes ($\phi = \pi$) corresponds to a table movement of

$$d = \frac{\lambda}{8}$$

At the HeNe laser wavelength, this movement is equivalent to 0.08 μm! In order to take advantage of these fringes, the detector must be able to determine accurately the position of both maxima and minima. In addition, the device must be capable of discerning the direction of motion. Drift of the laser can also affect measurements due to small wavelength shifts. With suitable precautions it is possible to measure lengths as long as 60 m with a resolution of 0.02 μm and an accuracy of 5 parts in 10^7.

8·4 multiple-beam interferometry

In the previous sections the interference of two beams was briefly discussed. In this section the interference produced by multiple passes of the incident beam in the interferometer is studied. This type of interference is common to a broad class of important devices and effects that are found in laser systems.

8·4·1 multiple interference in a plane-parallel transparent plate

Consider the plate shown in Figure 8-6; let a very narrow laser beam be incident on the plate. In general, the plate will reflect some light and transmit some in the manner shown. Each successive reflection and transmission grows progressively weaker than its predecessor. Let t be the fraction of amplitude transmitted and r the fraction reflected at each surface:

$$t = se^{-i\psi}, \qquad r = \rho e^{-i\psi}$$

In these expressions, ψ is the phase change occurring at the air-material interface; it may be found from the Fresnel formulas given in Section 6.1.1. Our treatment will be only of the transmitted light; in this case there are no phase changes of either the internal reflections or the transmitted waves ($\psi = 0$). The transmittance and reflectance of the material are given by

$$T = tt^* = s^2, \qquad R = rr^* = \rho^2, \qquad T + R = 1 \qquad (8\text{-}18)$$

The transmitted wavelets are collected by a lens and combined at the focal point. (A lens is not necessary if the incident light is near perpendicular to the plate.) The amplitude in the focal plane of the lens is found by summing the multiple transmitted waves,

$$A_n = A_0(t^2 + t^2r^2e^{-i\phi} + \cdots + t^2r^{2n}e^{-in\phi})$$

which can be written

$$A = \frac{A_0 t^2}{1 - r^2e^{-i\phi}} \qquad (8\text{-}19)$$

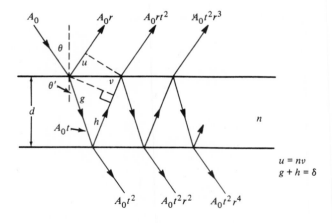

$u = nv$
$g + h = \delta$

Figure 8-6   Multiple reflections in a thin plate.

for a sufficiently large number of transmitted waves. The phase, ϕ, is the optical path difference in radians between adjacent transmitted waves. This difference is found from the geometry to be

$$\phi = \frac{4\pi n d}{\lambda} \cos \theta' \qquad (8\text{-}20)$$

where n is the index of refraction of the plate at the wavelength λ. The intensity is the only quantity detectable, and this is found by squaring the amplitude

$$I_t = AA^* = \frac{t^2 (t^*)^2 A_0^2}{1 + r^2 (r^*)^2 - r^2 e^{-i\phi} - (r^*)^2 e^{+i\phi}} \qquad (8\text{-}21)$$

Substitution of (8-18) yields

$$I_t = \frac{s^4 A_0^2}{1 - 2\rho^2 \cos \phi + \rho^4} = \frac{T^2 I_0}{1 - 2R \cos \phi + R^2} \qquad (8\text{-}22)$$

Equation (8-22) predicts a maximum transmitted intensity when the phase, ϕ, is multiple of 2π and a minimum when it is an odd multiple of π. This is mathematically expressed in a simplified form with the help of (8-20),

$$2nd(\cos \theta') = m\lambda \qquad \text{(bright fringe)}$$

and

$$2nd(\cos \theta') = (m + \tfrac{1}{2})\lambda \qquad \text{(dark fringe)} \qquad (8\text{-}23)$$

Let us consider two different illumination schemes and determine the shape of the observed fringes. The first scheme is illustrated in Figure 8-7. It is similar to that of Figure 8-6 except now the incident beam is extended, but collimated. Except for a possible increase in the observed intensity, there is no difference between the observed fringes produced by either an extended collimated source or a narrow beam; i.e., the interference pattern observed in the lens focal plane is a point with an intensity given by (8-22). But now, what if the source is monochromatic but extended and diffuse, such as an expanded laser beam passing through a ground glass? This second illumination scheme is shown in Figure 8-8. Each point on the

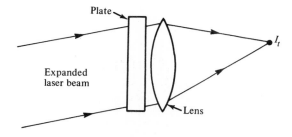

Figure 8-7 Fringe production with an expanded laser beam.

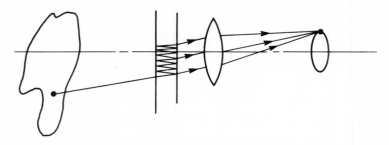

Figure 8-8   Circular fringe formation in a thin plate interferometer.

source will give rise to a ray that is incident on the plate exactly as shown in Figure 8-6.   In this case, (8-23) shows that for any given m, a bright point will appear in the focal plane of the lens.   Evidently, there are a number of points on the source which will satisfy this exact same condition but focus at a different point.   Therefore, there exists an ensemble of points in the lens focal plane constituting a bright *fringe*.   This fringe is the locus of points for which $\theta' = $ constant.   Perusal of (8-23) and Figure 8-9 will show that this locus is a circle whose center point lies on the optic axis of the lens.   Thus, each source point is associated with a bright or dark fringe of order m, and the fringe pattern of an extended source is a series of concentric rings called Fabry-Perot fringes (Figure 8-9).   The lens of Figure 8-7 or 8-8 may be the eye (provided the proper safety precautions are observed).   The plate must be thin (film) or the light incident near normal to the plate so that the transmitted waves arising due to multiple reflections do not spread appreciably and will pass through the pupil of the eye.   As a third and last point, consider the effect of the plate reflectance on the transmitted intensity.   We define a parameter,

$$F = \frac{4R}{(1 - R)^2} = \frac{4R}{T^2} \tag{8-24}$$

that in conjunction with (8-18) may be used to simplify (8-22) to give

$$I_t = \frac{I_0}{1 + F \sin^2 \phi/2} \tag{8-25}$$

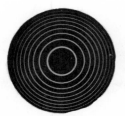

Figure 8-9   Fabry-Perot fringes.

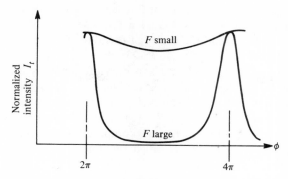

Figure 8-10   Influence of the parameter, F on Fabry-Perot fringes.

Figure 8-10 is a plot of the fringe intensity as a function of ϕ for small and large values of F.   Evidently, large values of F (high reflectance) result in narrow fringes.

8·4·2   the Fabry-Perot interferometer

In the preceding section, it was shown how a plane-parallel plate modified the intensity of transmitted light due to multiple interferences in the plate. Also, the high reflectances of the plate face narrowed the transmitted fringes, as observed in the focal plane of a lens.   This section shows how multiple interferences can be used in the Fabry-Perot interferometer to make a high resolution spectrum analyzer.

The Fabry-Perot interferometer is shown in Figure 8-11.   In this interferometer, the multiple reflections occur in the air space between two plates that have high reflectance inner faces.   The parallelism of the inner faces must be very good, a condition that may be achieved by the use of a very accurately made spacer.   In this or a similar form, the interferometer is commonly called a Fabry-Perot etalon and is meant to describe a fixed-plate separation.   A variation of this etalon is a plane-parallel plate of optical glass or fused quartz which has been coated for high reflectance.

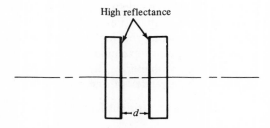

Figure 8-11   Fabry-Perot interferometer.

The description of the principles of this device is exactly that of the plane-parallel plate (Section 8.4.1). Only a few additional considerations are necessary to comprehend the utility of this device.

A comparison of (8-17) and (8-23) shows that the fringe spacing in both the Fabry-Perot and Michelson interferometers is the same for the same illumination scheme and air-spaced mirrors. However, the resolving power of the Fabry-Perot interferometer can be made much higher than the Michelson interferometer since the high reflectance of the mirrors cause fringes whose widths are very narrow compared to their spacing. In fact, we can define a quality index, called the finesse, that is related to the resolving power of the Fabry-Perot interferometer:

$$\text{Finesse} = \frac{\pi\sqrt{R}}{1-R} = \frac{\pi}{2}\sqrt{F} \qquad (8\text{-}26)$$

The finesse is the ratio of the fringe separation to the half width* of the fringe. It should be noted that the finesse is also related to the quality of the plates used in the interferometer. Quality is measured by flatness of the interferometer plates since this factor influences the plate separation at any point and, hence, the position of the fringes. This quality will influence the finesse and the *resolving power* of the instrument, as will be shown later. In practice, the finesse is more often limited by the plate flatness than by the reflectance of the plate faces. In fact, the finesse is approximately equivalent to the reciprocal of the plate flatness (in wavelengths). To complicate matters further, it is intuitively obvious that high reflectance precludes high transmission of light so that some compromise may be necessary between finesse and light detection.

At this point it may be useful to extend this description of the Fabry-Perot interferometer by considering the spectral analysis of a single transverse laser line. As indicated in Chapter 1, this laser line has a number of longitudinal modes spaced

$$\Delta v_c = \frac{c}{2\ell}$$

where ℓ is the cavity length, and c is the speed of light. The broadened line width of the laser beam is composed of a number of longitudinal modes of varying intensity. A typical structure is shown in Figure 8-12. If this structure is analyzed with a Fabry-Perot interferometer, each mode must be distinguished from the higher-order components of its neighbors. To clarify this point, examine the case of a laser beam normally incident to the interferometer. The medium between the interferometer plates is air, having an index of one, so that (8-23) reduces to

$$2d = m\lambda \qquad \text{(bright fringes)} \qquad (8\text{-}23')$$

---

* Half width is the width of the fringe at half the maximum intensity.

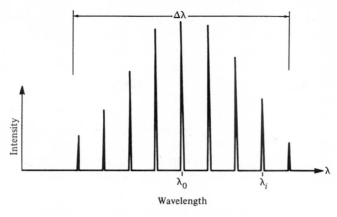

Figure 8-12   Longitudinal mode structure of a gas laser.

Provided (8-23′) is satisfied, the light transmitted by the interferometer will be a maximum and will have the same intensity profile as the incident beam. Small changes, Δd, in the plate spacing will alter the transmitted intensity as indicated by (8-20) and (8-22). In fact, if the spacing is continuously changed in one direction, the mode structure (Figure 8-12) of the laser will be observed as each longitudinal component, λ_i, sequentially satisfies (8-23′). When all of the modes have been observed in turn, the total change in the separation of the interferometer plates will be

$$\Delta d = \frac{m\,\Delta\lambda}{2} \tag{8-27}$$

The observation of the longitudinal mode structure is not uncomplicated, however. Each wavelength has higher-order components, m, which may also be detected along with each other wavelength and its components, thus greatly complicating the observation. Fortunately, this situation may be avoided by ensuring that higher-order components can occur only when the plate spacing is changed by an amount greater than Δd, as given by (8-27). Since the spacing between orders is $\lambda/2$, as found from (8-23′), the condition sought is

$$\frac{\lambda}{2} \geq \frac{m\Delta\lambda}{2}$$

or

$$\Delta\lambda \leq \frac{m}{\lambda} \tag{8-28}$$

By a simple transformation, (8-28) can be expressed in terms of frequency by

$$\Delta\nu \leq \frac{c}{2d} \tag{8-29}$$

a quantity called the free spectral range. The mirror spacing in the interferometer is then determined from (8-29). As an example, a 2 W argon-ion laser operating at 488 nm has a Doppler line width (in the frequency domain) of 2 GHz, dictating the Fabry-Perot spectrum analyzer to have a mirror separation,

$$d \leq 7.5 \text{ cm}$$

Now that the approximate mirror separation has been determined, the number of longitudinal modes "seen" or *resolved* can be found. Since the laser beam is incident at right angles to the interferometer plates, only one longitudinal mode will be seen for a fixed-plate separation. In order to "see" all the longitudinal modes, one of the mirrors must be moved through a distance given by (8-27), i.e., $\lambda/2$. If this is done rapidly, an oscilloscope can be used to simultaneously display all of the modes. In practical spectrum analyzers, the scanning mirror is driven by a piezo-electric device and the interferometer output is detected by a photosensor having fast time response. The display looks similar to that in Figure 8-12.

In addition, if the total number of modes is sufficiently large, a high finesse is required in order to resolve them. For normal incidence the resolving power is

$$\frac{\lambda_0}{\Delta\lambda_0} \simeq \frac{2Fnd}{\lambda_0} \qquad (8\text{-}30)$$

where λ_0 = the center wavelength,
$\Delta\lambda_0$ = the separation of modes,
n = the index of the medium between the interferometer plates,
d = the plate separation.

A Fabry-Perot interferometer with flat plates usually cannot be made with a finesse exceeding 50 if the aperture of the device is more than a few millimeters. In this case, the resolving power of an interferometer to examine the mode structure of an argon line at 488 nm would be about

$$\frac{\lambda_0}{\Delta\lambda_0} = \frac{2 \times 50 \times 7.5}{0.488 \times 10^{-4}} = 1.54 \times 10^7$$

Inasmuch as a typical argon laser is about 2 m long, the longitudinal modes are spaced by $\Delta v_c = 75$ MHz and the resolving power required to separate them is

$$\frac{\lambda_0}{\Delta\lambda_0} = 0.82 \times 10^7$$

Thus, a finesse of 50 is just barely sufficient to resolve the argon modes. The mode content of a typical argon laser line shown in Figure 8-12 could limit certain unequal path interference experiments by reducing the coherence length of the radiation (8-1).   For instance, the coherence length of the argon line used in the previous example ($\Delta v = 2$ GHz) is

$$\ell = \frac{\lambda^2}{\Delta\lambda} = \frac{(0.488 \times 10^{-3})^2 \text{ mm}^2}{0.17 \times 10^{-8} \text{ mm}} = 140 \text{ mm}$$

Now, just as the mode structure has been measured with a Fabry-Perot interferometer, it should be apparent that all but one of the longitudinal modes of a laser can be filtered by means of a fixed-plate Fabry-Perot interferometer, in this case a thick "etalon" usually of quartz,[4] inserted *in* the laser cavity.   The etalon is about 1 cm thick and acts to introduce sufficient losses so that only one longitudinal mode oscillates.

8·4·3   confocal, spherical mirror Fabry-Perot interferometers[3]

The Fabry-Perot interferometer with flat mirrors has limited usefulness where very high resolving power is required.   Attempts to use very narrow laser beams in order to reduce flatness requirements on the mirrors results in serious diffraction losses.   These effects can be minimized by the use of spherical mirrors in the interferometer.   This section is limited to the most useful of the spherical mirror Fabry-Perot interferometers: the confocal arrangement.

The confocal interferometer is shown in Figure 8-13.   Many spherical mirror interferometers that are not confocal require mode matching of the cavity to the laser beam.[5]   This means that only a single transverse mode may be coupled to the interferometer, and the laser beam axis must be carefully aligned to be collinear with the interferometer axis.   The benefit of spherical mirrors is that only a small portion of the mirror is active so that the finesse over this portion can be very high.   The confocal arrangement offers this advantage also but, in addition, it is mode degenerate so that several transverse laser modes may be excited simultaneously in the interferometer cavity.   This means that mode matching

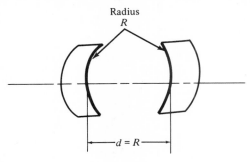

Figure 8-13   A confocal Fabry-Perot interferometer.

is not necessary, although the laser beam diameter should be the same as the aperture of the appropriate mode of the interferometer. This is simply accomplished with a fixed aperture and the interferometer is usually designed for fundamental mode operation. Although the confocal arrangement is less sensitive to alignment than the general spherical mirror interferometer, high finesse cannot be achieved unless alignment is correct. In this case a finesse of several hundred may be achieved. As a parting note, the free spectral range of this interferometer is

$$\Delta v = \frac{c}{4d} \qquad (8\text{-}31)$$

8·4·4 interference filters

With the body of information developed so far, it should be evident that fixed separation Fabry-Perot interferometers can be constructed that may be used to pass certain parts of the optical spectrum.   Such filters would be useful in isolating a certain spectral line such as the green line in a mercury discharge from other emissions, or isolating a laser line from tube fluorescence.

   In order to isolate a single color from broadband radiation, the resonances of the interference filter must be widely separated.   This means that the filter must transmit *low-order* fringes (see 8-23) and the light must be collimated.   Then, according to (8-23), the separation of the reflecting faces (multilayer dielectrics) must be very small, i.e.,

$$d = \frac{m\lambda_0}{2n} \qquad (8\text{-}32)$$

where n is the index of the material between the plates.   The reflecting faces are of high quality when multilayer dielectric films are used.   The filter takes the form shown in Figure 8-14.

   The peak transmission of the filter is given by (8-22) provided that reflectances of the filter and their separation are constant.   The half

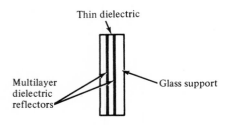

Figure 8-14   Interference filter.

TABLE 8-1 Typical Filter Specifications

Wavelength (nm)	Transmittance	Half Width (nm)
351.1	0.35	10.5
488.0	0.80	6.1
488.0	0.60	0.5
632.8	0.77	5.4
632.8	0.35	0.35

width of the transmitted fringe may be determined from (8-22), (8-23), and (8-26). For multilayer dielectric reflecting films the half width is approximately[2]

$$\Delta\lambda_0 \simeq \frac{\lambda_0}{F(m-1)} \tag{8-33}$$

As noted elsewhere, the transmittance of the filter decreases as the half width decreases. Some typical filter specifications are listed in Table 8-1.

8·4·5 antireflection films

These films are universally used in optical instruments to reduce light reflections from glass surfaces. Reflections usually degrade the performance of an optical system by reducing the contrast in the image and by reducing light transmission.

Consider a beam of monochromatic light that is incident nearly normal to a glass plate of index n_2, onto which has been deposited a thin layer of some other transparent material of index n_1 (see Figure 8-15). The problem is to find the condition under which the reflection from the air-film surface is cancelled by the reflection from the film-glass surface. The

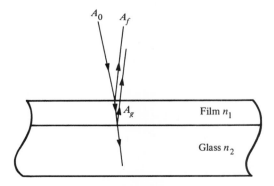

Figure 8-15 Antireflection film on glass.

amplitude of the reflected light is found from the Fresnel equations (6-2 through 6-5):

$$A_f = A_0\left(\frac{1 - n_1}{1 + n_1}\right) \quad \text{(air-film surface)} \tag{8-34a}$$

$$A_g = A_0\left(\frac{n_1 - n_2}{n_1 + n_2}\right) \quad \text{(film-glass surface)} \tag{8-34b}$$

where A_0 is the incident light amplitude and the film is nonabsorbing. Only two reflections are considered. Actually, multiple reflections will occur in the film but the result of this analysis is quite general. Now it is only necessary to find the optical thickness of the film that will cause the two reflections (8-34a,b) to be out of phase with each other so that they cancel. To do this, the total reflected amplitude is first written

$$A_R = A_f + A_g = A_0\left[\frac{1 - n_1}{1 + n_1} + \frac{n_1 - n_2}{n_1 + n_2}\cos\phi\right] \tag{8-35}$$

where ϕ is the phase difference between the two reflections and is identical to the phase term of (8-20) governing multiple reflections. If ϕ is required to be π, then the two reflections will be out of phase and will partially cancel. "Partially" is used because the amplitudes of the reflections (8-34a,b) are not equal. Mathematically,

$$\phi = \frac{4\pi n_1 d}{\lambda} = \pi \tag{8-36}$$

therefore,

$$n_1 d = \frac{\lambda}{4}$$

meaning that the optical thickness of the film should be one-quarter wavelength. In this case, the reflected amplitude reduces to

$$A_R = A_0\left[\frac{1 - n_1}{1 + n_1} - \frac{n_1 - n_2}{n_1 + n_2}\right]$$

Since the reflected intensity is our main concern,

$$I_R = I_0\left[\frac{2(n_2 - n_1^2)}{(n_1 + 1)(n_1 + n_2)}\right]^2 \tag{8-37}$$

Obviously, the condition for no reflection is

$$n_1 = \sqrt{n_2} \tag{8-38}$$

The practical realization of (8-38) is not as simple as this treatment.

Since most optical glasses have indices between $n_2 = 1.5$ and $n_2 = 1.9$, we should have antireflection films with indices between $n_1 = 1.22$ and $n_1 = 1.38$.   In practice there are only a few durable films that can be used for antireflection films.   The most commonly used materials are magnesium fluoride, $n_1 = 1.38$, and cryolite, $n_1 = 1.35$.   Since the index of refraction of both the nonreflecting film and the substrate vary with wavelength, it is evident that (8-38) cannot be satisfied with a wide spectrum even if (8-36) is satisfied.   As an example of these practical considerations, let us see the effects of a single layer of cryolite on the first crown glass element of a laser collimating lens to be used with an argon laser operating at 488 nm.   The crown has an index of 1.53, and the reflected fraction is

$$\frac{I_R}{I_0} = \left[\frac{2(1.53 - 1.35^2)}{(2.35)(2.88)} \right]^2 = 0.0073$$

or less than 1 percent for a single-layer film 90 nm thick.   In an uncoated condition the reflected fraction is found from (8-37), i.e.,

$$\frac{I_R}{I_0} = \left(\frac{1 - 1.53}{1 + 1.53} \right)^2 = 0.044$$

In a lens composed of, say, four compound elements, the light transmission for uncoated optics might be 0.7, a considerable reduction. Single-layer antireflection coatings can bring the transmission to a minimum of 95 percent.   The use of multilayer films can bring the transmission to 99 percent.

8·4·6   unequal path interferometry

The long coherence length of the laser, combined with high intensity, provides a great deal of flexibility in the use of two-beam and multiple-beam interferometers.   For instance, it is no longer necessary to design a two-beam interferometer (e.g., Michelson) with equal path lengths or multiple pass (e.g., Fabry-Perot) interferometers with small mirror separation.   The high illumination levels attainable in laser interferometers allow large beam areas, hence practical usefulness for testing or examining large objects.   However, greater care is required in the design of laser interferometers than in conventional interferometers because of the possibility of spurious fringe systems arising from multiple interferences in the optical elements, and diffraction patterns from dust and the like. This section briefly describes the unequal path Twyman-Green interferometer and its use in testing optical elements.

The Twyman-Green interferometer is shown in the schematic of Figure 8-16.   It can be seen that it is a modification of the Michelson

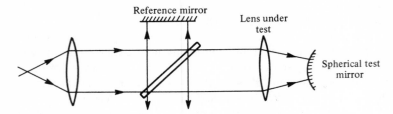

Figure 8-16   Twyman-Green interferometer (lens test).

interferometer (Figure 8-4).   The basic principle of the interferometer is to interfere a pseudo-collimated wave, arising from an optical element under test, with a collimated reference wave.   The objective lens under test is placed with its focal point coincident with the center of curvature of a well-corrected convex mirror.   If the lens is not perfect, the wave reflected from the mirror and emerging from the lens will not be plane. The phase errors are displayed as intensity variations when the aberrated wave interferes with the reference wave.   The displayed fringes are a contour map of the wavefront from the lens and indicate double the actual error due to double passage of the light through the lens.   The lens can be tested off-axis as well as on-axis.[6]   The Twyman-Green interferometer has been extensively used in optical shops as a means for testing and correcting lenses.   A modification of the interferometer for testing mirrors is shown in Figure 8-17.

It is perhaps more obvious in this case why the long coherence length of a laser is important.   If a long focal-length mirror is to be tested, it is not necessary to adjust path lengths to be nearly equal because of the long coherence length of the laser.   Therefore, the reference arm of the inter-ferometer need not be disturbed.   Figures 8-18a and 8-18b show a diagrammatic view of the curvature of a wavefront due to spherical aberration and the corresponding interference pattern.

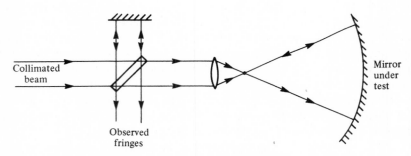

Figure 8-17   Twyman-Green interferometer (mirror test).

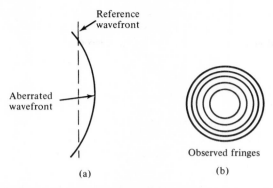

Figure 8-18   Observed wavefront—Twyman-Green interferometer.

Earlier it was mentioned that laser interferometers must be carefully designed to avoid spurious fringes arising from multiple interferences in the optics.   In spite of this care, however, instabilities may arise due to coupling of reflected light from the interferometer back into the laser cavity and reflections from the output mirror of the laser.   An interferometer for lens testing that avoids spurious reflections is shown in Figure 8-19.[25]   In this system, the incident light is plane polarized.   The optical component to be measured is located between the quarter-wave retardation plate* and the interferometer mirrors.   The quarter-wave plate serves to rotate the plane of polarization by 90° due to double passage of the light through the plate.   Since the polarization of reflected waves from the surfaces of all components *before* the quarter-wave plates

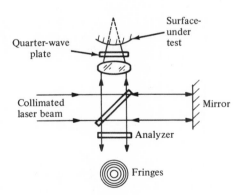

Figure 8-19   Technique to eliminate spurious reflections in an interferometer.

---

* See Glossary for description of these items.

have not been rotated, they can be filtered by insertion of an "analyzer" in the location shown in Figure 8-19. The analyzer is merely a polarizer with its axis oriented to block the spurious reflections.

8·5 holography

Holography, as no other topic in optics, has aroused and excited many people. This excitement arises chiefly from the capability of a hologram to produce three-dimensional images with the parallax properties of the original object. Actually, the science of holography, or wavefront reconstruction, began with a quest for an increase in the resolution of electron microscopes.[7] In this early work, the analysis of an object was to be made with the electron beam and the synthesis of the image by wavefront reconstruction in the optical domain. The practical accomplishment of the theoretical predictions has not been achieved due to the lack of a sufficiently intense coherent electron source. The first experiments in holography were made in the optical region, using filtered high-pressure mercury arcs. Since the hologram is the recorded interference pattern between a diffracted object wave and a separate coherent background or reference wave, it is apparent that the path difference between these two waves must be less than the coherence length of the light source. This was achieved by Gabor with the arrangement shown in Figure 8-20.

This arrangement proved only partially successful because the image is reconstructed in the presence of a strong background illumination associated with a "twin" image, located at a different plane, and a zero-order or undiffracted background. The advent of the laser provided the source enabling separation of the twin images and also the zero-order background. This was accomplished by an angular separation[8] of the object wave and the reference wave as depicted in Figure 8-21. This method, called *off-axis holography*, provided the impetus for a tremendous resurgence of interest in holography.

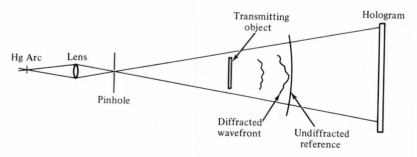

Figure 8-20   Recording a Gabor hologram.

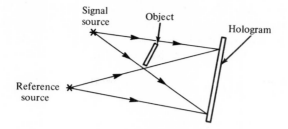

Figure 8-21   Recording an off-axis hologram.

8·5·1   elementary holograms—diffraction gratings and zone plates

Section 8.4 covered the interference of coherent waves. This section uses the concept of diffraction treated in Chapter 7 to describe the wave scattered from elementary objects and the interference of this wave with a phase-related reference wave.

Begin with the description of light diffraction at a grating (Figure 8-22). The grating may be visualized as an array of equally spaced slits. Light passing through any slit is scattered at the slit boundary; in the far-field or Fraunhofer region (7-8) or (7-19) the amplitude of the scattered wave is given by (7-12) or (7-36).

$$U(u) = c \, \frac{\sin kua}{kua} \tag{8-39}$$

where $2a =$ the slit width,
$\qquad k =$ the wave number,
$\qquad u =$ the angular coordinate shown in Figure 8-22.

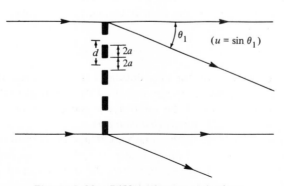

Figure 8-22   Diffraction at a grating.

In order to describe diffraction from the array of slits, we need only add the contributions of all the slits in the far field. Since each slit contributes a field identical to (8-39), only shifted in phase (which is indicative of the position of the slit), then the amplitude due to N slits is

$$U(u) = c \frac{\sin kua}{kua} [1 + e^{ikud} + e^{-ikud} + e^{i2kud} + e^{-i2kud} + \cdots e^{i(N/2)kud}]$$

$$= \frac{\sin kua}{kua} \times \frac{\sin N(kud/2)}{\sin(kud/2)} \tag{8-40}$$

and the intensity is

$$I(u) = [U(u)]^2 \tag{8-41}$$

Here, the phase factor, kud, describes the location of each slit pattern. The first term of (8-40) is the diffraction pattern of a single slit; the second term describes the interference of the waves emanating from all slits.

If the number of slits is large and the slit width very small, the diffraction term will be essentially unity over a broad region, and the only term of interest is the interference term. Close inspection of this term will show that there are a number of zeros and maxima; the principal maxima occur when

$$\frac{kud}{2} = m\pi \tag{8-42a}$$

where $u = \sin \theta_1$ as indicated in Figure 8-22, and m is an integer or order number. Equation (8-42a) then becomes

$$d \sin \theta_1 = m\lambda \tag{8-42b}$$

This equation describes the position of the primary intensity maxima or bright regions in the diffraction pattern. The pattern will include a number of secondary maxima of lower intensity.

As a final step, note that the previous treatment implies light incident normal to the grating. If the light is incident at an angle θ_2, we obtain the general result

$$d(\sin \theta_1 + \sin \theta_2) = m\lambda \tag{8-43}$$

Taking into consideration the convention that angles measured from the same side of the axis have the same sign, (8-43) is identical to the expression (8-11) governing maxima in the interference pattern of two plane waves. Equation (8-43) is called the *grating equation*.

At this point we leave further mathematical treatment of the diffraction grating to the references[1,2,3] and consider the physical implications of our development so far. Figure 8.23a shows the diffraction of a laser beam at a typical grating and what might be visually observed on a screen some

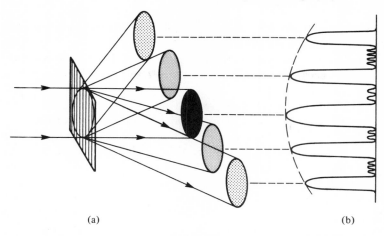

(a)   (b)

Figure 8-23   Observed intensity field from diffraction grating.

distance away.   Figure 8.23b shows the actual intensity profile.   Note that there are secondary maxima of greatly reduced intensity.   If the number of slits is large, these secondary maxima will be very small (as predicted by (8-40)) and ordinarily not observable with the simple arrangement of Figure 8.23a.   In addition, the principal maxima will be very narrow, i.e., of small angular width.   Inasmuch as a large number of slits may encompass several centimeters, the laser beam will have to be expanded if sharp diffraction orders are to be observed.   The observation screen usually is placed a fairly long distance away to separate these orders, since each diffracted order will be about the same diameter as the illuminating laser beam, and the angle between orders (as given by 8-43) may be small.

To make the fringes observable in a relatively short distance, a lens may be used.   The lens collects all of the light and concentrates it in a bright pattern at its focal plane, as shown in Figure 8-24.   Both Figures

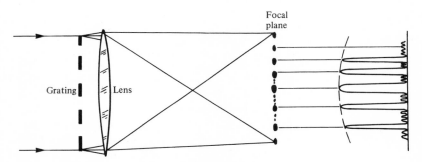

Figure 8-24   Fringes from grating in focal plane of lens.

8-23 and 8-24 show the intensity profiles.   Note modulation of the interference orders by the diffraction pattern of a single slit.   As mentioned previously, narrow slits will not appreciably affect the intensity of a number of interference orders since the diffraction intensity pattern is very broad for narrow slits.

The phenomena observed with a diffraction grating have been described without discussing the method of producing a grating.   For the purposes of this chapter we will not concern ourselves with the usual mechanical methods of making gratings, but with optical methods.   In Section 8.2.2 the interference produced by two plane waves at an angle to each other is covered (see Figure 8-1).   Equation (8-9) can be interpreted to indicate that the interference pattern is a periodic array of bright and dark fringes superimposed on a uniform background.   Diffraction gratings can be produced by photographing this interference pattern; thus the most elementary off-axis hologram is the creation of a plane-wave grating.   Since (8-11) describing the interference maxima is identical to the grating equation (8-43), it should be clear that the production of an elementary hologram by photographically recording the interference of two plane waves gives us the capability of reconstructing one of these waves (the signal) by illuminating the grating with the other (the reference). If the grating is two dimensional, i.e., has no thickness, then higher-order signals will be reconstructed, as previously discussed.   In practice, most holograms are made in photosensitive emulsions with appreciable thickness so that the recorded fringes are three dimensional in extent and lie in the volume of the emulsion.   These holograms are termed *volume holograms*.   This type of hologram will not support diffraction into many orders unless the angle between interfering beams is small, because of the Bragg effect.[9]   This effect is illustrated in Figure 8-25.

Since the bright fringes lie in the emulsion volume and on the angle bisector of the interfering beams, the photographic material will have its greatest exposure in these regions.   We can think of these recorded fringes as reflecting surfaces.   In order that all the waves reflecting from

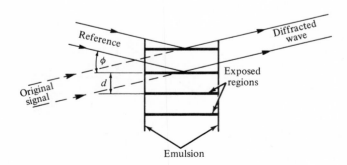

Figure 8-25   The Bragg effect.

these surfaces be in phase to produce the brightest reconstructed wave requires

$$2 \sin \phi = \pm \frac{\lambda}{d}$$

But this is a condition identical to the grating equation (8-43) used to specify the fringe spacing, i.e.,

$$2m \sin \phi = \sin \theta_1 + \sin \theta_2$$

Therefore, the first-order waves ($m = \pm 1$) will be efficiently reconstructed only when $\theta_1 = \theta_2$ or

$$\phi = \theta_1$$

A *conjugate* diffraction phenomenon can be produced with the hologram grating (see Figure 8-25). The hologram may be illuminated with a reference beam in the opposite direction, i.e., antiparallel (or conjugate) to the original reference beam. In this fashion a diffracted wave is produced that is antiparallel to the signal. This wave is termed the *real image wave*. When reconstructing with the identical geometry used to make the hologram, the diffracted wave is collinear with the original signal and is termed the *virtual image wave*. The real and virtual images are shown in the general case in Figure 8-26.

When a diffraction grating is illuminated, bright bands of light in prescribed directions or orders will be produced. Additionally, the production of a diffraction grating can be accomplished by interfering

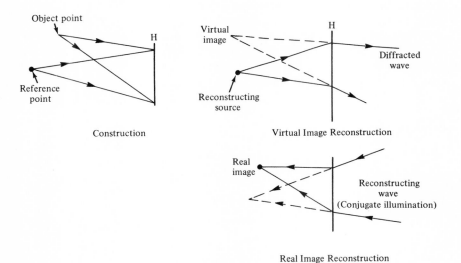

Figure 8-26   Construction and reconstruction of a holographic image.

two plane waves at a photographic plate, and this constitutes an elementary hologram with one beam called the signal and the other called the reference.   Now, consider another elementary hologram; that formed by a point source signal and a point reference source.   The hologram for this case may be called a zone plate in analogy with the well-known Fresnel zone plate.[10]   The construction of the hologram is shown in Figure 8-27a for the general case and in Figure 8.27b for an on-axis holographic zone plate that is used for mathematical development.

The intereference of spherical waves was covered for the general case in Section 8.2.2.   There it was found that the intensity at the observation plane (now this plane is called a hologram) varied sinusoidally (8-14) giving dark or bright fringes whose separation is governed by

$$\frac{2\pi x}{\lambda}\left[\frac{d}{R_o} + \left(1 - \frac{R_r}{R_o}\right)\sin\theta_1\right] = \pi(2m + 1) \qquad \text{(dark)}$$

$$\frac{2\pi x}{\lambda}\left[\frac{d}{R_o} + \left(1 - \frac{R_r}{R_o}\right)\sin\theta_1\right] = 2\pi m \qquad \text{(bright)}$$

These conditions are derived by finding the extrema of the argument of the cosine function in (8-14) and by substituting for S_1 and S_2 the appropriate distances from Figure 8-27 (R_r and R_o).   Note that the angle θ_1 has been replaced by $\sin\theta_1$, the more general expression.

For the situation of Figure 8-27b,

$$d = 0$$
$$x = R_r \sin\theta_1$$

so that bright fringes are found from

$$x^2\left(\frac{1}{R_r} - \frac{1}{R_o}\right) = m\lambda \qquad (8\text{-}44)$$

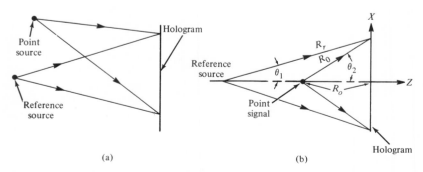

Figure 8-27   Geometry of hologram construction.

The term in parentheses is a constant:

$$\left(\frac{1}{R_r} - \frac{1}{R_o}\right) = \frac{1}{F} \qquad (8\text{-}45)$$

Finally, it is noted (Figure 8-27) that rotational symmetry exists about the Z axis, so that the bright fringes are concentric circles with radii

$$x = r = \sqrt{mF\lambda} \qquad (m = 1, 2, 3, \ldots) \qquad (8\text{-}46)$$

The photographic record of these fringes is called a *zone plate*. The circular zones alternate between dark and clear and get very close together as their radii increase. For instance, a zone plate constructed with $\lambda = 488$ nm and $F = 100$ mm has an inner zone diameter of 0.44 mm and is separated from the next zone by 0.1 mm. The fiftieth zone has a diameter approximately 3.12 mm but is separated from the fifty-first by only 0.016 mm. The zone plate has been known for some time and was probably one of the first computed holograms. Zone plates were usually produced by making greatly enlarged ink drawings of the zones and then photographically reducing them. However, it is difficult to draw a large number of zones accurately. A zone plate will form images in a fashion similar to a lens at positions determined by (8-45), which may be recognized as the familiar paraxial imaging formula of thin lens optics. The quantity F may be regarded as the focal length of the plate. The geometric imaging properties of a hologram may be determined by analogies to thin-lens optics. The next section will treat this problem from a purely geometric viewpoint.

8·5·2 paraxial imaging properties of holograms

In the previous section, some of the properties of a zone plate were derived by consideration of the interference of two spherical coherent waves. We saw that a zone plate is one type of elementary hologram—that of a point signal. Figures 8-26 and 8-27 show the construction and reconstruction of a point signal. The usefulness of a zone plate representation of a hologram will become clear when one realizes that any illuminated three-dimensional object may be considered to be an infinite ensemble of point sources. Each point will be recorded on the hologram as a zone plate. The position of the object point is a function of the phase relationship between the point signal and the reference signal at the hologram, and this relationship is recorded as intensity variations (produced by interference) that are the *zones* in the hologram. The faithful reconstruction of a three-dimensional image is dependent on the accurate recording of these zones and on a duplication of the recording geometry.

In order to specify fully the paraxial imaging properties of a hologram, the analysis of the previous section must be continued to include the reconstruction geometry. Figure 8-28 is a reproduction of Figure 8.27b and indicates that the construction of an elementary zone plate results in a series of concentric *fringes* whose radii are a function of the path difference $AB - BC$, i.e.,

$$AB - BC = m\lambda_r \quad \text{(bright fringes)} \tag{8-47}$$

In terms of Figure 8-28, (8-47) reduces to (8-44) reproduced here:

$$r^2\left[\frac{1}{R_r} - \frac{1}{R_o}\right] = m\lambda_r \tag{8-48}$$

where λ_r is the wavelength of the reference and object sources.

Now consider the reconstruction of this hologram. Suppose our reconstructing point source is located axially, at a distance R_c not the same as the original reference source. Evidently, there is a relationship equivalent to (8-47) for the reconstruction, and an image point located at R_i that will satisfy an equation similar to (8.48), i.e.,

$$r^2\left[\frac{1}{R_c} - \frac{1}{R_i}\right] = m\lambda_c \tag{8-49}$$

where λ_c is the reconstruction wavelength. Comparing (8-48) and (8-49), it is found that

$$\left[\frac{1}{R_c} - \frac{1}{R_i}\right] = \frac{\lambda_c}{\lambda_r}\left[\frac{1}{R_r} - \frac{1}{R_o}\right] \tag{8-50}$$

Now let us change (8-50) into a more general form that accounts for scale changes in the hologram produced by enlargement, etc., and for image formation by conjugate illumination.

Equation (8-50) describes the formation of a virtual image. The virtual image lies in the same space as the object and can be seen only by

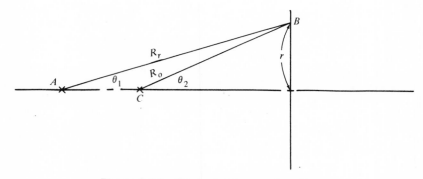

Figure 8-28   Fresnel zone construction.

looking through the hologram; it cannot be formed on a screen.   On the other hand, the real image lies in between the hologram and the viewer but can be seen at any location by forming the image on a diffusing screen.*   The formation of a real image occurs when conjugate illumination exists (see Figure 8-26).   This is mathematically expressed by a negative sign on the left side (8-49).   Finally, note that an enlargement of the hologram by a factor ε is tantamount to multiplying the zone radii by ε.   Taking these factors into consideration, (8-50) becomes

$$\frac{1}{R_i} = \frac{1}{R_c} \pm \frac{\lambda_c}{\lambda_r \varepsilon^2} \left[\frac{1}{R_r} - \frac{1}{R_o} \right] \tag{8-51}$$

where the positive sign indicates a real image and the negative sign a virtual image.   Although this expression was derived under paraxial assumptions, it is quite general and has been shown[11] to apply to nonparaxial situations. It clearly demonstrates the equivalence of holographic imaging to imaging with lenses and, in fact, (8-51) may be written as the familiar paraxial imaging equation,

$$\left[\frac{1}{R_i} + \frac{1}{R_c} \right] = \frac{1}{F}$$

where F is the "focal length" of the hologram,

$$F = \frac{\varepsilon^2}{\mu} \left[\frac{R_o R_r}{R_o - R_r} \right]$$

and μ is the wavelength ratio λ_c / λ_r.   In an analogous fashion, the coordinates of off-axis holograms are specified (Figure 8-29) by the expressions,

$$\frac{X_i}{R_i} = \frac{X_c}{R_c} \pm \frac{\mu}{\varepsilon^2} \left[\frac{X_r}{R_r} - \frac{X_o}{R_o} \right]$$

and

$$\frac{Y_i}{R_i} = \frac{Y_c}{R_c} \pm \frac{\mu}{\varepsilon^2} \left[\frac{Y_r}{R_r} - \frac{Y_o}{R_o} \right] \tag{8-52}$$

Subscripts i, c, o, and r refer to image, reconstruction, object, and reference coordinates.   The Cartesian coordinates X and Y have their origin at the hologram (Figure 8-28), and R is a radial distance from the origin.

As with a lens system, (8-51) and (8-52) merely describe the image position and do not indicate image quality.   In general, a wavelength change, or a hologram enlargement, or nonduplication of the reference beam will produce aberrations in the image.   The aberration coefficients

---

* Only a portion of the image will be in focus on the screen since the image is three dimensional.

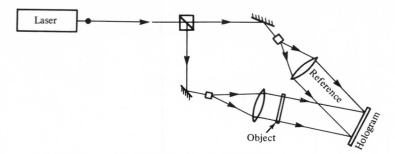

Figure 8-29   Typical hologram recording schematic.

are given in Ref. 11.   For high-quality imaging one must always ensure that the reconstructing source has the same wavelength and is in the same position as the reference source.

8·5·3   recording and reconstruction—off-axis holograms

So far, this presentation has been concerned largely with diffraction, the basic phenomena involved in the construction and reconstruction of a hologram.   Attention is now turned to the recording process and its influence on the reconstruction.   Whereas most of this discussion is applicable to holography in general, certain aspects of off-axis holography will be emphasized, since this recording scheme is by far the most important and widely used.   Figure 8-29 shows a plane view of a typical schematic for the construction of a hologram of a transmitting object.

The dot on the beam emerging from the laser is intended to indicate laser radiation polarized perpendicular to the paper.   This is the first important point regarding the recording geometry.   If the light is polarized in the plane of the paper, at least two serious problems are encountered. First, there could be a large reduction of the beam intensity at every surface due to polarizing effects as predicted by the Fresnel equations (6-2 through 6-5).   These effects do not occur with vertical polarization (light polarized at right angles to the plane of incidence; see Figure 8-30).   Second, only those components of the electric field oscillating parallel to each other can interfere.   One can see in Figure 8-30 that the vertical components of the incident, reflected, and transmitted waves are parallel, but the horizontal components are not.   It is easy to visualize a hologram made with horizontal polarization of the laser beams where the signal beam is at right angles to the reference beam; no interference occurs, thus producing a sterile hologram.

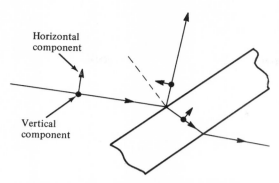

Figure 8-30 Polarization by reflection.

Now, assuming that the polarization of signal and reference is properly oriented, we can begin to examine the recording. For this purpose consider the situation of Figure 8-31; the interference of a point signal with a collimated reference beam. The signal may be written

$$E_s = A_s(x, y)e^{i(2\pi\phi(x, y))/\lambda}$$

where $\phi(x, y)/\lambda$ describes the phase at the position where the signal component strikes the hologram plane. Note that the amplitude, $A_s(x, y)$, of the signal varies over the hologram plane according to the distance r.

The reference beam is written

$$E_r = A_r e^{-i(2\pi x \sin \theta)/\lambda}$$

analogous to (8-8) where we describe the interference between two plane waves. The term $\sin \theta/\lambda$ has the dimensions of a spatial frequency.

As before, the quantity of interest is the total intensity, which is

$$I_t = (E_s + E_r)(E_s + E_r)^*$$

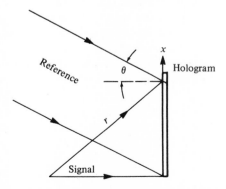

Figure 8-31 Hologram of a point signal.

where * indicates the complex conjugate.   Substituting for the amplitudes, the intensity † becomes

$$I_t = |E_r|^2 + |E_s|^2 + E_r^* E_s + E_s E_s^*$$

$$= I_r + I_s + 2\sqrt{I_s I_r} \cos 2\pi\left(\frac{x \sin \theta}{\lambda} + \frac{\phi}{\lambda}\right) \tag{8-53}$$

The first term of (8-53) is a constant and may be regarded as a bias intensity.   The second term, denoting the signal intensity, varies as $1/r^2$, where r is the distance from the signal to any point on the hologram.   The third term is the interference between the signal and reference that is now an intensity map of the signal.   The analogy of this interference to radio communication helps to elucidate the process.   The term $\sin \theta/\lambda$ may be regarded as a carrier frequency.   This carrier is frequency modulated (FM) by the signal term, ϕ/λ.   This is the way phase information is converted into intensity information.   The amplitude of the carrier is further modulated (AM) by the amplitude variations $[A_s(x, y)]$ of the signal.

By writing (8-53) in exponential form, the sidebands of the modulated signal are made evident:

$$I_t = I_r + I_s + \sqrt{I_r I_s}\, e^{i2\pi(x \sin \theta + \phi/\lambda)/\lambda} + \sqrt{I_r I_s}\, e^{-i2\pi(x \sin \theta + \phi/\lambda)/\lambda} \tag{8-54}$$

In order to faithfully record this total intensity (8-54), a linear recording medium is required.   For the time being, assume that the recording material is affected linearly only by the incident intensity:

$$\frac{dt_a}{dE} = \alpha \tag{8-55}$$

The terms of (8-55) are explained by Figure 8-32.

Linearity is obtained in certain restricted regions of most photographic emulsions.   In practice, no material is sensitive to the intensity alone but will include phase changes.   Below, phase holograms will be discussed where the intensity transmission of the emulsion is relatively insensitive to incident intensity variations.

If the photographic plate is developed so that it conforms to (8-55), i.e., the recording is linear, the resultant transmittance, t_a, can be expressed as

$$t_a(x, y) = A + \alpha[I_r + I_s + \sqrt{I_r I_s}\, e^{i2\pi(x \sin \theta + \phi)/\lambda}$$

$$+ \sqrt{I_r I_s}\, e^{-i2\pi(x \sin \theta + \phi)/\lambda}] \tag{8-56}$$

† The intensity as written in this chapter is not to be confused with photometric intensity which is luminous flux per solid angle.

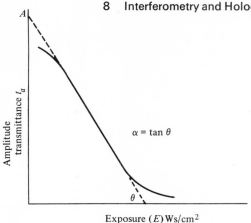

$\alpha = \tan \theta$

Figure 8-32   Exposure characteristic of recording medium.

The constants, A and α, are defined in Figure 8-32. This complex expression may be denoted by

$$t_a(x, y) = t_b + t_s + t_v + t_c \qquad (8\text{-}57)$$

where $t_b = A + \alpha I_r$ is the amplitude transmittance due to the "bias" of the reference beam, $t_s = +\alpha I_s$ is related to the "zero order" of the signal, t_v is a varying transmittance associated with the original signal wave, and t_c a varying transmittance associated with the conjugate of the signal.

Now, if this plate is illuminated with a beam identical to the original reference beam, the resultant transmitted wave will simply be the product of the plate transmittance and the reference amplitude:

$$U(x, y) = t_a(x, y)E_r$$

Making use of both (8-56) and (8-57), the transmitted field can be written in slightly more complicated form but one of great utility:

$$U = E_r[t_b + t_s + \alpha E_r^* E_s + \alpha E_r E_s^*]$$

$$= E_r t_b + E_r t_s + \alpha |E_r|^2 E_s + \alpha E_r^2 E_s^* \qquad (8\text{-}58)$$

Incorporated in this expression are the holographic image fields. The first term indicates a plane wave propagating in the same direction as the reference beam but with an amplitude reduced by t_b. The second term is the zero order of the signal; this term is usually small as a consequence of maintaining linear recording. The third term is the signal multiplied by a constant; this transmitted wave is the reconstructed signal wave or virtual image field. Note that, if the hologram is made with the geometry of Figure 8-31, the reconstructed image wave is diverging, in a fashion similar to images formed with a negative lens. In these situations the image is virtual, lying behind the hologram (lens), and viewed as if looking through a window with the dimensions of the hologram. Conversely, the hologram forms a "real image" similar to a positive lens; this image is indicated by the fourth term of (8-58), although complicated by the presence of the square of the reference beam. In volume holography, to be discussed below, one can see that if the hologram is illuminated by a beam identical to the reference beam but antiparallel to it, i.e., the conjugate, E_r^*, then the fourth term would read,

$$t_c = \alpha E_r E_r^* E_s^* = \alpha |E_r|^2 E_s^* = \alpha A_r^2 E_s^* \tag{8-59}$$

which is the *conjugate* signal of the real image, multiplied by a constant. This image can be focused in space and is viewed in front of the hologram, as illustrated in Figure 8-26. The real and virtual images are the twin images we spoke of earlier.

A greater insight into (8-58) is obtained by referring to the exponential forms of the signal and reference (8-54). By doing this, it may be concluded that the reference beam has a constant spatial frequency of

$$\beta = \frac{\sin \theta}{\lambda} \tag{8-60}$$

that is *modulated* by the phase variations of the signal. In analogy with radio communications, β is the carrier and the modulation technique is *FM*. Further, the spatial frequencies of the signal and reference are functions of angular coordinates as was elucidated earlier in the discussion of interferometry; therefore, in general, the reference beam, virtual image, and real image are all angularly separate. This does not mean that the images and the reference beam do not overlap. In practice it is usually easy to avoid overlapping by a careful geometric design of the location of the optical equipment. Now, let us see what angular separation means in terms of the total spectrum or bandwidth that is produced and what constraints this imposes on the recording medium. To find this spectrum, the Fourier transform is applied to the transmittance of the hologram plate (8-56 and 8-57). The general form of the transform is

$$f(u, v) = \int_{-\infty}^{\infty} E_s(x, y) e^{-i2\pi(ux + vy)} \, dx \, dy = \mathscr{F}[E_s(x, y)] \tag{8-61}$$

where u and v are spatial frequencies, and x and y are spatial coordinates. Thus,

$$\mathscr{F}[U] = [t_b] + \alpha \mathscr{F}[A_s^2] + \alpha A_r \mathscr{F}[E_s e^{-i2\pi x\beta}] + \alpha A_r \mathscr{F}[E_s^* e^{i2\pi x\beta}] \tag{8-62}$$

where A_r is the amplitude of the reference beam, and A_s is the amplitude of the signal beam. This expression is now written in succinct form with the aid of (8-61).

$$\mathscr{F}[U] = t_b \delta(u, v) + \alpha |f(u, v)|^2 + \alpha A_r f(u - \beta, v) + \alpha A_r f^*(-u - \beta, v) \tag{8-63}$$

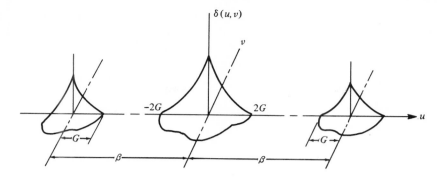

Figure 8-33   Frequency spectrum of off-axis hologram.

The spectrum of the signal has already been defined as $f(u, v)$. Now suppose that the highest signal frequency is G. Then, with the aid of Figure 8-33, (8-63) may be explained as follows: The first term, a delta function, is the spectrum of a plane wave and is indicated in Figure 8-33 as a spike at the origin. The second term of (8-63) is just the square of the signal spectrum; it has a maximum frequency of $2G$, the factor two arising from the exponential of $|f(u, v)|^2$. This is depicted schematically in Figure 8-33 as the "smear" about the origin. Note that in the figure there are two "sidebands" each located at the carrier frequency, β, from the origin. These displaced sidebands represent the signal spectra given by the last two terms of (8-63). Evidently, we can keep the sidebands isolated from the second term if

$$\beta \geq 3G$$

It can be seen that high resolution off-axis holography entails high spatial frequencies, imposing stiff requirements on the recording medium. The carrier frequency, β, could be reduced if the second term of (8-63) were absent. This can be done by reducing the signal amplitude well below that of the reference. This technique has another benefit; it helps to achieve linear recording when practical photographic emulsions are used. Then, the minimum reference frequency becomes

$$\beta \geq G$$

and the reference angle,

$$\theta_{\min} = \sin^{-1} G\lambda$$

8·5·4   recording media

At this point, the characteristics of a recording medium that are of most importance in the making of a hologram have been developed. They are: linearity, thickness, and spatial frequency bandwidth. By linearity is

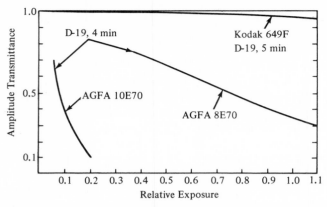

Figure 8-34   Characteristic curves of several photographic emulsions.

meant that the amplitude transmittance varies linearly with exposure. Holograms made with a material having this characteristic are called *absorption* holograms. Linearity in practical materials is realizable, although the region of linearity is somewhat restricted. The point is illustrated in Figures 8-34 and 8-35, showing the amplitude transmittance of several silver halide photographic emulsions of common use.

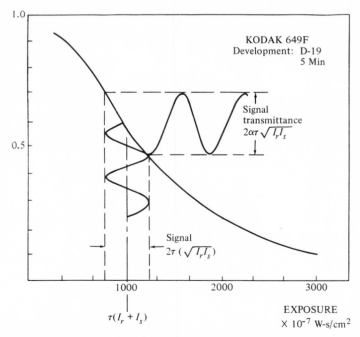

Figure 8-35   Recording a hologram on Kodak 649F. $\tau =$ **exposure time, $I_r =$ intensity of reference, $I_s =$ intensity of signal, $\alpha =$ slope.**

In Figure 8-35, the bias terms of (8-56) are drawn along with the interference or oscillatory terms. Obviously, the signal amplitude must be only a fraction of the reference beam amplitude if the recording is to be linear. In practice, the ratio of reference amplitude to signal amplitude may be greater than 10 : 1. This is the reason why the bias of the signal, given by the second term of (8-56), is often dropped. The hazards of large signal amplitudes are nonlinearities resulting in degraded images having either a surrounding haze[12] or ghosts. However, to casual observers of pictorial objects, these deficiencies are rarely noticed. For this type of object, the reference to signal amplitude ratio may be one since the result will be the brightest images. Linear recording is not without drawbacks. The interference of small signals with a strong reference background causes only a small amplitude modulation of the carrier so that the recorded interference pattern is of low "contrast." The result is that the reconstructing light wave is not efficiently diffracted, or coupled to the signal.

The *diffraction efficiency* is an important practical quantity and is commonly defined as

$$\eta = \frac{\text{first order image power}}{\text{reconstructing beam power}} \qquad (8\text{-}64)$$

The variation of diffraction efficiency versus beam intensity ratio is shown in Figure 8-36 for a typical absorption hologram. Note that the maximum diffraction efficiency is about 5 percent. Much higher diffraction efficiencies approaching 100 percent may be obtained with phase holograms,[13] and especially with thick phase holograms. In these holograms, the incident intensity variations produce localized changes in the index of refraction of the medium and/or changes in its thickness without any

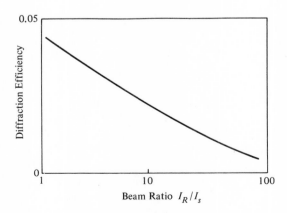

Figure 8-36 Diffraction efficiency versus beam intensity ratio, Kodak 649F spectroscopic emulsion.

alteration of the transparency.   Viewing such a hologram in diffuse room light, one sees only a clear plate.

One way of producing a partial phase hologram is to record in an absorption material, such as a silver-halide emulsion, and then bleach out the silver.   Efficiencies as high as 30 percent may be obtained by these methods,[14] but the images usually show a great deal of flare.   The flare arises due to scattering at the "relief" on the emulsion surface arising from a tanning action of the bleaching agent.   The flare may be considerably reduced by immersing the hologram in a liquid whose index of refraction matches that of the gelatin emulsion.   A suitable liquid is immersion microscope oil.   In order to achieve high diffraction efficiencies, a hologram that is to be bleached must be recorded at low transmittances, as shown in Figure 8-37, so that the recording process is nonlinear. Improved images may be obtained from bleached holograms by avoiding harsh treatment of the emulsion.[16]

A material that works as an almost perfect thick phase hologram with none of the objections of bleached holograms is dichromated gelatin.[17] The preparation and processing of this material are extremely simple. Reconstructed images show almost nonexistent "noise" due to scattering, and diffraction efficiencies of up to 96 percent have been measured for plane-wave gratings.   The recording characteristic of this material is shown in Figure 8-38.   This material has some drawbacks, as follows: First, it is orthochromatic and, for all practical purposes, insensitive above 514.4 nm.   Second, its sensitivity is very low; about ten times below Kodak 649F.   Third, the emulsion is sensitive to humidity levels above 50 percent.

A useful comparison of exposure times for various materials is shown in Table 8-2 for a typical recording scheme using an argon laser operating at 488 nm.

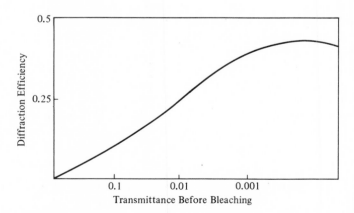

Figure 8-37   Diffraction efficiency of bleached holograms.[14]   **(With permission of American Institute of Physics.)**

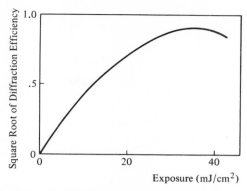

Figure 8-38 Response of dichromated gelatin at 488 nm.[17] (*With permission of American Institute of Physics.*)

Mention has been made of "volume" holograms. This type of hologram has a thickness much larger than the wavelength. The recorded interference pattern or fringes lie throughout the emulsion as illustrated in Figure 8-25, so that the image reconstruction is dominated by the Bragg effect; i.e., unless the Bragg condition is satisfied, the reconstructing wave will not be efficiently coupled to the image wave. This is graphically depicted in Figure 8-39a where the amount of departure, $\Delta\theta_r$, from the Bragg angle, θ_r, for extinction of the image, is given in terms of the emulsion thickness, t.

Figure 8-39b shows experimentally measured attentuation versus the angle of reconstruction for Kodak 649F emulsion. This discussion of the effects of emulsion thickness is very important because, in all likelihood, most of the holograms today are "volume holograms" made in thick media. For instance, Kodak 649F spectroscopic emulsion, a commonplace hologram recording medium, is about 15 μm thick. Therefore, for $\lambda = 488$ nm, $t = 30\lambda$ at 488 nm, and extinction of the image occurs at only 4° on either side of the Bragg angle (Figure 8-39a). The experimental results depicted in Figure 8-39b verify these calculations. Further complicating this point is the fact that photographic films shrink in thickness during normal processing so that the fringes in the emulsion may become angularly reoriented as indicated in Figure 8-40.

In this case, the image quality can be severely degraded, and the image brightness reduced, especially if the signal wavefront is not planar. Attempts to adjust the reconstruction beam angle to compensate for the

TABLE 8-2   Typical Exposure Times

	Dichromated Gelatin	Kodak 649F	Agfa 8E70
Exposure time, s	50	0.5	0.05

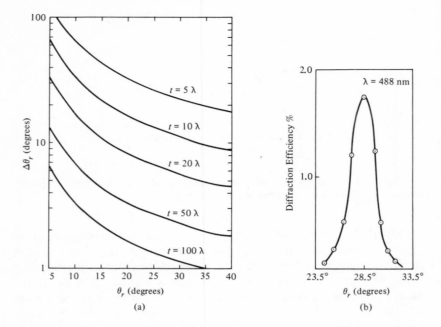

Figure 8-39 (a) Orientation sensitivity of Bragg holograms.   Curves are for total extinction.[12]   (b) Experimental measurement of orientation sensitivity.   Kodak 649F emulsion (t $\simeq$ 15 μm) at λ = 488 nm.   ((a) is with permission of John Wiley and Sons, Inc.)

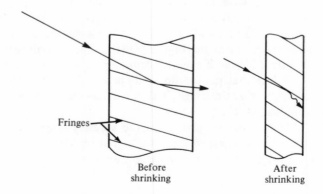

Figure 8-40   Effect of emulsion shrinkage.

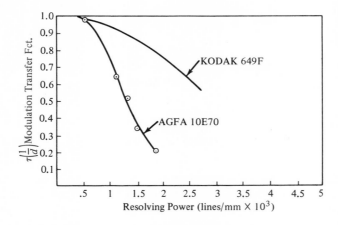

Figure 8-41   Response of two holographic emulsions.

angular fringe shift only introduces aberrations into the image.[11]   There are several ways around this problem: First, the emulsion may be swelled to its original thickness.[4]   This method is not satisfactory where the highest resolution is required or where a great degree of permanency is required.   Second, the recording film may be placed at right angles to the angle bisector of the signal and reference beams.   In this case, the fringes will lie at right angles to the plane of the emulsion and they will not be angularly shifted during shrinking.   Third, processing techniques or emulsions can be used that do not shrink.

To conclude this brief account of recording media, mention should be made of resolving power requirements.   The bandwidth of the recording process for off-axis holograms was seen to be quite high.   In fact, spatial frequencies of several thousand lines per millimeter are not uncommon. Most photographic emulsions do not resolve above about 200 lines/mm. However, there are fine-grain photographic plates that can resolve thousands of lines per millimeter.   The response of two of these is given in Figure 8-41.   The response is defined as the normalized diffraction efficiency of a plane-wave grating formed in the emulsion with a fringe frequency, v.   It is a measure of the *contrast* of the recorded interference fringes and their ability to diffract light into the image.

8·5·5   *other practical considerations*

Beam Uniformity   We have seen how the diffraction efficiency and image quality depend on the beam ratio I_r/I_s.   It is particularly important that the reference beam be fairly uniform over the hologram. There are a number of ways to achieve beam uniformity.   In the following,

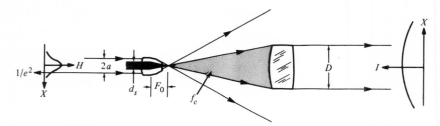

Figure 8-42   Beam expansion using low f/number objective.

a laser beam with Gaussian intensity distribution is assumed.   The first and easiest method is to sample the laser beam.   This is graphically illustrated in Figure 8-42 for a beam expander configuration.   Evidently, a laser beam can be expanded to almost any diameter just by using a telescope in reverse.   The amount of expansion is determined by the focal lengths of the lenses.   However, if the f/number of the largest (colli-mating) lens is greater than the expanding lens, as shown in Figure 8-42, the expanded intensity distribution will not be the same as the laser beam (Gaussian).   This is because only a portion of the expanded beam passes within the aperture of the collimating lens.   In fact, we can project the expanded beam diameter back through the expanding lens to find the "active" diameter d_s (Figure 8-42) of the laser beam.   In this manner we can find the maximum amount of power emerging from the system and the uniformity.   The power emerging is

$$P_0 = 2\pi \int_0^{d_s/2} I_r r \, dr = P_1[1 - \exp(-d_s^2/2a^2)] \tag{8-65}$$

where P_1 = the laser power ($P_1 = I_0 \pi a^2/2$),
    I_r = the intensity distribution [$I_r = I_0 \exp(-2r^2/a^2)$],
    r = a radial dimension,
    a = the beam radius at which the intensity drops to $1/e^2$.

The ratio, Δ, of the intensity at the beam edge to that at the center is given by:

$$\Delta = \frac{I_r(d_s/2)}{I_r(0)} = \exp(-d_s^2/2a^2) \tag{8-66}$$

Comparison of (8-65) and (8-66) shows that the percentage of power conserved by the optical system is

$$\frac{P_0}{P_1} - 1 = \Delta \tag{8-67}$$

a simple but very useful relationship.   Figure 8-43 shows the intensity at the expanded beam edge as a function of the laser beam radius for two expanding lenses of different focal lengths.   Obviously, good intensity

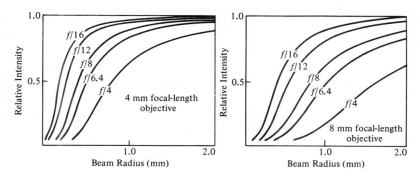

Figure 8-43   Intensity at expanded beam edge as a function of expansion optics.

uniformity across the expanded beam requires wasting a large fraction of the incident laser power as indicated by (8-67).   A technique not nearly as wasteful but more difficult to accomplish is to filter the Gaussian; i.e., reduce the high intensity in the beam center until it matches the intensity level near the beam edge as shown in Figure 8-44.   The intensity of the laser beam is

$$I_r = \frac{2P_1}{\pi a^2} \exp(-2r^2/a^2) \tag{8-68}$$

and therefore a filter whose intensity transmittance is given by

$$T = \exp[2(r^2 - r_0)/a^2)] \tag{8-69}$$

is needed.   The r_0 term is introduced to limit the transmittance to values less than unity.

The power transmitted by this filter is given by:

$$P_t = \text{(area of the filter)} \times \text{(transmitted intensity)}$$

$$= (\pi r_0^2)\left(\frac{2P_1}{\pi a^2}\right)\exp(-2r_0^2/a^2)$$

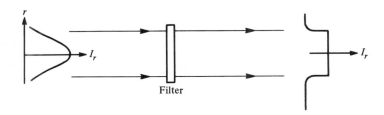

Figure 8-44   Effect of absorption filter with inverse Gaussian transmittance.

The power transfer is maximized when

$$r_0 = a/\sqrt{2}$$

Thus,

$$P_{max} = \pi r_0^2 \frac{2P_1}{\pi a^2} \exp(-2r_0^2/a^2)\Big|_{r_0 = a/\sqrt{2}} = 0.37P_1$$

A filter of this type may be produced in an approximate fashion on fine-grain photographic film.   However, the substrate must be plane-parallel to avoid multiple interferences in the plate, thus restricting this method to small diameter filters.   There are methods that can convert the Gaussian distribution to a cylindrical distribution with insignificant power loss.   One of these[18] uses two aspheric glass elements: the first to redistribute the power to produce the uniform intensity, and the second to correct the phase so that the emerging wavefront is plane (Figure 8-45a).

Another method is to produce the desired redistribution using variable index glasses, i.e., glass whose index of refraction grades in the proper manner from the optical axis to the edges.   Two elements would be required with plane-parallel faces (Figure 8-45b).

<u>Coherence Length Extension</u>   It is sometimes desirable to extend the coherence length of a laser, particularly when a high-power gas laser is the source.   This is because the spectral line will be relatively broad in a high-power laser and there will be many longitudinal modes (i.e., wavelengths).   In other cases, we may be interested in forming a hologram of a large three-dimensional object, giving a variety of widely different signal path lengths from each portion of the object.   Measurement of the optical paths is frequently done with a graduated tape, which is convenient but not very accurate.   There are other reasons for desiring a long coherence length, but the ones given are representative.

A *coherence length extender* in its commonly advertised form is nothing more than a fixed separation Fabry-Perot interferometer that is placed in the laser cavity.   The thickness of the "etalon" is selected to

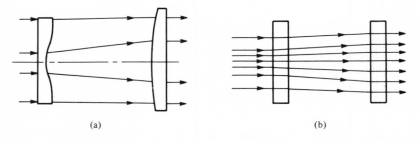

(a)   (b)

**Figure 8-45   Devices for changing Gaussian intensity distribution.
(a) Aspheric elements (U.S. Patent 3,476,463).   (b) Graded index glass.**

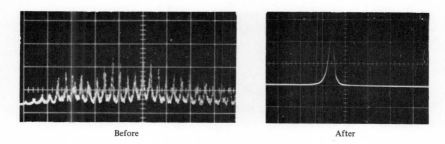

Before   After

Figure 8-46   Effect on mode structure of inclusion of Fabry-Perot etalon in laser cavity.

allow one or a few longitudinal modes to pass and the others to be reflected. In this manner the effective line width of the laser is narrowed and the coherence length extended according to (8-1), repeated here,

$$\ell = \frac{\bar\lambda^2}{\Delta\lambda} \tag{8-1}$$

HeNe lasers usually do not require coherence extenders except for making holograms of large objects. A 50 mW HeNe laser has a coherence length of about 30 cm. High-power argon-ion lasers are a different story. The coherence length at 488 nm is typically only 6 cm. In this case, the tuning of a coherence length extender (etalon) can be a troublesome procedure unless a scanning spectrum analyzer* is available. Figure 8-46 shows the spectrum of a 1 W laser beam at $\lambda = 488$ nm with and without a coherence length extender.

Detectors   Except in those cases of extremely low light levels that might result when a low-power HeNe laser beam is expanded, the use of a photomultiplier for intensity measurements is usually not required. In addition, the photomultiplier tube requires a complicated, bulky power supply and meter. It is also affected by magnetic and electric fields, a point that cannot be overemphasized considering the common use of large cast-iron optical tables and the possibility of RF excited lasers. Cadmium-sulfide cells serve quite well especially for HeNe radiation. They are compact and convenient with little electronics required. However, they are nonlinear with intensity and somewhat unstable. Vacuum phototubes have good stability and linearity and are convenient to use (see Chapter 9).

Finally, it might be mentioned that it is usually important to be able to measure the intensity and uniformity of the reference beam at the hologram. If the reference beam is diverging it may be difficult and

---

* A moving mirror confocal Fabry-Perot interferometer.

inconvenient to measure the intensity if the detector and housing are physically large because of possible interference with other optical equipment, such as the photographic plate holder.

Losses at Optical Components
This discussion is chiefly of reflection and absorption losses. Reflection losses usually occur at glass-air interfaces, such as uncoated lenses. These unwanted reflections can be troublesome for two reasons:

1. They reduce the power intensity (W/cm^2) at the hologram, thereby increasing exposure time. As an example, an uncoated air-spaced doublet lens will have a loss due to reflection of about 20 percent.
2. They can result in unwanted signals at the hologram. For instance, an uncoated back surface of a beamsplitter will produce a low-level "ghost" of the intended beam. In the case of an uncoated lens, reflections at each surface produce real and virtual point sources. These arise since each spherical surface acts as a partial mirror. The imaged point sources will interfere and produce interference fringes at the hologram; they usually appear in the reconstructed image, particularly if they are present in the reference beam.

Reflections can be significantly reduced by coating transmitting optical elements with an antireflection film. Quite often lens elements are used that were not optimally designed for the wavelength of interest. In these cases it is sometimes fruitful to eliminate lenses and replace them with mirrors. However, front surface metallized mirrors develop absorption losses in time. A typical absorption loss in the surface is about 15 percent.

Optical Component Damage
High-power unexpanded laser beams will damage cement used in compound lenses and in prism beamsplitters. For instance, a 1 W argon laser beam will melt cement in microscope objectives and prism beamsplitters and burn holes in absorption type neutral density filters. In addition, *pinhole spatial filtering* becomes somwhat more difficult due to heating of the metal foil when the filter is slightly detuned.

Signal Redundancy
It is very desirable to spread the signal over as much of the hologram area as possible. This reduces the requirements on the photographic film by limiting the signal variations to fall within the linear dynamic range of the emulsion and to provide redundancy of the signal. A hologram recorded in this manner will be insensitive to system perturbations, such as dust or scratches on the hologram, and can be useful in increasing the resolution of the hologram.

In the case of three-dimensional objects, the aforementioned redundancy is achieved by virtue of the *diffusing* nature of most holo-

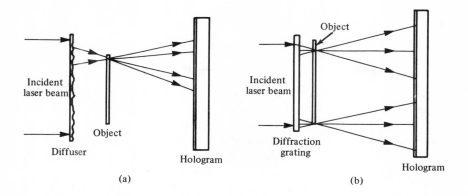

Figure 8-47   Methods of achieving signal redundancy.

graphic subjects.   For two-dimensional transparencies, a ground glass may be used behind the subject (Figure 8-47a).   Unfortunately, the reconstructed image is "noisy" because a speckle pattern is observed in the image background.   One might say that the resolution is limited by a high noise level.   Microimages are affected by this background, but pictorial subjects do not suffer as much because of the limited resolution of the eye and the nature of the subject.

Redundancy can also be achieved by use of a diffraction grating, as shown in Figure 8-47b.

Spatial Filtering   Noise generated by dust on the output mirror of the laser, beamsplitters, and expanding lenses is intolerable for practically all holograms, including pictorial or three-dimensional holograms. Since a dust particle is essentially an amplitude impulse, the spectrum of the impulse consists of high spatial frequencies.   In other words, the light is scattered into large angles as shown in Figure 8-48.   An expanding lens (microscope objective) will display these scattered light waves over a

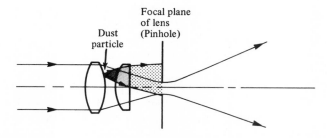

Figure 8-48   Removal of optical noise with spatial filter (pinhole).

broad area at its focal plane.   On the other hand, a collimated laser beam is focused to a spot on the optical axis no smaller in diameter than

$$d_0 = \frac{1.27F\lambda}{d_L} \tag{8-70}$$

when the incident beam is Gaussian distributed in intensity.   The symbol F refers to the lens focal length, and d_L is the laser beam diameter at the $1/e^2$ points.   In Chapter 7, the Fourier transforming property of lenses is discussed and it is shown that the spectrum of an incident light wave is displayed at the lens focal plane.   If the incident light wave is a laser beam, the spectrum consists of a large zero-order term, corresponding to the focused spot.   Spread around this zero-order term are the high spatial frequency components of low intensity.   If a small pinhole is put at the focal plane of the lens so that only the zero-order or focused spot passes, the beam is *spatially filtered* to exclude high frequencies, i.e., we have a low-pass filter.   The pinhole can be twice as large in diameter as that given by (8-70) without significantly affecting filtration, since noise due to dust, etc., is composed of very high frequencies.   For example, a $40\times$ microscope objective ($F = 4$ mm) used to filter a 1 mm HeNe laser beam requires a pinhole approximately $d_0 = (2)(1.27)(4)(0.63)/1 = 6$ μm in diameter. Pinholes above 3 μm in diameter are readily available.

<u>Stability</u>   The question of stability is graphically outlined by the following question: Can holograms be made of moving objects or with moving optical equipment?   The answer is yes, but under a specified condition.   The condition is that during the recording process, the interference fringes generated by the signal and reference may move only a small fraction of their separation.   Any large movements will cause a smearing, and either the fringes will not be recorded or they will be of low contrast which leads to low diffraction efficiency.   The tolerable amount of fringe movement is determined from the resolution that is desired in the hologram.   For instance, an angle of 90° between the signal and reference beams will produce a fringe separation of one-half wavelength.   If the fringe separation is not to change by one tenth of this, then the object and the optical equipment must be stable *during the exposure time* to within $\lambda/20$.   Obviously, shorter exposure times will allow greater rate of movement of the fringes.   The use of Q-switched ruby lasers will give exposure times as short as 25 ns; therefore, holograms of good quality can be made with objects moving at speeds of about 5 m/s.

Inasmuch as most work in holography involves the use of a CW laser, exposure times are usually greater than 1 s and sometimes are several minutes.   Time-exposure holography requires stability between all components including the object.   This means that all components must be rigid, fixed relative to each other, and not subject to vibrations.   This is usually accomplished by mounting all equipment on a stable platform that is isolated from all disturbances, including acoustic.   The best platforms (tables) have good isolation from the building and are well damped; in addition, they do not vibrate (ring) in response to acoustic noise.   In some cases, it is desirable to have a system light in weight.   This can be accomplished by use of a composite construction of several materials.   However, the platform must be rigid.

Early holographic practice was to "float" a block of granite or cast iron on a bed of partially inflated inner tubes.   These systems are not very well damped and will tend to oscillate for fairly long periods in response to impulsive forces applied to the table top.   For instance, a $4' \times 10'$ ribbed cast-iron table weighing $1\frac{1}{2}$ tons, (supported by 16 aircraft tire inner tubes inflated to 4 psi) will have a total displacement of one tenth the wavelength of a HeNe laser 23 s, after an impulse is applied to the top.   This means that if the table is used to mount holographic equipment, it should be allowed to stabilize for about 30 s before any exposures are made, even though all the equipment is rigidly fastened to the table.   This is a tolerable amount of time and massive tables of this type are quite useful for holography.   Because of their weight, they do not move appreciably when leaned upon, making them convenient working surfaces.   However, the floor loading is fairly high.   Granite blocks have an advantage over cast iron in that granite will not support "ringing."   Therefore, it is not subject to acoustic forces such as the "click" of a shutter.   However, it is easier to provide clamping means for optical equipment on a cast-iron table.

In recent years tables specifically designed for holography and precision optical work have become available (Figure 8-49).   They employ air bearings which give excellent isolation from floor vibrations.   A variety of table tops can be supplied, from granite to aluminum honeycomb structures.   However, the buyer should ensure that the top has high inertia to prevent continuous oscillations in response to acoustic noise.   This quality is not always supplied with certain types of composite table tops. The result is good floor isolation but continuous platform movement.

8·5·6   applications of holography

Although holography has stirred the imagination of many people, industrial applications are not legion.   It has been said that holography has provided a use for the laser; now we are searching for a use for holography. At present, holography remains largely a laboratory tool.   The reason is that good quality holographic images are consistent only with high stability of the holographic camera.   In addition, practical exposure times are limited by the power of the laser.   Hence, it is most convenient to carry on experiments or processes on a stable table using CW gas lasers.

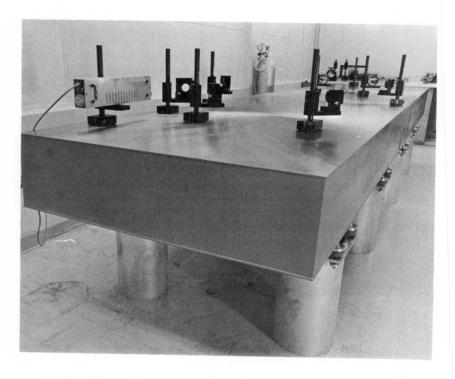

Figure 8-49 *Optical table of composite construction with air piston supports. (With permission of Modern Optics, Inc.)*

Although Q-switched ruby lasers have ameliorated this condition some-what,[19] it is not likely that we will see many applications outside the laboratory in the near future. In spite of this situation, there are many exciting applications of holography in information storage, optical data processing, interferometry, microscopy, and even displays. In the next few pages, a brief account is given of some of these applications.

Holographic Interferometry   In this application, the holographic image is made to interfere with an object or another holographic image. The amount of disparity between them is displayed as a pattern of inter-ference fringes. The scheme is illustrated in Figure 8-50. The hologram is constructed in the usual manner. During reconstruction, the object is illuminated as before, and the scattered object light is superposed on the

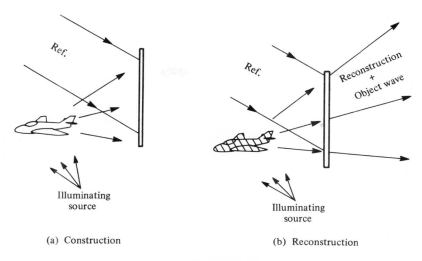

(a) Construction

(b) Reconstruction

Figure 8-50   Principle of holographic interferometry.

reconstructed virtual image wave.   Any phase variations between the two superimposed waves will result in interference that appears as a contour map of the difference.   Holographic interferometry affords great advantages over interferometry or other more conventional measurement techniques.   First, three-dimensional objects can be examined in one step without the need for sectioning or restricting the object field; this is due to the large depth of field of a hologram.   Second, object deformations can be viewed in real time; i.e., changes in the object shape are continuously displayed as a changing interference pattern.   These points are to be kept in mind while considering the following three applications of holographic interferometry: the testing of large mirrors and lenses, generation of contours on objects of arbitrary shape, and holographic interference microscopy.

The Testing of Large Optics   In one method,[26] large mirrors are tested in their mounts by a two-step process: first, a laser beam is focused to a spot by the mirror and a hologram is made of this spot; second, the hologram is reconstructed in a laboratory environment and the usual optical tests (knife-edge, etc.) performed on the reconstructed spot as if the mirror were actually there.   The advantage is that the effects of the mirror and environment may be measured; the environment and certain operating conditions are difficult to achieve in the laboratory.   Also, the reconstructed virtual image wave may be made to interfere with a spherical wavefront as indicated in Figure 8-51.   The displayed fringes are the mirror aberrations.

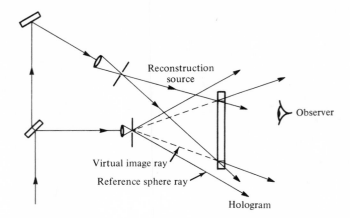

Figure 8-51 Setup for common path hologram interferometry.[26]
(*With permission of American Institute of Physics.*)

In another variation, a reconstruction of the real image can be used to perform a Foucault or knife-edge test on a mirror or lens. The results of a test on a 100 mm focal length, $f/1$ lens are shown in Figure 8-52. The knife-edge was inside the reconstructed focus; the lens has spherical aberration.

Another technique[27] used to test unworked mirror blanks utilizes the interference between the original object wave (alternatively, the reconstructed wave) and the wave from the same object after it has been deformed by thermal or mechanical means. The technique requires that the hologram be placed back in its original position after development and, further, that holograms emulsion shrinkage must be avoided or compensated. The hologram is constructed as shown in Figure 8-53a; an interferogram of a heated mirror blank is shown in Figure 8-53b. The circular fringes show that the curvature of the mirror blank has changed uniformly.

Contour Generation   By using certain techniques, to be discussed shortly, it is possible to cause interference between two images of an object in such a way that the fringes are displayed as contour lines.[20] The benefits of such a technique are obvious: the automatic mapping of objects.

One method of generating contours is to make a multiple hologram in which there are two successive exposures corresponding to two positions of the object illuminating source (signal). By changing the position of the illuminating source in between exposures, there will be a phase difference between the two object waves. Figure 8-54a shows the recording scheme. In Figure 8-54b the loci of the interference fringes is shown.

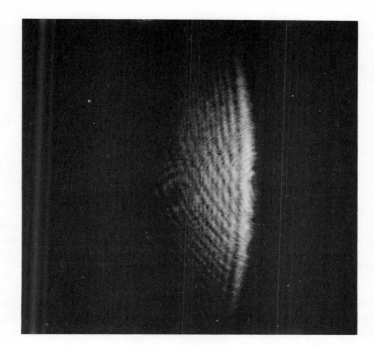

Figure 8-52   Knife-edge test on reconstructed focus of a 100 mm f/1 positive lens.   Knife edge inside focus; curved edge indicates presence of spherical aberration.

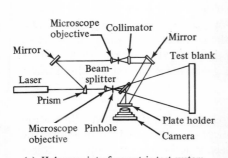

(a) Hologram interferometric test system.

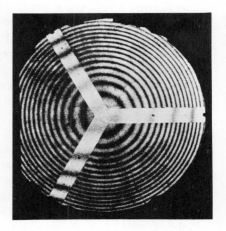

(b)   Interferogram of 70 cm fused silica mirror blank taken when blank was 26°C above room temperature

Figure 8-53   (With permission of American Institute of Physics.)[27]

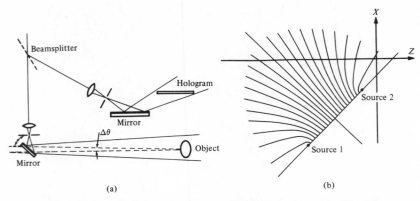

Figure 8-54 (a) Experimental arrangement for recording contour holograms using the two-source method ($\Delta\theta$ represents the notation of the mirror between exposures). (b) Loci of interference for the two-source hologram.

It should be evident upon examination of these figures that the object must be side-lighted in order to obtain contour planes that lie parallel to the hologram. Using (8-16) and Figure 8-2, the distance between contours is found to be

$$s = \frac{\lambda}{2 \sin(\Delta\theta/2)}$$

Figure 8-55 is a photograph of the virtual image of a mandrel showing contour lines produced by the two-source method. The stainless-steel mandrel is ellipsoidal in shape and is used to make reflectors for infrared heating applications. The mandrel was sprayed with a flat white lacquer to increase the diffuse reflectance of the surface. The minor diameter of the ellipsoid is 75 mm and the contours are 2 mm apart. It should be noted that the contours may also be generated by using an illuminating source having two wavelengths.[20]

Holographic Interference Microscopy In this third illustration of holographic interferometry, a microscope is used to magnify the object; interference takes place between a reference field and the object in the same way as previously indicated in the testing of mirror blanks. In one method,[28] a hologram is made of a clean glass slide that is positioned in the object plane as shown in Figure 8-56. The hologram is located near the image plane of the microscope objective.

After development, the hologram is carefully placed in its original position and re-illuminated with the reference beam. At the same time, an object specimen is placed on the microscope stage and is illuminated

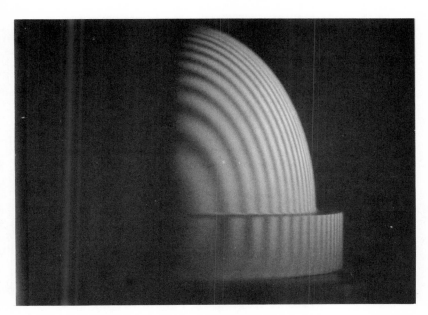

Figure 8-55   Photograph of a virtual holographic image of an ellipsoidal mandrel showing contour lines produced by the two-source method. The contour lines indicate a displacement of 2 mm.

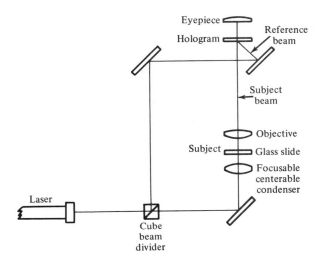

Figure 8-56   Transmitted light holographic interference microscope.[28] *(With permission of American Institute of Physics.)*

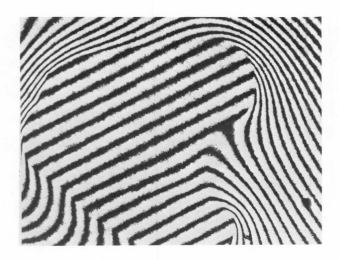

Figure 8-57 Oil smear photographed on holographic interference microscope—oblique section interference.[28] *(With permission of American Institute of Physics.)*

with the laser.   Evidently, the reconstructed image wave of the clear slide will be superimposed onto the specimen wave and the phase differences will result in interferences.   Therefore, the viewed display will be fringes that are contours of constant phase difference.   The effect is illustrated in Figure 8-57.

Correction of Lens Aberrations   The aberrations of a simple lens may be corrected, using a hologram, for one pair of object and image points[21] (conjugates).   The advantage of this technique appears to be the possibility of achieving good quality lenses in an inexpensive way.   Although this is true to a certain extent, the actual performance of a corrected lens leaves a lot to be desired, chiefly due to the properties of the hologram.   For instance, monochromaticity of the reconstructing source is a necessity, although the high temporal coherence of the laser is not required.   Second, the hologram also adds aberrations of its own when the reconstructing source is not located at the position of the reference source.   This is important when imaging extended objects.   Nevertheless, the corrected lens generally exhibits better performance over a given angular field than the lens alone.   To elaborate on these statements, consider the schematic of a general aberration correction arrangement as shown in Figure 8-58a.   In the diagram the signal source is shown located on the optical axis of the simple lens.   In this case, the wave emerging from the lens has spherical aberration; i.e., the wavefronts, or surfaces of constant phase, do not conform to the contour of a sphere.   If the aberrated wave interferes with a spherical reference wave of the correct

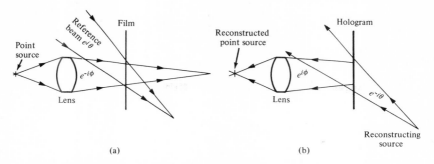

(a)   (b)

Figure 8-58   **(a)** *Construction of corrector hologram.*   **(b)** *Reconstruction of the conjugate aberrated field.*

curvature, then the aberration is recorded in the form of a hologram.   In the reconstruction process, the hologram is illuminated with the *conjugate* to the reference beam so as to produce the *real reconstructed image* (Figure 8-58b).   Since this real image wave is the conjugate of the aberrated wave that originally emerged from the lens, the lens will convert this wave into a perfectly spherical wavefront so that the lens is limited only by diffraction at its aperture.   It is to be emphasized that this condition is true only for the original object and image points.   For other points, i.e., off-axis objects and images, the performance of the corrected lens degrades, but it does not degrade in the same manner as the lens alone.   Figure 8-59 makes this comparison for an 8 cm focal-length lens.

Figure 8-59 is a chart of the approximate cutoff resolving power of each system.   Although this chart is a measure of the lens performance in the presence of those hologram and lens aberrations that influence image clarity, such as spherical aberration and coma, there is no indication of the effects of distortion or curvature of field, which influence image position only.   In Figure 8-60a, the image curvature of a planar object is shown in a qualitative way.   It is seen that the chief contributor to this degradation is the hologram.   Figure 8-60b shows the image distortion occurring

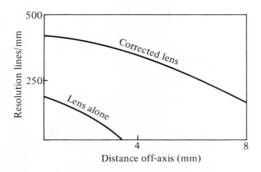

Figure 8-59   *Comparison of lens resolution with and without corrector.*

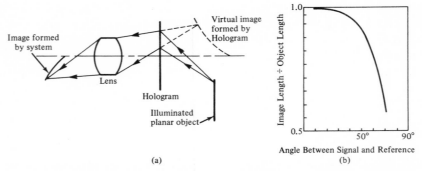

Figure 8-60 **(a) Images of a planar object formed by lens-corrector system. (b) Hologram-corrector image distortion.**

to object lengths in the plane of Figure 8-60a. This is solely a consequence of the off-axis character of the recording scheme (Figure 8-58a).

In summary, it may be said that the overall quality of a holographically corrected lens is improved over the lens alone provided one is interested only in image clarity.

Optical Memories   Optical memories are attractive because of the huge information storage capacity of photographic materials. In addition, the access may be made random and at high speed by rapid switching of a light beam. A schematic of one type of optical memory, a holographic memory, is shown in Figure 8-61. This system is being investigated by Bell Telephone Laboratories. In order to have a capacity that is competitive with existing disc memories, the information must be stored in page form, each page consisting of a number of bits of information. Selection of a particular page may be at random and is accomplished by reconstructing from the holographic store. The reconstructing laser

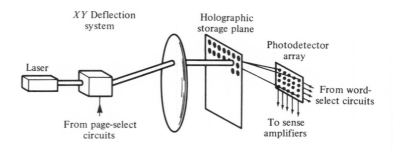

Figure 8-61   Random-access holographic memory being developed in Bell Telephone Laboratories, Inc.   (With permission of Laser Focus 6, 36 (February 1970).)

beam is moved to the proper position by means of an acoustic beam deflector.[29]   The chief problem with holographic memories seems to be material in nature; i.e., one would like to have not only permanent memories but also read-write types.   It is this latter need that will require significant research and development before a useful material is obtained.

Volume Imaging and Displays   The initial excitement over holography was the result of the display of three-dimensional images and the parallax properties of these images.   In addition, the semidiffuse nature of such objects as figurines, toy trains, ship models, etc., allowed the clear demonstration of the redundancy built into the hologram; i.e., the ability to reconstruct most of the image from a fragment.   If one could collect all the holograms made throughout the world since 1963, most likely the majority would be of the display type.   However, the first industrial application of holography was in *volume imaging*, where the three-dimensional application character of the image was of great interest.   This application was the measurement of the size and distribution of aerosol particles.[30]   Although the details of this application will not be elaborated here, a companion application will be described in detail.   Consider an object whose surface contour is to be measured as a function of Cartesian coordinates.   The holographic real image of this object is a duplicate of the object and is localized in space.   If this image can be measured, then an optical, noncontact method of storing and retrieving dimensions results. A basic schematic of the idea is shown in Figure 8-62.

Two problems must be solved to make this measurement technique viable.   First, the image contour must be discernible from the rest of the light pattern in the image and, furthermore, it must be sufficiently localized in space.   This means that the image contour must be set apart from the

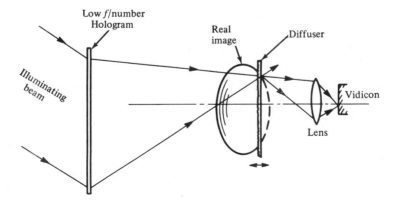

Figure 8-62   Measurement of the three-dimensional contour of an object by examination of the holographic real image.

background of light that is forming other parts of the image, and the contour must be sharply imaged. This problem is solved by:

1. Painting the object with a discernible matrix such as a grid, and
2. Constructing the hologram so that it has a low f/number and, therefore, a very restricted depth of focus.

The second problem is that there must be some way to measure automatically the Cartesian coordinates. This is obtained by cross-sectioning the image with a diffusing screen, as shown in Figure 8-62. The contour of the object at that longitudinal cross section is then displayed on the screen and may be electronically scanned with a television system, and the contour coordinates measured in terms of the video signal.

In order to achieve good definition of a particular cross-sectional contour and to restrict this contour to a small longitudinal region (small depth of focus) for reasons of good resolution, the hologram must image with a low f/number. The depth of focus of a diffraction limited optical system is

$$D = 4f^2\lambda$$

This is the longitudinal region about the image plane for which one obtains no appreciable degradation of the image quality. In the system described here, geometric limitations on off-axis recording of the hologram prevent the attainment of very low f/numbers. This is because the object will shadow the reference beam. Practically speaking, the useful depth of focus will be around 50 μm.

An area that may eventually prove quite useful is holographic displays for simulation and training. In a training situation involving visual displays, it is necessary to transmit a sufficient number of accurate visual cues to the trainee, so that he will react in a similar fashion to the real situation. Quite often, the visual display is an image of a model scene. The image is transmitted either electronically or optically to a viewing screen. The display changes in accordance with the trainee's response and the characteristics of the vehicle that is being simulated. For instance, suppose that a pilot is to be trained to land a jetliner on a commerical airfield. The pilot is to see a lighted runway looming before him and the position of that runway must change according to changes in the response of the aircraft under direction of the pilot. The essential parts of the simulator are shown in Figure 8-63a. The scale of the model scene is limited by the physical size of the imaging probe. The model is likely to be fairly large and movement of the probe or scene in six degrees of freedom is necessary to simulate the flight characteristics of a jetliner. This system can be simplified if a hologram is made of the model scene. The schematic is shown in Figure 8-63b. The hologram is shown mounted on a servo system. This requires a "thin" hologram so that Bragg

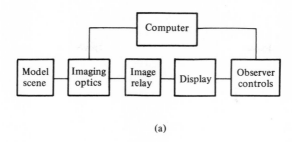

(a)

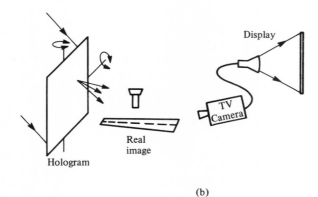

(b)

Figure 8-63   (a) Block diagram of real-time simulator.   (b) Schematic of real-time holographic display.

losses do not limit the angular motion of the hologram to only a few degrees.   In addition, the real image has to be used if the simulator is to "land" on the airfield.

Microimaging   The advantages of using holography to do micro-imaging are not as immediately clear as the previous applications.   The requirements of microimaging are fairly straightforward: to produce the highest quality images at or near the limit of optical resolution.   An industrial use of this is in the production of microelectronic circuits. Here, a camera containing the optical system is used to project an image of some circuit array onto a photoresist covered substrate such as silicon. The array contains many fine features and the subsequent processing of the microelectronic circuit may involve about ten sequential overlayed image projections and chemical processings.   Each of these images is required to mate properly with its predecessor.   The optical system should be as close to diffraction limitation as possible.

Recently, there has been a decided effort to design lenses for projection printing of silicon integrated circuits.   The lenses must be designed for ultraviolet wavelengths (because of photoresist sensitivity), and a high degree of correction must be achieved over the field.   In practice, image quality degrades from the center to the edges of the image field.   Therefore, there is a limit to the size of the image field commensurate with a given limiting resolution of the lens.   This can be expressed as a *space-bandwidth-product*,

$$\text{SBP} = (\text{limiting resolution})(\text{field size})$$

which is given here in a one-dimensional form.   The product for an area would be the square of that given above except for a constant.

The SBP is a measure of the amount of information that can be passed by the optical system, i.e., the total amount of detail that can be transmitted. The SBP for a well-designed lens operating over a 50 mm image field at a wavelength of 436 nm approaches 25,000.   Larger field sizes usually require lenses of longer focal length so that the angles that the rays make in the image space do not get too large (the aberrations of a lens are related to higher powers of the image angle).   However, longer focal-length lenses can have high space-bandwidth products, but usually with lower limiting resolution.

The advantage of a hologram is that it can exceed the SBP of a lens, especially for large field sizes.   There are a number of parameters that influence the attainment of good image quality using a hologram.   Each of these will be evaluated in the following discussion along with those factors affecting the use of holography in microelectronic production.   A typical schematic of a holographic microimaging setup is illustrated in Figure 8-64.   The *size of the reference reconstructing sources* (shown as pinholes) influences the resolution in the reconstructed image.   The pin-

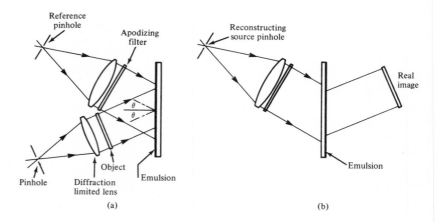

Figure 8-64 **(a) Holographic recording of microimages.   (b) Real-image reconstruction.**

hole is used to spatially filter the laser beam,* in order to remove "noise" generated by dust on the optics, fluorescence of the laser, etc., that would reduce image quality if allowed to remain.   If the pinhole diameter is less than the diffraction limit of the collimating lens, then the lens influences the image resolution and the pinhole has no effect.   If the pinhole is larger than the diffraction limit of the lens, then the limiting image spot size is given by[31]

$$R_i \left[\frac{\delta_r}{R_r} + \frac{\delta_c}{R_c} \right]$$

where δ_r and δ_c are the pinhole diameters of the reference and reconstructing sources and the other parameters are identified on page 469. Thus, high resolution can be attained by use of small pinholes and low f/number collimating lenses.

Also of interest is the effect of the *bandwidth* of the illuminating and reconstructing laser sources.   Referring to the section in this chapter on diffraction gratings, one can deduce the effect of bandwidth on a diffraction grating (plane-wave hologram) by assuming the source wavelength to have some spread, $\Delta\lambda$.   The spread may be the Doppler broadened line of a gas laser transition.   When the hologram is reconstructed, there will be a spread in the diffracted light since each wavelength component will be satisfying the grating equation (8-11).   When the same laser is used to construct and reconstruct, the angular spread is given, approximately, by

$$\Delta\theta \simeq \frac{\Delta\lambda}{\lambda}$$

A typical HeNe laser has a broadened line width of about 0.002 nm; thus

$$\Delta\theta \simeq 3 \times 10^{-6} \text{ rad}$$

This is much smaller than the diffraction limit of most holograms.   Only when the hologram is quite large ($\simeq 25$ cm) is the image resolution limited primarily by the laser bandwidth.   The hologram size for an argon-ion laser is smaller.   However, with the use of a coherence length extender, the bandwidth of a gas laser can be greatly reduced to the point where the image resolution is insignificantly affected.

Hologram Aberrations   Aberrations must be reduced to a nonexistent level if the hologram is to have a large SBP.   The alignment of a hologram within the reconstruction beam is a crucial factor in the elimination of hologram aberrations.   The situation is illustrated in Figure 8-65a for the general case of a spherical reference beam.   The emulsion is shown facing the reference source.   If the glass is facing the source, the diverging light must pass through the glass thickness before reaching the film.

---

* See section in this chapter on Spatial Filtering.

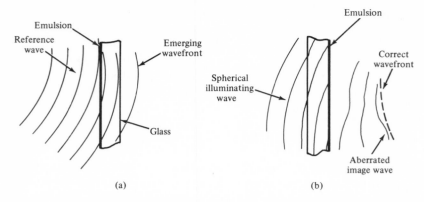

Figure 8-65 *(a) Spherical reference wave propagating through a photographic plate. (b) Image reconstruction showing effect of substrate glass.*

This can introduce spherical aberration and astigmatism. However, these aberrations are introduced into the real image anyway, since the reconstructing beam must converge through the glass as shown in Figure 8-65b. This problem is avoided by using a collimated reference and signal beam. Collimation has other, more significant benefits. First, spherical aberration and coma are absent in the image. Second, the longitudinal position of the hologram is not critical since the curvature of the wavefront is zero and, therefore, a constant everywhere.

References

1. F. A. Jenkins and H. E. White, *Fundamentals of Optics*, 3rd Ed., McGraw-Hill Book Co., New York (1957).
2. M. Born and E. Wolf, *Principles of Optics*, Rev. Ed. 4th Ed., Pergamon Press, Inc., New York (1970).
3. M. Francon, *Optical Interferometry*, Academic Press Inc., New York (1966).
4. L. H. Lin and C. V. LoBianco, "Experimental Techniques in Making Multicolor White Light Reconstructed Holograms," *Appl. Optics* 6, 1255 (July 1967).
5. R. L. Fork, D. R. Herriott, and H. Kogelnik, "A Scanning Spherical Mirror Interferometer for Spectral Analysis of Laser Radiation," *Appl. Optics* 3, 1471 (1964).
6. F. Twyman, *Prism and Lens Making*, Hilger, Hilger and Watts, Ltd., London (1957).
7. D. Gabor, "Microscopy by Reconstructed Wavefronts," *Proc. Phys. Soc.* A197, 454–487 (1949). Also, D. Gabor, "Microscopy by Reconstructed Wavefronts: II," *Proc. Phys. Soc.* B64, 449–469 (1951).
8. E. N. Leith and J. Upatnieks, "Reconstructed Wavefronts and Communication Theory," *J. Opt. Soc. Amer.* 52, 1123 (1962).

9. J. W. Goodman, *Introduction to Fourier Optics*, p. 244, McGraw-Hill Book Co., New York (1968).

10. Ora E. Myers, Jr., "Studies of Transmission Zone Plates," *Am. J. Phys.* **19**, 359 (1951).

11. Edwin B. Champagne, "Nonparaxial Imaging, Magnification, and Aberration Properties in Holography," *J. Opt. Soc. Amer.* **57**, 51 (1967).

12. H. M. Smith, *Principles of Holography*, Interscience Publishers, Inc., New York (1969).

13. H. Kogelnik, "Reconstructing Response and Efficiency of Hologram Gratings," *Proc. Symp. Modern Optics*, Polytechnic Press, New York (1967).

14. J. Upatnieks, and C. Leonard, "Diffraction Efficiency of Bleached, Photographically Recorded Interference Patterns," *Appl. Optics* **8**, 85 (1969).

15. C. B. Burckhardt and E. T. Doherty, "A Bleach Process for High-Efficiency, Low-Noise Holograms," *Appl. Optics* **8**, 2479 (1969).

16. K. S. Pennington and J. S. Harper, "Techniques for Producing Low-Noise, Improved Efficiency Holograms," *Appl. Optics* **9**, 1643 (1970).

17. L. H. Lin, "Hologram Formation in Hardened Dichromated Gelatin Films," *Appl. Optics* **8**, 963 (1969).

18. J. L. Kreuzer, "Coherent Light Optical Systems Yielding an Output Beam of Desired Intensity Distribution at a Desired Equiphase Surface," U.S Patent 3,476,463, November 4, 1969.

19. R. G. Zech, "Pulsed Laser Holography," Spring Meeting of Optical Society of America, San Diego, Calif., March 11, 1969.

20. B. P. Hildebrand and K. A. Haines, "Multiple-Wavelength and Multiple Source Holography Applied to Contour Generation," *J. Opt. Soc. Amer.* **57**, 155 (1967).

21. J. Upatnieks, A. Vander Lugt, and E. Leith, "Correction of Lens Aberrations by Means of Holograms," *Appl. Optics* **5**, 589 (1966).

22. E. H. Linfoot, *Recent Advances in Optics*, Oxford University Press, London (1955).

23. G. B. Parrent, Jr., and G. O. Reynolds, "Space Bandwidth Theorem for Holograms," *J. Opt. Soc. Amer.* **56**, 1400 (1966).

24. Mil-Hdbk-141, *Optical Design*, Section 21, U.S. Government Printing Office (October 1962).

25. J. H. Bruning and D. R. Herriott, "A Versatile Laser Interferometer," *Appl. Optics* **9**, 2180 (1970).

26. B. P. Hildebrand, K. A. Haines, and R. Larkin, "Holography as a Tool in Testing of Large Aperture Optics," *Appl. Optics* **6**, 1267 (July 1967).

27. W. Van Deelen and P. Nisenson, "Mirror Blank Testing by Real-Time Holographic Interferometry," *Appl. Optics* **8**, 951 (May 1961).

28. K. Snow and R. Vandewarker, "An Application of Holography to Interference Microscopy," *Appl. Optics* **7**, 549 (March 1968).

29. E. I. Gordon, "A Review of Acousto-optical Deflection and Modulation Devices," *Proc. IEEE* **54**, 1391 (October 1966).

30. B. J. Thompson, J. H. Ward, and W. R. Zinky, "Application of Hologram Techniques for Practice Size Analysis," *Appl. Optics* **6**, 519 (1967).

31. Edwin B. Champagne and Norman G. Massey, "Resolution in Holography," *Appl. Optics* **8**, 1879 (September 1969).

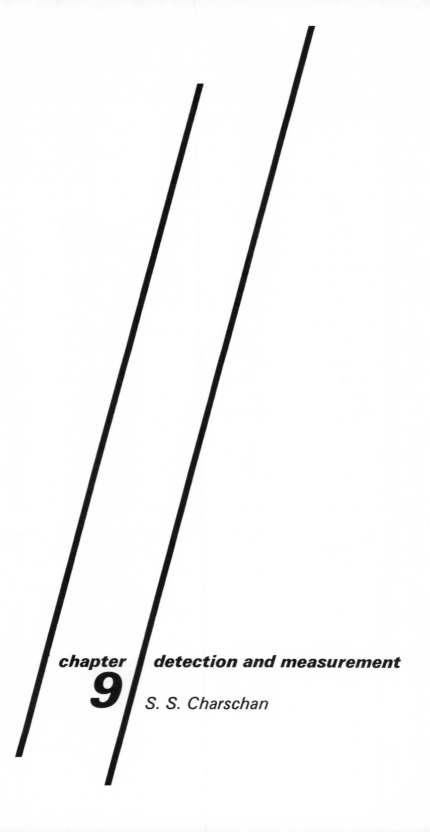

chapter 9 **detection and measurement**

S. S. Charschan

9·0 introduction

Many kinds of detectors are commonly used to analyze the spectral distribution and measure the output energy and power of laser radiation. In the visible spectrum, patterns can be observed on a sheet of paper or recorded on photographic films.[1] At other frequencies, phosphors can be caused to luminesce. However, in most cases, quantitative measurements are required.

Detectors which are commonly used to measure the radiant energy emanating from lasers may be separated arbitrarily into two general types. The first type, *quantum detectors*,[2] are those devices that will produce measurable outputs when the sensing elements are struck by photons and free electrons (or holes) are produced. Such detectors are quantum counters in the sense that the interaction involves a single photon of radiant energy and the output is proportional to the number of photons. The second type, *heat detectors*, are those devices that produce some measurable indication of change in the physical states of the sensing elements when they absorb radiated energy.[3] Thermal radiation detectors, being energy integrators, respond only to the intensity of the absorbed radiant power. Both types of detectors are square-law devices; their output signals are proportional to the input radiant power.

Figure 1-14 shows various lasers, their frequencies and photon energies. This chapter relates the various types of detectors to the frequencies they are normally used to detect.

For short wavelengths (λ between 400 nm and 1200 nm) phototubes offer the advantages of amplification by electron multipliers and higher speed. Semiconductor detectors (which also are quantum detectors) are useful over the entire range. Intrinsic semiconductors are available for energies greater than 0.2 eV; whereas doped semiconductors, which require cooling, detect wavelengths in the infrared. Heat detectors provide wide coverage, although they have less speed and sensitivity than quantum detectors.

Having described briefly the various types of detectors currently available, we must consider the conditions under which they may be used, their limitations, and the relative merits of various alternatives.

9·1 terminology and definitions

The fundamental physical phenomenon that determines many aspects of our subject is the fact that electromagnetic radiation interacts with matter in "quanta" called *photons*. The photon energy is given by

$$E = \frac{hc}{\lambda} \text{ ergs} = \frac{hc}{\lambda} (1.6 \times 10^{-12}) \text{ eV} \qquad (9-1)$$

where h, Planck's constant, is 6.5×10^{-27} erg-s; c, the velocity of light in free space, is 3.0×10^{10} cm/s; and λ is wavelength.   Thus 1 mJ of radiation energy at a wavelength of 400 nm (blue light) corresponds to 2×10^{15} photons.

Light is defined as electromagnetic radiation that stimulates the visual senses.   Therefore, the acronym "laser" strictly defines a coherent radiation source emitting in the visible region.   However, the term "laser" is now being used in the broadest sense to denote sources with outputs ranging from the ultraviolet to far infrared.   The ultraviolet region extends, in wavelength, from below the visible region (380 nm) to the X-ray region at about 10 nm.   The infrared extends from the approximate upper region of the visible (780 nm) to the radio band beginning at about 780×10^5 nm.

Radiometry deals with the measurement and specification of radiation. However, when the human eye is used as a detector of radiation, the phenomena is described in terms of the luminous intensity, and we speak of the study of photometry.   This chapter is limited to radiometry.

9·1·1   quantities of radiometry

The basic quantity in radiometry is the radiant power of the source, the radiant flux (Φ).   The watt is a typical unit of radiant flux (International System (SI) Unit).

$$\text{Flux} = \Phi \quad \text{W} \tag{9-2}$$

The flux density (irradiance) of a unit area of a receiver is dimensionally identical to the flux per unit area emitted by the source (emittance).   A typical unit is the watt per square meter.

$$\text{Irradiance } (M) = \frac{d\Phi}{dA} \quad \text{W/m}^2 \tag{9-3}$$

$$\text{Emittance } (E) = \frac{d\Phi}{dA} \quad \text{W/m}^2 \tag{9-4}$$

where dA is the infinitesimal area over which the flux, $d\Phi$, is measured. In measuring irradiance, the spectral characteristics of the light source, the detector, and any intervening optics must be defined.

With a point source, the irradiance drops inversely with the square of the distance (r).   This factor of proportionality is called *radiant intensity* (I).

$$\text{Irradiance } (H) = \frac{d\Phi}{dA_n} = \frac{I}{r^2} \tag{9-5}$$

where A_n is the component of the area element normal to the flux propagation. The solid angle, measured in steradians, subtended by an infinitesimal area element, dA_n, at a point distance r, is

$$d\Omega = \frac{dA_n}{r^2} \qquad (9\text{-}6)$$

where Ω is referred to as the solid angle. Thus, we have

$$\text{Intensity } (I) = \frac{d\Phi}{d\Omega} \qquad \text{W/sr} \qquad (9\text{-}7)$$

i.e., the intensity is the amount of flux radiated per steradian. In general, a source can be considered a point if we are far enough away from it. If

TABLE 9-1   Standard Units, Symbols, and Defining Equations for Fundamental Photometric and Radiometric Quantities[a]

Quantity[a]	Symbol[a]	Defining Equation[b]	Commonly Used Units	Symbol
Radiant energy	$Q, (Q_e)$		Erg	
			Joule[e]	J
			Kilowatt-hour	kWh
Radiant density	$w, (w_e)$	$w = dQ/dV$	Joule per cubic meter[e]	J/m^3
			Erg per cubic centimeter	erg/cm^3
Radiant flux[c]	$\Phi, (\Phi_e)$	$\Phi = dQ/dt$	Erg per second	erg/s
			Watt[e]	W
Radiant flux density at a surface				
Radiant exitance (Radiant emittance)[d]	$M, (M_e)$	$M = d\Phi/dA$	Watt per square centimeter	W/cm^2
Irradiance	$E, (E_e)$	$E = d\Phi/dA$	Watt per square meter, etc.[e]	W/m^2
Radiant intensity	$I, (I_e)$	$I = d\Phi/d\omega$ (ω = solid angle through which flux from point source is radiated)	Watt per steradian[e]	W/sr
Radiance	$L, (L_e)$	$L = d^2\Phi/d\omega \, (dA \cos\theta)$ $= dI/(dA \cos\theta)$ (θ = angle between line of sight and normal to surface considered)	Watt per steradian and square centimeter Watt per steradian and square meter[e]	$W/sr\ cm^2$ $W/sr\ m^2$
Emissivity	ε	$\varepsilon = M/M_{blackbody}$ (M and $M_{blackbody}$ are, respectively, the radiant exitance of the measured specimen and that of a blackbody at the same temperature as the specimen)	One (numeric)	

Note: The symbols for photometric quantities are the same as those for the corresponding radiometric quantities (see above). When it is necessary to differentiate them the subscripts v and e, respectively, should be used, e.g., Q_v and Q_e.

[a] Quantities may be restricted to a narrow wavelength band by adding the word spectral and indicating the wavelength. The corresponding symbols are changed by adding a subscript λ, e.g., Q_λ for a spectral concentration or a λ in parentheses e.g., $K(\lambda)$, for a function of wavelength.
[b] The equations in this column are given merely for identification.
[c] Φ_i = incident flux; Φ_a = absorbed flux; Φ_r = reflected flux; Φ_t = transmitted flux
[d] To be deprecated
[e] International System (SI) unit
With permission of the Illuminating Engineering Society.

an error of 10 percent in the irradiance can be tolerated, the source can be as large in diameter as one tenth the distance. Of course, this depends on the physical characteristics of the source and the angular location of the observer.

When the area of the radiating source is not negligible, the intensity per unit area may be of interest. This is called *radiance* or *angular emittance* (L) and is expressed as

$$\text{Radiance } (L) = \frac{dI}{dA_n} = \frac{d^2\Phi}{d\omega\, dA_n} \qquad \text{W/sr m}^2 \qquad (9\text{-}8)$$

For pulsed radiation, the time integral of the flux is used to express the quantity of radiant energy (Q).

$$\text{Radiant energy } (Q) = \int_0^t \Phi\, dt \qquad \text{J} \qquad (9\text{-}9)$$

See Table 9-1 for a summary of the units, symbols, and defining equations.[4]

9·1·2   detector terminology and performance criteria

The pertinent characteristics of photon detectors have been given in different ways in the literature. This variation, which often leads to confusion, is primarily due to the diverse backgrounds and nomenclature of contributors who are optical engineers, material scientists, infrared physicists, or communications engineers.

Responsivity   For detectors with an electrical output the responsivity, R, is simply defined as the ratio of the rms value of the detected voltage to the rms power incident on the detector.

$$R = \frac{\text{rms output voltage}}{\text{rms input power}} \qquad (9\text{-}10)$$

To be useful, this transfer function is usually linear over an appreciable range.

The responsivity of an individual photodetector (with fixed detector area, A, and detecting time constant, τ) depends upon five key parameters.

$$R = R(\lambda, f, P_a, T, g) \qquad (9\text{-}11)$$

where λ is the wavelength of the source; f is the signal frequency (usually a mechanical chopper) used to enable low-drift, high-gain amplification of small signal voltages; P_a is the ambient background radiation; T is the absolute temperature; and g is the gain parameter.

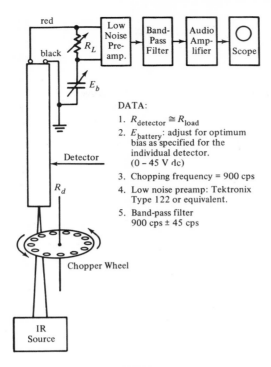

red

black

R_L

Low Noise Pre-amp.

Band-Pass Filter

Audio Amp-lifier

Scope

E_b

DATA:

1. $R_{\text{detector}} \cong R_{\text{load}}$
2. E_{battery}: adjust for optimum bias as specified for the individual detector. (0 – 45 V dc)
3. Chopping frequency = 900 cps
4. Low noise preamp: Tektronix Type 122 or equivalent.
5. Band-pass filter 900 cps ± 45 cps

Detector

R_d

Chopper Wheel

IR Source

Figure 9-1   Typical (infrared detector) laboratory test setup.   (With permission of Raytheon Company.)

Figure 9-1 is a typical infrared detector laboratory test setup, and Figure 9-2 shows response curves.

Responsivity is usually measured when the detector is operated under maximum detectivity conditions while being irradiated with a blackbody source at 500°K.   Therefore, the measured value of responsivity is of little value in determining the power sensitivity of the detector to monochromatic laser light.   The spectral responsivity R_λ of the detector may be obtained by comparison with a radiation thermopile.

Noise-Equivalent Input   Noise-equivalent input, NEI, is a measure of the minimum irradiance, H, per unit area of detector required to produce a signal-to-noise ratio of unity.

$$\text{NEI} = \frac{H}{(\Delta f)^{1/2}} \frac{V_n}{V_s} \quad \text{W/cm}^2 \text{ Hz}^{1/2} \qquad (9\text{-}12)$$

For specification purposes, noise bandwidth (Δf) is normalized to 1 Hz. Noise data are conveniently taken at 4 Hz and the noise voltage divided by 2 (the square root of the bandwidth employed for measurement). NEI depends upon operating conditions, just as responsivity.

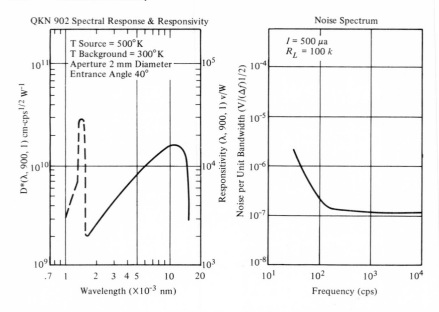

Figure 9-2   Response curves for an infrared detector (QKN 902-Raytheon).   (With permission of Raytheon Company.)

<u>Noise-Equivalent Power</u>   Noise-equivalent power, NEP, is a measure of the minimum power that can be detected.   It is the product of NEI and the area of the sensitive surface, and, therefore, NEP is a performance measure of a specific detector.

$$NEP = (NEI)A = \frac{HAV_n}{V_s(\Delta f)^{1/2}} \quad W/Hz^{1/2} \quad (9\text{-}13)$$

The conditions of measurement affect the NEP as they do NEI.   If manufacturers' values are used for NEP, it is essential that due note be taken of the condition under which the NEP was measured.   Standard conditions for its measurement employ a blackbody source operated at 500°K, and modulating frequencies of 90, 400, or 900 Hz.

Under certain conditions, the use of the NEP as a criterion for selecting the best detector for a receiving application can lead to the wrong choice even though the best possible signal-to-noise ratio is obtained.   As the bandwidth requirements increase, the thermal noise power can no longer be ignored.   The NEP does not take into account this thermal noise because it is specified for 1 Hz bandwidth where the dark current noise in photodiodes is always greater than the thermal noise.   The best detector to discriminate against background noise is the detector with the highest quantum efficiency, whereas the best detector to discriminate against internal noise is the detector with the best NEP.

The NEP is often written as NEP (500°K, 400, 1) which indicates that this is the detector noise equivalent power for a 500°K source, a 400 Hz chopping frequency, and a 1 Hz bandwidth.   Note that a lower NEP means an increase in the detecting capability.

Detectivity   The reciprocal of NEP is denoted as detectivity, D. The term (no longer widely used) associates a large number with a corresponding higher detector sensitivity.   Detectivity expresses the rms signal-to-noise voltage ratio obtained per watt of incident radiant power.

Detector D^* and D_λ^* For fundamental reasons, detector noise is usually proportional to the sensitive area of a detector.   The D^* of the detector, conceptually related to detectivity and originally introduced to remove the dependence of NEP on the detector's sensitive area,[5] is related to NEP by the expression

$$D^* = \frac{A^{1/2}}{\text{NEP}}   \text{cm Hz}^{1/2}/\text{W} \tag{9-14}$$

where A is the sensitive area of the detector reduced to 1 cm^2, and a Δf of 1 Hz.

The use of D^* has met wide industry acceptance as a figure of merit, and it is presently used more than NEP to specify the detector's sensitivity. Because D^* is spectrally dependent, its value is frequently quoted as a specific function of wavelength D_λ^*.

The theoretical limitations of sensitivity in terms of D^* are based on Planck's radiation law.   The detectivity will be ultimately limited by the background and the signal fluctuations.

A background-limited photoconductive detector, which is called a BLIP detector, has its D^* value given by

$$D_\lambda^* = \frac{1}{2h} \frac{\varepsilon^{1/2}}{J_B} \tag{9-15}$$

where J_B is the background irradiance in photons/cm^2/s, and ε is emissivity.

Figure 9-3 is a plot of energy distribution of blackbodies for different temperatures.[6]   It can be seen that as long as one can reduce the background temperature, D^* will increase until the background photons are of the same value as the signal photons, at which point consideration must be given to the signal photon noise.

As with NEP, it is common practice to report D^* in the form D^* (500°K, 900, 1) equals a value.   These refer to the value of D^* for a 500°K blackbody, as measured at a 900 Hz chopping frequency, and a 1 Hz noise bandwidth.

The value of D^* is independent of the detector frequency response for what has been denoted[7] Class I detectors, which include photoemissive

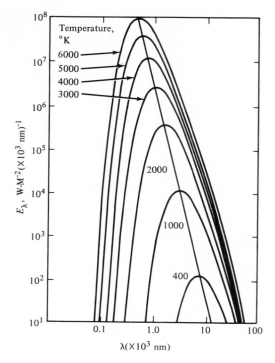

Figure 9-3   Energy distribution of blackbodies.[6]   **(With permission of IEEE, Inc.)**

devices and some photoconductive devices. In Class II detectors, $D*$ varies as the square root of the inverse of the frequency response. Lead sulfide detectors are of the Class II type.

A figure of merit, M, is also introduced for the two classes. For Class I detectors, M is defined as the ratio of the measured value of $D*$ to the value of $D*$ for an ideal detector at the temperature $300°K$. M is given by

$$M_1 = [5.52 \times 10^{-11} \text{ W/cm Hz}^{1/2}]D* \qquad (9\text{-}16)$$

For Class II detectors, M_2 was defined as the ratio of $D*$ to the value of $D*$ for a detector that accords with Haven's limit. Haven's limit is an engineering estimate of the maximum possible detectivity of a thermo-couple or bolometer. M_2 is given by

$$M_2 = [6 \times 10^{-11} \text{ W·s/cm}]D*/s^{1/2} \qquad (9\text{-}17)$$

The figures M_1 and M_2 are dimensionless; they are plotted in Figures 9-4 and 9-5.

The relative $D*$ can be improved in most detectors by limiting the angular field of view of the sensitive area of the detector. The narrower

the viewing angle, the fewer the background photons admitted and, therefore, the higher the detectivity.   Although a $1/(\sin \theta/2)$ improvement of a
factor of 5 is predicted theoretically if the cone angle θ is decreased to 20°,
the actual improvement is only about 2.5.   This gain may nonetheless be
significant in low-power, laser-gain measurements where the detector is
operated D^* BLIP (a background limited photoconductive detector).

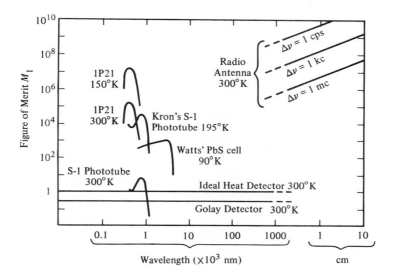

Figure 9-4   Figure of merit M_1.   (With permission of IEEE, Inc.)

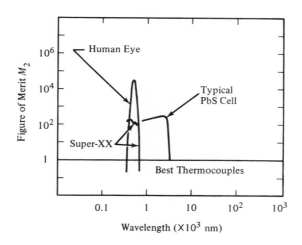

Figure 9-5   Figure of merit M_2.   (With permission of IEEE, Inc.)

9·2   laser detectors

Lasers have been developed which span the range of wavelengths from sub-millimeter to the vacuum ultraviolet wavelengths, and with power output capabilities ranging from milliwatts to tens of gigawatts. The scope of the problem of determining laser output is apparent from the enormous wavelengths and power range to be covered.

There are several basic types of laser output to be detected, namely, CW, pulsed, Q-switched, and mode-locked. CW lasers (gas or solid state) have outputs typically in the range of 10^{-3} to 10^3 W. In the case of pulsed lasers, pulse durations of 10^{-1} to 10^{-6} s with peak powers of several megawatts and total output energy of several hundred joules may be encountered. In Q-switched laser operation, the output pulses are usually less than 500 ns in duration with peak powers as high as a gigawatt. Mode-locked operation of CW, pulsed, and Q-switched lasers has resulted in pulse durations as short as 10^{-12} to 10^{-13} s, with peak powers as high as 10^{10} W. The enormous range of laser-pulse widths, output powers, and energies greatly complicates the measurement problem. It is unlikely that any one method or instrument can be used to measure the output power and energy of all lasers.

9·2·1   detector considerations

Laser output detectors ideally should satisfy the following conditions:

1. The response should be uniform over the area of the receiving aperture.
2. The response should be independent of the direction of the incident radiation so that it has the same response to the highly collimated laser beam as it has to the radiation from the calibrating source.
3. The response should be linear so that energy from the relatively weak calibrating source, incident for perhaps 1 s, and the energy from the pulsed laser, incident for 10^{-6} s or less, can be compared.
4. The detector should not be damaged by high powers.

Unless the detector is an absolute, i.e., the constant of the device is known theoretically, the detector must be calibrated. Calibration is usually the case. Because the detector may have a more or less complicated wavelength response, it must be calibrated at the laser wavelength. This may be accomplished by the use of a thermopile calibrated at the laser wavelength, or a standard lamp whose spectral radiance is known.

There is a broad range of detectors available, each with attributes that make it particularly suitable for certain applications. The problem is that meaningful comparisons can be made only after considering many parameters and the total system. For instance, *speed* is not simply a function of the device's parameters.   Often a load of more than 10,000 Ω will cause the switching speed to be a function of the RC time constant—the capacitance being that which is due to the photodevice and to any external components.

Another factor that is sometimes confusing is the *gain* inherent in some of the photosensitive devices.   For instance, the phototransistor's built-in gain provides obvious circuitry advantages.   However, the gain of a photo-transistor decreases as the light level increases.

Sensitivity is also an important parameter.   The important point is that sufficient light flux must impinge on the photodevice's active area to provide a usable output.   The factors that affect this parameter are initial source intensity, distance from the source to the detector area, the type of intervening optics, and the matching of source and detector characteristics.

One of the least flexible properties is *spectral response*, where the choice is somewhat limited by the material from which these photo-detectors are fabricated.

9·2·2   noise considerations

Energy or signal in industrial applications is generally high—hence, in most cases noise is of secondary importance.   The primary problems are electronic circuitry and its associated time constants.   However, it is advisable to review briefly the causes of noise and the limitations these pose on the detector performance, because the minimum energy that can be detected, or the accuracy of a measurement, is greatly affected by noise.

Since radiation exists from all objects above absolute zero, a review of blackbody radiation theory, as discussed in Chapter 2, may be helpful for a better understanding of the treatment of noise.   A more elaborate discussion of noise is available in the literature.[8]

Internal Receiver Noise   In practice, one deals with imperfect devices rather than with ideal ones.   It is therefore necessary to consider the internal noise contributions of the various receiving elements.   The types of noise contributed by the receiving device are dark current, flicker, recombination, thermal agitation noise, modulation noise, and contact noise, with each receiving device possessing its own particular noise producers.

Dark Current   In photoemissive devices, dark current is the major factor that prevents the achievement of the theoretical limits of sensitivity.   The dark current can have three causes:

1. Thermionic emission from the cathode and other tube elements
2. Ohmic leakage
3. Regenerative effects

Thermionic emission from the cathode can be computed from the Richardson law. If the applied plate voltage is sufficiently high to cause all emitted electrons to move to the anode (no space charge), the thermionic current density is given in mks units by

$$i_t = 1.2 \times 10^6 T^2 e^{-\phi q/kT} \tag{9-18}$$

where T is the temperature in degrees Kelvin, ϕ is the work function of the emitting metal in volts, q is the electron charge, and k is Boltzmann's constant. This thermionic emission can be reduced considerably by cooling the cathode.

Ohmic leakage results from the imperfect insulating properties of the tube's components. Although usually negligible, it is the predominant source of dark current at low voltage operating conditions.

Regenerative effects caused by the impact of positive ions upon the cathode and by field emission are, in general, less important than leakage current and thermionic emission. These effects can be reduced by reducing the applied voltage and by cooling. Static charges on the glass wall are usually avoided by coating the walls of the photomultiplier tube with a conductive layer.

Random fluctuations in dark current constitute the major internal noise of vacuum phototubes where anode and cathode terminations are at opposite ends of the tube. The thermionic emission random fluctuations are determined by the shot noise formula given by

$$i_N^2 = 2q i_t \Delta f \tag{9-19}$$

where Δf is the bandwidth of the receiver, and q is the electronic charge.

Thermal Noise   Thermal noise, also known as Nyquist or Johnson noise, is a natural result of the laws of radiation. This is the familiar frequency independent noise arising from thermal fluctuations in the motions of electrons within a resistive element. It can be shown that the open-circuit, mean-square noise voltage for some resistance R is given by

$$v_n^2 = 4kT \Delta f R \tag{9-20}$$

and the mean-square noise current, since $i_n = v_n/R$, is given by

$$i_n^2 = \frac{4kT \Delta f}{R} \tag{9-21}$$

The value of kT at room temperature is $1/40$ eV. The noise voltage for room temperature will then be

$$v_n = 1.28 \times 10^{-10} (R \Delta f)^{1/2}$$

The noise current for room temperature will be

$$i_n = 1.28 \times 10^{-10} \left(\frac{\Delta f}{R}\right)^{1/2}$$

For Johnson noise to predominate in photomultiplier tubes, RI must be less than $0.05/G$ V, where R is anode resistor, I is anode current, and G is gain.

Flicker Noise At low frequencies, flicker noise, which has also been denoted in the literature as $1/f$ noise, is dominant. Flicker noise results from an excess of material dependent shot noise on the cathode in vacuum tubes. This type of noise decreases with increasing frequency. An empirical expression fitting the measured data is of the form

$$i_N^2 = \frac{AI\alpha\,\Delta f}{f^\beta} \qquad (9\text{-}22)$$

where I is the total current, and $\alpha \simeq 2$, $\beta \simeq 1$, and A is a proportionality factor. At low frequencies the flicker noise appears as excess shot noise.

Noise in Semiconductors Noise in semiconductors is due to various mechanisms in both surface and bulk properties. The relative noise level as a function of frequency for the different noise sources in a photoconductor is shown in the literature.[9]

The dominant noise, at frequencies above those at which significant contact noise occurs, is due to the photocurrent and is denoted often as generation-recombination noise. The output noise can be given in the form

$$i_n^2 \simeq 4qIG\,\Delta f \qquad (9\text{-}23)$$

where G is the photoconductive gain. The frequency distribution of this noise is determined by the free carrier lifetime for a trap-free photoconductor.

At low frequencies the dominant noise has been found to be current noise, which is very similar to flicker noise in electron tubes. Both have a $1/f$ response, where $\beta = 1.0$ for flicker noise, and $\beta = 1.0$ to 3 for current noise.[10]

When the photoconductor contains traps, the photocurrent noise has its frequency response determined by τ_0, which is the lifetime of a trapped carrier before it returns to its recombination center with $\tau_0 > \tau$. This time, τ_0, also determines the post-detection frequency response of the photoconductor. The effect of the traps has been to reduce the detector bandwidth from that determined by the lifetime of a free carrier to that determined by the lifetime of a trapped carrier.

It can be shown[9] that the thermal noise component is ever present and flat with frequency, although overshadowed in many cases by the other noise sources in semiconductors.

Generation-recombination (GR) noise has been called shot noise because of the similarity with electron-tube random fluctuation. Also, as in electron tubes, dark current noise is often called shot noise. However,

GR noise is due to fluctuations in the number and lifetime of thermally generated carriers.

Current noise also has been called contact noise, modulation noise, and excess noise, as well as "one over f" noise. Current noise has been attributed to many causes, but they are all associated with potential barriers.

Contact noise has often been confused with modulation noise, although both make up current noise. Contact noise, as its name implies, has its source at the contacts. Modulation noise has its physical location, at least in part, near the surface of the crystal.

Radiation Fluctuations   A review of blackbody theory clarifies that both quantum fluctuations and wave interference fluctuations exist. It should be noted that quantum fluctuations only become important for very low light levels, whereas wave interference fluctuations cause conventional thermal noise. A detailed development of each of the two noise types, in electrical engineering terminology, is available in the literature.[11]

The radiation falling on a detector can be pictured as a stream of quanta whose arrival rate is subject to statistical fluctuations. In general, the rms fluctuation in the power radiated over the entire spectrum by a blackbody at temperature T will be proportional to $\sqrt{T^5 \, \Delta f}$.

Effective Noise Temperature   With low numbers of detected photons, one deals with the probability of detection. And, since thermal noise exists even without the signal, sufficient signal must be received to overcome the noise that is present. The quantum noise produced by the signal will also be less than the signal. Thus, in contrast to the statements that optical detectors are "noisy," it can be said more correctly that they are quantum limited in detection capabilities.

Miscellaneous Noise Sources   Miscellaneous noise sources include some that are amazingly hard to cure and can cripple the performance of the most elaborate system. Among these are:

Microphonics, or noise arising from mechanical vibrations. A frequent offender is small-diameter coaxial cable, the capacitance of which may change during flexing.

Extra temperature noise due to the boiling of a cryogenic fluid within a Dewar. Careful design of the detector mount can decouple the element from some of these fluctuations.

Capacitor noise due to random breakdown and healing of the dielectric films. It is best to avoid electrolytic capacitors in low-level amplifier stages. Dc coupling from the detector is preferable if very low chopping frequencies are used. The reader is referred to the literature for more extensive treatment of laser noise, including nonlinear effects.[11-13]

9·2·3   measurement devices

Table 9-2 summarizes measurement devices by energy and power classifications.[14]   Although energy (time-integrated measurements) and power (time-resolved measurements) are distinctly different but related quantities, the terms are, unfortunately, sometimes loosely used.   This is undoubtedly because some of the techniques that have been traditionally used to measure these quantities from blackbody radiators can be used to measure either one.   For instance, although most photoelectric detectors and radiation thermopiles are basically designed to measure instantaneous power, they can also be used to measure the total energy in a pulse by electronically integrating the output, providing the detector time constants are much shorter than the pulse lengths involved.   Conversely, many calorimeters and virtually all photographic methods are basically total energy measuring techniques, but they can also be used for measuring power if the time history of the radiation is known or measured independently.

Table 9-3 lists representative commercially available instruments. The listings are separated into quantum detectors and heat detectors, in an order which is subsequently followed in discussing and detailing background theory and operation on a device level.

TABLE 9-2   Summary of Devices for Energy and Power Measurements[a]

Device	Range of Operation	Typical Response Time (s)	Surface Damage[b]
Energy (J)			
Cone calorimeters	10^{-2}–2×10^3	1–20	10–20 mW/cm² in 50 ns
Metal disc calorimeter	10^{-2}–10	10	50 mW/cm² in 50 ns
Rat's nest calorimeter	10^{-3}–10	10^{-4}	—
Wire calorimeter	10^{-3}–0.5	10	10 mW/cm² in 50 ns
Liquid calorimeter	1–500	10–60	—[c]
Torsion pendulum	0.5–500	60	—
Integrating photocurrent	10^{-8}–10^{-3}	1	1 mW/cm²
Thermopile	10^{-6}–1	10^{-1}	300 mW/cm²
Copper sphere	5×10^{-4}–10	180	—
Power Density (W/cm²)			
Phototube	10^{-8}–10^{-3}	3–10 ns	1 mW/cm²
Photodiode	10^{-4}–6	0.3–4 ns	10 W/cm²[d]
Nonlinear crystal	10^3–10^{12}	10^{-5}	10^{12} W/cm²[e]

[a] Used with permission of IEEE, Inc.
[b] Surface damage may occur at the indicated power density.
[c] Local boiling of the liquid should be avoided.
[d] Above this power, the response of this device is nonlinear.
[e] Breakdown of quartz at roughly this power density.

TABLE 9-3 Representative List of Commercially Available Laser Measuring Instruments (as of July 1970)

Type	Manufacturer	Model No.	Spectral Response (nm)	Sensitivity	Power Rating	Energy Rating	Aperture (sq cm)	Rise Time	Decay Time	Bandwidth
1. QUANTUM DETECTORS										
	EG & G	580A-D	200-1150	0.13 A/W	7×10^{-9}– 4.5 W/cm²	0.7 J/cm²	12.97	1 ns		
Photoemissive	Cintra	101	400-1200		10^{-10}–40 W/cm²		1.6			40 KHz
	Int. Light Inc.	IL600/610	200-1150	0.089 A/W	200 W					
	Raytheon	1A 31	350-1020					0.3 ns		1 GHz
	Korad	K-D1	300-1150	0.002 A/W	1 μW-10 GW	0.01-100 J	3.0	0.3 ns		1.1 GHz
Photovoltaic	Optics Tech.	615	400-1150		0.03-1 W		4.1			50 KHz
	Spectra Physics	401 C	450-1150		0.02-0.1 W					20 KHz
	Jodon	450 B	400-1150		0.02-0.1 W		5.0			50 KHz
Photo-conductive	EG & G	560 B	350-1130	0.5 μA/μW	0.25 W Peak 2×10^{-3} avg.		0.07	5 ns	20 ns	
	United Aircraft		300-1100	400 μA/μW	15 kW at 1060		5.0			1350 MHz
2. HEAT DETECTORS										
"Rats nest" Thermopile	Westinghouse	D1	100-40,000	625 μV/J	250 mW	.1-5 J/cm²	5.0	0.1 ms	20 s	
Calorimeter	Eppley Labs.			0.8 mV/mW	5×10^8 W/cm²		0.1	2 s		
	Korad (Control Data)	K-J3	530-1060	5 μV/J		0.1-500 J	5.0			
Cone thermopile	Coherent Radiation	201	300-30,000	40 μV/W	10^{-1}-200 W/cm²		5.25	1 s		
Pyroelectric	Laser Precision Corp.	KT 1000	5000 to mm	200 V/W at 1 KHz	500 mW avg.		0.8	1 ns		

9·3   detection techniques

To be practical, all discussions of laser detection and measurement must lead up to optical detection techniques. This section, therefore, clarifies terminology and emphasizes the how-to-use aspect.

9·3·1   direct photodetection

Direct photodetection consists of detecting the incident energy within the spectral response of the detector, with the resultant detected signal following the amplitude variations induced by the incoming signal modulation. The detector is a photon detector and, thus, responds to individual photons at a particular quantum efficiency for every wavelength. In direct photodetection, all optical frequency and phase information is lost. Similarly, the detector cannot respond to frequency or phase modulation of the optical carrier. It will reproduce amplitude variations of the incident power as long as the rate of the variations is less than the frequency response of the detector.

The direct photodetector can make no distinctions between signal photons or nonsignal (background noise) photons that are within the relatively broad spectral response characteristics. It has no special arrival angle requirement, except that the photon be intercepted by the photosensitive area. Thus, in order to achieve spectral discrimination (if it is required), we must insert an optical filter. Similarly, if we are to achieve spatial filtering, we must reduce the field of view.

The advantage of direct photodetection by itself is its simplicity. In many cases, this means reduced cost, weight, size, and power consumption over other techniques.

The most fundamental limit in direct detection appears to be the photoemissive cathode's quantum efficiency, which is generally lower than in a solid-state detector. When the known quantum efficiency is taken into account, it appears that either technique is capable of approaching within a factor of two the ideal limiting detectable energy of about 3×10^{-19} J in the visible spectrum.

Of the two most promising techniques for the detection of low-level radiation, a heterodyne system offers a detection threshold which is lower than that of direct detection by a factor of two. Furthermore, since a variety of solid-state detectors can be used for heterodyning, additional advantages are obtained in the infrared region of the spectrum because the quantum efficiencies of these devices are much higher than those of a photoemissive cathode.

On the other hand, the heterodyne process is inherently narrow band, and detection is limited to a frequency range centered on the reference wavelength. This disadvantage is not encountered in the direct detector, which detects energy over a wide range of optical spectrum and is relatively simple to operate.

Many laser applications depend on a detector's ability to respond to vanishingly small quantities of radiation. In such applications, which include deep space communications, Doppler shift velocity measurement, and Raman and Brillouin spectroscopy, it makes economic sense to consider such sophisticated techniques as optical heterodyning, photon counting, and synchronous detection.

9·3·2   *heterodyning or photomixing*

The advantage that is usually looked for as a justification for using photomixing or addition of a quantum amplifier is sensitivity, i.e., ability to detect a weaker signal than can be detected with direct photodetection. This may take the form of greater background rejection or discrimination.

Photomixing as a receiving technique was immediately considered for lasers, and, in the first flush of enthusiasm, it was assumed that the improvement in receiver sensitivity would be similar to that obtained at radio frequencies by using a superheterodyne receiver instead of a crystal local oscillator. Although no such improvement is possible in general, there are certain advantages to using photomixing as a receiving technique as compared to direct photodetection. There are also a number of additional complexities to utilization of a photomixing system.

Photomixing, as in radio-frequency heterodyning processes, is a form of coherent detection, whereas direct photodetection can be regarded as incoherent.

It is well known[61-64] that when detecting coherent radiation with a detector whose current response is proportional to the input power, enhancement of the signal-to-noise ratio is achieved by optical heterodyning, i.e., by mixing the weak CW signal of frequency v_S with a more intense local oscillator of frequency v_L and power P_L.

From a practical point of view, the most striking result for a heterodyning process is that, since the reference bias can be used to overcome equivalent background interference, quantum detectors with inherently higher quantum efficiency (η) can be used, the reference acting as a form of internal gain. Hence, the *p-i-n* diode with a quantum efficiency of 0.7 has an NEP more than an order of magnitude lower than an S-20 photomultiplier in the red.

In order to overcome background fluctuations, a large value of reference power must be used. For example, to overcome the Johnson noise of an amplifier with a 3 db noise figure, a reference power of 2.4 mW

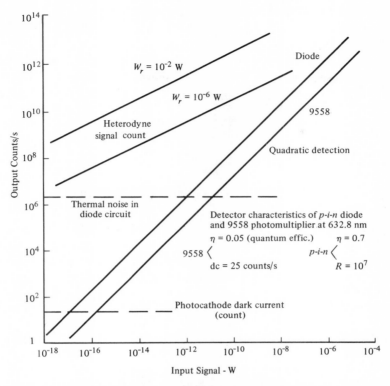

Figure 9-6   Comparison of the heterodyne performance of a p-i-n diode and a quality photomultiplier.

must be employed ($\eta = 1$, $R = 50\ \Omega$). A fortunate feature of the *p-i-n* diode is its ability to handle large power levels without fatigue. A comparison of the heterodyne performance of a *p-i-n* diode and a quality photomultiplier is indicated in Figure 9-6. Analysis of the relative advantage and discussion of the ideal heterodyne detector are readily available in the literature.[65,66]

9.3.3   energy and power measurements

All previous discussions have clarified the various definitions, considerations, and parameters for laser detection and measurement. CW and pulsed lasers of a variety of frequencies understandably, therefore, may require a variety of detection systems. The following examples can serve as guides to the engineers becoming involved in laser technology:

For measurement of CW argon laser, see Figure 9-7.

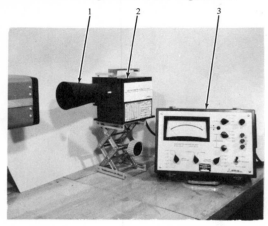

1. Hooded filter diffuser.
2. Detector head – S20 response.   } Radiometer
3. Indicator unit.   E.G.& G. Model 580.

Figure 9-7   Measurement of CW argon laser (488.0 nm).

For measurement of pulsed and Q-switched CO_2 laser, see Figure 9-8.

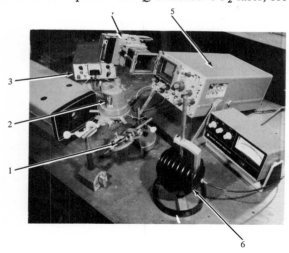

1. Coherent Radiation Laboratories, Ge partial reflector, Cat #WI-01 trans.
   95.8%, absorption 2.8%
2. Philco Ford, gold doped Ge detector – GPC 215,
3. Kepco, 0–50V dc supply
4. Tektronix camera Model C31
5. Tektronix, Model 454 oscilloscope
6. Coherent Radiation Laboratories, Model 201 power meter

Figure 9-8   Measurement of pulsed and Q-switched CO_2 laser (10.6 $\times$ 10^3 nm), 50 W TEM$_{00}$.

For measurement of YAG laser Q-switched pulse, see Figure 9-9.

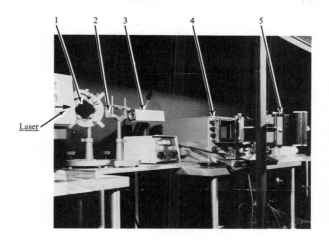

1. Baird Atomic, optical interference filters.
2. Ground glass diffuser
3. E.G.& G. Lite Mike Model 560B
4. Tektronix, Model 454 oscilloscope
5. Tektronix, Model C31 camera

Figure 9-9   Measurement of YAG laser (1060 nm) Q-switched pulse.

For measurement of high-power CO_2 laser, see Figure 9-10.

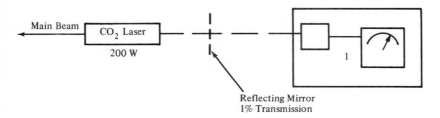

1. Disc-type thermopile system − 201 CRL

Figure 9-10   Measurement of high-power CO_2 laser (10.6 × 10³ nm).

For measurement of water-vapor laser, see Figure 9-11.

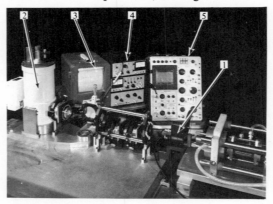

1. Princeton Applied Research Chopper, Model 125
2. Texax Instruments, Inc., Bolometer (Pyroelectric Detector)
3. Varian Associates, 2 channel chart recorder
4. Keithley Instruments, Inc.
   Model 823 nV amplifier
   Model 822 phase-sensitive detector
   Model 821 phase shifter
5. Tektronix, 549 storage oscilloscope

Figure 9-11   Measurement of water-vapor laser (119×10^3 nm).

For measurement of pulsed ruby laser energy and power, see Figure 9-12.

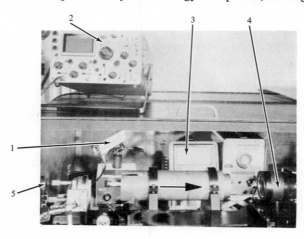

1. E.G. & G. Lite Mike Model 506 B
2. Tektronix, Model 454 oscilloscope
3. Ballentine dc μV meter

Figure 9-12   Measurement of pulsed ruby laser (694.3 nm) energy and power.

For velocity measurement of heterodyned CO_2 laser (Michelson interferometer setup), see Figure 9-13.

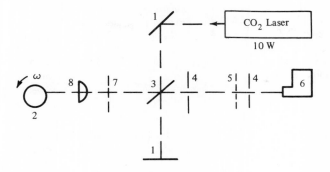

1. Aluminum front surface mirror
2. Off-center wheel
3. Beamsplitter – Irtran II, Kodak
4. Iris
5. Polarizer – germanium, Perkin Elmer
6. Au doped Ge detector – GPC 215, Philco Ford
7. Ge attenuator
8. Lens – Irtran II, Kodak

Figure 9-13 Velocity measurement of heterodyned CO_2 laser (Michelson interferometer setup).

9·4   quantum detection devices

Quantum or photodetectors depend on the action of light quanta on a single electron rather than on the absorption and distribution of energy over an entire macroscopic body.   A photodetector counts the number of quanta of radiation absorbed, in contrast to the thermal detector which responds to the total energy.

Quantum detectors may be selected for operation in a number of modes.   For instance, photoemissive detectors emit electrons, and photoconductive detectors increase in electrical conductivity when radiated. Photovoltaic detectors yield an electrical voltage at the output terminals when the sensing element is irradiated.   Other device types, such as photoelectromagnetic, quantum amplifiers and photoparametric solid-state detectors are also available.

Since a direct detector for low light levels does not have a signal output sufficiently large to overcome amplifier noise, preamplification is necessary.   The most versatile device for this purpose is the photomultiplier tube, which provides a relatively noise-free amplification factor as high as 10^8.   One of the most useful features of such a tube is the wide handwidth (typically 100 MHz), which allows it to resolve individual

TABLE 9-4   Summary of High-Frequency Photodetectors Using the External Photoelectric Effect[a]

Photodetector	Current Multiplication M[b]	Equivalent Resistance R_{eq} (Ω)	Figure of Merit $M^2 R_{eq}$ (Ω)	Comments
High-speed vacuum photodiode	1	50	50	Useful for very high input light levels, and very high frequencies
Photoklystron	1	140	140	Not much better than photodiode, and much worse than TWP. Likely not to be used except, perhaps, at very high frequencies
Traveling-wave phototube (TWP)	1	10^7	10^7	Very useful in heterodyne operation, but not as good a direct detector as multipliers
Dynamic crossed-field electron multiplier (DCFEM)	10^7	50	5×10^{15}	Very sensitive and potentially capable of very high frequency operation, but need for a microwave pump source will probably limit its application compared to other photomultipliers listed below
Static crossed-field photomultiplier	2×10^5	50	2×10^{12}	Very sensitive and seems best choice for most baseband applications

[a] With permission of IEEE, Inc., Ref. 2.

[b] The values quoted are those that have been experimentally observed. With further development all of the multiplying detectors should provide sufficient gain to achieve noise-in-signal limited operation with GHz bandwidths.

TABLE 9-4   Summary of High-Frequency Photodetectors Using the External Photoelectric Effect^a (cont.)

Photodetector	Current Multiplication M^b	Equivalent Resistance R_{eq} (Ω)	Figure of Merit $M^2 R_{eq}$ (Ω)	Comments
Electrostatic, cancellation-in-pairs photo-multiplier	10^3	50	5×10^7	Can be very sensitive. Suitable for large area cathodes if desired, and can use multigap or helical output circuits. Noise and stability problems are still to be ironed out
TSEM-type multiplier TWP	64	10^5	6×10^7	A very sensitive band-pass detector. Capable of very high (>10 GHz) frequency response. However, (1) signal-to-noise ratio is limited by low current density capability of the TSEM films, and (2) very high voltages are required to achieve large multiplication factors
Reflection dynode multiplier TWP	10^3	10^4	10^{10}	A very sensitive, wide-dynamic-range band-pass detector; probably a best choice for most band-pass applications

photon events. Hence, photon events rather than the average photo-electric current can be registered on an electron counter. However, even the newer semiconductor cathodes, in general, limit operations to between 400 and 1200 nm.

Table 9–4 summarizes and comments on photoemissive photodetectors, those discussed and others.

Table 9-5 gives a brief description and summarizes pertinent comments on a variety of solid-state photodetectors.

TABLE 9-5   Brief Description and Features of Photodetectors[a]

Type	Brief Description	Pertinent Comments
Photoconductive cells	Light sensitive resistors Typical materials cadmium sulfide, lead selenide, etc.	Generally used to control large amounts of power Large area film devices have highest sensitivity of any photo sensor Millisecond response time Peak spectral response range from 520 nm to 740 nm to allow matching of emitter characteristics Wide dynamic range
Photovoltaic	n on p or p on n construction with one very thin layer Silicon and selenium most common materials	Converts radiation to electricity directly, no bias required Large areas possible for high power output and 2 μs rise time Silicon devices have much higher output than selenium
Photodiodes	Light sensitive diode capable of operating in the photovoltaic mode or with a reverse bias to achieve higher sensitivity, faster speeds, etc.	Typical rise time of 0.1 μs with nanosecond response times possible For low dark current (increased sensitivity) guard-ring construction is used Devices designed to become totally depleted under a given reverse bias exhibit nanosecond response times Using p-i-n construction provides <1.0 ns response, a quantum efficiency linear over 6 decades and a negligible noise current Biasing near avalanche breakdown point provides a gain increase of over 100 and high gain-bandwidths. NEP is 100 times that of non-avalanche photodiodes
Phototransistors	Light sensitive transistors with either two or three terminals	Bipolar rise times are typically 2 μs PhotoFET's rise times are typically 30 ns Darlingtons have high gain, but response time limited to 50 μs Plastic units now available for $\simeq 60$ ¢ PhotoFET's must be biased off for light sensing operation PhotoSCR's used to drive high power loads

[a] With permission of *Electro-Optical Systems Design*, Ref. 15.

TABLE 9-5   Brief Description and Features of Photodetectors[a] **(*cont.*)**

Type	Brief Description	Pertinent Comments
Photodiodes (Schottky)	Cold formed metal-semiconductor Schottky barrier has *p-i-n* construction	5 ns response time Not being diffused means that majority carrier lifetimes are not degraded, thus ensuring high quantum efficiency and minimum noise current Very low leakage ($<10^{-7}$ A/cm^2) allows powers as low as 10^{-13} W to be detected Very large areas possible

9·4·1   photoemissive devices (photoelectric devices)

Devices such as ordinary phototubes, photomultipliers, and traveling-wave phototubes are all photoemissive devices; i.e., they depend on the photoemissive characteristics of particular materials.   The photoemissive materials are placed on a cathode, forming a photocathode.   The photo-cathode will eject electrons when light falls upon it.

The absorption of a quantum of electromagnetic radiation at the surface of a suitably prepared metal or alloy may give rise to the ejection of an electron if the energy is greater than some threshold value, as discussed in Section 2.2.2.

In a semiconductor such as a compound of antimony and cesium, photons must provide sufficient energy to move an electron from the Fermi level across the energy gap and leave it with a surplus to overcome the surface forces, if it is to be emitted as a photoelectron.   In $Cs_3 Sb$, the electron affinity is between 0.4 and 0.6 eV, and the energy gap is about 1.4 eV; therefore the long wavelength threshold corresponds to an energy around 1.9 eV, i.e., 660 nm.   The fact that the work function is lower than that of a normal metal makes it easier for some of the free electrons to escape from the surface.

Above the photoelectric threshold, the quantum efficiency for the photoelectric process, that is to say, the ratio of photoelectrons to incident photons, varies with photon energy.   The variation, although complex in detail, follows the general form shown in Figure 9-14, rising to a maximum as the excess energy provided to the electron increases, and falling off in a manner determined by the optical absorption of the photon surface and of any window interposed.

Table 9-6 lists typical combinations of photosensitive surfaces and window materials that can provide the basic spectral response designations standardized by Electronic Industries Association.

TABLE 9-6   Spectral Responses for Devices with Related Photocathode Characteristic Values[a]

Device S-Number	Photocathode Type and Envelope	Conversion Factor (k) (lumens/W)	Typical Luminous Sensitivity (μA/lumen)	Maximum Luminous Sensitivity (μA/lumen)	λ_{max} (nm)	Typical Radiant Sensitivity (mA/W)	Typical Quantum Efficiency (percent)	Typical Photocathode Dark Emission at 25°C (A/cm²)
S-1	AgOCs Lime-glass bulb	93.9	25	60	800	2.35	0.36	900×10^{-15}
S-3	AgORb Lime-glass bulb	286	6.5	20	420	1.86	0.55	—
S-4	CsSb Lime-glass bulb	977	40	110	400	39.1	12	0.2×10^{-15}
S-5	CsSb Lime-glass bulb	1252	40	80	340	50.1	18	0.3×10^{-15}
S-8	CsBi 9741 glass bulb	755	3	20	365	2.26	0.77	0.13×10^{-15}
S-9	CsSb Semitransparent, Lime-glass bulb	683	30	110	480	20.5	5.3	—
S-10	AgBiOCs Semitransparent, Lime-glass bulb	508	40	100	450	20.3	5.6	70×10^{-15}
S-11	CsSb Semitransparent, Lime-glass bulb	804	60	110	440	48.2	14	3×10^{-15}
S-13	CsSb Semitransparent, Fused-silica bulb	795	60	80	440	47.7	13	4×10^{-15}
S-17	CsSb Lime-glass bulb, Reflecting substrate	664	125	160	490	83	21	1.2×10^{-15}
S-19	CsSb Fused-silica bulb	—	40	70	—	22	11	0.3×10^{-15}
S-20	SbKNaCs (Multialkali) Semitransparent, Lime-glass bulb	428	150	250	420	64.2	18	0.3×10^{-15}
S-21	CsSb Semitransparent, 9741 glass bulb	779	30	60	440	23.4	6.6	—

[a] With permission of RCA Corporation, Ref. 16.

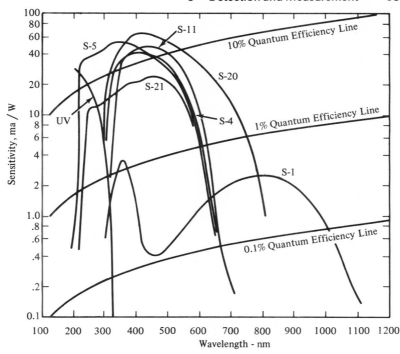

Figure 9-14   Typical absolute spectral response characteristics of photoemissive devices.   The S-number is the designation of the spectral response characteristic of the device and includes the transmission of the device envelope.[16]   (With permission of RCA Corporation.)

Because the process of photoemission is extremely fast, the current from the photocathode can accurately follow the changes in intensity associated with even the fastest pulsed lasers.   The spread in the transit times of the photoelectrons between the photocathode to the anode is the ultimate limit, although the capacity associated with external circuitry usually limits the response before this point is reached (unless great care is taken).   The transit time spread is decreased approximately with the square root of the applied voltage per stage, as is done in the use of photo-multipliers.   Well-designed photomultipliers can have rise times of the order of a few nanoseconds, and photodiodes a fraction of a nanosecond.

<u>Phototubes</u>   Vacuum photodiodes are used in applications where the radiation flux level is relatively high and spectral sensitivity from the ultraviolet to the near infrared is required.   Relatively large areas are available; for example, 1.75 in. diameter for ITT Model 114A, with an S-20 photocathode.   The response time is limited by the transit time of the electrons and is typically about 0.5 ns.   Dark current is high, being of the order of 5 nA at room temperature.   In general, phototubes have a moderate sensitivity of 0.025 A/W, as typified by the RCA 1P42.   They are stable and do not change their characteristics readily.

For quantitative measurements the usual precautions must be observed: the phototubes must be used within their peak and average current limitations; they must be shielded against magnetic and electrostatic fields; and accurately determined voltages from well-regulated power supplies must be used to set phototube gain.

Several precautions should be observed in applying the photoelectric technique of energy measurement. Due to the nonuniform sensitivity of the photocathode, it is necessary that a large fraction of the surface be illuminated. Errors will be introduced in the measurements if the anode of the photocell casts a shadow on the cathode. (This effect can be eliminated by properly orientating the photocell or using a planar photocell.) Because the instantaneous output of the phototube is proportional to the instantaneous intensity or power of the light incident on the photocathode, it is possible to measure the energy in the laser pulse by integrating the phototube output with respect to time. This can be done either by measuring the area under the output-versus-time characteristic or by integrating electronically. The maximum energy in a fixed pulse length that can be measured directly is limited by the power level (incident upon the photosensitive surface) at which response ceases to be linear. The limiting power level of most vacuum photocells is of the order of 1 W; hence the energy limitation is of the order of millijoules for millisecond pulse lengths, and attenuators must usually be employed.

A direct measurement of the energy can be made by a self-integrating circuit, i.e., a circuit that integrates the photocurrent. The principle of a simple photocurrent integrating circuit[17] is demonstrated in Figure 9-15. The capacitance C is charged up to a voltage V by closing the switch S to the power supply (battery). This switch is opened before a measurement is taken. When an incident light pulse causes a current pulse through the phototube Ph, a charge Q is removed from the capacitance C. The charge Q is the integral of the photocurrent in the pulse time and proportional to the integrated luminous flux, i.e., the energy of the light pulse.

The arrangement shown in Figure 9-15 has been assembled using a sensitive electrostatic voltmeter, and an RCA 6570 vacuum phototube

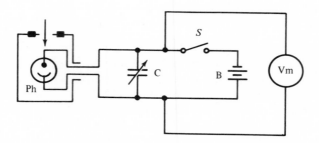

Figure 9-15   Photocurrent integrating circuit.[17]   (With permission of IEEE, Inc.)

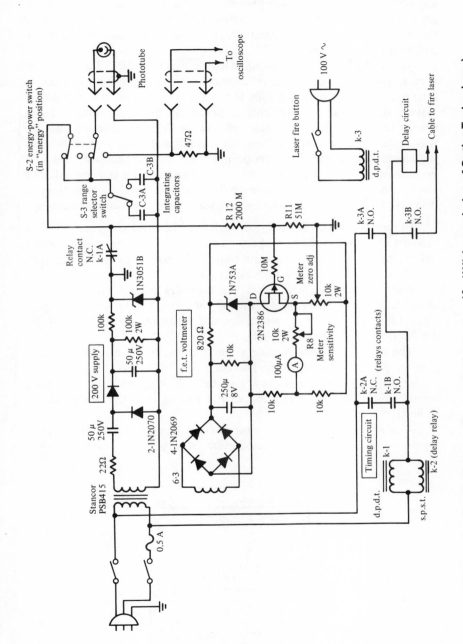

Figure 9-16 Circuit diagram of a monitoring system.[18] (*With permission of Optics Technology.*)

mounted in a metal housing with a compur shutter in order to prevent any stray light from hitting the phototube. The shutter is opened only for the moment of the laser pulse. Therefore, the amount of energy entering the meter is the product of intensity, time interval the shutter is opened, and area of the iris opening.

A system [18] designed to monitor laser pulses from 10^{-4} J to 10^3 J uses a clear glass plate beamsplitter and several high-density glass filters as attenuators. Figure 9-16 details the circuit diagram of the monitoring system showing all components required, including a timing circuit needed to tie into the laser system. A Cetron CE-22V vacuum phototube was chosen because of its "end-on" configuration, which eliminates the shadowing effect of the anode upon the cathode surface, and also because of its S-1 spectral response. Tests have shown that the CE-22V photocathode surface can receive up to 0.8 mJ per total cross section, or 0.48 mJ/cm^2, at 694 nm without losing linearity in its light current response.

Photomultipliers Photoemissive devices have been the most widely used detectors in the visible range as a result of the photomultiplier, which has made possible large post-detection gains (power gains, for example, of 120 db) through electron multiplication.

Photoemissive surfaces form the cathodes of the photomultiplier tubes which conveniently amplify the current arising from electron emission. These tubes vary in size, in sensitivity, and in intrinsic noise which limits the detection of very weak signals.

The most important consideration in the selection of a photomultiplier for photon counting is the photocathode. It should have the maximum possible quantum efficiency, and the multiplier structure of the tube should utilize as large a fraction as possible of the electrons from the cathode.

A single stage of secondary emission may be used in a photocell, as in Figure 9-17, to multiply the photocurrent by a factor of about 5, but the

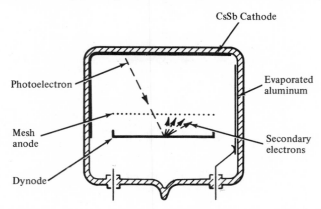

Figure 9-17   A single-stage multiplier photocell.   (With permission of EMI Electronics Ltd.)

main application is found in multistage tubes, since n stages give a total gain of g^n. The design problem in a secondary emission multiplier is to ensure that electrons strike a dynode (secondary emission elements are called *dynodes*), at a region where the electric field is directed away from the surface and toward the next dynode.

A typical multiplier phototube used in laser detection may have 16 stages, an end window effective photocathode diameter of 0.1 in., with an S-1 or S-20 spectral response. Detection and amplification of low-level light are achieved with multiplier phototubes within a configuration of three basic elements: a photocathode, a system of dynode multipliers, and a collector (see Figure 9-18). Light impinging on the photocathode

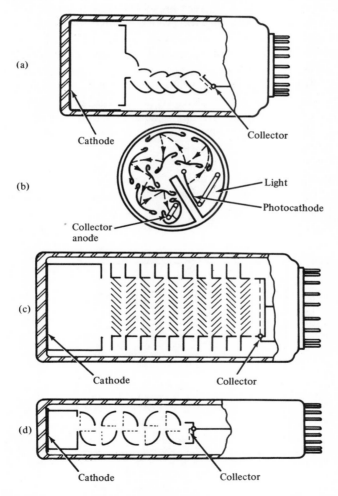

Figure 9-18   Electrostatic dynode systems.   (a) Focused structure. (b) Compact focused structure.   (c) Venetian-blind structure.   (d) Box-and-grid structure.   (With permission of EMI Electronics Ltd.)

stimulates emission which is directed to the first dynode, and secondary emission caused at the first dynode is equivalent to an amplified signal. The process is repeated through each dynode and is collected at the anode, which serves as the signal output electrode.

The time spread in a photomultiplier tube sets an upper limit to the frequency response, which may be taken to be approximately $1/\pi\tau$ Hz. Hence, a venetian-blind dynode tube with $\tau = 6$ ns has an upper frequency limit of about 50 MHz. At the lower end of the frequency spectrum, the photomultiplier tube responds with highest gain since the secondary emission multiplier is, in effect, a linear dc amplifier for small input currents.

A photomultiplier has a dark current in the absence of any external illumination. This dark current appears as events which are similar to, but not identical to, photoelectric events. Signal events are most likely to be one-electron events (referred to the photocathode), whereas a large fraction of the dark-current events may involve more than one electron. This feature appears as a difference in pulse-height distributions at the photomultiplier tube's output, where the noise pulses can be discriminated against by a gating circuit that rejects large pulses and establishes a lower threshold.[19] The gate parameters to determine optimum performance are ascertained from experimental pulse-height distributions with this technique called *photon counting*.

Photon-counting techniques[20] minimize the influence of detector noise in order to approach the performance of an ideal direct detector. In this application the photomultiplier is invariably used because it provides the low noise preamplification needed to overcome circuit noise. In addition, the pulse-height characteristics of certain photomultiplier types

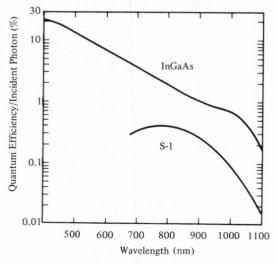

Figure 9-19   Spectral dependence of photoresponses of a photo-cathode prepared with alloy of indium, gallium, and arsenic, compared with that of a good S-1 photosurface.[22]   (With permission of Laser Focus.)

are particularly valuable for some applications. Furthermore, since the limiting dark current of good photomultiplier tubes originates in thermal emission from the photocathode and is proportional to its size, considerable advantages can be obtained by using tubes with small cathode areas and by cooling the photocathode to dry-ice temperatures.

For precise measurements, the temperature of many photomultipliers must be controlled or known, because the gain can increase with temperature (0.3 percent/°C for 1P21 tubes). In addition, the quantum yield of photocathodes can increase slightly with temperature near the long wavelength end of their spectral response characteristic.

A result[22] of particular significance in laser detection has been achieved with an $In_{0.16}Ga_{0.84}As$ alloy. The spectral dependence of the photo response of a photocathode prepared from this material is shown in Figure 9-19 and compared with that of a good S-1 photo surface. The

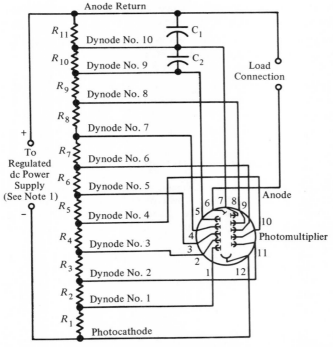

Figure 9-20   Typical voltage divider arrangement.[21a]   *(With permission of RCA Corporation.)*

C_1: *0.02 µF, 20%, 500 V (dc working), ceramic disc*
C_2: *0.01 µF, 20%, 500 V (dc working), ceramic disc*
R_1: *910,000 Ω, 2 W*
R_2 *through* R_{11}: *470,000 Ω, 1 W*

Note 1:   Adjustable between 500 and 1500 V dc.
Note 2:   Capacitors C_1 and C_2 should be connected at tube socket for optimum high-frequency performance.
Note 3:   Component values are dependent upon nature of application and output signal desired.

$In_{0.16}Ga_{0.84}As$ surface has much higher sensitivity at all wavelengths, and an order of magnitude improvement in quantum efficiency is obtained at 1060 nm. In addition, this improvement in efficiency is accompanied by a reduction in dark current by almost two orders of magnitude.

Photomultiplier Circuits   In a standard photomultiplier circuit, a number of dynode voltages are required. The simplest circuit to obtain these voltages is a resistive voltage divider, as shown in Figure 9-20.[21a] The operating voltage applied to the voltage divider is of the order of 1 kV.

The voltage for each stage will be between 70 and 150 V. Higher voltages are frequently applied to the first stage to improve the collection of emitted photoelectrons. Collection efficiency over 95 percent has been achieved.

Under normal low and medium level input signal conditions, the circuit shown in Figure 9-20 will operate properly without introducing nonlinearities in the circuit. Since the gain of photomultiplier tubes varies considerably with supply voltage, stabilized sources are required to keep the gain constant. A variation of supply voltage by a few percent can change the gain by as much as 50 percent.

Typical Vacuum Phototube and Photomultiplier Characteristics   In order to illustrate what is commercially available, Tables 9-7 and 9-8 are reprinted.[21b]

TABLE 9-7   6570 Vacuum Photodiode[a]

SIDE-ON type having S-1 response, wavelength of maximum spectral response is 800 ± 100 nm. This type makes use of a semicylindrical photocathode, and has a direct interelectrode capacitance of 3 picofarads. It weighs approximately 1.3 ounces and has a nonhygroscopic base.

Maximum Ratings (Absolute-maximum values):

Anode-supply voltage (dc or peak ac)	500 max	V
Average cathode-current density	25 max	μA/sq in.
Average cathode current	5 max	μA
Ambient temperature	100 max	°C

Typical Characteristics:

Anode-supply voltage	250	V
Radiant Sensitivity (at 800 nm)	0.0028	A/W
Luminous sensitivity[b]	30	μA/lumen
Maximum luminous-sensitivity difference along cathode length[c]	4.5	μA/lumen
Anode dark current (at 25°C)	0.013 max	μA

[a] With permission of RCA Corporation.
[b] With light input of 0.1 lumen from a tungsten-filament lamp operated at a color temperature of 2870°K. Range of luminous sensitivity is 20 to 40 μA/lumen.
[c] With light input of 0.1 lumen (same conditions as above) and a light spot 1/2 in. in diameter.

TABLE 9-7   6570 Vacuum Photodiode (*cont.*)

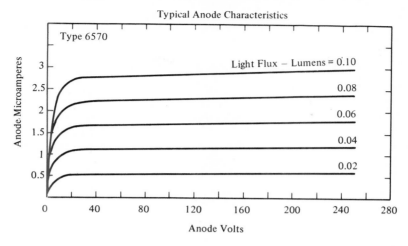

9·4·2   *photovoltaic devices*

"In a photovoltaic cell a junction of two different materials produces a contact potential.   The two materials may be a semiconductor and a metal or they may be an *n*-type and a *p*-type semiconductor.   The silicon solar cell is this latter type of photovoltaic cell.   An *n*-type silicon wafer is formed with a *p*-type layer on one surface.   The operation of such a cell is illustrated in Figure 9-21.   The *p*-type material is shown at the left and the *n*-type material at the right.

"For the *p*-type, the Fermi level lies near the bottom of the forbidden gap; for the *n*-type, it is near the top.   When the two types of silicon are

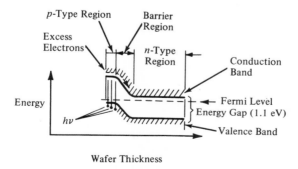

Figure 9-21   Energy model of a silicon solar cell.[21b]   **(With permission of RCA Corporation.)**

TABLE 9-8   7102 Multiplier Phototube[a]

TEN-STAGE, head-on, flat-faceplate type having S-1 response. Wavelength of maximum response is 800 ± 100 nm. This type makes use of silver-magnesium dynodes and a flat-circular, silver-oxygen-cesium, semitransparent photocathode. (This type may also be ordered with copper-beryllium dynodes.) Window material is Corning No. 0080 lime glass or equivalent. Tube weighs approximately 2 ounces and has a nonhygroscopic base. For outline and terminal-connection diagram, refer to type 6199.

Direct Interelectrode Capacitances (Approx.):

Anode to dynode No. 10	4	pf
Anode to all other electrodes	7	pf

Maximum Ratings (Absolute-Maximum Values):

Supply Voltage (dc or peak ac):

Between anode and cathode	1500 max	V
Between anode and dynode No. 10	250 max	V
Between consecutive dynodes	200 max	V
Between dynode No. 1 and cathode	400 max	V
Average anode current	10 max	μA
Ambient temperature	75 max	°C

Typical Anode Characteristics

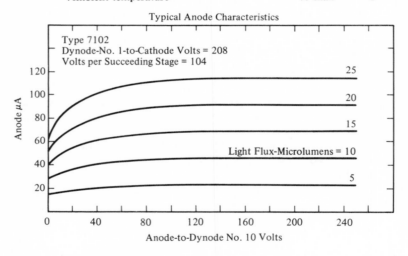

Type 7102
Dynode-No. 1-to-Cathode Volts = 208
Volts per Succeeding Stage = 104

Light Flux-Microlumens = 10

Anode μA

Anode-to-Dynode No. 10 Volts

Typical Characteristics:

Dc supply voltage[b]	1250	V
Radiant sensitivity (at 800 nm)	420	A/W
Cathode radiant sensitivity (at 800 nm)	0.0027	A/W
Luminous sensitivity:		
At 0 cps[c]	4.5	A/lumen
With dynode No. 10 as output electrode	2.7	A/lumen

[a] With permission of RCA Corporation.
[b] Dc supply voltage (E) is connected across a voltage divider which provides 1/6 of E between cathode and dynode No. 1, 1/12 of E for each succeeding dynode stage, and 1/12 of E between dynode No. 10 and anode.
[c] With light input of 10 microlumens from a tungsten-filament lamp operated at a color temperature of 2870°K. Range of luminous sensitivity is 1 to 30 A/lumen at 1250 V.

TABLE 9-8 7102 Multiplier Phototube (*cont.*)

Cathode luminous sensitivity:

With tungsten light source	30	μA/lumen
With infrared source	0.036	μA
Current amplification	150,000	

Equivalent anode-dark-current input:

At a luminous sensitivity of 4 A/lumen	5 max	μ lumen
At 800 nm	55 max	pw

Equivalent noise input:

Luminous	0.15	n lumen
Infrared	1.7	pw

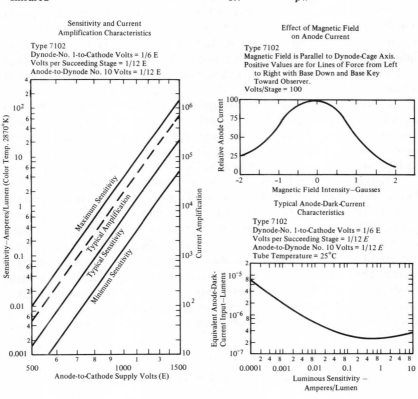

Sensitivity and Current
Amplification Characteristics

Type 7102
Dynode-No. 1-to-Cathode Volts = 1/6 E
Volts per Succeeding Stage = 1/12 E
Anode-to-Dynode No. 10 Volts = 1/12 E

Effect of Magnetic Field
on Anode Current

Type 7102
Magnetic Field is Parallel to Dynode-Cage Axis.
Positive Values are for Lines of Force from Left
to Right with Base Down and Base Key
Toward Observer.
Volts/Stage = 100

Typical Anode-Dark-Current
Characteristics

Type 7102
Dynode-No. 1-to-Cathode Volts = 1/6 E
Volts per Succeeding Stage = 1/12 E
Anode-to-Dynode No. 10 Volts = 1/12 E
Tube Temperature = 25°C

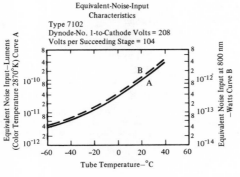

Equivalent-Noise-Input
Characteristics

Type 7102
Dynode-No. 1-to-Cathode Volts = 208
Volts per Succeeding Stage = 104

in intimate contact, a potential adjustment takes place across the boundary. Electrons flow from the *n*-type material to the lower vacant levels of the *p*-type material and holes flow across the boundary in the opposite direction. When the Fermi levels are at the same height, the current ceases to flow, as shown in the potential energy model. A contact potential equal to the original difference in Fermi levels exists; the *p*-type material is negative. When the area in the neighborhood of the junction is illuminated, hole electron pairs are created. The minority carriers (holes in the *n*-type silicon and electrons in the *p*-type silicon) flow across the junction and constitute the current developed by the cell."[21b]

Photovoltaic cells possess several advantages. External power supplies are not needed. The cell output is extremely stable with respect to time. Short-circuit current is directly proportional to illumination intensity and illuminated cell area, and a compact, highly portable power meter can be made for routine measurements of the CW power output of a laser.

A broad selection of photovoltaic photon detectors of such materials as silicon, indium arsenide, and indium antimonide are commercially available in a wide variety of package choices. Detectors that required no cooling may be packaged on standard transistor headers. Others such as InSb and InAs are available in glass Dewars for liquid nitrogen cooling.

The responsivity of selenium cells is well suited to power measurements in the near ultraviolet, whereas silicon solar cells lend themselves to power measurements in the near infrared. Their response peaks at approximately 870 nm, and they require no additional apparatus except a voltmeter for indication of their response. With cooling, detectors such as InSb are useful out to 5500 nm, as shown in Table 9-9. A plot of current-voltage characteristics of a solar cell with white light intensity as a parameter shows that the open-circuit voltage is a logarithmic function of light intensity. The short-circuit current or the current through a sufficiently low ohmic load, however, is directly proportional to light intensity. There-

TABLE 9-9 Typical Photovoltaic Devices

Material	Spectral Response, nm	Operating Temperature	Detectivity[a]	Response Time, μs
Si	500–1100	−65°C–140°C	2×10^{12}	1
InAs	1000–3600	300°K	2×10^{9}	1
InAs	1000–3600	5–77°K	2×10^{11}	1
InSb	1000–5500	5–110°K	$0.5–1 \times 10^{11}$	1

[a] Measured using an unfiltered tungsten filament bulb operating at a color temperature of 2800°K, chopped at a rate of 1 kHz, 50 percent duty cycle, and an amplifier with bandwidth normalized to 1 Hz.

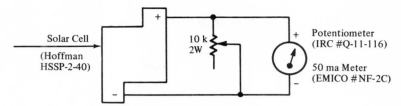

Figure 9-22 Simple light meter.

fore, the voltage developed across a low ohmic load can be made linear to light intensity over a wide range. It can be shown that a high ohmic load of 200 Ω to 1000 Ω does not give a linear response over a wide range; loads of 10 Ω to 100 Ω, however, will give a linear response over five or more orders of magnitude of intensity.[23]

The photovoltaic operating mode results in a very low photodiode generated shot noise, lower sensitivity at the longer wavelengths, and a shorter frequency response due to higher junction capacity.

Representative photovoltaic and photocell devices and their characteristics are listed in the literature.[24]

A simple light meter is illustrated schematically in Figure 9-22.

A packaged optical power measurement device incorporates a silicon detector and guarantees ±5 percent accuracy at 6328 over a 0.020 to 100 mW range. Measurements at other wavelengths are possible using the supplied correction graph. A schematic drawing of the sensing unit optical system is shown in Figure 9-23.

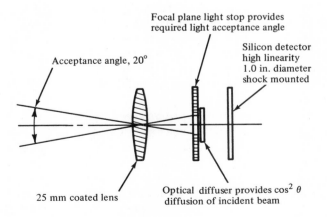

Figure 9-23 Schematic drawing of sensing unit optical system. (With permission of Jodan Engineering Association, Inc.)

9.4.3   photoconductive devices

The same kind of energy-state model that applies to photovoltaic cells also applies to photoconductors.

When, as previously described, the junction of a semiconductor is illuminated and a connection is made to both sides of the junction, a current will be seen to flow during the period of illumination. The current will also flow if an external bias is applied in the reverse direction at the *p-n* junction.

Because of the relatively low mobility of carriers in semiconductors, space charge usually limits the currents to low values. The effect of the charge is greatly increased by the presence of trapping centers. In some cases, the space-charge fields of trapped holes result in the ejection of electrons from the negative terminal, or space-charge fields of trapped electrons result in the ejection of holes from the positive terminal. In either case, a secondary current is generated. As a result of such secondary processes, it is possible to have a quantum efficiency greater than one; i.e., one photon results in the movement through the semiconductor of more than one electron. Time delays are observed in the photocurrent which are associated with the time spent by current carriers in traps or recombination.

In the photoconductive mode, the diode acts as a current generator and will continue to deliver essentially the same amount of ac signal current into any load for a fixed signal source of radiation. However, precautions should be taken to ensure that the diode has sufficient voltage across it to keep it from saturating. In general, it is advisable to maintain at least 10 V across the diode.

The photodiode dark current under reverse bias increases with increasing area. Surface leakage current is dependent on surface defects, cleanliness, bias voltage, and surface area. Bulk leakage current is dependent on active area, the silicon resistivity, and bias voltage. Both the surface leakage current and the bulk leakage current are temperature dependent. A good approximation for the temperature coefficient of dark current is that the dark current doubles for every 10°C increase in operating temperature.

We can distinguish three primary types of photoconductive devices: junction photodiodes, point-contact photodiodes, and surface-barrier photodiodes. Any reverse biased *p-n* junction is potentially useful as a photodetector, although the most common configuration is the surface illuminated *p-i-n* structure.[25] The main advantage of the *p-i-n* configuration is the freedom allowed in the choice of the depletion layer thickness, which is determined primarily by the high-resistivity intermediate region. For values of α (the optical absorption constant) less than 10^4 cm^{-1}, the *p-i-n* structure offers the best frequency response; for greater values, the *p-n* structure is preferable.[26]

Photodiodes can also be made using a point-contact geometry.[27] Here, the active volume is very small, typically a cube a few microns on a side. As a result, both the drift time and capacitance are extremely small and the device is particularly suited to very high modulation frequencies (operation to more than 50 GHz has been reported).

A depletion layer can also be realized by using the barrier formed by a metal semiconductor contact (the Schottky surface barrier photodiode). To avoid large reflection and absorption losses when the diode is illuminated through the metal contact, the contact must be made very thin and anti-reflection coated. When this is done, good quantum efficiencies can be obtained—70 percent in a silicon device.[28]

Optimum power conversion dictates that the resistivity of the silicon be as low as possible in order to keep resistive power loss to a minimum as current is drawn from it. However, photodiodes made on high resistivity silicon (> 100 Ω-cm) have high speed and a broad spectral response only slightly dependent on the lifetime of the carriers.[29] The resistivity and bias voltage determine the photodiode junction depletion depth, junction capacity, sensitivity profile, series resistance, response time, and dark current.

Figure 9-24 presents typical relative spectral response curve for two resistivity ranges.[30] The absolute sensitivity at peak wavelength is 0.52

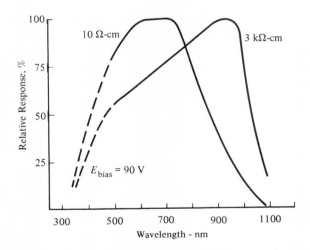

Figure 9-24 Typical relative spectral responses for photodiodes fabricated from two bulk silicon resistivities.[30] *(With permission of Electro-Optical Systems Design.)*

A/W for the 3000 Ω-cm material and 0.35 A/W for the 10 Ω-cm material. Improved monochromatic sensitivity of 10 to 30 percent may be obtained by the application of an antireflective coating to the photodiode sensitive area.

The *planar diffused*, oxide passivated photodiode exhibits low leakage current, low noise, high sensitivity, and excellent stability characteristics. With the addition of a guard ring structure, surface leakage currents have been eliminated and bulk leakage current has become the predominant contributor to the photodiode generated shot noise.   The reverse biased photodiode signal current is linear over 5 to 9 decades of irradiance.   It is limited at high irradiance levels by the permissible power dissipation quoted for the device, provided that the load plus series resistance is not current limiting.

A typical biasing circuit for a guard-ring structured, planar diffused photodiode is presented in Figure 9.25.

Because the photodiode performs as a current source in the photo-conductive mode, it may be preferable to operate the photodiode into an operational amplifier.   Figure 9-26 shows how the guard-ring structured photodiode is used with an operational amplifier.

The open-loop voltage gain of a typical operational amplifier is on the order of 10^4 which, in conjunction with a 1 MΩ feedback resistance, would produce a low-frequency input impedance of 100 Ω.   The photo-diode dark current flows through the feedback resistor and produces a dc offset voltage at the amplifier output terminals.   This offset voltage can be compensated by delivering a current to the summing mode that is equal to the dark current.[30]

Schottky barrier silicon photodiodes have an enhanced blue response. The spectral response, the inherent response time, the temperature characteristic, and the linearity of the photodiodes are independent of active area size.   However, larger area photodiodes have proportionately large capacitances and somewhat greater leakage currents than smaller ones;

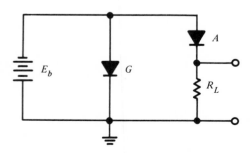

Figure 9-25   Typical bias current.   Photodiode is at A. G **is guard-ring diode.**[30]   **(With permission of Electro-Optical Systems Design.)**

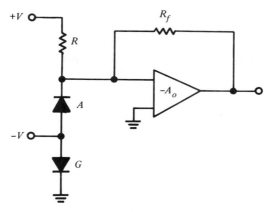

Figure 9-26 Photodiode used with an operational amplifier. (With permission of Electro-Optical Systems Design.)

therefore, large size is a limitation for fast response. A compromise may be in order since sophisticated optics may be required to focus the light on the smaller active areas.

If the front barrier is improperly formed, excess noise and leakage current can result. However, the leakage currents in the guarded Schottky structure are lower than in the *p-n* planar structure because the lifetime in the diffused device is reduced during the diffusion processing.[31]

A typical Schottky photodiode used as a detector in laser systems (the *p-i-n*-5 by UDT) is mounted in a TO5 can and has a 0.035 cm^2 active area. Sensitivity at 850 nm is 0.5 $\mu A/\mu W$, with a rise time of 30 ns and a typical dark current of 0.1 μA. An NEP of 2×10^{-13} W/Hz$^{1/2}$ was measured on a 4000 Ω-cm n silicon for a 1 cm diameter detector at 100 Hz. Figure 9-27 illustrates the typical spectral response for *p-i-n* photodiodes, and Figure 9-28 shows the equivalent circuit for both the planar diffused and Schottky barrier devices.

The most promising solid-state detector with internal current gain is the *avalanche photodiode*. Gain is achieved by impact ionization of carriers. When photons are injected into a photodiode biased to the avalanche region, there is a multiplication of the signal over the usual bias voltage signal. This multiplication (M) is due to the created electron-hole pairs colliding with the lattice and creating more electron-hole pairs under the influence of the large biasing field.

Typical photocurrent gains are 100 to 200 times that of conventional nonavalanche diodes. This limits the need for noise amplifying cascade amplifiers that sacrifice bandwidth. Gain bandwidth products can be as high as 100 GHz.[32] Avalanche diode response is essentially flat to

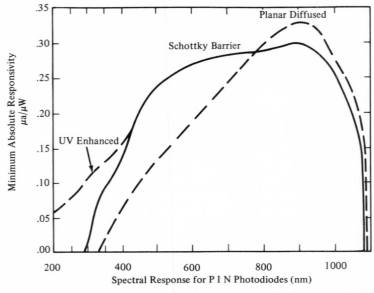

Figure 9-27   Spectral response for p-i-n photodiodes, in nanometers. (With permission of United Detector Technology.)

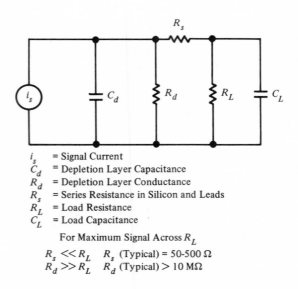

i_s = Signal Current
C_d = Depletion Layer Capacitance
R_d = Depletion Layer Conductance
R_s = Series Resistance in Silicon and Leads
R_L = Load Resistance
C_L = Load Capacitance

For Maximum Signal Across R_L

$R_s \ll R_L$ R_s (Typical) = 50-500 Ω
$R_d \gg R_L$ R_d (Typical) > 10 MΩ

Figure 9-28   Equivalent circuit for p-i-n photodiode.   (With permission of United Detector Technology.)

frequencies of several gigahertz, assuring excellent performance as a detector of amplitude modulated laser waves.

A circuit analysis of the avalanche effect[33] reveals that the detected signal power bandwidth product is a constant. The NEP is found to vary directly with the bandwidth, in a pulse-type system. Avalanche operation increases the signal power by M^2 and decreases the NEP by M at high frequencies.

The avalanche photodiode can be considered as a solid-state replacement to the commonly used photomultiplier tube in many applications. Its signal-to-noise ratio, frequency response, and stability, exceeds that of the S-1 PMT, and it has other inherent advantages of small size, low power, high reliability, and room-temperature operation. It can be made with high quantum efficiencies, is small and rugged, and is not subject to damage from high light levels. On the other hand, the avalanche process is an unavoidably noisy one, and the possible gains are not nearly as high as those available in photomultipliers; therefore, additional amplification stages must be used. However, with present-day transistors, this is not a major problem.[34]

For laser pulse widths of the order of 100 ns, an avalanche photodiode with a quantum efficiency of about 50 percent compares favorably with a photomultiplier having a quantum efficiency of 10 percent. Moreover, the optimum gain for the avalanche photodiode is low—of the order of 20 or less—so that gain stability should not be a problem.

Operating data and specifications on an avalanche photodiode (AV-102 by EG & G) are as shown in Figure 9-29.

It is necessary to maintain bias regulation of ± 0.005 V in order to obtain a constant avalanche gain and stable signal-to-noise improvement. However, the optimum bias voltage varies with temperature by approximately 60 mV/°C. Therefore, unless ambient temperature is also highly regulated, constant voltage operation is not desirable.

The circuit in Figure 9-30 offers a solution: the photodiode is operated from a constant current source utilizing a zener diode and an n-p-n transistor. The output load (R_L) is ac coupled to the diode by a capacitor (C_c). A potentiometer in series with a fixed resistor is connected to the emitter of the transistor and can be adjusted for an appropriate value of resistance (R), necessary to provide a constant current (I_A) to the photodiode.[35]

Table 9-10 summarizes some of the characteristics of representative depletion-layer photodiodes. Tabulations of commercially available photodiodes and details of various characteristics are readily available from the literature.[36]

n-p-n silicon *phototransistors* and *photoFETs* are becoming increasingly available in various configurations and at low cost. Here, too, specific information is readily obtainable[36] from the suppliers, especially on the wide variety of integrated circuitry and packaging.

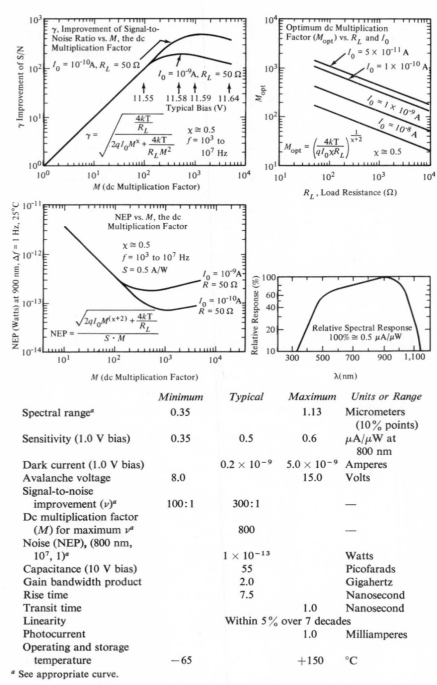

	Minimum	Typical	Maximum	Units or Range
Spectral range[a]	0.35		1.13	Micrometers (10% points)
Sensitivity (1.0 V bias)	0.35	0.5	0.6	$\mu A/\mu W$ at 800 nm
Dark current (1.0 V bias)		0.2×10^{-9}	5.0×10^{-9}	Amperes
Avalanche voltage	8.0		15.0	Volts
Signal-to-noise improvement (ν)[a]	100:1	300:1		—
Dc multiplication factor (M) for maximum ν[a]		800		—
Noise (NEP), (800 nm, 10^7, 1)[a]		1×10^{-13}		Watts
Capacitance (10 V bias)		55		Picofarads
Gain bandwidth product		2.0		Gigahertz
Rise time		7.5		Nanosecond
Transit time			1.0	Nanosecond
Linearity		Within 5% over 7 decades		
Photocurrent			1.0	Milliamperes
Operating and storage temperature	-65		$+150$	°C

[a] See appropriate curve.

Figure 9-29   Operating data and specifications—avalanche photo-diode AV-102.   (With permission of EG & G, Inc.)

TABLE 9-10 Characteristics of Representative Depletion-Layer Photodiodes[a]

Photodetector	Wavelength Range (nm)	Diameter of Active Area	$C(pF)$	$R_{eq}{}^{b}$ Ω	$M_{opt}{}^{d}$	$M_{opt} \times R_{eq}$ Ω	Comments
Ge p-i-n	600 to 1600	150	2	120	1	120	Can be made to have very low series resistance and optimum depletion layer width
$GaAs_xP_{1-x}$-GaAs Heterojunction	770 to 880	60	0.2	1250	1	1250	Capable of very high frequency operation. Relatively narrow wavelength range
Si point contact	400 to 1000	5	0.15	250[c]	10	25	Capable of very high frequency operation. Very small active area
Si surface barrier	400 to 1000	140	0.4	600	1	600	Relatively simple to fabricate
Si avalanche	400 to 1000	40	1	250	100	25000	Has highest gain-bandwidth product of all solid-state detectors
Ge avalanche	600 to 1600	40	1	250	25	150	Most sensitive wide-band infrared detector available

[a] With permission of IEEE, Inc., Ref. 2.
[b] A bandwidth $B = 1$ GHz has been assumed.
[c] Determined by the finite shunt resistance (~ 1 kΩ) of the diode. The bandwidth, determined by the capacitance, is then about 2 GHz.
[d] Based on a 6 dB noise figure for the following amplifier.

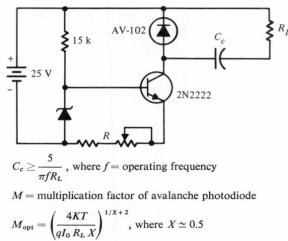

$C_c \geq \dfrac{5}{\pi f R_L}$, where f = operating frequency

M = multiplication factor of avalanche photodiode

$M_{opt} = \left(\dfrac{4KT}{qI_0 R_L X}\right)^{1/X+2}$, where $X \simeq 0.5$

$V_z \simeq$ Zener voltage, 2–10 V

$V_{EB} \simeq 0.8$ V

$I_A = I_0 M = M(I_{dark} + I_{signal} + I_{background})$

$R = \dfrac{V_z - V_{EB}}{I_A}$

Figure 9-30   Avalanche circuit and operating parameters.[35]   *(With permission of EG & G, Inc.)*

9·4·4   *infrared quantum detectors*

Infrared quantum detectors have proved very effective in applications requiring great sensitivity and high speed of response. The photoconductor employed depends upon the wavelength of interest. Figure 9-31 shows the infrared spectrum with principle detectors.

For the very near infrared (long wave limit of 1.8×10^3 nm), germanium junction photodiodes are used. At somewhat longer wavelengths (3.5×10^3 nm), lead sulfide and indium arsenide have suitable responses. For still longer wavelengths (7×10^3 nm), PbTe, PbSe, and InSb are the most frequently used photoconductors. Except for relatively low sensitivity InSb junction devices, detectors employing these materials require liquid nitrogen cooling.[37] Extrinsic photoconductors of appropriately doped germanium are used for longer wavelengths, to beyond 100×10^3 nm, depending upon the activator employed. Such cells require considerable cooling to reduce thermal excitation of carriers. The sensitivity of these detectors depends upon their cooling, the level of background radiation, and the configuration of the detector.

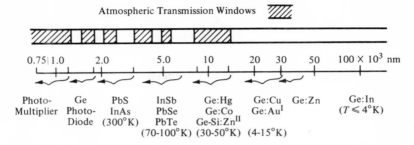

Figure 9-31 Infrared spectrum with principal detectors.[37] (With permission of RCA Review.)

For particular regions of the spectrum one can do considerably better with a photoelectric detector than with an uncooled thermal detector and also achieve a much more rapid response. Here the NEP depends on the area A of the detector element, being roughly proportional to $A^{1/2}$. Thus, for the PbS region one may have an NEP of about 10^{-12} W/Hz$^{1/2}$ for a detector having an area of 1 mm^2 cooled with solid CO_2, with a time constant of about 10^{-3} s. One may use a detector with a shorter time constant with some deterioration of performance. For the intermediate infrared, one of the extrinsic detectors operated at the optimum temperature can furnish an NEP of the order of 3×10^{-12} W/Hz$^{1/2}$ for a detector of area 1 mm^2 with a time constant in the order of 10^{-6} s. Figure 9-32 shows the spectral response of various infrared detectors.[38]

We can calculate a limiting D^* for a detector if we know its long wavelength limit and the spectral distribution of blackbody radiation. The limiting $D^*(\pi)$ as a function of wavelength for a detector (having unit quantum efficiency) and a 2π solid angle of view is shown in Figure 9-32. If the angular aperture of the system, θ, is less than 180°, then

$$D^*(\theta) = D^*(\pi)(\sin \theta/2)^{-1} \qquad (9\text{-}24)$$

The response times vary considerably among these detectors. Many are faster than 1 s, and zinc doped germanium at 5°K has a response time better than 10 ns.

Cooling improves detectivity by a significant amount. For example, note PbS in Figure 9-32. Some words about cooled detectors are, therefore, in order.

"The envelope must be of Dewar construction in order to permit cooling of the detector. It must be provided with a window, transparent in the region in which the detector material shows sensitivity. Figure 9-33 shows sample envelopes used for PbTe and Ge detectors. An average detector has a room temperature resistance of about 30 kΩ and a resistance of about 50 MΩ when cooled to liquid nitrogen temperature.

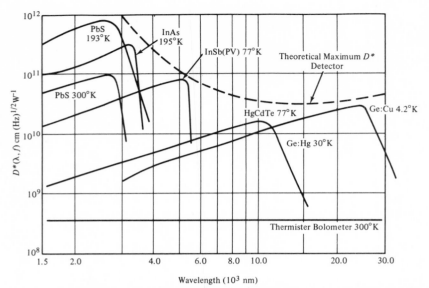

Figure 9-32 *Spectral detectivity curves for typical infrared detectors. All devices represented are photon detectors with exception of the thermistor bolometer which is a thermal detector.* D^* *values shown were not all taken at the same chopping frequency.*[38] (**With permission of Electro-Optical Systems Design.**)

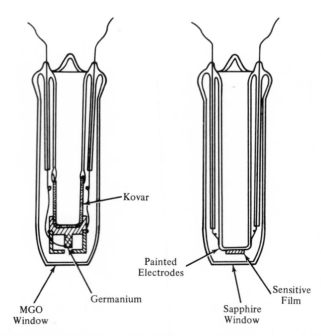

Figure 9-33 *Germanium and lead-telluride detector assemblies.*[39] (**With permission of Journal of the Optical Society of America.**)

Detector resistance may deviate by an order of magnitude in either direction from this value."[39]

One typical infrared detector is copper activated germanium which is sensitive in the $1-30 \times 10^3$ nm region. However, due to an external barium fluoride filter, peak sensitivity is achieved in the 11×10^3 nm region (see Figure 9-34). The QKN 902 (Raytheon) shown in this figure is a long wavelength, photoconductive detector, sensitive in the $2-15 \times 10^3$ nm region, which makes it useful for passive detection of room temperature targets. The detector has a time constant of less than 0.1 μs permitting fast scan rates and high resolution. The detector element is mounted in a compact self-contained, all metal Dewar providing 9.0 h of unattended operation. It is vibration isolated to minimize microphonics.

In spite of major advances in photoelectric detection, conventional thermal detectors are still used. One reason for this is that many of the photoelectric detectors cover only a very limited region of the spectrum. Thus, if wide spectral coverage is required, a multiplicity of detectors is needed. Also, except for wavelengths of the near infrared and for shorter wavelengths, the more sensitive detectors require cooling, ultimately with liquid helium for the long wave end of the infrared spectrum.

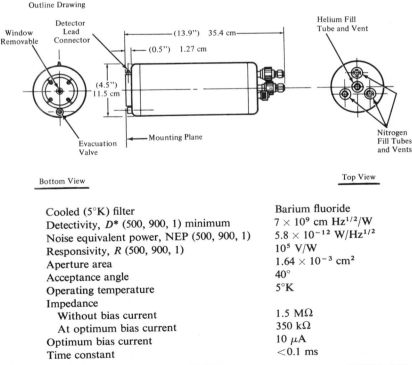

Cooled (5°K) filter	Barium fluoride
Detectivity, D^* (500, 900, 1) minimum	7×10^9 cm Hz$^{1/2}$/W
Noise equivalent power, NEP (500, 900, 1)	5.8×10^{-12} W/Hz$^{1/2}$
Responsivity, R (500, 900, 1)	10^5 V/W
Aperture area	1.64×10^{-3} cm^2
Acceptance angle	40°
Operating temperature	5°K
Impedance	
Without bias current	1.5 MΩ
At optimum bias current	350 kΩ
Optimum bias current	10 μA
Time constant	<0.1 ms

Figure 9-34 Copper actuated germanium detector (QKN 902— Raytheon). (With permission of Raytheon Company.)

9·5   heat detectors

All bodies are subject to heating by radiation.   The energy flux and spectral power density associated with a radiator are related to its temperature by such equations as Planck's law, the Stefan-Boltzmann law, Wein's distribution and displacement laws, and the Rayleigh-Jeans equation. Although these are derived for ideal (blackbody) radiators, the behavior of real objects can be inferred using an empirical sensitivity factor.

In total radiation devices, the measured variable is usually the temperature rise of a standard blackbody absorber exposed to the object under test.   The radiation thermopile detects a quantity proportional to the amplitude of the optical wave squared, i.e., power.   Most systems employ thermocouples, resistance wire, or thermistors, although some units are pneumatic.   Thermopile devices can be made sufficiently stable to permit usage as primary calibration standards.   General requirements are that the energy collector must withstand the localized sample of the laser beam, disperse the energy quickly over an extended energy absorbing area, and minimize reradiation, reflection, and conduction losses before the temperature reaches equilibrium and is measured.

When uniform spectral response is required from a detector over a wide range of wavelengths, a thermal detector must be used.   Care must be taken, however, to make sure that the detector is uniformly absorbent over the entire wavelength range required.

Temperature transducers employ a number of readout instruments, the most common of which are sensitive circuits of the microvoltmeter or Wheatstone bridge type.   The overall accuracy and sensitivity of the temperature change detector are dependent upon the combined transducer and circuit.   Precision instrumentation includes regulating apparatus that essentially frees the instrument from its environment.   This includes temperature compensation, regulated sources of supply voltage, isolation from induced sources of noise, and compensation for lead resistance, as well as thermally induced voltages.

A variety of calorimeters for measuring the power and energy of pulsed and CW laser radiation have appeared.[40,41]   This discussion will be limited to a few of the more common measuring devices used in industry.

9·5·1   bolometers

Bolometers are radiant power detection devices which depend on measuring the temperature change in resistance of a material due to the heating effect of absorbed radiation.   The resistance change is a measure of the radiant power absorbed from radiation at all wavelengths.

Since heat may be lost before equilibrium is reached, an error may be introduced in the determination of the total energy absorbed.   This type of error is minimized in the *rat's nest wire calorimeter*, which was developed specifically to measure the energy in the output of a ruby laser.[42]

In the rat's nest calorimeter the incident beam impinges on and is absorbed in a bundle of fine enameled copper wire (bolometer unit). The change in resistance of the wire is a measure of the total energy absorbed and, since the change in resistance is independent of the volume distribution of heat in the wire, there is no need to wait for temperature equalization.   It is also easier to measure this change in resistance than to measure the small change in the output voltage of a thermocouple. Since this is a calorimetric device, relatively insensitive to wavelength of the incident radiation, it can measure the radiation from any source in the visible and infrared regions of the spectrum.

The bolometer at the heart of the rat's nest calorimeter consists of approximately 1000 ft (980 Ω) of No. 40 B & S gauge enameled copper wire loosely and randomly packed into a 50 ml beaker silvered on the inside.   Two similar bolometer units, one active and one dummy, are arranged in a conventional bridge circuit (Figure 9-35).   The active bolometer unit receives the radiant energy to be metered, and the dummy minimizes galvanometer drift resulting from changes in ambient temperature.

In application, the laser beam is directed to the calorimeter wherein it is reflected, scattered, and absorbed, causing a rapid rise in the resistance

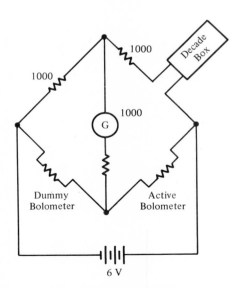

Figure 9-35   Bridge circuit of rat's nest calorimeter.[42]   **(Reprinted by special permission from the February 1963 issue of Electronics, Fig. 1. Copyright © 1963 by McGraw-Hill Publications, New York.)**

of the insulated bundle of wire.   The resistance change is directly proportional to laser energy if the wire size is uniform and the temperature
coefficient of resistance and specific heat of the wire are independent of
temperature.

Although the simple relation described above implies that the calorimeter is capable of absolute calibration, it turns out that there are several
sources of error that must be considered.   These include the effect of the
0.0003 in. layer of insulating varnish on the wire, which increases the heat
capacity as much as 29 percent, Fresnel reflection at the calorimeter
window (approximately 8 percent), and backscattering of energy from the
wire bundle (approximately 18 percent).   Applying these corrections, the
energy equation becomes approximately

$$U = 2.38 \, \Delta R \qquad J \tag{9-25}$$

The inherent time constant is on the order of 10^{-4} s so it can be used
with a fast detector or recorder if desired.   Repetitive use will build up a
temperature differential between the active and dummy bolometers and,
if a slow detector like a galvanometer is used, drift will ultimately limit
the accuracy of measurement.   Application of this calorimeter is restricted on the high side by damage to the insulation at about 10 J/cm^2.
Its use to measure the output of Q-switched lasers is not recommended.

An example of *a bolometer using a platinum ribbon* sensitive element
which is in a permanently evacuated, nonhygroscopic AgCl tube is
illustrated in Figure 9-36.   Its virtue, for the precision needs of laser

Detectivity	$D^* = 6 \times 10^8$ cm (Hz)$^{1/2}$ watt
Spectral Sensitivity	Uniform from 1 μm to 26 μm
Thermal time constant	16 ms
Resistance	40Ω (nominal)

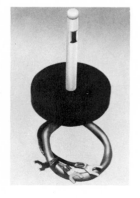 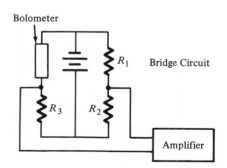

Figure 9-36   Bolometer.   (With permission of Baird Atomic.)

measurement, is its flat response over a wide spectral range. The bolometer may be calibrated at 1×10^3 nm and then used with confidence at 10.6×10^3 nm or at any other useful wavelength out to 26×10^3 nm.

In the most common type of bolometer system, the radiation impinging on the bolometer is chopped mechanically at the rate of 10 Hz and the bolometer is used as a variable resistor in a simple bridge circuit. The voltage resulting from unbalance of the bridge is amplified by a very high-gain, low-noise amplifier tuned at 10 Hz. The final output may be indicated on a voltmeter.

Although bolometers are of three types—metal, semiconductor, and superconductor—no discussion of the latter two will be included because industrial uses are limited, primarily by the need for liquid helium cooling. Further discussion is readily available in the literature.[43,44,45]

9·5·2   thermopile devices

In 1830, L. Nobili used a device, based on Seebecks' discovery of the thermoelectric effect in 1826, to measure small differences in temperature. This became known as a *thermocouple*. A number of such thermocouples in series were used by M. Melloni in 1833 as a radiation detector, which was called a *thermopile*. The thermopile was made from a number of junctions (generally antimony-bismuth), alternate ones being exposed to the radiation. This sets up a temperature difference between these and the remaining junctions and so creates a thermoelectric electromotive force (emf). This instrument was much more sensitive than the thermometers previously used and became the most widely used detector of infrared radiation for the next half century. By its means Melloni greatly extended the range of observations on the infrared spectrum. Detailed analysis and discussion are available in the literature.[46]

A typical *thermopile* is shown in Figure 9-37 and consists simply of a

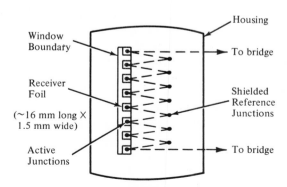

Figure 9-37   Radiation thermopile.

series connection of a number of low mass junctions mounted on a blackened receiver.   Radiation absorbed by the receiver causes the junction temperature to rise.   The active and reference junctions are maintained within the same enclosure at the same temperature, the reference junctions being shielded from the radiation to be measured.   Radiation falling on the active junctions raises their temperature slightly with respect to that of the reference junctions.   Variations of the ambient temperature do not greatly affect performance.

Normally carbon-black coated silver receivers are used with bismuth-silver couples for sensitivity, or with copper constantin for ruggedness. Gold-blacks or platinum-blacks are also used to obtain the highest response speeds, which can be further improved by reducing the area and weight of the element at some sacrifice of sensitivity and ruggedness.   Typical thermopiles (Eppley) reach 90 percent of their maximum emf within 2 s but should not be used for the measurement of radiation intensities greater than 1 W/in.^{2} (0.115 W/cm^2).

Evacuated enclosures having infrared transmitting windows are frequently employed to improve detectivity by reducing convection losses. The value of D^* for a well-constructed radiation thermocouple is 1.4×10^9 cm Hz$^{1/2}$/W.   Thus, it is about an order of magnitude from the photon noise limit for thermal detectors.

The simplest method of evaluating thermopile outputs, and the one requiring the least expensive equipment, is by reading galvanometer deflections.   However, if accurate absolute measurements are required, this method requires frequent calibration of the thermopile by means of a standard lamp.

A typical thermopile calibration sheet is shown in Table 9-11.

The device used to measure pulsed energies should have a sufficiently long time constant for true integration and ease of observation and high damage thresholds.   These conditions are fulfilled by the *ballistic thermopile*[47] (or Mendenhall-Wedge ballistic calorimeter) shown in Figure 9-38. The receiver in this thermopile is a polished carbon cone in which the radiation is reflected down toward the apex of the cone and out again.   In this process, the incoming rays undergo multiple bounces causing the energy to be almost totally absorbed.

Note the identical reference cone package in the same calorimeter so that drift due to ambient temperature variations are minimized.

A Model 118 "Cone" (TRG) can only take 1 W CW, but has a maximum energy rating of 1000 J for a 4 cm diameter aperture.   Additional specifications are: sensitivity of 22 mV/J, 90 s rise time, about 2.5 min decay time, ± 2 percent accuracy.

Since the laser output pulse is very short compared with any thermal time constants of the calorimeter, the integration time for the device is sufficiently long to yield accurate results for pulse durations of the order of 1 s or less.

TABLE 9-11   Thermopile Calibration Sheet[a]

Type: Circular
Elements: Bismuth silver
No. of junctions: 8
Coating: Lampblack

Resistance: 11.4 Ω
Type of case: Air with slide
Window: 1 mm quartz
Shutter opening: 13/32 in. dia.

The emf developed by this thermopile, with the window and shutter opening as above and exposed at ATMOSPHERIC PRESSURE, under standard conditions, at an ambient temperature of 25°C and relative humidity of 37 per cent to radiation of three different intensities from a standard lamp calibrated by the National Bureau of Standards was as follows:

Intensity of Radiation ($W\ cm^{-2}$)	Emf (μV)	$\mu V/\mu W/cm^2$
42.1×10^{-6}	4.81	0.1143
62.2×10^{-6}	7.13	0.1146
87.0×10^{-6}	9.93	0.1141

From this series of measurements this thermopile is calculated to develop a mean emf of 0.114 $\mu V/\mu W/cm^2$.

[a] With permission of the Eppley Laboratory, Inc.

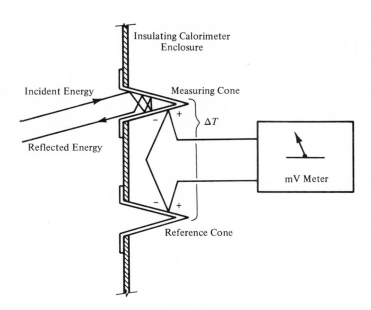

Figure 9-38   Mendenhall cone-type laser calorimeter.

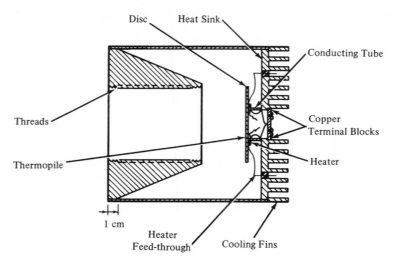

Figure 9-39   Cross section of the disc calorimeter. A laser beam incident on the disc is converted to heat which sets up a temperature gradient in the conducting tube. The gradient is sensed by the thermopile.[49]   (With permission of The Review of Scientific Instruments.)

The advent of lasers capable of producing many watts of power resulted in the development of *disc* and *cone flow thermopiles.*[48]

An improved disc calorimeter, which can be calibrated, is shown in Figure 9-39[49] and is reported to be accurate to ±2.5 percent in the 1–30 W range. The instrument is constructed of aluminum alloy 6061 with a vapor blasted, black anodized finish. The main parts are the disc, conducting tube, thermopile, and a calibrating electric heater. In order to avoid the thermal resistances of mechanical connections, the disc, conducting tube, and heat sink with its vertical cooling fins are machined from a solid block of aluminum. The front surface of the disc is painted with a special flat black paint.

TABLE 9-12   Electrical Calibration Data for the Disc Calorimeter[49]

Power, V^2/R (W)	Response (μV)	Sensitivity, S_d ($\mu V/W$)
1.005	83.20	82.76
4.914	405.2	82.46
9.930	811.2	81.69
14.94	1212.0	81.11
19.71	1598.0	81.08

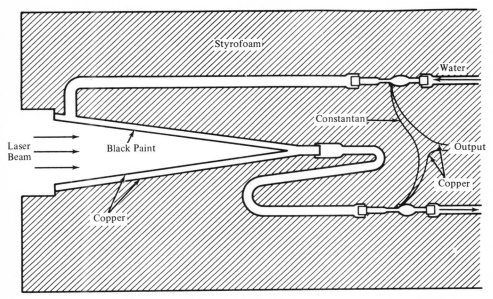

Figure 9-40 Schematic of the cone-flow power meter showing construction details.[48]

The ΔT, which is generated along the tube, is measured by a four-junction series-connected copper constantan thermopile of 0.13 mm wire (No. 36 gauge).

On the back side of the disc, at a 3 mm distance from the cylinder, is a ledge on which is wound a heater wire of 0.13 mm manganese wire (No. 36 gauge). It has a resistance of approximately 90 Ω and is connected to feed-throughs by 18 gauge copper wire. This heater allows one to electrically calibrate the instrument by joule heating (see Table 9-12).

The *cone flow* meter shown in Figure 9-40 has proven accurate to 3 percent for the range of 1 to 5 kW of CW laser power.

Incident laser power increases the temperature of water flowing through the double cone. Flowing water in contact with the inner, heat-absorbing cone maintains its temperature near room temperature, making radiation and convection negligible. A commercial version (Model 213 by CRL) has a response time of less than 1 s, a 38 mm aperture, and a water-cooled absorption head capable of dissipating 1 kW on a continuous basis.

9.5.3 pyroelectric detectors

Some calorimeters utilizing surface absorption of the energy do not measure the change in temperature of the absorber with an independent sensor, but measure the change in some temperature sensitive characteristics of the absorber, such as resistance or pyroelectric current. A promising and relatively new approach to the problem of infrared detection is to make use of the pyroelectric effect. This effect occurs in certain classes of materials, called ferroelectrics, which possess a permanent electric polarization that is highly dependent on temperature. A miniscule variation in the material's temperature causes a finite change in this polarization, producing a change in the potential difference across the detector. Unlike other thermal detectors, pyroelectric devices are capacitive rather than resistive. As a result, their impedance falls with frequency, giving rise to very high electrical frequency response. This peculiarity accounts for their excellent high-frequency performance.

Because the detector operates at room temperature, is small and

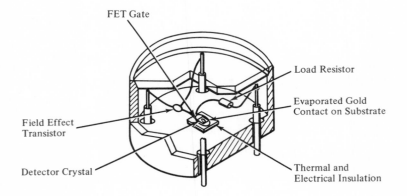

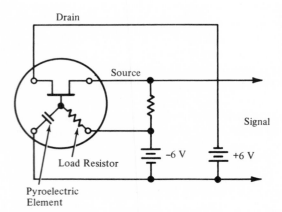

Figure 9-41   Pyroelectric (TGS) detector with integral Field Effect Transistor (FET) amplifier.   FET matches high impedance of TGS crystal, increases signal level, and reduces output impedance, cutting line noise pickup.[54] (Commercially available from Barnes Engineering.) (With permission of Electro-Optical Systems Design.)

compact, has a fast response time, and has high sensitivity, it is a convenient device for use with CO_2 and other far-infrared lasers. Pyroelectric detectors were described in 1962[50] when it was shown that, if radiation is absorbed on one electrode of a barium titanate capacitor, the change in polarization induced by heating causes the ferroelectric to respond to the incident radiation with a rise time of 5 μs. The minimum detectable flux was estimated to be 100 μW/cm^2.

It should be noted that detectors of this type possess no true steady-state responsivity as uninterrupted exposure to a strong source of infrared radiation produces heating of the ferroelectric and degradation of the output signal. It is necessary, therefore, when studying continuous sources, to chop the incident radiation.

Pyroelectric detectors have been used to resolve the output of lasers up to wavelengths of 337×10^3 nm (HCN).[51] CO_2 lasers, Q-switched at 200 Hz with 1 μs pulse lengths have been measured with a pyroelectric detector.[52] Studies[53] have also shown that the detector is linear with respect to incident radiation flux over the range of 0–60 W/cm^2 and gives an output of 1.3 mV/W/cm^2 when shunted with a 1 MΩ resistor.

The medium most widely used in triglycine sulfate, or TGS. Figure 9-41 is a pictorial view and schematic of a commercial TGS detector that provides good absorption from short wavelengths out to at least 600×10^3 nm, and which has been used at modulation frequencies as high as 1000 Hz.

More recent commercial designs possess the mechanical and chemical advantages of the perovskites and exhibit responsivities comparable to many TGS detectors.[55] High sensitivity models exhibit responsivities up to 500 V/W at 1 kHz. High-power models, on the other hand, exhibit saturation powers of 200 mW average, and remain functional up to 1 W. The minimum detectable power (NEP) of (KT1000 Laser Precision) detectors with 0.2×0.2 mm areas measures 3×10^{-9} W.

9·6   attenuation and beam-sampling techniques

To protect detectors from overload or damage, as well as to extend the range of all types of devices for measuring laser output, it is frequently necessary to reduce the intensity of radiation incident on the detector. In such cases it is necessary to attenuate a laser beam to bring the energy or power of the beam within the dynamic range of a particular detector. Alternatively, if a well-calibrated attenuator is available, it is possible to measure the range over which a detector follows some prescribed response law or the deviations from that law.

For this purpose, a variety of attenuators have been developed: neutral density filters, integrating spheres, coarse diffraction gratings, and diffuse reflectors. Other beam-sampling techniques will also be reviewed.

9·6·1   neutral density filters[56]

At relatively low intensities neutral-density filters are commonly used as attenuators. They are suitable concentrations of absorbing material in a transparent medium such as gelatin or glass. The spectral-absorption characteristics of the material are relatively independent of wavelength, at least within the visible spectrum. Hence they are gray or black in appearance, depending on their total absorption. Care should be exercised in using these filters over narrow wavelength bands because the transmission characteristics of typical filters may vary as much as 2:1 over the visual spectrum. For this reason, as well as the fact that the surface reflections from inside stacks of such filters can interact to make the total insertion loss of the array greater than the sum of the individual insertion losses, each filter or stack of filters must be calibrated at the particular wavelength being studied if precise measurements are required.

Of these attenuators, the neutral density filter is most susceptible to damage by very high-power laser beams. However, a cell filled with a solution which is absorbing at the laser wavelength may be used in place of the neutral density filter.

9·6·2   optical interference filters (see Chapter 8)

Optical interference filters have several advantages over glass or gelatin absorption filters:

a. Narrow passbands
b. Sharp cutoffs
c. Symmetrically shaped passbands
d. Resistance to moisture

The peak wavelength of an interference filter is a function of the angle of incidence of the radiation impinging on the filter. For small angles of incidence, this dependence is given by the equation

$$\lambda_\phi = \lambda_0\left(1 - \frac{\sin^2 \phi}{n^2}\right)^{1/2} \qquad (9\text{-}26)$$

where λ_ϕ = peak wavelength,
λ_0 = peak wavelength when ϕ is zero,
ϕ = angle of incidence,
n = effective index of refraction of the spacer.

The peak wavelength of an interference filter is also a function of the temperature of the filter. The peak wavelength will shift about 0.1 nm for each 5.5°C change in temperature.

Figure 9-42 gives some pertinent definitions.

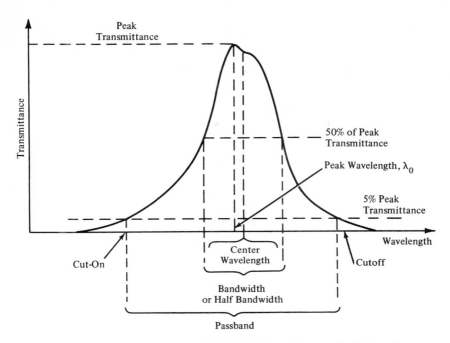

Figure 9-42 Some graphical definitions for optical interference filters. (With permission of Baird Atomic.)

Interference filters are the "most neutral" of all types of neutral density filters. They have less variation of density as a function of wavelength than any other neutral density filter. They have two limitations, however, which must be kept in mind whenever they are used.

1. They have a slight diffusing effect which tends to blur any image formed from light which has passed through the filter.
2. The rated density is the average density for a beam of light, $\frac{1}{2}$ in. in diameter, passing through the filter. At any given point of the filter surface, the filter is either totally opaque or highly transparent, the only absorption being due to the substrate.

Each filter consists of opaque parallel lines or two perpendicular sets of parallel lines etched on a 1 in. by 1 in. square substrate. These filters are obtainable on fused silica, quartz, or IRTRAN substrates for use at various wavelengths.

9·6·3 silicon attenuators[57]

Since radiative recombination of excess carriers in an indirect band-gap material is a very inefficient process, experiments have shown[10] that the use of silicon as a "wavelength converting" attenuator is feasible. Ruby radiation was absorbed on the front surface of a polished silicon wafer 0.10 cm thick, mounted directly on the window of an S-1 photomultiplier. An 1100 nm recombination radiation emitted from the rear surface was then measured by the photocurrent in the detector.

Although the Si used had a lifetime of 400 μs, the photomultiplier current clearly reproduced laser pulses down to 2×10^{-8} s (the limit of the electronic equipment used).

This technique enables the display of the rapid spiking action of a ruby laser on an oscilloscope.

The chemical inertness, high melting point, and elemental nature of silicon eliminate the bleaching problems found in compounds. Attempts to obtain quantitative data relating the dependence of the attenuation factor on the beam intensity and semiconductor characteristics showed that tight control over the flash-lamp voltage and laser-rod temperature was essential.

9·6·4   integrating spheres[58]

The integrating sphere attenuator is essentially a sphere with two small openings. The laser beam enters one of these, is scattered and rescattered from the inner surface, then emerges from the second opening. The attenuation factor is given approximately by the ratio of the area of the exit hole to the total surface of the sphere.

9·6·5   diffraction grating[59]

In the diffraction grating attenuator, the monochromatic laser radiation is deflected into a direction determined by the order of the diffraction. The ratio of the intensity of the diffracted beam to that of the beam incident on the grating is given by diffraction theory (Chapter 7). The degree of attenuation achieved depends upon the grating constant and the spectral order being observed. Considerable attenuation can be obtained if the grating is coarse. For plane polarized light, the efficiency of the grating depends upon whether or not the electric field of the plane polarized light is parallel or perpendicular to the grooves. It can be shown that, in a slit grating, the ratio of the illumination in the mth order to that in zero order is

$$\frac{I_m}{I_0} = \frac{1}{m^2 \pi^2} \tag{9.27}$$

Only about 10 percent of the light appears in the first order, about 2 percent in the second order, and so on.

9·6·6   *diffuse reflectors*[60]

One of the simplest as well as one of the more reliable attenuator techniques takes advantage of the I/R^2 decay of radiation scattered from a diffuse Lambertian surface.

A convenient diffusing and attenuation scheme involves the use of a magnesium carbonate or aluminum oxide block (see Figure 9-43).   In this configuration, the irradiance in the plane of the photodiode is related to the power incident on the diffusing block by

$$H = \frac{P \cos \theta}{\pi R^2} \, \rho \qquad (9.28)$$

where the distance R between the diffuser and the detector is large compared to the illuminated spot size, ρ is the reflectivity of the diffuser, and θ is the angle of incidence.

The diffuse, white scattering target can be made of a variety of materials, many of which have been developed and tested for use in integrating spheres.   These include barium sulfate, magnesium oxide, and magnesium carbonate coatings, although opal glasses and white pyroceramics may withstand higher power densities and have more durable mechanical properties and higher reflectivities in the near infrared.

9·6·7   *beamsplitters*

Beamsplitters, by themselves, provide a useful technique for attenuating a laser beam, and if the surfaces are optically flat and the material homogeneous, the spatial coherence of both portions of the beam are unaffected by the beamsplitter.

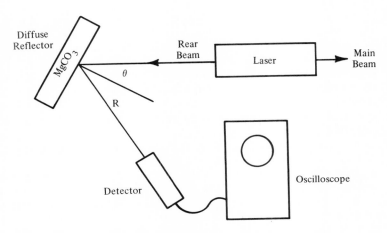

Figure 9-43   Attenuation by a diffuse reflector.

Glass and fused silica beamsplitters are frequently used as Fresnel reflectors to sample a portion of the beam. In its basic form a beamsplitter is a flat plate of transparent dielectric material, which, for use in the visible or near infrared, is usually made of quartz and, for use in the infrared, is frequently made of germanium. Because these beamsplitters will affect the radius of curvature of the wavefront, they must be smooth, extremely flat, and have negligible wedge if coherence is to be preserved. It has been found that thin celluloid beamsplitters consisting of pellicles (see Glossary) approximately 8 μm thick can be used to attenuate the beam without damage to the thin film.

References

1. G. Bird, R. Jones, and A. Ames, "The Efficiency of Radiation Detection by Photographic Films," *Appl. Optics* 8, No. 12, 2389 (December 1969).
2. L. K. Anderson and B. J. McMurty, "High-Speed Photodetectors," *Proc. IEEE* 54, No. 10, 1335 (October 1966).
3. R. A. Smith, "Detectors for Ultraviolet, Visible and Infrared Radiation," *Appl. Optics* 4, No. 6, 631 (June 1965).
4. "Nomenclature and Definitions for Illuminating Engineering," *USA Standard* Z7.1, 32 (1967).
5. R. C. Jones, "Phenomenological Description of the Response and Detecting Ability of Radiation Detectors," *Proc. IRE* 47, 1495 (September 1959).
6. T. P. Merritt and F. F. Hall, Jr., "Blackbody Radiation," *Proc. IRE* 47, 1435 (September 1959).
7. R. C. Jones, "Phenomenological Description of the Response and Detecting Ability of Radiation Detectors." *Proc. IRE* 47, 1495 (September 1959).
8. M. Ross, "Receiving Devices," *Laser Receivers*, John Wiley and Sons, Inc., New York (1966).
9. A. Rose, *Concepts in Photoconductivity and Allied Problems*, John Wiley and Sons, Inc., New York (1963).
10. T. G. Maple *et al.*, "Variation of Noise with Ambient in Germanium Filters," *J. Appl. Phys.* 26, 26 (1955).
11. B. M. Oliver, "Thermal and Quantum Noise," *Proc. IEEE* 53, 436 (1965).
12. H. Hanken, "Theory of Coherence of Laser Light," *Phys. Rev.* 13, 329 (1964).
13. J. A. Fleck, Jr., "Nonlinear Laser Noise and Coherence," *J. Appl. Phys.* 37, 188 (1966).
14. G. Birnbaum and M. Birnbaum, "Measurement of Laser Energy and Power," *Proc. IEEE* 55, No. 6, 1026 (June 1967).
15. R. D. Compton, "The 'Now' Field of Optoelectronics," *Electro-Optical Systems Design*, p. 26 (May 1970).
16. R. W. Engstrom, "Absolute Spectral Response Characteristics of Photosensitive Devices," *RCA Rev.* 21, 184–190 (1960).
17. E. J. Schiel, "Photoelectric Energy Meter for Measuring Laser Output," *Proc. IEEE* 51, 365 (1963).

18. R. A. Epstein and R. Rockwell, "Monitor for a Pulsed Laser System," *Optics Tech.* **1**, No. 5, p. 245 (November 1969).
19. G. A. Morton, "Photon Counting," *Appl. Optics* **7**, No. 1, 1 (January 1968).
20. H. Carleton and M. Brady, "Detectors for Low Light Levels," *Laser Focus*, p. 33 (December 1969).
21a. *RCA Electron Tube Handbook*, HB-3 (November 1969).
21b. *RCA Phototubes and Photocells*, Technical Manual PT-60 (1963).
22. E. Savoye and J. Tietjen, "Bright Outlook for Infrared Detectors," *Laser Focus*, p. 34 (January 1970).
23. E. J. Schiel and J. J. Bolmerich, "Absolute Measurement of GaAs Diodes Radiation Using Solar Cells," *Proc. IEEE* **51**, 218 (1963).
24. "Opto-Electronic Product Directory," *Electro-Optical Systems Design* **3**, No. 5 (May 1971).
25. K. M. Johnson, "High-Speed Photodiode Signal Enhancement at Avalanche Breakdown Voltage," *IEEE Trans. on Electron Devices* **ED-12**, 55 (1965).
26. G. Lucovsky *et al.*, "Coherent Light Detection in Solid-State Photodiodes," *Proc. IEEE* **51**, 166 (1963).
27. M. DiDomenico, Jr., and O. Svelto, "Solid-State Photodetection: A Comparison between Photodiodes and Photoconductors," *Proc. IEEE* **52**, 136 (1964).
28. E. Ahlstrom and W. W. Gaertner, "Silicon Surface Barrier Photocells," *J. Appl. Phys.* **33**, 2602 (August 1962).
29. R. L. Williams, "Fast High-Sensitivity Silicon Photodiodes," *J. Opt. Soc. Amer.* **52**, No. 11, 1237 (November 1962).
30. E. L. Danahy, "The Real World of Silicon Photodiodes," *Electro-Optical Systems Design*, p. 36 (May 1970).
31. P. Wendland, "Silicon Photodiode Revisited," *Electro-Optical Systems Design* (August 1970).
32. L. K. Anderson and B. J. McMurty, "High-Speed Photodetectors," *Proc. IEEE* **54**, No. 10, 1335 (October 1966).
33. K. M. Johnson, "High-Speed Photodiode Signal Enhancement at Avalanche Breakdown Voltage," *IEEE Trans. on Electron Devices* **ED-12**, 55 (1965).
34. R. J. McIntyre, "Comparisons of Photomultipliers and Avalanche Photodiodes for Laser Applications," *IEEE Trans. on Electron Devices* **ED-17**, No. 4, 347 (April 1970).
35. "AV-102 Silicon Avalanche Photodiode," *EG & G Electronic Products Div.*, Data Sheet AV-102 (February 2, 1969).
36. "Opto-Electronic Product Directory," *Electro-Optical Systems Design* **3**, No. 5 (May 1971).
37. G. A. Morton, "Infrared Detectors," *RCA Rev.* **26**, 4 (1965).
38. Staff Report, "Infrared Detection—Seeing the Invisible," *Electro-Optical Systems Design* **2**, No. 6, 34 (June 1970).
39. W. Beyen *et al.*, "Cooled Photoconductive Infrared Detectors," *J. Opt. Soc. Amer.* **49**, No. 7, 686 (July 1959).
40. H. Heard, "Measurement of Energy and Power," *Laser Parameter Measurement Handbook*, p. 93, John Wiley and Sons, Inc., New York (1968).
41. A. Bernstein and L. Carrier, "Development of Devices for Measuring Optical Radiation," *Technical Documentary Report No. RTD TDR-63-3015*, Project No. 8814, Periodical AD 420 574.

42. R. M. Baker, "Measuring Laser Output with RAT's Nest Calorimeter," *Electronics* **36**, No. 36, 36 (February 1963). Reprinted by special permission from the February, 1963 issue of *Electronics*, Figure 1, copyrighted © 1963 by McGraw-Hill Publications, New York, New York.

43. R. A. Smith, "Detectors for Ultraviolet, Visible and Infrared Radiation," *Appl. Optics* **4**, No. 6, 631 (June 1965).

44. J. Siekman and R. Morijn, "A Simple Power-Output Meter Specially Designed for Continuous Laser Beams," *Phillips Res. Repts.* **23**, 375 (1968).

45. P. W. Kruse *et al.*, *Elements of Infrared Technology*, John Wiley and Sons, Inc., New York (1962).

46. R. A. Smith *et al.*, *The Detection and Measurement of Infrared Radiation*, 2nd Ed., Oxford University Press, Oxford, England (1968).

47. T. Li and S. Sims, "A Calorimeter for Energy Measurements of Optical Lasers," *Appl. Optics* **1**, No. 3, 325 (May 1962).

48. "Laser Power and Energy Measurements," *NBS Tech. Note 382* (October 1969).

49. D. Jennings and E. West, "A Laser Power Meter for Large Beams," *Rev. Sci. Instr.* **41**, 565 (1970).

50. J. Cooper, "Minimum Detectable Power of a Pyroelectric Thermal Receiver," *Rev. Sci. Instr.* **33**, 92 (1962).

51. J. Ludlow *et al.*, "Infrared Radiation Detection by the Pyroelectric Effect," *J. Sci. Instr.* **44**, 694 (September 1967).

52. M. Kimmitt *et al.*, "Use of a Pyroelectric Detector to Measure Q-Switched CO_2 Laser Pulses," *Proc. IEEE* **56**, 1250 (1968).

53. W. Dudley, "A Simple Room Temperature Detector for Use with CO_2 Lasers," *J. Sci. Instr.* **44**, 629 (1967).

54. *Electro-Optical Systems Design*, p. 30 (June 1970).

55. W. Doyle, "Pyroelectric Detectors," *Laser Focus*, p. 34 (July 1970).

56. A. L. Glick, "A Method for Calibration of Laser Energy Output," *Proc. IRE* **50**, 1835 (August 1962).

57. K. Kessler, E. Passaglia, and N. Winogradoff, "Research on Laser Standards and Materials at the National Bureau of Standards," *NBS Tech. Note 449* (June 1968).

58. E. J. Schiel, "Photoelectric Energy Meter for Measuring Laser Output," *Proc. IEEE* **51**, 365 (1963).

59. R. Gerharz, "Attentuation of Laser Light by a Diffraction Grating," *Proc. IEEE* **52**, 438 (April 1964).

60. R. C. Leite and S. Porto, "A Simple Method for Calibration of Ruby Laser Output," *Proc. IEEE* **51**, 606–607 (April 1963).

61. G. Lucovsky *et al.*, "Coherent Light Detection in Solid-State Photodiodes," *Proc. IEEE*, p. 166 (January 1963).

62. A. E. Siegman and S. E. Harris, "Optical Heterodyning and Optical Demodulation at Microwave Frequencies," presented at the Symposium on Optical Masers, Polytechnic Institute of Brooklyn, April 16–19, 1963.

63. M. Teich, "Infrared Heterodyne Detection," *Proc. IEEE* **56**, No. 1, 37 (January 1968).

64. E. Leiba, "The First Demonstration of Photomixing with Pyroelectric Detectors at 300 Hz," *Comptes Rendus* **268**, 31 (1969).

65. R. Dixon and E. Gordon, "Acoustic Light Modulators Using Optical Heterodyne Mixing," *Bell System Tech. J.* **47**, 367 (1967).
66. H. Carleton and M. Brady, "Detectors for Low Light Levels," *Laser Focus* p. 33 (December 1969).

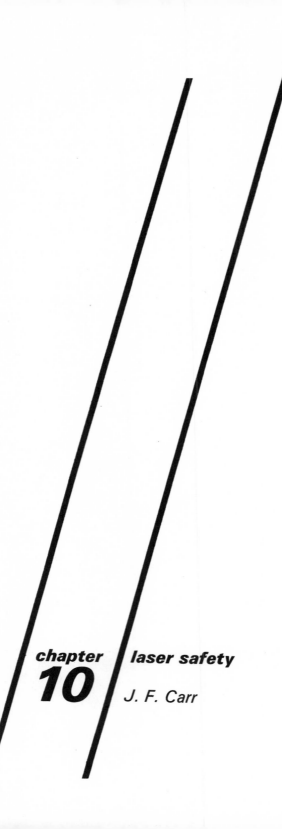

**chapter
10** | **laser safety**

J. F. Carr

10·0 introduction

As laser manufacturing tools enter production jobs, engineering consideration on how to safely install and use these machines becomes of paramount importance. New and unique hazards arise that are quite unlike the usual hazards of a production machine. For instance, if a punch press operator overcomes an interlock system, he usually places only himself in danger. However, if someone defeats the interlock system on a high-power laser, he not only endangers himself, but other personnel in the area may also be injured by laser radiation.* Thus, it is vital that engineers and managers specifying a laser tool for an application be aware of what lasers can and cannot do, what hazards are involved, and what precautions should be taken.

In previous chapters the reader has been told how and why lasers work, what their characteristics are, how they interact with materials, and how they can be used in manufacturing applications. The reader should also understand the effect of laser radiation on human beings. This chapter describes laser hazards and how to avoid them in both manufacturing and laboratory situations. Research into the effects of laser radiation on human beings is discussed and the use of this information in preparing safety procedures is presented. The development of standards and codes, as well as safety procedures of individual companies, is discussed in light of experience gained in the laboratory and in manufacturing.

10·1 why the laser is a unique hazard

Radiation from a laser is both spatially and temporally coherent. Two major safety problems resulting from these characteristics are: (1) the laser beam can traverse great distances with little change in the radiation characteristics, and (2) extreme intensities can be obtained. This last point can be easily understood by comparing the effects on the eye of a 100 W frosted incandescent light bulb and a 1 mW CW HeNe laser.

Figure 10-1 shows in cross section how the eye images a light bulb and a laser beam. To calculate the power density at the retina, we need to know two parameters—the power density at the cornea and the image size on the retina. For an extended source (one that the eye can resolve) the retinal image size is given by

$$d_r = af/r \qquad (10\text{-}1)$$

where a is the object size, f is the image focal length of the eye (usually $f = 17$ mm), and r is the distance from the object to the eye. The retinal power density is given by

$$I_r = I_c \frac{d_c^2}{d_r^2} = (\text{corneal irradiance}) \frac{\text{corneal area}}{\text{retinal area}} \qquad (10\text{-}2)$$

* As used throughout the chapter, radiation is electromagnetic radiation.

579

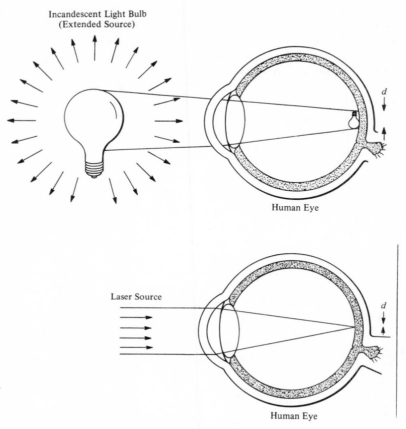

Incandescent Light Bulb
(Extended Source)

Human Eye

Laser Source

Human Eye

Figure 10-1   Comparison between extended source image and laser source image on the retina.

where I_c is the corneal power density, and d_c is the pupil diameter. We have assumed that the pupil of the eye is fully illuminated and that a round source is used.

Assuming a frosted light bulb 8 cm in diameter isotropically radiating 10 W in the visible portion of the spectrum, located 50 cm from the eye, we obtain

$$I_r = 2.1 \text{ mW/cm}^2 \qquad \text{light bulb}$$

For a laser with a Gaussian energy distribution, the laser radiation is imaged to a minimum spot by a perfect eye. This is the worst case situation and is of most concern in evaluating hazards and eye damage. From classical optics the minimum spot size that can be obtained from a lens is determined by its diffraction limit. Thus, if an eye could perform as a diffraction limited optical system, the minimum spot size would be

$$d_r = 1.27\lambda f/D \qquad \text{diffraction limited} \qquad (10\text{-}3)$$

where D is the pupil diameter, f is the focal length of the eye, and λ is the wavelength of the incident light (see Chapter 7).

Assuming a 1 mW HeNe laser this gives

$$I_r = 16 \times 10^3 \text{ W/cm}^2 \qquad \text{laser—diffraction limited spot}$$

It is clear from this simplified analysis that even a 1 mW laser supplies power densities on the retina many orders of magnitude greater than those of normal light sources.   This ability of the laser to be focused to extremely small spots of extreme power densities is one of the major hazards.

10·2   laser hazards

It has long been apparent that the beam emerging from a laser could be harmful to the eye.   Experience has shown that reflected and scattered laser light, nonlinear interactions, and other optical effects can be hazardous.   We also know what is not hazardous.   The problem of clarifying the separating region between these two is a major topic of investigation.

10·2·1   research on laser hazards

The human eye is a sensitive light detector and is quite susceptible to laser radiation damage at the retina due to focusing of the eye, or at the cornea due to absorption of radiation not transmitted by the eye (Figure 10-2).   Most research on laser hazards has been aimed at

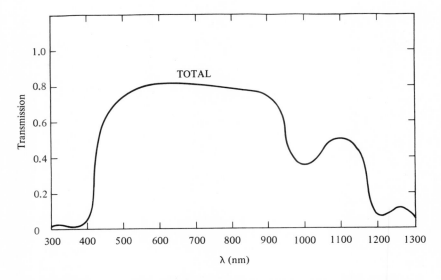

Figure 10-2   Transmission of light through ocular media.[14]

determining retinal and corneal damage thresholds.   Transmission characteristics and general absorption properties of the eye are shown in
Figure 10-3.

Starting in the early 1960's research has primarily concentrated on
damage to mammalian eyes with some research also examining damage to
the skin.   Most studies employed either rabbits or monkeys as subjects,
with some work being performed on humans.   A typical eye damage

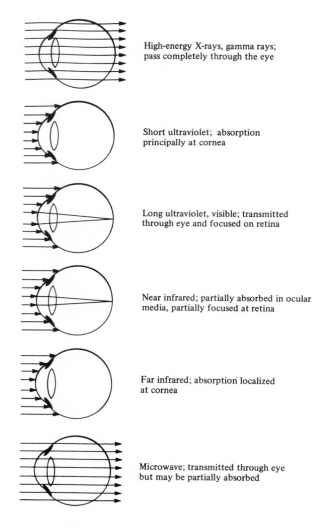

**Figure 10-3   Absorption properties of the eye for electromagnetic
radiation.**

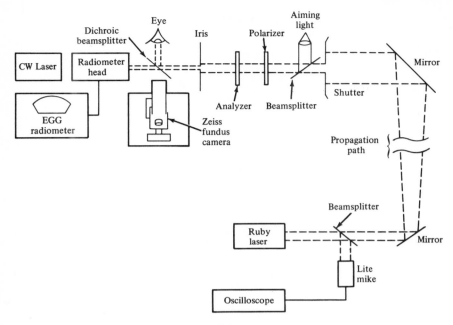

Figure 10-4   Experimental arrangement for retinal damage studies.[4]

experimental setup is shown in Figure 10-4. Experiments and experimental procedures for examination of both eye and skin damage are explained in great detail in reports presented by several groups.[1,2,3,4]

Although most experimental results are from rabbits or monkeys, it seems reasonable, based on past experience with other light sources such as carbon arcs and limited human data, to tentatively set human exposure limits based on these results. Indeed, some figures have been set by various groups. It is satisfying to note that all these figures on safe exposure levels, regardless of who proposes them, use essentially the same source of data. A lively debate on how to interpret the results, how to analyze them statistically, and how to add safety factors has gone on for several years. Data are now supplied in many forms, such as corneal irradiance, corneal intensity, retinal intensity, and so on, creating some confusion. Because the eye is an active optical system and because eyes vary in their responses to light, it is quite difficult to set truly accurate and safe exposure levels. Several "safe exposure levels" have been recommended by various groups (Table 10-1). A large difference in levels has occurred because different interpretations of the data were used and different safety factors were employed. However, it now has been determined that the data from these several sources, when properly adjusted to take account of the different procedures and test animals, give essentially the same results for damage thresholds.

TABLE 10-1   Permissible Exposure Levels Specified By Several Groups

(a) COMPARISON OF RECOMMENDED VALUES—EYE

Group	Q-Switched 694.3 nm 1 ns–1 μs J/cm²	Non-Q-Switched 694.3 nm 1 μs–0.1 s J/cm²	CW 400–750 nm 0.1 s W/cm²
ACGIH	1×10^{-7}	1×10^{-6}	1×10^{-5}
Army-Navy	1×10^{-7}	1×10^{-6}	1×10^{-6}
Air Force	5×10^{-7}	4×10^{-6}	1×10^{-3}
British (calculated)	21×10^{-7}	21×10^{-7}	25×10^{-5}

(b) COMPARISON OF RECOMMENDED VALUES—SKIN EXCLUDING EYE

Group	Pulsed 1 ns–1 μs J/cm²	Pulsed 1 μs–0.1 s J/cm²	CW 5 s W/cm²
ACGIH	0.1	0.1	1
Army-Navy	0.01	0.1	0.1

10·2·2   biological effects of laser radiation

Laser radiation is partially reflected, transmitted, and absorbed when incident on biological matter. The degree of each depends upon the properties of the tissues involved. This section summarizes the results obtained by many groups on the effects of laser radiation on various tissues.

Retinal Effects   The effect of laser radiation upon retinal tissue may be a temporary change without pathological reactions; or it may be more severe, varying from small indistinguishable lesions to gross damage of the retina. The mildest observable effect may be simple reddening. With increasing energy, lesions may occur, progressing from endema to charring with hemorrhaging and secondary effects about the lesion.[5] With very high energy, gases form which can disrupt the retina and may create small explosions in the eye.[4]

Within the retinal area the most critical area for vision is the fovea (Figure 10-5). This area is about 1 mm in diameter and contains the highest density of cone cells, resulting in the highest image resolution of the eye. Minimal damage (smallest area of functional loss of vision) in

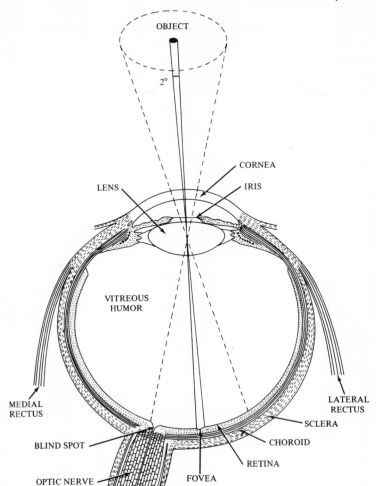

Figure 10-5   Structure of the human eye.[15]   *(From "Movements of the Eye," by E. L. Thomas.   Copyright © August 1968 by Scientific American, Inc.   All rights reserved.)*

the peripheral field of the retina may go undetected since the brain compensates, up to a certain point, for small-area vision losses.   The fovea, however, is much more susceptible to damage than the para-macular region of the retina, and even small area losses result in severe impairment of vision.   Thus, damage to the fovea is always assumed when trying to establish safe exposure levels.

<u>Corneal and Skin Effects</u>   Ultraviolet radiation (200–400 nm) is absorbed at the cornea and can cause painful damage.   It can cause conjunctivitis and erythema to the face and other exposed tissues.   Depending on the wavelength of the ultraviolet radiation, photochemical reactions

can also be induced.[6]   The general effect of ultraviolet radiation is that of a severe sunburn.

Infrared radiation is also absorbed by the cornea and by the skin and is converted to heat, with the overall effect being a heating of the tissue on a localized basis.   Many tissues are quite sensitive to thermal changes and can be damaged when even slight temperature changes occur.   Infrared radiation has been shown to cause lens opacities.

Although the above effects are generally to be protected against when a laser is used, it is interesting to note that they can also be usefully employed in medicine.   A variety of laser radiation effects are utlized in several medical applications.   Lesions are purposely formed, such as in welding detached retinas; localized heating is used in removing tattoos;[7] and large skin areas are burned in the study of skin cancer.[8]   A variety of medical studies involving lasers are underway.   For the industrial user, the work is of interest in how it shows the effect of the laser on biological matter.

10·2·3   specular and diffuse hazards

The hazards to the eye and skin from specular reflections of a laser beam are essentially identical to those of the unreflected beam.   A diffuse reflection or transmission of a laser beam, however, alters the basic character of the laser radiation by destroying both the directionality and spatial coherence of the incident beam.   An easy way to understand the difference is to consider what a mirror and a piece of ground glass do to light.   When light strikes a mirror or specular surface, it reflects such that the angle of incidence equals the angle of reflection.   Ground glass, however, scatters light that strikes it, causing both the directionality and intensity of the light to be greatly altered.   In many cases when diffuse or semispecular surfaces are involved, the change imparted to the laser radiation is insufficient to reduce the hazards to a safe level.

A perfect diffuser[9] reflects all incident light into a hemisphere with a radially symmetric distribution.

$$I = I_0 \cos \theta \qquad \text{Lambert's law} \qquad (10\text{-}4)$$

where θ is the angle from the surface normal, and I_0 is the intensity at $\theta = 0$.   The imaging of a perfect diffuse spot source by an eye (Figure 10-6) has two important aspects.

1. The retinal power density is unaltered regardless of how far away the surface is from the viewer, provided the eye can resolve the surface spot size.   Although the power radiated into the eye decreases as the inverse square of the distance from the surface to the eye, the image size on the retina simultaneously becomes smaller.   Therefore, the power density at the retina does not change.
2. The retinal power density is unaltered regardless of viewing angle.

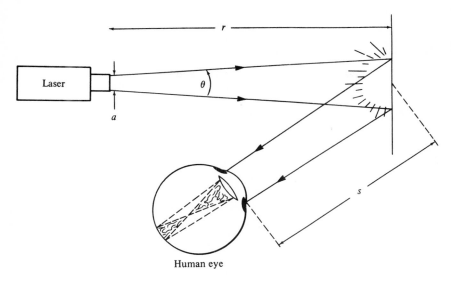

Figure 10-6   Viewing reflection from diffuse surface.

In most cases a practical diffuser will not follow Lambert's law,[10] but will have some different characteristic energy distribution associated with the reflected or transmitted light.   In these cases it is necessary to evaluate the radiation scattering characteristics of the surface and determine the radiation patterns of the scattered light.   As an example, consider the effects of ground glass on a laser beam.   For ground glass, with and without a silicone coating, significantly different distributions are obtained (Figure 10-7).   In one case, the energy is spread out into a 40° cone; in the other case, a narrow 10° cone with a much greater intensity occurs.   Clearly, the hazards presented by each surface vary significantly.

Many surfaces commonly found in laboratories or manufacturing locations are diffuse or semispecular in nature; therefore, it is important to evaluate the hazard potential of each.   A series of experiments were run to measure the radiation patterns of several common laboratory surfaces when irradiated by a 1 W argon-ion laser.   The apparatus used (Figure 10-8) measured the reflected energy at a constant radius as a function of angle.   Results obtained are plotted in Figures 10-9, 10-10, 10-11, and 10-12.   The illumination at any distance, r, from the sample is calculated from

$$E_r = E_{36 \text{ cm}} \frac{(36)^2}{r^2} \text{ W/cm}^2 \qquad (10\text{-}5)$$

These calculations (10-5) assume that the spot produced by the laser beam on the surface closely approximates a point source.

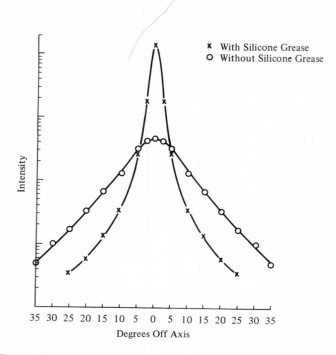

Figure 10-7   Scattered light distribution from ground glass.

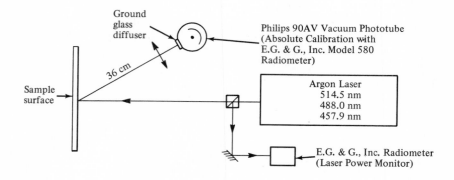

Figure 10-8   Experimental arrangement to measure reflected light distribution from various surfaces.

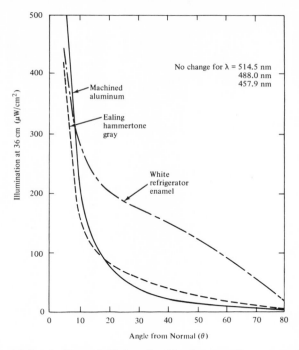

Figure 10-9   Reflected light distribution, various samples.   Light normally incident, 1 W.

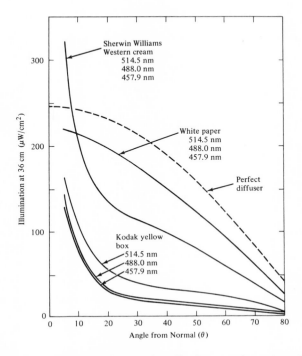

Figure 10-10   Reflected light distribution, various samples.   Light normally incident, 1 W.

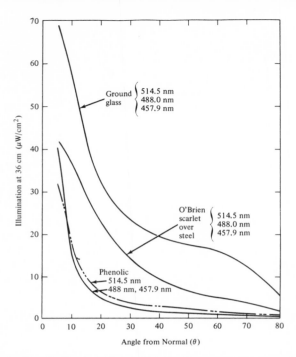

Figure 10-11 Reflected light distribution, various samples. Light normally incident, 1 W.

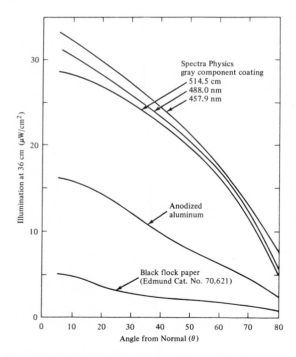

Figure 10-12 Reflected light distribution, various samples. Light normally incident, 1 W.

The results in Figures 10-9, 10-10, 10-11, and 10-12 show that sufficient power is reflected by several normally used surfaces to present an ocular hazard at near distances.   Hence installing a laser must not only involve consideration of specular surfaces, but also examination of diffuse or semispecular surfaces to determine potential problems.

10·2·4   eye and skin exposure levels

Establishing safe eye and skin exposure levels for the wide spectral range covered by lasers has proven to be a difficult task.   Research has probed a variety of hazard areas, some in depth and some superficially, and has produced a wealth of data.   Results indicate apparent exposure levels that should be safe for specific lasers.   Although uncertainty about these results exist due to the multitude of variables (e.g., subject, retinal pigmentation, researchers, etc.), enough correlation of the data has occurred to set conservative exposure levels.

In considering damage to human tissue by laser radiation, two important factors have to be realized.   The first is that tissues vary in their tolerance to thermal and nonthermal phenomena and, secondly, the eye is an optical system.   The optical properties of the eye magnify the sensitivity of the retina to damage.   For example, assume that the retina can tolerate X W/cm^2, the cornea $2X$ W/cm^2, and the skin $3X$ W/cm^2.   Now assume that a laser beam with intensity X W/cm^2 is incident on the cornea. Clearly neither the skin nor the cornea will be damaged.   However, focusing by the eye will reduce the irradiated area by a factor of about 10,000, giving a retinal intensity of $10,000X$ W/cm^2.

Most of the research into retinal damage has been to determine the thresholds for damage.   Definitions of threshold damage vary, but the most commonly accepted definition for threshold retinal damage is: *the energy density required to produce, within some given time after exposure, a clinically visible retinal lesion.*

Some data show that damage to the retina may occur for subthreshold values.[11]   However, for even extreme damage to the retina, there is good reason to believe that the retina can and does repair itself.[12]   For minimal corneal lesions due to CO_2 radiation there are strong biological regenerative powers that repair much or all of the damage.[5]   Thus, we are faced with several almost contradictory results that make establishing exposure levels quite difficult.

10·2·5   possible and probable new hazards

As the public use of lasers increases, more and more people will become involved with laser radiation.   An example of a possible future use is the "laser cane"[13] for the blind, which contains three small laser radars to

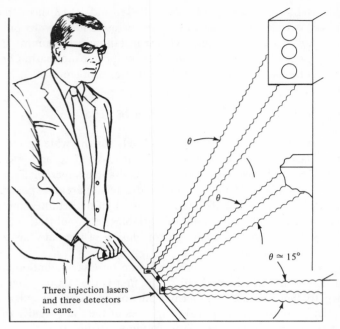

θ

θ

$\theta \simeq 15°$

Three injection lasers
and three detectors
in cane.

Figure 10-13   Laser cane.

warn a blind person of obstacles. As can be seen (Figure 10-13), the laser radiation spreads out over a relatively wide solid angle and thus people passing near the user will probably be exposed to some of the highly diverging laser radiation.

Another area of hazard investigation is concerned with chronic effects of laser radiation. The effects of exposure to subthreshold radiation over extended periods are under study and the results are of great interest for many users. As high repetition rate Q-switched and pulsed lasers are introduced into manufacturing and to the general public, and as CW lasers become widely used in construction and in the home, these questions become quite important.

Another hazard is the effect of ultraviolet radiation. This has been studied for many years utilizing sources other than lasers. Ultraviolet wavelengths induce photochemical reactions and can cause mutations in biological cells (DNA absorbs ultraviolet below 290 nm). Many other proteins and molecules can be altered by this short wavelength radiation. It is currently recommended that ultraviolet exposure be limited as specified by the American Medical Association's 1948 Council of Physical Medicine. This council concluded that for radiation at 253.7 nm, exposure for 7 h or less should be 0.5 μW/cm^2 and for 24 h per day should be 0.1 μW/cm^2 or less.

When lasers are introduced into consumer products, the possibility of accidents occurring will increase if proper precautions are not observed. Consumer products wear out, are broken, or are altered by the user. Consumers often are unaware or may not sufficiently care about dangers. Thus, the engineer must make his products tamperproof in order to fulfill his obligations to society in a responsible manner.

10·2·6   associated hazards—equipment and materials

A complete analysis of each laser installation is necessary to determine all the hazards possible. The following list, although not complete, contains most of the possible hazards associated with using a laser.

a. Voltage sources and leads
b. X-radiation from high-voltage sources
c. Ozone generation from high-voltage sources and ultraviolet radiation
d. Ungrounded electrical equipment, including laser heads and work stations
e. Toxic materials
f. Combustible materials
g. Chemically active materials
h. Cryogenic fluids
i. Inert purging gases
j. Flash-lamp explosion
k. Radiation other than the laser beam may also be hazardous
l. Violent interactions can occur during the interaction of laser radiation and materials. Explosions, fires, chemical reactions, brilliant plumes, and toxic material emission may occur
m. Mechanical items may break. High-speed mechanical scanners, Q-switches, choppers, and so forth, can fatigue and break
n. Interlocks may fail
o. Accidental discharging of the laser can occur
p. Ultraviolet and infrared beams cannot be seen
q. Fallible human beings operate lasers

10·3   safety programs

In general, safety programs are designed to prevent accidents from known hazards. Although the details of any safety program vary according to the hazards, the overall forms depend on two basic precepts: first, that individual control (e.g., engineering control) is proper and sufficient to control the hazards; and second, that a strict operating procedure provides the necessary control of the hazards.   In developing laser safety programs for industry, commerce, and government, one will find that both precepts will be used.   For the industrial applications toward which this book is aimed, one will also find that both approaches are proper and necessary. The application of either approach will be greatly influenced by several factors, the main one being the standard safety policies of individual organizations.   Generally, however, individual control within some overall procedural framework prevails in research and development, whereas rigid, formal operating procedures are used in other areas.

Regardless of the philosophy and the pertinent details used to formulate a safety program, the key to successful implementation is the training of the personnel involved.   It is essential that all the people involved with using a laser in industry be well informed concerning laser hazards and the subsequent control measures required.   The specific details covered in this training process will depend on the personnel (e.g., the laser system operator, the engineer, the supervisor, and the manager).   The goal of each particular training program should be a minimum knowledge sufficient to permit an appropriate, realistic understanding of the tool with which the individual is working.   Clearly a machine operator has no need to understand laser physics, but he should understand that a laser can cause eye injury and that laser beams can traverse great distances and still be harmful.

10·3·1   hazard evaluation and measurement

Laser hazard evaluation can be separated into two broad categories—those hazards related to the laser beam itself and those associated hazards of an electrical or chemical nature.   In general, the associated hazards are well covered in national codes, such as the National Electrical Code.   The hazards specific to laser radiation have been described in Section 10.2.

Evaluation and measurement of laser radiation hazards can follow a number of procedures.   The laser can be considered separately, as an integral part of a system, or as to how it is operated.   Of the several possibilities the most useful and practical procedure is to evaluate the complete system of which the laser is an integral part.   Thus, pulsed laser welders are evaluated rather than pulsed lasers.   High-power CW lasers in a laboratory setup are evaluated rather than just high-power CW lasers. The hazards associated with a particular laser emitting its radiation into the open are well known.   But these hazards will be controlled in some way by the installation of the laser into a total system whether it be a factory or a laboratory, and it is the evaluation and control of the total system that is important.

There are several instruments available to measure the energy and/or power associated with the main beam (see Chapter 9).   No instrument has yet been specifically developed to help implement measurement of radiation levels that will be set under state and federal laws. It is possible to use presently available instruments to determine intensities, etc. Some equations and calculations useful in determining intensities are given in Appendix 10-A.

10·3·2 manufacturing

For the purposes of this section, we can define a manufacturing use of a laser as one where the laser is part of a piece of equipment producing some product. Some typical application areas are discussed and problem areas are pointed out. (Note that Chapters 4 through 8 cover applications in great detail.)

a. High-Power Pulsed Lasers In general, the large ruby and Nd:glass and pulsed CO_2 lasers form this group. The most common applications are welding, drilling, cutting, or scribing. Some typical values for the pulsed output are a few joules in a few milliseconds for welding, a few joules in a few hundred microseconds for drilling and cutting, and less than a joule in 200 ns for scribing. In all cases, the peak powers obtained exceed several hundred watts and, in some instances, megawatt powers may be involved. An interesting comparison to keep in mind when using energy as a parameter is that a joule is given by

$$1 \text{ J} = 1 \text{ kg} \times 1\left(\frac{m}{s}\right)^2$$

Hence, 20 J is 20 kg $-$ (m/s)^2 or roughly equivalent to a 2 lb brick moving at 10 mph.

In most cases the interaction of a high-power pulse with materials generates a brilliant plume, often sufficiently bright to present an occular hazard itself. The material ejected in the plume may contain toxic or harmful constituents. Reflected radiation from the workpiece may present a specular or diffuse hazard (see Section 10.2.3). Secondary effects such as harmonic generation, shock waves, and chemical reactivity of the work material could produce a hazard. The engineer should examine the complete system to determine what may or may not occur. Normally, a high-power laser system should be fully contained within a light-tight enclosure.

b. High-Power CW Lasers To individuals concerned with applying the laser, "high power" is a relative term describing the power output of a given laser. A "high-power" HeNe supplies approximately

0.1 W, whereas a "high-power" CO_2 might have a 1000 W output. Thus the term as presently used is nonspecific and clearly related to the type of laser. A useful definition for "high power" that is becoming widely accepted is that a "high power" laser is any laser that can produce a diffuse hazard. For analyzing hazard potential, it is also useful to distinguish between high and low power on an application basis.

Three high-power CW lasers are in use: CO_2 with powers to 1000 W, Nd:YAG with up to 250 W, and noble gas-ion lasers at a maximum of 35 W. Under development are multi-kilowatt CO_2 and Nd:YAG lasers operating at 10.6×10^3 nm and 1.06×10^3 nm, respectively, and a 100 W argon-ion laser operating in the ultraviolet and visible. The 10.6×10^3 nm radiation is not transmitted by the eye. The radiation heats the skin and the cornea. It is interesting to note that 0.1 W/cm^2 at 10.6×10^3 nm incident on the skin does not produce a sensation of heat, whereas 0.5 W/cm^2 can be quite painful. The normal total irradiance at the earth's surface from the sun is approximately 0.1 W/cm^2.

Neither 10.6×10^3 nm nor 1.06×10^3 nm radiation can be seen, although the latter is transmitted through the eye to the retina. As invisible beams, they are quite susceptible to being accidentally intercepted if they are in the open. Several watts in a fairly narrow beam, 5–20 mm in diameter, will quickly burn the skin. The probability of damaging the eye is very high.

As with any high-power laser, the manufacturing use of a high-power CW laser should be in a light-tight, well-ventilated enclosure. There should be no access to the interior of the enclosure during operation.

A comment on precautions that may be necessary: kilowatt lasers will melt firebrick, steel, and most other material. The main beam must be closely confined and controlled so that specular and/or diffuse reflections will not damage the enclosure or associated equipment.

c. High Repetition Rate Pulsed
For pulse trains with repetition rates above 10 Hz, the eye does not have time to relax thermally. Thus, not only do the hazards of peak powers occur, but also average power hazards similar to CW damage may occur. Because high repetition rate lasers are used in the majority of manufacturing applications, they are of special concern.

Scribing of semiconductors and ceramics with repetitively pulsed or Q-switched Nd:YAG and CO_2 lasers involves a large number of laser systems in production situations. The high-speed drilling of materials, particularly ceramics and other refractory materials, is also coming into production usage. Large ruby and Nd:glass lasers pulsed at 1–20 Hz and CO_2 lasers pulsed at much higher rates, 100 Hz to 1000 Hz, are being used in some applications.

The precautions to be taken, again, are the enclosure of the laser and associated equipment in a light-tight, properly ventilated enclosure.

d. Low-Power Pulsed and CW Lasers   One of the uses of the laser that will bring it into contact with the general public and large numbers of workers is its great utility as a measuring device.   Long-range interferometers, long- or short-range alignment, spatial filtering, surface inspection, scanning television systems, and surveillance are a few of the multitude of applications for low-power systems.   It is these lasers which may involve chronic exposure to subthreshold radiation.   In most cases it is impractical and unnecessary to enclose fully the laser and associated equipment.   The procedure to follow is to carefully control and monitor the beam path.   One should also make sure that transient and nonoperating personnel are kept out of the controlled area and that the operator understands and controls the tool he is using.

Common sense plays a critical role in laser safety.   The individual given control of a laser must understand his responsibility for the laser's safe use.

Designing an Installation   The variety of possible laser applications leads to a variety of laser installations.   Specific rules and regulations about "laser installations" are not widely applicable.   A general check list of important items to note when designing a laser installation follows:

A. Application (e.g., welding, drilling, alignment)
B. Laser type (e.g., pulsed, CW, HeNe, ruby)
C. Installation location (e.g., factory, laboratory)
D. Electric requirements
E. Ventilation requirements (e.g., toxic fumes)
F. Water requirements
G. Operator requirements (e.g., qualifications and training)
H. Enclosure type and necessary controls

    1. Fully enclosed
       a. Shielding material
       b. Interlocks
       c. Barriers to laser radiation

    2. Not fully enclosed
       a. Type of area controls
         i. Barriers to passage of visitors, etc.
         ii. Operator controls (gates, doors, etc.)
         iii. Other controls (e.g., gates, doors)
       b. Interlocks for laser controls

I. Person responsible for control
J. Cryogenic liquids
K. Ionizing radiation, plasmas
L. Explosive materials
M. Other high-intensity light sources

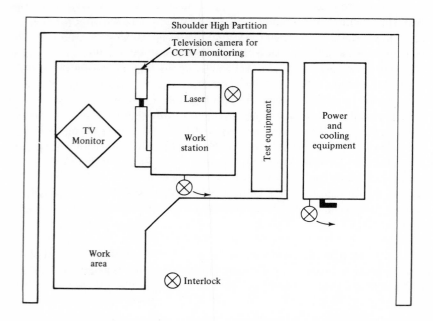

Figure 10-14   High-power laser installed in a large production area.

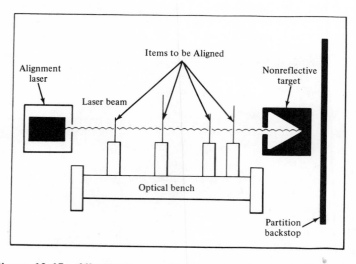

Figure 10-15   Alignment use of a laser in a factory.   This is a controlled area; i.e., all reflections are eliminated and the access is controlled.

In order to give potential laser-system users a grasp of what is involved, two hypothetical installations will be described.   One will consist of a high-power pulsed ruby laser to be used in a processing room.   The second will utilize an alignment (HeNe) laser in an assembly room.

In Figure 10-14 an overall schematic of the high-power pulsed system is given.   Specific safety features are noted.   Figure 10-15 shows the alignment situation in which the safety features are apparent.

The first industrial use of the laser occurred at Western Electric's Buffalo Plant in 1965, where diamond wire drawing dies are drilled with a high-power pulsed ruby laser (Figure 10-16).   No industrial experience was available to draw upon in designing the installation, and thus every possible hazard, both known and potential, was considered.   The result was a fully enclosed laser (with CCTV monitoring of the workpiece) placed in a room (with only the laser and its operator) monitored with another CCTV.

Another industrial laser application involved the adjustment of precision carbon deposited resistors at Western Electric's Merrimack Valley Works.   Again, a fully light-tight enclosure surrounded the pulsed ruby laser and the work stage.   CCTV allowed remote control of the workpiece (Figure 10-17).   However, there is no monitoring of the room, as in the first example.

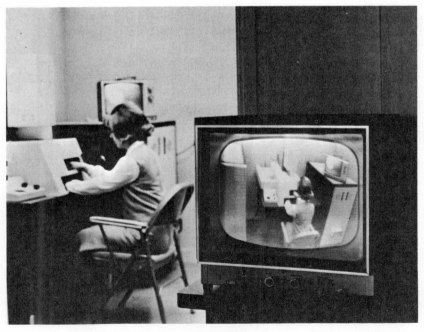

Figure 10-16   Diamond drilling installation at Western Electric's Buffalo Plant.

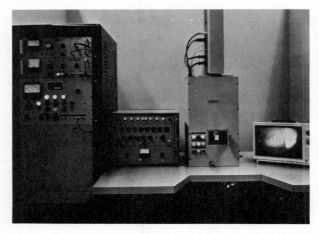

Figure 10-17   Carbon deposited resistor adjustment laser installation.

A later industrial application involves a pulsed ruby laser welder at Western Electric's Oklahoma City Works. The laser welder is situated in a large production room with shoulder high partitions on three sides to limit access to the operator's area (Figure 10-18). Note that all three of these systems have maintained the complete safety of the operator and other people while allowing progressively greater flexibility in location of the laser and use of the laser's potential as a manufacturing tool.

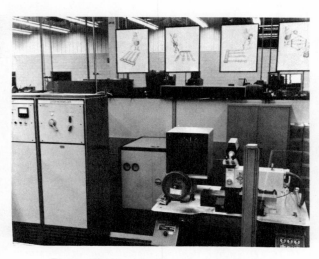

Figure 10-18   Laser welder installation.

10·3·3   research and development

Lasers in laboratories are used in hundreds of different ways with each researcher having a particular need.   To prescribe a rigid safety procedure is unnecessary and restrictive.   For instance, in a laboratory it is often impossible to enclose fully a high-power laser.   Operating a laser often involves hand adjustment of the laser cavity; also high-speed photographs of laser pulses usually must be taken with no enclosure.   These situations can be performed safely with proper laboratory design and proper training of individuals in the use of safety equipment.   Protective eye wear and clothing, warning lights, door interlocks, explosion shields, and radiation shielding are some of the safety items that can be used in a laboratory.

Laboratory Design   A laser laboratory should be designed to minimize hazards to workers in that laboratory and eliminate hazards to any transient personnel.   A researcher or technician knows what to watch for, but a visitor does not.   The following list contains a number of requirements that should be met.

a. Control the laser beam path
b. Eliminate or reduce reflective surfaces
c. Determine radiation coverage area
d. Use interlocks wherever possible
e. Keep transient personnel out of radiation area
f. Keep sufficient protective equipment available, e.g., eye wear for all personnel and visitors
g. Maintain safety equipment and ensure quality over extended periods
h. Use common sense

Schematic illustrations of laboratory layouts are shown in Figure 10-19.

10·3·4   protective equipment

Protective equipment can mean anything from eye wear to a micro-switch interlock.   For this section we will limit the meaning to personal items.

Hazard Evaluation   In most manufacturing applications, there will be no radiation or associated hazards, since the lasers will be fully enclosed. In the rare case when this is not so, special precautions are required.   The user must determine if any eye hazard will exist.   He must examine the possibilities for specular or diffuse reflections, light leaks, plume generation, secondary radiation sources such as flash lamps or glow discharges, and then he must determine whether these will be harmful.

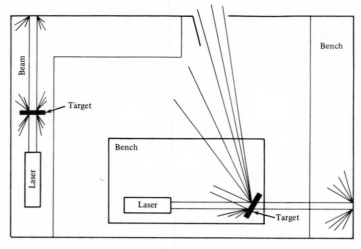

(a) Unsafe Design

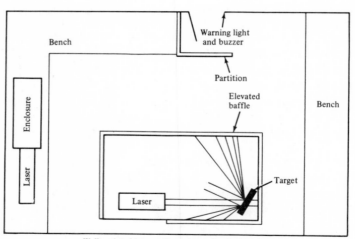

Walls painted in complementary color for laser light

(b) Better Design

Figure 10-19   Laboratory design.

TABLE 10-2   Requirements for Laser Safety Eye Wear

---

1. Clear and permanent identification of the optical density, wavelength band for the given optical density, and the lasers in this band should be placed conspicuously on the front and sides of the eye wear. If the characteristics of the front and sides differ, the difference should be clearly marked.
2. Visibility and fresh air circulation should be as great as possible.
3. Information should be supplied on how the laser radiation is attenuated, whether by reflection, absorption, or scattering.
4. Data on lifetime and aging characteristics of the eye wear should be given.
5. Effects such as bleaching, cracking, thermal effects, chemical reactivity, etc., should be given.
6. Saturation characteristics of the optical density, if any, should be given.

Eye Wear   A variety of safety glasses and goggles are available that are designed to reduce laser radiation levels to extremely low intensities. Since a number of problems and faults in design and construction have been found in the past, a list of requirements (Table 10-2) has been developed that should ensure the integrity and safety of laser safety eye wear. These requirements are meant to fulfill two needs: (1) to eliminate the possibility of someone accidentally using the wrong eye wear; and (2) to reveal any adverse characteristics or qualities in the eye wear material and design.

One of the most important items in Table 10-2 is the specification on appropriate marking and identification. The optical density and the lasers covered by the goggles (e.g. ruby, HeNe, Nd:YAG, Nd:glass, or GaAs) should be permanently and obviously written on the lenses and the holder. A chart similar to Table 10-3, which lists attenuation in the commonly used forms, should be included with each pair of goggles for

TABLE 10-3   Attenuation

Optical Density (O.D.)	Decibel (db) Attenuation	Attenuation Factor
1	10	10
2	20	10^2
3	30	10^3
4	40	10^4
5	50	10^5
6	60	10^6
7	70	10^7
8	80	10^8

TABLE 10-4 Laser Eye Protection Goggles[a] (Based on Manufacturers' Information)

Optical density = $\log_{10}$ (1/transmittance)

Manufacturer or Supplier	Catalogue Number	Argon 488 nm	HeNe 632.8 nm	Ruby 694.3 nm	GaAs 840 nm	Nd 1060 nm	CO₂ 10600 nm	UV <400 nm >300 nm	Coated Filter	Approx. Cost $	No. of Glass Filters and Thickness of Each	Visible Light Transmission %	Useful Range nm
American Optical Co.	SCS-437[b]	0.15	0.20	0.36	1	5	High	No	No	55	1, 3.5 mm	90	1060
	SCS-440												1060
	580, 586[b]	0.2	2	3.5	4	2.7	—	>0.2	No	35, 25[b]	1, 3.5 mm	27.5	—
	581, 587[b]	0.6	4.1	6.1	5.5	.3	—	>1.6	No	35, 25[b]	1, 3.5 mm	9.6	632.8
	584	0	1	5	13	11	High	>0.6	No	55	2, 2 mm	46	1060
	585	0.3	2	8	21	17	High	>0.6	No	55	2, 2 mm	35	694.3-1060
	598[b]	13	0	0	0	—	—	>14	No	25[b]	1, 3 mm	23.7	455-515
	599	11	0	0	0	—	—	>14	No	35	1, 2.5 mm	24.7	455-515
	680	0	1	0	0	0	50	No	No	35	1, 2.7 mm	92	1060
	698	13	1	4	11	8.5	High	>14	No	55	2, 2 & 3 mm	5	1060 and 530
Bausch & Lomb	5W3754	15	0.2	0	0	0	≦35	20	Yes	39	1, 7.9 mm	4.3	330-530
	5W3755	4	0	0	0	0.1	≦35	10	Yes	39	1, 7.9 mm	57	400-460
	5W3756	0.8	12	15	5.6	4.8	≦35	3	Yes	39	1, 6.4 mm	6.2	600-800
	5W3757	0.9	4.5	7.7	12	5.7	≦35	2	Yes	39	1, 7.1 mm	4.7	700-1000
	5W3758	1.9	1.8	2.2	4.8	7.5	≧35	2	Yes	39	1, 7.6 mm	3	1000-1150
Control Data Corp.	TRG-112-1	—	5	12	30	30	—	No	No	50	1, 6 mm	22	694.3
	TRG-112-2	10	0	0	0	0	—	No	No	50	1, 6 mm	31	488
	TRG-112-3	5	2	6	15	15	—	No	No	50	2, 3 mm	5	694.3-488
	TRG-112-4	—	—	—	—	—	High	No	No	50	1, 5 mm	92	10600
Fish-Schurman Corp.	FS650AL/18	0.34	3.8	10	>10	>10	—	No	No	30	1, 6 mm	30	694.3, 840, 10600
Glendale Optical Co.	NDGA[c]	1	0.5	2	16	16	High	>20	No	25	Plastic	60	840, 1060
	R[c]	0.4	2.2	6.3	0.4	0.0	High	5	No	25	Plastic	19	694.3
	NH[c]	0.4	5	2.5	0.6	0.5	High	>10	No	25	Plastic	19	632.8
	A[c]	15	0	0	0	0	High	>12	No	25	Plastic	59	488, 514.3
	NN[c]	0	0	0	0	0	High	>12	No	25	Plastic	70	332, 337
Spectrolab	—	8	5	9	13	12	0	8	Yes	115	2, 3.2 mm	<15	Broadband

[a] With permission of W. J. Schreibeis, Bell Telephone Laboratories, Murray Hill, N.J.   [b] Spectacle type.   [c] Available in goggles or spectacle type.

CAUTION

1. Goggles are not to be used for viewing of laser beam. The eye protective device must be designed for the specific laser in use.
2. Few reliable data are available on the energy densities required to cause physical failure of the eye protective devices.
3. The establishment of engineering controls and appropriate operating procedures should take precedence over the use of eye protective devices.
4. The hazard associated with each laser depends upon many factors, such as output power, beam divergence, wavelength, pupil diameter, specular or diffuse reflection from surfaces, etc.

use as a convenient, quantitative check list.   The factors in Table 10-3 can be easily related thus:

$$O.D.(\lambda) = \log_{10} A_\lambda$$

$$\log_{10} A_\lambda = \log_{10} \frac{1}{T_\lambda}$$

$$A_{db}(\lambda) = 10 \log_{10} A_\lambda$$

$$10 \log_{10} A_\lambda = 10 \log_{10} \frac{1}{T\lambda}$$

where $O.D.(\lambda)$ = optical density (bels) at λ,
  A_λ = attenuation at λ,
  T_λ = transmission at λ,
  $A_{db}(\lambda)$ = decibel attenuation at λ.

In many instances it is important that a safe level of laser radiation be transmitted by the eye wear.   Proper alignment of measuring and aligning tools and holographic setups usually can be performed only if the laser radiation can be seen.   Thus a variety of eye wear should be made with optical densities that cover a range.   Most safety eye wear comes with an optical density of 10 or more and completely blocks the laser radiation. Representative laser eye wear available from various manufacturers is presented in tabular form in Table 10-4.

As important as having safe eye wear is its proper use.   Before an individual uses or gives someone else safety eye wear to use, he should check that the appropriate wavelength(s) are blocked sufficiently, that the proper optical density is being used, and that the eye wear is in good condition.   He should know where the laser radiation will go and what other precautions may be necessary.

10·4   *medical surveillance**

The procedures and recommendations contained in this section are essentially those proposed by the American National Standards Institute's Standards Committee on Laser Safety.   This committee consisted of the leading experts in all areas of laser safety, and the recommendations stem from the combined efforts of the individuals best known in each field.

---

* This section and Appendix 10-B closely follow the treatment rendered by H. Christian Zweng, M.D., of the Stanford University Medical Center.   The material, used with Dr. Zweng's permission, was presented at the "Laser Safety Conference and Workshops" at the College of Medicine, Univ. of Cincinnati, January 31 1968.

Medical surveillance of personnel working with lasers has a twofold purpose. The first is the protection of the individual from any deleterious effects of laser radiation, and the second is the protection of the employer afforded by appropriate documentation on the individual's health. Since only two organs, the eye and the skin, have been found to be affected by laser radiation, a medical program for laser safety need only include, at this time, ophthalmological and dermatological examinations. Only qualified medical personnel—those aware of laser injuries—should carry out these programs.

The following sections clarify who should be kept under medical surveillance for laser hazards, what procedures should be used, and how often examinations should be performed—by classifying according to the risks involved.

A. Those who run a high risk of exposure to laser energy sufficient to do eye and/or skin damage (e.g., workers in research and development laboratories).
B. Those who are routinely in laser environments but who are ordinarily fully protected by safety features built into machines and procedures (e.g., industrial laser workers, military crews operating laser equipment, etc.).
C. Minimal risk personnel. Those whose work makes it possible, but unlikely, that they are exposed to laser energy sufficient to damage their eyes and/or skin (e.g., management, secretarial, and maintenance personnel in industrial plants where lasers are being used, large bodies of military personnel who are in areas where lasers are to be used, as on maneuvers, etc.).

Medical eye examination procedures can now be specified for each category. The protocol for group A is given in Appendix 10-B. For group B, items 1, 2, and 8 (with mydriatic instead of cycloplegic) of Appendix 10-B will be used. Also, if the best corrected visual acuity in either eye is less than 20/20, or if any pathology is seen, the potential worker is advised to have a complete eye examination. If any eye pathology (not based on refractive error) is found, Protocol A is to be employed. With group C, only item 2 in Appendix 10-B need be included.

The time between eye examinations can also be determined according to the risk classification.

Group A
1. On entry into a laser environment.
2. On discharge from laser environment.
3. Immediately after suspected laser eye exposure.
4. When any visual functional complaint is noted.
5. At *one*-year intervals during time in a *laser* environment (no photograph to be taken).

Group B
1. On entry into a laser environment.
2. On discharge from a laser environment.
3. Immediately after suspected laser eye exposure.
4. When any visual functional complaint is noted.
5. At *five*-year intervals during time in a laser environment (no photograph to be taken).

Group C
None

Medical surveillance for skin damage should be determined according to the risks involved.   Known thresholds for skin damage are several orders of magnitude above those for eye damage.   Thus the health officer in charge should determine if such an examination is required.   The recommended protocol is given in Appendix 10-C*.

10·5   government regulations

10·5·1   federal

On October 18, 1968, the United States Congress passed the Radiation Control for Health and Safety Act of 1968, public law 90-602.   This legislation stipulates that the Secretary of Health, Education and Welfare "shall . . . develop and administer performance standards for electronic products. . . ." as well as fulfill several other requirements.   He is "authorized to (1) (A) collect and make available . . . the results of . . . research and studies relating to the nature and extent of the hazards and control of electronic product radiation; and (B) make such recommendations relating to such hazards and control as he considers appropriate. . . ."

Since the passage of this law, the Secretary of HEW has delegated the Bureau of Radiological Health of the Environmental Control Administration of the Public Health Service as the responsible agency for enforcing the law and for prescribing appropriate regulations.   The B.R.H. is investigating the laser areas as well as the other electronic product areas seeking to determine what the hazards are and what safety procedures and regulations are necessary.   At this time, all interested parties are reviewing the same topics for the purpose of generating information and promulgating recommendations for the government.   Among these groups are the American National Standards Institute, whose Z-136 Committee is developing broad-based recommendations for the safe use of lasers, and the

---

* The material in Appendix 10-C is used with the permission of Leon Goldman, M.D., of the Children's Hospital Research Foundation, Cincinnati, Ohio.

Electronics Industries Association, whose laser subdivision has collaborated with the Bureau of Radiological Health in establishing reporting procedures for laser products.

Meanwhile, since June 27, 1970, the Federal Government has required every laser manufacturer to maintain records, make reports on the first purchases of lasers which exceed specific power/energy levels, and report incidents in which radiation injuries occur or are alleged to have occurred.

10·5·2 state

Several states (e.g., New York, Illinois, Pennsylvania, Massachusetts) have passed or are considering legislation requiring the registration of some or all lasers within the state. In addition, some states may also have other regulations concerning lasers and their use. Thus, any laser users should consult with state officials to determine whether germane state regulations exist.

References

1. S. Fine *et al.*, "Interaction of Laser Radiation with Biological Systems, I. Studies on Interaction with Tissues," *Fed. Proc.* **24** (1), Suppl. 14: S-35 (1965).
2. L. Goldman, "Comparison of the Biomedical Effects of the Exposure of Human Tissue to Low and High Energy Lasers," *Ann. N.Y. Acad. Sci.* **122**, 802 (1965).
3. W. T. Ham, Jr. *et al.*, "Effects of Laser Radiation on the Mammalian Eye," *Trans. N.Y. Acad. Sci.* **28** (4), 517 (1966).
4. A. Vassiliadis *et al.*, "Investigations of Laser Damage to Ocular Tissue," *Air Force Avionics Lab. TR-67-170* (1967).
5. A. Vassiliadis *et al.*, "Investigations of Laser Damage to Ocular Tissues," *Final Report Contract F33615-67-C-1752*, U.S. Air Force, School of Aerospace Medicine, Aerospace Medical Division (AFSC), Brooks Air Force Base, Texas.
6. D. G. Cogan and V. E. Kinsey, "Action Spectrum of Keratitis Produced by Ultraviolet Radiation," *Arch. Ophthalmol.* **77**, 670 (1967).
7. R. B. Yules *et al.*, "The Effect of Q-Switched Ruby Laser Radiation on Dermal Tattoo Pigment in Man," *Arch. Surg.* **95** (August 1967).
8. L. Goldman *et al.*, "The Biomedical Aspects of Lasers," *J. Am. Med. Assoc.* **188**, 302 (1964).
9. T. Walsh, *Photometry*, 2nd Ed., Constable & Co., London (1953).
10. M. Born and E. Wolf, *Principles of Optics*, Rev. Ed. 4th Ed., Pergamon Press, Inc., New York (1970).
11. W. J. Geeraets, J. Burkhart, and D. Guerry, IV, "Enzyme Activity in the Coagulated Retina: A Means of Studying Thermal Conduction as a Function of Exposure Time," *Acta Ophthalmol.*, Suppl. **76**, 79 (1963).

12. H. C. Zweng, "Accidental Q-Switched Laser Lesions of Human Macula," *Arch. Ophthalmol.* **78**, 596 (1967).
13. "VA Optimistic about Safety of Laser Cane for the Blind," *Laser Focus* **5**, No. 13, 24 (July 1969).
14. E. A. Boettner and J. R. Wolter, "Transmission of the Ocular Media," MRL-TDR-62-34 (May 1962).
15. E. L. Thomas, "Movements of the Eye," *Sci. American* **219**, No. 2, 90 (August 1968).

Appendix 10·a   sample calculations

(U.S. Army & Navy Publication TB MED 279 NAVMED P-5052-35, 24 FEBRUARY, 1969)

A. Symbols

Q = level of radiation leaving the laser (CW output measured in watts; pulsed output measured in joules).

r = range from the laser to the target (cm).

r_1 = range from the laser target to the viewer (cm).

E, H = radiant exposure (H) or irradiance (E) at range, r, measured in J/cm^2 for pulsed lasers and W/cm^2 for CW lasers.

E_0, H_0 = emergent beam radiant exposure (H_0) or irradiance (E) at zero range (units as for E, H).

a = diameter of emergent laser beam (cm).

ϕ = emergent beam divergence measured in radians.

e = base of natural logarithms.

μ = atmospheric attentuation coefficient (cm^{-1}) at a particular wavelength.

f = effective focal length of eye (1.7 cm).

θ_{min} = minimum angle subtended by the minimal retinal spot size (radians).

d_e = diameter of the pupil of the eye (varies from approximately 0.2 to 0.8 cm).

D_e = diameter of the exit pupil of an optical system (cm).

D_L = diameter of laser beam at range r (cm).

D_0 = diameter of objective of an optical system (cm).

d_{min} = diameter of minimal spot on retina (cm).

R = spectra reflectance of a diffuse object.

P = magnification or power of an optical system.

G = ratio of retinal energy or power density received by optically aided eye to retinal energy or power density received by unaided eyes.

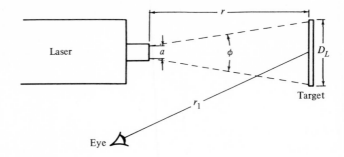

Graphical representation of symbols used.   (With permission of the American Conference of Governmental Industrial Hygienists.)

B.   Formulas and Calculations

1. Beam irradiance (E) or radiant exposure (H) for nondiverging beam at range, r, which is attenuated by the atmosphere is

$$H = H_0 e^{-\mu r}, \qquad E = E_0 e^{-\mu r} \tag{A-1}$$

Note: The attenuation coefficient, μ, varies from 10^{-4}/cm in thick fog to 10^{-7} in air of very good visibility.   The Rayleigh scattering coefficient at 694.3 nm is 4.8×10^{-8} cm^{-1}, and 1.8×10^{-8} cm^{-1} at 500 nm. The effect of aerosols in even the cleanest atmospheres usually raises μ at 694.3 nm to at least 10^{-7} cm^{-1}.

2. Average radiant exposure at range, r (direct circular beam) is the total energy in the beam at that range divided by the area of the beam at that range:

$$H = \frac{Q_e^{-\mu r}}{\pi \left[\dfrac{a + r\phi}{2}\right]^2} = \frac{1.27 Q_e^{-\mu r}}{(a + r\phi)^2} \tag{A-2}$$

Note: Accurate only for small ϕ; i.e., accuracy better than 1 percent for angles below 0.17 rad (10°) and better than 5 percent for angles less than 0.37 rad (21°).

Example: To find the radiant exposure at 1 km (10^5 cm) of a 0.1 J ruby laser which has a beam divergence of 1 mrad (10^{-3} rad) and an emergent beam diameter of 0.7 cm (use $\mu = 10^{-7}$ cm^{-1}).

$$H = \frac{1.27(0.1)e^{-(0.01)}}{(0.7 + (10^5)(10^{-3}))^2} = \frac{(1.27)(0.1)(0.99)}{(0.7 + 100)^2} = 1.25 \times 10^{-5} \text{ J/cm}^2$$

3. Minimum beam diameter at range r:

$$D_L = a + \phi r \qquad \text{for small } \phi \tag{A-3}$$

Example: To find the diameter of a laser beam at 1 km where the emergent beam diameter is 10 cm and the beam divergence is 0.1 mrad:

$$D_L = 10 \text{ cm} + (10^{-4} \text{ rad})(10^5 \text{ cm}) = 10 + 10 = 20 \text{ cm}$$

4. Maximum reflected radiant exposure from diffuse reflector:

$$H = \frac{QR}{\pi r_1^2} \qquad (\text{for } r_1 \gg D_L) \qquad \text{(A-4)}$$

Example: To find the maximum reflected radiant exposure from a diffuse matte of reflectance 0.6 which would return a distance of 10 m to the operator of a 0.1 J laser:

$$H = \frac{(0.1 \text{ J})(0.6)}{(3.14)(10^3 \text{ cm})^2} = 1.91 \times 10^{-8} \text{ J/cm}^2$$

5. Limiting angle for extended object:

$$\theta_{min} = d_{min}/f \qquad \text{(A-5)}$$
$$= 0.6 \text{ mrad} \qquad \text{for } d_{min} = 10 \ \mu\text{m}.$$

6. Ratio G of radiant exposure irradiance at the retina when viewing is aided by an optical system, as opposed to viewing by the naked eye:
   a. Direct viewing and specular reflection (or diffuse spot unresolved by eye and optical system):

$$G = \frac{D_0^2}{d_e^2} \qquad \text{for } d_e \geq D_e \qquad \text{(A-6)}$$

and

$$G = \frac{D_0^2}{D_e^2} = P^2 \qquad \text{for } d_e \leq D_e \qquad \text{(A-7)}$$

   b. Indirect viewing of a diffuse reflection; extended objects only (i.e., object subtends angle greater than 0.6 mrad when magnified):

$$G = \frac{D_0^2}{P^2 d_e^2} \qquad \text{for } d_e \geq D_e \qquad \text{(A-8)}$$

and

$$G = \frac{D_0^2}{P^2 D_e^2} = 1 \qquad \text{for } d_e \leq D_e \qquad \text{(A-9)}$$

Example: The laser operator of preceding example desires to view the diffuse reflection of the laser flash through a pair of 10 × 50 binoculars (i.e., $P = 10$ and $D_0 = 50$ mm). For night viewing find the relative hazard to this man's eyes. Since the exit pupil is $D_0/P = 0.5$ cm, (A-8) estimating d_e to be 0.7 will give

$$G = \frac{(5 \text{ cm})^2}{(10)^2(0.7 \text{ cm})^2} = \frac{25}{(100)(0.49)} = 0.51$$

The hazard is equivalent to a corneal radiant exposure on the naked eye of: $(0.51) (1.91 \times 10^{-8} \text{ J/cm}^2) = 9.7 \times 10^{-9} \text{ J/cm}^2$.

Example: A laser operator views a specularly reflected beam at a point where the beam energy density measures 2×10^{-9} J/cm². If he were to view the beam through a pair of 7×50 binoculars, what would be the relative hazard compared with unaided viewing? The magnification, P, of the binoculars is 7 and, if inserted in (A-7), will provide the simplest solution:

$$G = P^2 = 7^2 = 49$$

Thus, the operator would be viewing a level 49 times greater than by the naked eye, or a corneal radiant exposure of nearly 10^{-7} J/cm².

appendix 10·b   eye examination protocol*

1. **Ocular History:** The patient's past eye history and family eye history are reviewed. Any current complaints which he now has about his eyes are noted. The patient's general health status should be inquired about with emphasis on diseases (hypertension, diabetes) which can give ocular problems.
2. **Visual Acuity:** Tested and recorded in snellen figures for distance with and without lenses down to 20/15. The visual acuity at near is tested at 35 cm and recorded in Jaeger test figures with and without lenses, if any.
3. Determination of patient's lens correction with a lensometer.
4. **External Ocular Examination:** This includes examination of brows, lids, lashes, conjunctiva, sclera, cornea, iris and pupillary size, equality, and regularity.
5. **Amsler Grid:** The Amsler grid sheet is presented to each eye separately and any distortion of the grid is noted by the patient and drawn by him.
6. **Visual Fields:** The peripheral visual field is charted with a 1 mm white target at 33 cm distance and a central visual field involving the fixation area is charted with a 1 mm red target at 1 m.

The pupils are then dilated by the instillation of a cycloplegic drop in each eye. The remainder of the examination is carried out with the eye under this medication.

---

* This appendix follows the treatment rendered by H. Christian Zweng, M.D. The material is used with Dr. Zweng's permission.

7. **Cycloplegic Refraction:** This is to measure the patient's total refractive error and the new visual acuity of the patient must be noted if
   the visual acuity is improved over the patient's old lenticular prescrip-
   tion, or if he has no lenses at the time of the examination. This
   examination shall be carried on in all personnel whose visual acuity in
   either eye is less than 20/15.
8. **Examination of the Ocular Fundus with an Ophthalmoscope:** In the
   recording of this portion of the examination the points to be covered
   are: the presence or absence of opacities in the media, the sharpness
   of the outline of the optic nerve, the color of the optic nerve, the size
   of the physiological cup if present, the ratio of the size of the retinal
   veins to that of the retinal arteries, the presence or absence of a well-
   defined macula and the presence or absence of a foveolar reflex, and
   any other retinal pathology that can be seen with a direct ophthalmoscope. Even small deviations from normal should be described and
   carefully localized.
9. **Examination by Slit Lamp:** The cornea, iris, and lens are examined
   with this biomicroscope and carefully described.
10. **Measurement** of intraocular pressure.
11. **Photograph of the Posterior Pole of the Fundus:** This includes the area
   of the macula and head of the optic nerve and is to be taken in color
   film. Positive color photograph should be mounted in the patient's
   chart. Also, all areas of the retina which show any pathology outside
   the posterior pole should also be photographed.
12. **Examination of the Retina with the Slit Lamp and the Goldman 3-Mirror
   Lens:** This examination allows all of the retina, including the periphery, to be surveyed with binocularity, high magnification, and excellent illumination to give a very definitive examination of the retina.
13. **Special examinations,** such as ERG, fluorescence angiography, etc.,
   shall be done as indicated on recommendation of the examiner.

appendix 10·c medical surveillance for possible skin damage from exposure to lasers*

1. As with any surveillance procedure, special laser medical record
   forms should be used.
2. For the skin section, the basic divisions of this form should be:
   A. History
   B. Examination
   C. Recommendations

---

* Appendix 10-C is used with the permission of Leon Goldman, M.D., of the Children's
Hospital Research Foundation, Cincinnati, Ohio.

3. A. History—data should be requested on:
   1. Atopy
   2. History of exposure to X-ray, nuclear radiation, ultraviolet sources, high-intensity visible or infrared sources, cutting oils, arsenic, penicillin, sulfa
   3. Presence or absence of reactions to drugs and chemicals
   4. Photodermatitis
   5. Intensity of exposure to sun
   6. Skin cancers—type, location, and treatment
   7. History of previous skin disorders
   8. History of extensive or severe thermal burns

   B. Examination:
   1. Skin color as to
      a. Caucasian—light, medium, dark
      b. Negro—light, medium, dark
      c. Oriental—light, medium, dark
      If special instrumentation is available for precise analysis of skin color, these should be used and data recorded.
   2. Presence or absence of these changes as observed under normal light and Wood's light on exposed and unexposed skin—body charts may be used
      a. General skin type—normal (N), seborrheic (S) or ichthyotic (I)
      b. Pigmentation—type, severity, distribution
      c. Depigmentation—type, severity, distribution
      d. Keratoses—actinic, seborrheic—type, distribution, patterns
      e. Skin malignancies—type, size, distribution patterns
      f. Skin disorders—type, distribution patterns
   3. Photographs if indicated—black and white, color, and under Wood's light

   C. Recommendations—with skin protection—include details with area control and personnel control as regards, gloves, clothing, protective creams, templates, etc.:
   1. No laser exposure
   2. Limited laser exposure
   3. Laser exposure with ordinary precautions

   D. Annual examination—complete

   E. Final examination—on leaving laser work—complete

   F. Analysis of effectiveness of the skin surveillance program

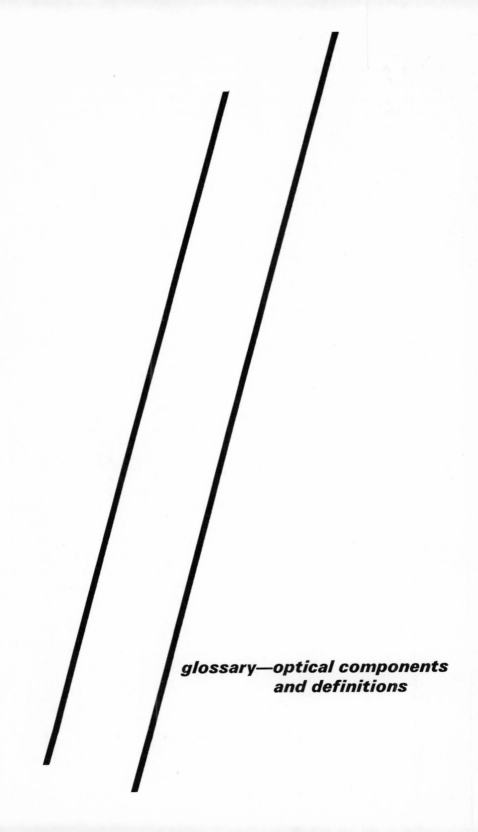

*glossary—optical components
and definitions*

Axicon   A conical lens usually of the configuration shown in the diagram. An axicon followed by a conventional lens can focus a laser beam to a ring whose radius is dependent on the index of refraction and apex angle of the axicon, and on the spherical lens focal length.   The width of the ring depends on the quality and numerical aperture of both elements.

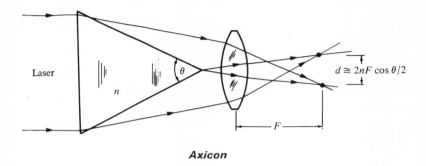

Axicon

Back Focal Length   The distance from the last glass surface of a lens to the focal point.

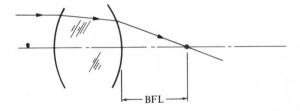

Back focal length

Beam Expander   Any combination of optical elements that will increase the diameter of a laser beam; an inverted telescope, i.e., a short focal-length lens followed by a long focal-length lens and separated by the sum of the focal lengths.   In this case, the expanded beam will be larger by the ratio of the output

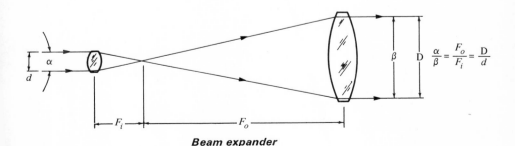

Beam expander

lens focal length to the input lens focal length (F_o/F_i) provided that the f/number of the output lens is equal to or smaller than the input lens f/number. The angular divergence of the output beam will be reduced by the multiplicative factor (F_i/F_o).

Beamsplitter   An element used to amplitude-divide a light beam as shown in the diagram.   The element is coated with a partially reflecting film, such as a thin metal layer or a multilayer dielectric coating depending on the wavelength or efficiency required.   See **pellicle beamsplitter**.

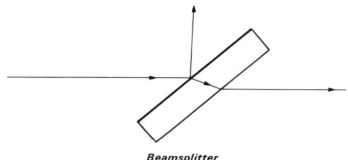

Beamsplitter

Brewster Window   The optical element forming the ends of the active laser medium enclosure.   The windows are set at Brewster's angle to the incident laser beam as shown in the diagram.

   In this case, the parallel component, E_p, of the electric field is not reflected at the window surfaces.   The perpendicular component, E_s, has losses at the window and tends not to propagate.   The output is thus plane polarized with a parallel field component.   Brewster windows are usually made of fused silica.

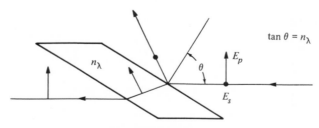

Brewster window

Brightness   A term denoting the visual sensation.   This term is often confused with the photometric term luminance.   Luminance is often called "photometric brightness," which is further confusing.   Under certain conditions, the visual sensation(s) may be related to the luminance by

$$S = \log L + c$$

Catadioptric   An optical system using both reflective and refractive optics. See **Schmidt system** for an example.

Collimator   A line system that reduces the angular divergence of a laser beam.   See **beam expander.**

Corner Cube Reflector   A prism of optical quality glass having three mutually orthogonal faces (corner).   An incoming ray of light is reflected antiparallel to the direction of the incident, i.e., it is *retroreflected.*

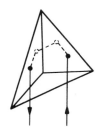   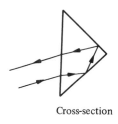

Cross-section

Corner cube reflector

Depth of Field/Focus   The depth of field of an optical system is the longitudinal object space (ΔZ) over which an acceptably clear image can be obtained in the image plane.   By "acceptably clear" is meant a tolerable blur in the image, i.e., an object point is imaged as a blur of diameter, c.   As can be seen from the diagram, the tolerable blur also determines a region in the image space ($\Delta Z'$) over which an acceptable image may be formed.   This region is termed the *depth of focus* and is related to the depth of field by the *longitudinal* magnification of the system,

$$\Delta Z' = \Delta Z M_{\text{long}}$$

If $\Delta Z'$ is small compared to the focal length, then

$$\Delta Z' = \Delta Z M_{\text{lat}}^2$$

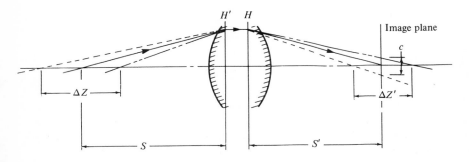

Depth of field/focus

where M_{lat} is the familiar lateral magnification of the system.   The depth of field of a lens is given by

$$\Delta Z = F\left[\frac{SF - fc(S - F)}{F^2 - fc(S - F)} - \frac{SF + fc(S - F)}{F^2 + fc(S - F)}\right]$$

where f is the f/number of the lens at infinity.

For a diffraction limited lens, the depth of focus is

$$\Delta Z' = 4f^2\lambda$$

where λ is the wavelength.

Diffraction Grating   A device useful for analyzing the spectrum of light. It consists of alternately opaque and transparent strips, usually on a glass substrate.   The spacing between opaque strips can be quite small, of the order of 1 μm.   A collimated beam of light incident on a grating will be divided into a number of collimated beams upon transmission according to

$$d(\sin\theta + \sin\theta') = m\lambda \quad \text{(grating equation)} \qquad m = \pm 1, \pm 2, \ldots$$

The intensity of each beam is modulated by the diffraction pattern of a single transparent strip.   See Chapter 8, Ref. 1.

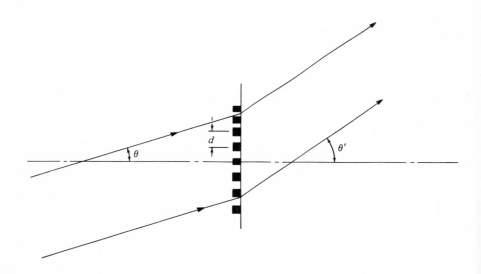

Diffraction grating

Diffraction Limited   An optical system free of aberrations and limited only by diffraction at the aperture is said to be diffraction limited.   A diffraction limited spherical lens with a circular aperture will focus a monochromatic beam of uniform intensity to a "spot" called the Airy disc of diameter

$$d_u = 2.44f\lambda \qquad \text{where } f \text{ is } f/\text{number}$$

A laser beam with a Gaussian distributed intensity cross section will be focused to a spot diameter (to the $1/e^2$ points) of

$$d_g = 1.27 f \lambda$$

A diffraction limited lens imaging spatially incoherent light (diffused laser light) is a low-pass filter of spatial frequencies, i.e., the lens will not image a closely spaced bar pattern (alternate black and white bars) whose frequency in the image plane is greater than

$$\nu_m = \frac{1}{\lambda f}$$

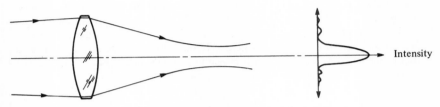

Intensity

Diffraction limited

Etalon   Originally, a hollow glass cylinder used as an accurate spacer between the reflectors of a Fabry-Perot interferometer. Now, commonly used to designate a very flat plane-parallel plate.

Exposure   The product of illumination and time, commonly in units of meter-candle seconds (mcs), useful for determining the exposure time of photographic emulsions to light of certain illuminating levels.

Focal Length   The distance from the secondary nodal point (see Chapter 8, Ref. 1) of a lens to the primary focal point.   In a thin lens, where the thickness is less than one tenth the diameter, the focal length is the distance between the lens and the focal point.

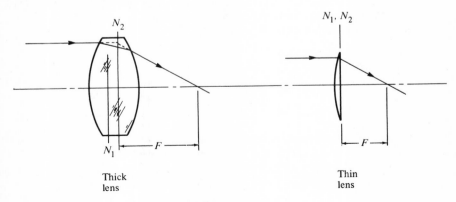

Thick
lens

Thin
lens

Focal length

f/Number The f/number is related to the image cone of an optical system and is defined

$$f = \frac{1}{2 \tan \theta}$$

When the lens is focused at infinity, the *infinity conjugates* f/number is given by

$$f = \frac{F}{d}$$

where F is the lens focal length, and d is the diameter of the aperture at the secondary nodal point.

If the lens is thin, d is the diameter of the clear aperture. Low f numbers designate "fast" lenses that might be used in low light-level photography or in high light-level situations where short exposure times are desired. However, fast lenses have short depths of field. If the lens is diffraction limited, a low depth of focus f/number lens will image fine details, i.e., it has higher resolving power than a high f/number lens (see **diffraction limited**).

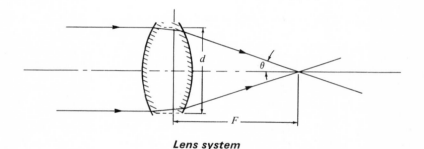

Lens system

Fresnel Lens A lens composed of circular zones, each having a prismatic cross section approximating the curvature of a spherical lens of the same focal length. By this means, the f/number may be made very low and the lens is useful in collecting light. The first use of this technique was probably in glass searchlight lenses for lighthouses, although now they are made of plastic and are commonly found in Vu-Graph projectors.

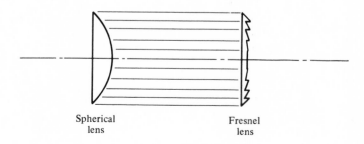

Spherical   Fresnel
lens   lens

Glan-Taylor Prism A polarizing prism made of natural calcite crystal with end faces perpendicular to the incident light. The angular aperture of this prism is very large, i.e., the angle of incidence of a light beam can vary over a large tolerance, but the design is very costly of calcite.

It is useful in transmitting ultraviolet, and the input and output beams can be made very nearly collinear.

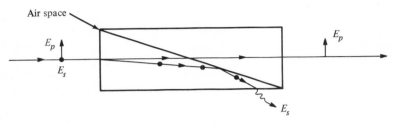

Glan-Taylor prism

Glan-Thompson Prism A Glan-Taylor Prism with cemented components.

Half-Wave Retardation Plate See **retardation plate**.

Interference Filter A thin piece of optical material, with high reflectance faces, that acts as a fixed-separation-Fabry-Perot interferometer (see Section 8.4.1). The reflecting faces may be metallic; however, multilayer dielectric interference films can be used that not only greatly reduce absorption losses but narrow the transmitted waveband to fractions of a nanometer.

Kerr Cell A device usually containing a liquid such as nitrobenzene that will advance or retard the two electric field components of a light beam when a strong electric field is applied. Replaced by the Pockels cell in most applications (see **modulator**).

Littrow Prism A prism that can be used for lossless coupling of energy into some material or, alternatively, can be used with one reflecting face as a wavelength selector in a laser cavity. The prism apex angle is the Snell component of the Brewster angle.

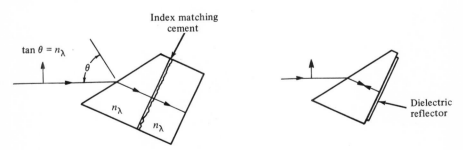

Littrow prism

Luminance   A photometric term designating the *photometric intensity* per unit projected area of a light source.   The light source may be a secondary source such as an illuminated object.

$$\text{Luminance } (L) = \frac{\text{light flux}}{\text{solid angle} \times \text{projected area}} = \frac{\text{intensity}}{\text{area}}$$

The units of luminance are lamberts defined as $1/\pi$ candle/cm², although at present the foot-lambert ($1/\pi$ candle/ft²) is much more widely used in the United States.

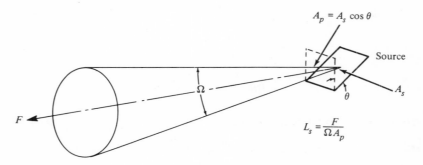

Luminance

MacNeille Prism   A prism beamsplitter in which the parallel component of the field is almost entirely transmitted and the perpendicular component almost entirely reflected.   This device is very useful for isolating a laser beam from unwanted reflections.

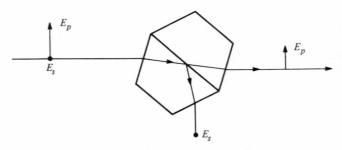

MacNeille prism

Meter-Candle Second   A unit of exposure defined as

$$\text{mcs} = \frac{\text{lumens}}{\text{square meter}} \times \text{second} = \frac{\text{luminous flux}}{\text{unit area}} \times \text{time}$$

The luminous flux falling on a unit area of some surface is usually called the illumination (E) and is more commonly measured in foot-candles (lumens/ft^2).

Modulator   A device consisting of a Pockels cell and auxiliary polarizing devices depending on whether phase or amplitude modulation is desired.   For amplitude modulation of a polarized laser beam, the following arrangement may be used.   The Pockels cell is a piezoelectric crystal which will retard one field component when a voltage is applied.   In the off condition, no light is transmitted due to the orientation of the analyzer.   An applied voltage (V_a) will allow transmission of one component of the field which is aligned to the analyzer and at right angles to the input polarization.   Under this condition, the transmitted intensity is

$$T = \sin^2 \frac{\pi V_a}{2V_0}$$

where V_0 is the voltage necessary for maximum transmission (half-wave voltage). If it is desired to operate the cell in a linear fashion between intensity and applied voltage, the modulator must be biased to the midpoint of the approximately linear region of T either by a voltage $V_b = \frac{1}{2}V_0$ or by insertion of a quarter-wave plate.

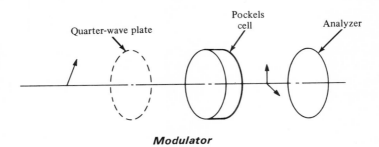

Quarter-wave plate
Pockels cell
Analyzer

Modulator

Pellicle Beamsplitter   A very thin ($\simeq 8$ μm), transparent, stretched plastic membrane that can be coated with multilayer dielectrics to act as a partial reflector.   The thin membrane aids in the elimination of ghost images that may occur with thick glass beamsplitters and also greatly reduces aberrations that can occur in conventional beamsplitters.

Photographic Speed   A number used to compare the average sensitivities of different photographic emulsions.   This number is very useful in estimating the exposure of the emulsion.   There are approximately eight different photographic speed systems in use today.   The most familiar is the ASA.   The diagram shows the criteria for determining the speed of an emulsion for two systems: The ASA and the relative sensitivity (S_A).

The relative sensitivity is used to compare spectrographic emulsions such as Kodak 649F, an emulsion frequently used in holography.

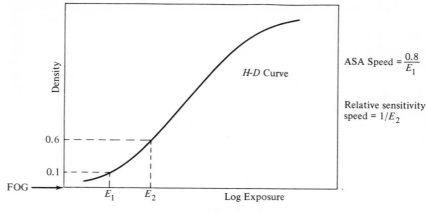

$$\text{ASA Speed} = \frac{0.8}{E_1}$$

Relative sensitivity
speed $= 1/E_2$

Photographic speed

Q-Switch; Acoustic   A solid or liquid material in which acoustic waves
are generated with a pressure transducer.   The waves cause index of refraction
variations so that the material acts as a diffraction grating.   When activated,
the laser beam is diffracted at the Bragg angle.   When not activated, the cell
acts as a plane-parallel plate.

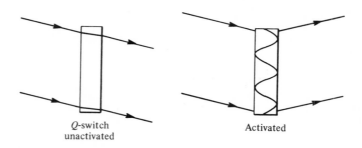

Q-switch; acoustic

Quarter-Wave Plate   See **retardation plate**.

Rayleigh Scatter in a Medium   Diffusion of radiation in the course of
its passage through a medium containing particles with sizes which are small
when compared with the wavelength of the radiation.

Reflectance   The ratio of reflected radiant power to incident radiant power.

Reflecting Objectives   A reflecting system applicable to the ultraviolet or
infrared spectral regions because of difficulty in finding suitable refracting
materials for these regions.

The basic construction is shown in the figure and consists of two nearly concentric mirrors. The central obscuration modifies the diffraction pattern of the image, somewhat reducing the contrast of coarse targets and improving the contrast of fine details. For use in laser processing the opening in C_1 should ideally be equal to the beam waist diameter.

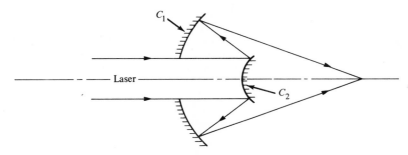

Reflecting objectives

Retardation Plate   A thin piece of optical material, usually mica or quartz, in which the perpendicular component of the electric field is retarded in phase over the parallel component. When the retardation is 180°, the device is called a "half-wave plate"; when 90°, the device is called a "quarter-wave plate."

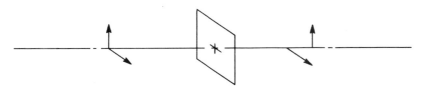

Retardation plate

Second Harmonic Generator   A nonlinear crystal used to double the frequency of the incident wave. For efficient conversion from the fundamental frequency to its second harmonic, both waves will have to propagate through the material with the same speed. Most common crystals used for this purpose are ADP, KDP, $LiNbO_3$, $LiIO_3$, and $Ba_2NaNb_5O_{15}$.

Solid Angle   The angle, measured in steradians, subtended by an area (A) at a distance (R) from a point and commonly written

$$\Omega = \frac{A}{R^2} \text{ sr}$$

This approximation holds sufficiently well when $A \ll R^2$. For a circular area, the exact expression is

$$\Omega = 2\pi(1 - \cos \theta)$$

For purposes of calculating energy collected by a lens from a point source, the following equation may be useful.

$$\Omega = 2\pi\left(1 - \frac{2f}{\sqrt{4f^2 + 1}}\right)$$

One can see that lenses with low f/numbers (fast lenses) will subtend relatively small solid angles when compared to a sphere ($\Omega = 4\pi$) showing the difficulty of collecting a major fraction of the power radiated by an isotropic light source.

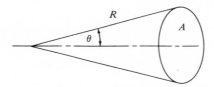

Solid angle

Schmidt System   A catadioptric system consisting of a spherical lens and an aspheric corrector plate as shown in the diagram.   The unique feature of this objective is that the correction of aberrations is very good at large apertures owing to the placement of the corrector at the center of curvature of the mirror. The corrector serves the function of parabolizing the spherical mirror.

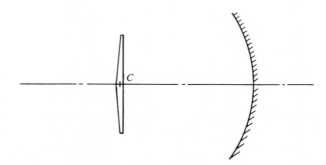

Schmidt system

Simple Lens   A lens consisting of only one element.   This type of lens is frequently used for focusing high-power lasers since it is inexpensive and not easily damaged.   However, for these applications, a simple lens may have an intolerable amount of spherical aberration.   In order to minimize spherical aberration when using collimated laser radiation, a simple lens should be situated with its optical axis on the laser beam axis and should have the configuration shown in the diagram.

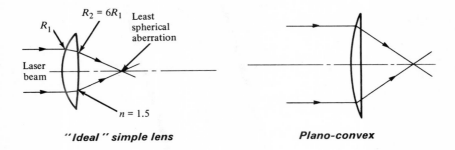

"Ideal" simple lens   Plano-convex

Since it may be difficult to find any more information than the focal length of a lens, it will generally suffice to choose a plano-convex lens of the required focal length.

Specular Reflection   A mirror-like reflection.   It is also known as regular reflection.

Transmittance   The ratio of transmitted radiant power to incident radiant power.

Wave Number   The number of wavelengths in 1 cm:

$$\nu = \frac{1}{\lambda}$$

where ν is the frequency in inverse centimeters.

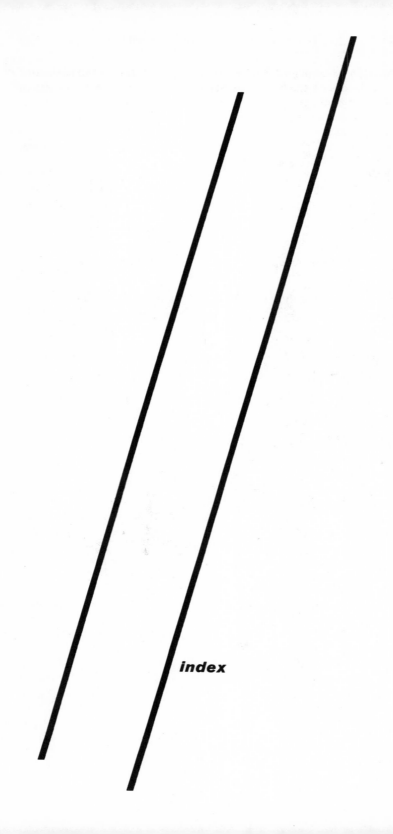

index

index

Absorption: coefficient, 107, 112, 161, 325; free carrier, 325; intrinsic, 325; metals, 116; of the eye, 581; semiconductors, 118; under intense radiation, 129

Absorptivity: defined, 128; in laser annealing, 301; of common metals, 146; of dielectric materials, 307

Acrylic plastic. *See* Plastic

Airy; diffraction pattern, 388

Alignment: in an assembly room, 599; in holographic setups, 605; in a zone melter, 308; instruments, aerospace industry, 368; uses of low-powered lasers, 597

Alloy systems: metallurgy of, 177

Alumina (aluminum oxide): absorption of CO_2 laser radiation, 249; laser cutting of, 284–285; laser fracture of, 277, 278, 279; properties of 250, 252, 310

Alumina drilling: analysis of thermal stress, 252–256; aspect ratio of holes, 247; energy required for, 252; hole profile, 256; penetration depth, 253, 255

Amplification, 4; through stimulated emission, 6

Amplitude division, 443

Analyzer, 327, 328, 329

Annealing: definition of, 300; by laser, 306

Antireflection film, 455, 456; cryolite, 457; magnesium fluoride, 457

Anti-Stokes component. *See* Stokes

Anti-Stokes line. *See* Stokes

Aperture: for hole drilling, 230

Aperture position, diffraction, 386

Argon laser: energy levels, 45; typical CW power, 45, 46, 59; wavelengths, 46, 59

Attenuation: of laser radiation, 308; of laser safety goggles, 603, 605; of zone refining gases, 310

Avalanche photodiodes: characteristics of, 554

Band: conduction, 97; gap, 96; theory of solids, 91; valence, 97

Beam: alignment, 368; expander, 230; expansion, 617; propagation, non-Gaussian example, 149; shaping, 207; splitters, as optical attenuators, 573, 574; uniformity, 482, 483, 484; waist, definition, 141

Beam diameter: applied to focusing, 298; defined (radius), 139, 297; illustration of, 297; in laser zone melter, 307; measurement of, 144

Beryllium copper, 214

Blackbody: equivalent temperature of laser, 305; radiation, 78

Bolometers: description of, 560–561

Boltzmann distribution, 7

Bond: interatomic, 86, 87

Boron fiber composite: laser cutting, 285

Bragg effect, 464

Brillouin: scattering, 123

Brillouin: zone, 95

Calorimeter: disc type, 566; cone flow type, 567; Mendenhall wedge ballistic, 564; pyroelectric type, 567; rat's nest, 561

Capacitor: fabrication by laser, 262, 263; trimming by laser, 262

Carrier concentration: measurement of, 335

Cataphoresis: in HeCd laser, 49

Cavity—laser: dumping, description of, 28; losses, 13; mirror configurations and stability, 20

Character recognition: two dimension, 427

Chemical reactions: by lasers, thermally induced, 310

Clapeyron equation: statement of, 154, 181

CO_2 laser: cutting applications, 282; lenses for, 195; output characteristics, 47, 48, 59; pulsed, 250; Q-switched and mode locked, 48; TEA laser characteristics, 59. *See also* Lasers, CO_2

Coherence: length, 30, 128, 437; length extension, in gas laser, 484,

191 - 226

X8